Manual

of Pulmonary Function Testing

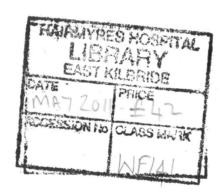

NINTH EDITION

Manual
of **Pulmonary
Function Testing**

GREGG L. RUPPEL
MEd, RRT, RPFT, FAARC
Adjunct Professor, Division of Pulmonary, Critical
Care, and Sleep Medicine
Director, Pulmonary Function Laboratory
Saint Louis University Hospital
Saint Louis, Missouri

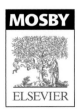

MOSBY

ELSEVIER

11830 Westline Industrial Drive
St. Louis, Missouri 63146

MANUAL OF PULMONARY FUNCTION TESTING, NINTH EDITION   ISBN: 978-0-323-05212-2

Notice

Knowledge and best practice in this field are constantly changing. As new research and experience broaden our knowledge, changes in practice, treatment and drug therapy may become necessary or appropriate. Readers are advised to check the most current information provided (i) on procedures featured or (ii) by the manufacturer of each product to be administered, to verify the recommended dose or formula, the method and duration of administration, and contraindications. It is the responsibility of the practitioner, relying on their own experience and knowledge of the patient, to make diagnoses, to determine dosages and the best treatment for each individual patient, and to take all appropriate safety precautions. To the fullest extent of the law, neither the Publisher nor the Author assumes any liability for any injury and/or damage to persons or property arising out of or related to any use of the material contained in this book.

The Publisher

Library of Congress Control Number: 2007940429

Publisher: Jeanne Wilke
Managing Editor: Billi Sharp
Senior Developmental Editor: Mindy Hutchinson
Publishing Services Manager: Patricia Tannian
Project Manager: Claire Kramer
Cover Design: Paula Catalano
Text Design: Paula Catalano

Printed in China

Last digit is the print number: 9 8 7 6 5 4 3 2

Working together to grow
libraries in developing countries

www.elsevier.com | www.bookaid.org | www.sabre.org

ELSEVIER   BOOK AID International   Sabre Foundation

For Carol, Paul, Katie, and Karen

Contributors

David A. Kaminsky, MD
  Associate Professor
  Pulmonary and Critical Care
  University of Vermont
  Attending Physician
  Medicine, Pulmonary, and Critical Care
  Fletcher Allen Health Care
  Burlington, Vermont

Carl Mottram, BA, RRT, RPFT, FAARC
  Director
  Pulmonary Function Laboratories and Pulmonary
    Rehabilitation
  Associate Professor of Medicine
  Mayo Clinic College of Medicine
  Mayo Clinic
  Rochester, Minnesota

Jack Wanger, MS, RRT, RPFT
  PRA International
  Lenexa, Kansas

Deborah K. White, BS, RPFT, RRT
  St John's Mercy Medical Center
  Respiratory Therapy Department
  St. Louis, Missouri

Reviewers

Kevin Shane Keene, MBA, MS, RRT-NPS, CPFT
Director of Clinical Education
East Tennessee State University
Johnson City, Tennessee
Consultant, Tennessee Board of Respiratory Care
Nashville, Tennessee

James A. Knight, EdD, RRT
Director
Clinical Education
Division of Respiratory Care
Long Island University
Brooklyn, New York

J. Kenneth Le Jeune, BSE, MS, RRT, CPFT
Program Director
Respiratory Education
University of Arkansas Community College–Hope
Hope, Arkansas

Ralph C. Lucki, MA, RRT
Respiratory Care Program Director
Health Sciences Division Chair
West Virginia Northern Community College
Wheeling, West Virginia

Michael R. McCumber, EdD, RRT
Director
Respiratory Care Associate of Science Program
Chair of Allied Health
Daytona Beach Community College
Daytona Beach, Florida

Stanley M. Pearson, MSED, RRT, C-CPT
Program Director and Assistant Professor
Respiratory Therapy
C-ASA, School of Allied Health
Southern Illinois University–Carbondale
Carbondale, Illinois

Bill Pruitt, MBA, RRT, CPFT, AE-C
Senior Instructor
Cardiorespiratory Care
College of Allied Health
University of South Alabama
Mobile, Alabama

Candace S. Schladenhauffen, MS, RRT-NPS, RPFT
Chair
School of Health Sciences
Ivy Tech Community College Northeast
Fort Wayne, Indiana

Robert D. Tarkowski, MS, RRT, RPFT
Director of Clinical Education
Assistant Professor
Respiratory Care Program
Gannon University
Erie, Pennsylvania

Christopher Tino, BS, RRT
Respiratory Therapy Program
Luzerne County Community College
Nanticoke, Pennsylvania

LaVerne Yousey, MSTE, RRT
Professor of Respiratory Care
Program Director
Respiratory Care Programs
Department Head
Allied Health Department
University of Akron
Akron, Ohio

Foreword

You have certainly made the best choice for a book about pulmonary function testing (PFT) if you're preparing for the CPFT or RPFT examination. I've had the pleasure to recently work with Gregg Ruppel on the NBRC board of directors. He knows more about the technical aspects of the various tests and instruments than anyone else I know; he explains it clearly, and he keeps up-to-date. For this version, he has assembled a world-class group of experienced respiratory therapists to write or edit each chapter.

If you are a pulmonary physician who is the medical director of a PFT laboratory, this book is also an essential resource. You need to know the techniques, analyzers, transducers, and instruments for each test to understand what can go wrong and to communicate effectively with your laboratory staff. The American Thoracic Society PFT boiler-plate manual of procedures is also necessary for each PFT laboratory, but it does not explain how each instrument works, nor does it help you to select new equipment. Pulmonary physiologists will also find this book useful as they select and use instruments for both animal and human studies that need lung function testing.

Take this book home and read it chapter by chapter for the first time. Then take it to your office and keep it as a reference.

Paul Enright, MD
Research Professor of Medicine
The University of Arizona
Tucson, Arizona

Preface

The primary functions of the lung are oxygenation of mixed venous blood and removal of carbon dioxide. Gas exchange depends on the integrity of the entire cardiopulmonary system, including airways, pulmonary blood vessels, alveoli, respiratory muscles, and respiratory control mechanisms. A few pulmonary function tests assess individual parts of the cardiopulmonary system. However, most lung function tests measure the status of the lungs' components in an overlapping way.

This ninth edition describes the most common pulmonary function tests, their techniques, and the pathophysiology that may be evaluated by each test. Topics covered include the following:

- Basic tests of lung function, including spirometry, lung volume measurements, diffusing capacity, and blood gas analysis
- Ventilation and ventilatory control, cardiopulmonary exercise tests, and pediatric and infant pulmonary function testing
- Specialized test regimens that focus on bronchial challenge, exhaled nitric oxide measurements, forced oscillation techniques, metabolic studies, disability determination, and preoperative evaluation
- Pulmonary function testing equipment and quality assurance

Distinctive Features

The ninth edition includes many of the features from the previous editions:

- Learning objectives for entry-level and advanced practitioners are again included at the beginning of each chapter.

- Each test section includes criteria for acceptability and repeatability, as well as interpretive strategies with criteria that are organized to help those who perform pulmonary function tests adhere to recognized standards.
- Some criteria are based on the clinical practice guidelines of the American Association for Respiratory Care.
- The interpretive strategies are presented as a series of questions that can be used as a starting point for test interpretation.
- Case studies are included in most chapters as examples of the performance and interpretation of specific tests.

As in previous editions, each chapter includes self-assessment questions. The questions in this edition are new and are divided into entry-level and advanced categories. The answers may be found in Appendix A. A selected bibliography at the end of each chapter is arranged according to topics within the chapter, including standards and guidelines. Reference equations and sources for reference values are again included in the appendixes, along with information on the use of reference values. Sample calculations for lung volumes, plethysmography, diffusion, and exercise tests can also be found in the appendixes.

Changes to This Edition

The ninth edition elaborates on material presented in the first eight editions. The following changes to this edition reflect suggestions of the users of previous editions, as well as new developments in pulmonary function testing.

- Test criteria are based largely on the most recent recommendations of the American Thoracic Society (ATS) and European Respiratory Society.
- Chapter 10 includes updated information on spirometers designed for use in primary care practice, along with blood gas analyzers and exhaled gas analyzers.
- Chapter 11 addresses calibration, quality control, quality assurance, and safety issues, as well as the current equipment recommendations of the ATS and European Respiratory Society and safety guidelines from the Centers for Disease Control and Prevention.

Using This Book

This manual is intended to serve as a text for students of pulmonary function testing and as a reference for technologists and physicians. Because of the wide variety of methods and equipment used in pulmonary function evaluation, some tests are discussed in general terms. For this reason, readers are encouraged to use the selected bibliographies provided. The presentation of indications, pathophysiology, and clinical significance of various tests presumes a basic understanding of cardiopulmonary anatomy and physiology. Again, readers are urged to refer to the General References included in the selected bibliographies to refresh their background knowledge of lung function. The terminology used is that of the American College of Chest Physicians (ACCP)–ATS Joint Committee on Pulmonary Nomenclature. In some instances test names reflect common usage that does not follow the ACCP-ATS recommendations.

Evolve Ancillaries

Evolve is an interactive learning environment designed to work in coordination with *Manual of Pulmonary Function Testing*, ninth edition. Included on Evolve are an instructor's manual with key terms, chapter objectives, instructional chapter outlines, suggested activities, and general discussion questions; a test bank in ExamView containing approximately 400 questions; an electronic image collection consisting of images from the textbook; and approximately 30 case studies. Instructors may use Evolve to provide an Internet-based course component that reinforces and expands the concepts presented in class. Evolve may be used to publish the class syllabus, outlines, and lecture notes; set up "virtual office hours" and e-mail communication; share important dates and information through the online class calendar; and encourage student participation through chat rooms and discussion boards. Evolve allows instructors to post examinations and manage their grade books online. For more information, visit http://evolve.elsevier.com/Ruppel/ or contact an Elsevier sales representative.

Gregg L. Ruppel, MEd, RRT, RPFT, FAARC

Acknowledgments

My thanks to Drs. William Kistner, John Winter, and James Wiant for their encouragement in the development of the original text. My special thanks to Drs. Roger Secker-Walker, Susan Marshall, and Gerald Dolan for comments and constructive criticisms in the preparation of the revised editions. Special thanks also go to Ronald Gilmore and Jack Tandy for their contributions to the illustrations in previous editions. A note of thanks also to Thomas Anderson, MEd, RRT; David Shelledy, MA, RRT; Patricia Dent, BS, MS, RPT; and Barbara Disborough, MA, RRT, for their reviews of and suggestions for the fourth edition. Louis Metzger, RPFT; Donald Barker, BS, PA, RPFT; David Hoover, RRT, RPFT; Randall Krohn; James Kemp, MD; Alan Hibbett, RPFT; and Michael Snow, RPFT, all provided guidance and suggestions for the fifth edition. Cesar Keller, MD, and Deborah Stanger, RD, provided insight for case studies for the sixth edition. Robert Brown, RRT, RPFT, and Deborah White, RRT, RPFT, suggested significant changes for the seventh edition. Both Carl Mottram, RRT, RPFT, and Deborah White, RRT, RPFT, contributed to the eighth and ninth editions. Jack Wanger, RRT, RPFT, contributed the chapter on lung volumes, and David Kaminsky, MD, contributed the chapter on spirometry and material on forced oscillation techniques for the ninth edition. Philip Quanjer, MD, PhD, provided insight and guidance regarding predicted values and interpretive strategies. I am deeply indebted to all these individuals for their support.

My appreciation for photos and illustrations provided for this and previous editions goes to the following companies:

Abbott Critical Care Systems
Aerocrine, Inc.
Biochem International, Inc.
Hans Rudolph, Inc.
HealthScan Products, Inc.
I-STAT Corporation
Jones Medical Instrument Co.
Marquette Medical Systems
Masimo Corporation
Medical Graphics, Inc.
Morgan Scientific, Inc.
ndd Medical Technologies, Inc.
Nonin Medical, Inc.
nSpire Health, Inc. (Ferraris Respiratory)
Respironics, Inc.
Radiometer America, Inc.
Spirometrics Medical Equipment Company
VIASYS Healthcare
Vitalograph, Inc.
Warren E. Collins, Inc. (Ferraris Medical Inc.)

Contents

Manual

of **Pulmonary Function Testing**

Chapter 1

Indications for Pulmonary Function Testing

CHAPTER OUTLINE

OBJECTIVES

After studying this chapter you will be able to:

Entry-level
1. Categorize pulmonary function tests according to specific purposes
2. List indications for spirometry, lung volumes, and diffusing capacity
3. Identify at least one obstructive and one restrictive pulmonary disorder
4. Relate pulmonary history to indications for performing pulmonary function tests

Advanced
1. Identify three indications for exercise testing
2. Name at least two diseases in which air trapping may occur
3. Describe the use of a technologist-adapted protocol for pulmonary function studies

KEY TERMS

body plethysmograph	hyperventilation	oximetry
bronchial challenge	hypoventilation	pulse oximetry
capnography	maximal expiratory flow volume	resting energy expenditure (REE)
diffusing capacity (DLCO)	(MEFV)	spirometry
edema	maximal voluntary ventilation	vital capacity (VC)
forced vital capacity (FVC)	(MVV)	
hypercapnia		

This chapter provides an overview of pulmonary function testing. Common pulmonary function tests are introduced, and the indications for each test are discussed. Diseases that commonly require pulmonary function tests are described, and guidelines regarding patient preparation and assessment are presented. Adequate patient preparation, physical assessment, and pulmonary history help the tests provide answers to clinical questions. The importance of patient instruction in obtaining valid data is discussed. These topics are developed more fully in subsequent chapters.

PF TIP

Pulmonary function data are usually grouped into categories (see Figure 1-1). The patient's demographic data (age, height, gender, race, weight) are usually at the top of the report. The PFT data are presented in several columns. These columns show the predicted (expected) values, the lower limit of normal (LLN) or upper limit of normal (ULN), measured values obtained during testing, and the percent of predicted values for each test (actual/predicted × 100). Be sure to identify which column is actual and which is predicted.

PULMONARY FUNCTION TESTS

Many different tests are used to evaluate lung function. These tests can be divided into categories based on the aspect of lung function they measure (Box 1-1). Although the tests can be performed individually, they are often performed in combination. Figure 1-1 shows a sample pulmonary function test report that includes spirometry, lung volumes, diffusing capacity, and airway resistance measurements in a format that is commonly used. Determining which tests to do depends on the clinical question to be answered. This question may be explicit, such as "Does the patient have asthma?" or less obvious, such as "Does this patient, who needs thoracic surgery, have any pulmonary disease that might complicate the procedure?" In either case, indications for specific tests are useful (see Boxes 1-2 through 1-6).

Airway Function Tests

The most basic test of pulmonary function is the measurement of **vital capacity (VC)**. This test simply measures the largest volume of air that can be moved into or out of the lungs. In the mid-1800s, Hutchinson developed a simple water-sealed spirometer that allowed measurement of what he named *vital capacity*. Hutchinson popularized the concept of using VC to assess lung function, and the names he gave to several other lung compartments are still used today. He observed that VC was related to the standing height of the patient. He also developed tables to estimate the expected VC for a healthy patient. The VC was usually graphed on chart paper, which allowed subdivisions of the VC to be identified (see Chapter 2).

Forced vital capacity (FVC) is an enhancement of the simple VC test. During the 1930s, Barach

BOX 1-1	Categories of Pulmonary Function Tests

A. Airway function
  1. Simple spirometry
     a. VC, expiratory reserve volume (ERV), inspiratory capacity (IC)
  2. Forced vital capacity maneuver
     a. FVC, FEV_1, FEF, PEF
        (1) Prebronchodilator and postbronchodilator
        (2) Prebronchochallenge and postbronchochallenge
     b. MEFV curves $\dot{V}max_x$
        (1) Prebronchodilator and postbronchodilator
        (2) Prebronchochallenge and postbronchochallenge
  3. Maximal voluntary ventilation (MVV)
  4. Maximal inspiratory/expiratory pressures (MIP/MEP)
  5. Airway resistance (Raw) and compliance (C_1)
B. Lung volumes and ventilation
  1. Functional residual capacity (FRC)
     a. Open-circuit (N_2 washout)
     b. Closed-circuit/rebreathing (He dilution)
     c. Thoracic gas volume (V_{TG})
  2. Total lung capacity (TLC), residual volume (RV), RV/TLC ratio
  3. Minute ventilation, alveolar ventilation, and dead space
  4. Distribution of ventilation
     a. Multiple-breath N_2
     b. He equilibration
     c. Single-breath techniques
C. Diffusing capacity tests
  1. Single-breath (breath holding)
  2. Steady state
  3. Other techniques
D. Blood gases and gas exchange tests
  1. Blood gas analysis and blood oximetry
     a. Shunt studies
  2. Pulse oximetry
  3. Capnography
E. Cardiopulmonary exercise tests
  1. Simple noninvasive tests
  2. Tests with exhaled gas analyses
  3. Tests with blood gas analyses
F. Metabolic measurements
  1. Resting energy expenditure (REE)
  2. Substrate utilization

observed that patients with asthma or emphysema exhaled more slowly than healthy patients. He noted that airflow out of the lungs was important in detecting obstruction of the airways. Barach used a rotating chart drum (kymograph) to display VC changes as a spirogram. He even evaluated the effects of bronchodilator medications using the forced vital capacity traced as a spirogram.

In 1947 Tiffeneau described measuring the volume expired in the first second of a maximal exhalation in proportion to the maximal volume that could be inspired (FEV_1/IVC) as an index of airflow obstruction (i.e., the Tiffeneau index). Around 1950, Gaensler began using a microswitch in conjunction with a water-sealed spirometer to time FVC. He observed that healthy patients consistently exhaled approximately 80% of their FVC in 1 second, and almost all the FVC in 3 seconds. He used the forced expired volume in the first second (FEV_1) to assess airway obstruction. In 1955, Leuallen and Fowler demonstrated a graphic method used to assess airflow. They measured airflow between the 25% and 75% points on a forced expiratory spirogram. This measure was described as the maximal midexpiratory flow rate (MMFR). This and similar measurements have been used to describe airflow from both healthy and airflow-obstructed patients. To standardize terminology, the MMFR is now referred to as the forced expiratory flow 25%–75% ($FEF_{25\%-75\%}$).

In addition to displaying FVC as a volume-time spirogram, it can also be represented by plotting airflow against volume. In the late 1950s, Hyatt and others began using the flow-volume display to assess airway function. The tracing was termed the **maximal expiratory flow volume (MEFV)** curve. By combining the forced expiration with an inspiratory maneuver, a closed loop can be displayed. This figure is called the flow-volume loop (see Chapter 2).

Peak expiratory flow (PEF) is measured with either a flow-sensing spirometer or a peak flow meter. In the 1960s, Wright and McKerrow popularized the use of peak flow to monitor asthmatic patients. Peak flow can be readily assessed from the flow-volume loop as well. Recently, portable peak

Name:	Public, John Q.	**Age:**	65	**Sex:**	Male
ID:	123456789	**Height:**	71.5	**Race:**	White
Doctor:	Smith	**Weight:**	237	**Date:**	6/7/2007

	Pre-drug				Post-drug		
	Pred	**LLN**	**Actual**	**%Pred**	**Actual**	**%Pred**	**%Chg**
SPIROMETRY							
FVC (L)	4.86	3.89	4.00	82			
FEV_1 (L)	3.63	2.81	2.90	80			
FEV_1/FVC (%)	75	65	73				
$FEF_{25\%-75\%}$ (L/sec)	2.87	1.20	2.16	75			
FEFmax (L/sec)	9.17	6.75	6.21	68			
MVV	126	101	108	86			
MIP	−104	−76	−59	57			
MEP	202	155	111	55			
LUNG VOLUMES							
SVC (L)	4.86	3.89	4.42	91			
TLC Pleth (L)	7.31	5.77	7.89	108			
RV Pleth (L)	2.59		3.47	134			
RV/TLC Pleth (%)	35		44	126			
V_{TG} (L)	4.14		4.01	97			
ERV (L)	1.55		0.54	35			
IC (L)	3.17		3.87	122			
DIFFUSION							
D_{LCO} (ml/min/mm Hg)	26.3	20.0	20.3	77			
D_{LCO}corr (ml/min/mm Hg)	22.9	17.4	20.3	89			
D_L/V_A (ml/min/mm Hg/L)	3.6		3.3				
V_A (L)	7.31		6.18	85			
Hb (g/dl)			10.7				
AIRWAY RESISTANCE							
Raw (cm H_2O/L/sec)	1.25		1.13	90			
sGaw (L/sec/cm H_2O/L)	0.22	0.12	0.20	91			

Technologist's comments:
  Spirometry meets ATS/ERS criteria and MVV, MIP, MEP were all acceptable.
  Lung volumes by plethysmography were acceptable and repeatable.
  D_{LCO}: Meets ATS/ERS criteria; corrected for 10.7 Hb.

Interpretation:
  All maneuvers were performed acceptably.
  Spirometry is within normal limits with no evidence of obstruction. The patient's maximal inspiratory and
    expiratory pressures are both below the lower limit of normal.
  Lung volumes by plethysmography show a moderate increase in the residual volume and RV/TLC ratio consistent
    with air trapping.
  Diffusing capacity, using a predicted value corrected for Hb, is within normal limits.
  Airway resistance and conductance are normal.
  Impression: Essentially normal spirometry, but with decreased maximal pressures. Some evidence of air trapping.
    Normal diffusing capacity. Recommend clinical correlation of decreased respiratory muscle function.

FIGURE 1-1   Sample Pulmonary Function Test Report. Patient information is usually listed at the top. Lung function tests are grouped by category in the left column. The first data column contains patient's predicted (expected) values. The second column lists the lower limit of normal (LLN) for the specified variable. The third column contains the measured values obtained during testing. The fourth column contains the percent of predicted value for each test (actual/ predicted × 100). The next three columns are blank on this report because the patient was not retested after bronchodilator. These columns would be used to display the measured, percent of predicted, and percent change following administration of a bronchodilator. Following the tabular data are sections containing the technologist's comments and the physician's interpretation and impression.

flow meters that allow monitoring at home, as well as in the hospital or clinic, have been developed.

The FVC, FEV_1, and other flows, along with flow-volume loops, are all used to measure response to bronchodilator medications (see Chapter 2). Tests are performed before and after inhalation of a bronchodilator, and the percentage of change calculated. The same tests may be used to assess airway response after a challenge to the airways. These tests are referred to as **bronchial challenge** or bronchial provocation tests. The challenge may be in the form of a nonspecific inhaled agent (e.g., methacholine) or a physical agent (e.g., exercise). In either case, airflow is assessed before and after the challenge. The percent change (normally a decrease) after challenge is calculated (see Chapter 9).

Maximal voluntary ventilation (MVV) was described as early as 1941. Cournand and Richards originally called it the maximal breathing capacity (MBC). In the MVV test, the patient breathes rapidly and deeply for 12–15 seconds. The volume of air exchanged is expressed in liters per minute. The MVV gives an estimate of the peak ventilation available to meet physiologic demands.

Measurement of respiratory muscle strength is accomplished by assessing maximal inspiratory pressure (MIP) and maximal expiratory pressure (MEP). This is done using either a pressure transducer or a simple aneroid manometer. MIP and MEP are important adjuncts to spirometry for monitoring respiratory muscle function in a variety of pulmonary and nonpulmonary diseases.

Airway resistance (Raw) measurements date back to the development of the **body plethysmograph** in the early 1950s. Comroe, Dubois, and others perfected a technique that provided estimates of alveolar pressure. The patient sits in an airtight box called a plethysmograph (see Chapter 10). The plethysmographic method allows calculation of the pressure drop across the airways related to flow at the mouth (see Chapter 2). This technique originally required complicated monitoring and recording devices. Microprocessors have simplified the measurement of the required signals so that plethysmography is now widely used. The same equipment can also be used to rapidly and accurately measure thoracic gas volume (V_{TG}).

Lung compliance is measured by passing a small balloon into the esophagus to measure pleural pressure. Intrapleural pressure can then be related to volume changes to estimate the distensibility of the lung (see Chapter 2). Other less invasive techniques are available but not widely used.

Lung Volume and Ventilation Tests

Measurement of lung volume dates back to the early 1800s, well before Hutchinson's development of spirometry. Various techniques have been used to estimate the volume of gas remaining in the lung after a complete exhalation. Davy used a hydrogen dilution technique to estimate residual air. This technique was later improved by Meneely and Kaltreider using helium (He) instead of hydrogen. Around the same time, Darling, Cournand, and Richards began using oxygen breathing to wash nitrogen (N_2) out of the lungs. The collection and analysis of the volume of exhaled N_2 allowed the functional residual capacity (FRC) to be estimated. Using simple spirometry combined with FRC determinations allows total lung capacity (TLC) and residual volume (RV) to be calculated. The other commonly used method for measuring lung volumes uses the body plethysmograph to measure V_{TG} or FRC. Estimation of lung volumes from chest radiographs is possible but is not widely used. Lung volume can also be estimated from computerized tomography (CT) scans, but such measurements are seldom performed just for the purpose of measuring lung volume.

Closed-circuit (He dilution) and open-circuit (N_2 washout) techniques are both widely used to measure FRC. Besides determining lung volumes, each technique provides some limited information about distribution of ventilation within the lungs. The pattern of N_2 washout can be displayed graphically. The time required for He to equilibrate during rebreathing provides a similar index of the evenness of ventilation. In the early 1950s and 1960s, Fowler developed a single-breath N_2-washout technique. This method plotted N_2 concentration in expired gas after a single breath of 100% oxygen. The single-breath N_2 washout also provides limited information about gas distribution in the lungs. It also allows estimates of the lung volume at which airway closure occurs when the patient exhales completely (see Chapter 3).

Measurement of resting ventilation requires only a simple gas-metering device and a means of collecting expired air. Portable computerized spirometers allow minute ventilation, tidal volume (V_T), and breathing rate to be readily measured in almost any setting. Determination of alveolar ventilation or dead space (wasted ventilation) requires measurement of arterial partial pressure of carbon dioxide ($PaCO_2$) in addition to total ventilation. Alternately, the partial pressure of carbon dioxide (PCO_2) can be estimated from expired CO_2. The availability of blood gas analyzers and exhaled CO_2 analyzers makes these measurements routine.

Diffusing Capacity Tests

The basis for the modern single-breath **diffusing capacity (DLCO)** test was described by August and Marie Krogh in 1911. They showed that small but measurable differences existed between inspired and expired gas containing carbon monoxide (CO). This change could be related to the uptake of gas across the lung. Although they used the method to test a series of patients, they did not employ the single-breath technique for clinical purposes. Around 1950, Forrester and colleagues revisited the method. They developed it as a tool to measure the gas exchange capacity of the lung. About the same time, Filley and others were promoting other techniques using CO to measure diffusing capacity. Most of these techniques allowed patients to breathe normally, rather than hold their breath. These methods are called steady-state techniques. Each method has certain limitations. However, the single-breath technique is the most widely used and standardized in the United States and Europe (see Chapter 5).

Blood Gases and Gas Exchange Tests

Measurement of gases (O_2 and CO_2) in the blood began with volumetric methods used since the early 1900s. In 1957, Sanz introduced the glass electrode to measure pH of fluids potentiometrically. In 1958, Severinghaus added an outer jacket containing a bicarbonate buffer to the glass electrode. The electrode-buffer was separated from the blood being analyzed by a membrane that was permeable to CO_2. This allowed the pressure of CO_2 in the blood to be measured as a pH change in the electrode. In 1956 Leland Clark covered a platinum electrode with a polypropylene membrane. When a voltage was applied to the electrode, O_2 was reduced at the platinum cathode in proportion to its partial pressure. These three electrodes (pH, PCO_2, and partial pressure of oxygen [PO_2]) were the basic measurement device in blood gas analyzers for many years. Miniature electrodes gradually replaced the traditional electrodes. Today, blood gas analyzers use a variety of electrochemical techniques (see Blood Gas Analyzers, Chapter 10) to measure not only pH, PCO_2, and PO_2, but also the various fractions of Hb, such as O_2Hb and COHb. Similar methods to measure electrolytes (K^{++}, Na^{++}, Cl^-) are also included in many blood gas analyzer systems. Transcutaneous electrodes, using techniques similar to the classical blood gas electrodes, are available for measurement of O_2 and CO_2 tensions ($tcPO_2$ and $tcPCO_2$).

Blood **oximetry** was developed during World War II to monitor the effects of exposure to high-altitude flight. During the 1960s, spectrophotometric analyzers that could measure the total hemoglobin (Hb), along with oxyhemoglobin (O_2Hb) and carboxyhemoglobin (COHb) levels, were perfected. Blood oximetry testing is commonly combined with blood gas analysis so that both can be accomplished with a single instrument. **Pulse oximetry** was developed in the 1970s as a result of efforts to monitor cardiac rate by using a light beam to sense pulsatile blood flow. It was quickly discovered that the pulse could be sensed, and changes in light absorption could also be used to estimate arterial oxygen saturation. Modern microprocessors have allowed pulse oximeters that are very small and portable, with some devices capable of measuring COHb in addition to O_2 saturation.

Capnography, or monitoring of exhaled carbon dioxide, was developed in conjunction with the infrared gas analyzer (see Chapter 10). This sensitive and rapidly responding analyzer allows exhaled CO_2 to be monitored continuously. Most critical care units, operating rooms, and emergency departments use some combination of blood gas analysis, pulse oximetry, and capnography for patient monitoring. Blood gas analysis is an integral part of routine pulmonary function testing because it is the definitive test of the basic functions of the lung.

Exhaled nitric oxide (eNO), while not a measure of blood gas or gas exchange, has emerged as an important parameter for assessing inflammatory changes in the lungs. Asthma, chronic obstructive pulmonary disease (COPD), and other pathologies characterized by inflammation of the airways or lung tissue, can be monitored by analyzing trace amounts of NO in exhaled gas.

Cardiopulmonary Exercise Tests

Exercise tests commonly use a treadmill or cycle ergometer to impose an external workload that stresses the cardiovascular and musculoskeletal systems. The simplest types of exercise tests are those in which the patient performs work and only noninvasive measurements are made. Such measurements include heart rate and rhythm monitoring using an electrocardiogram (ECG). Other simple, noninvasive measurements are blood pressure and respiratory rate monitoring. Analysis of exhaled gas is noninvasive, but the patient does have to breathe through a mouthpiece or mask. Ventilation and tidal volume (V_T) can be estimated by collecting the exhaled air. Analysis of expired gases permits oxygen consumption and CO_2 production to be measured. When invasive measures (blood gas analysis, arterial catheters, pulmonary artery catheters) are used, the entire range of physiologic variables that affect exercise can be monitored. Computerized exhaled gas analysis allows sophisticated measurements to be made rapidly while the patient continues to exercise (breath-by-breath gas analysis). Simple exercise tests such as the 6-Minute Walk Test (6MWT) have become popular because the distance walked correlates well

with more sophisticated exercise measurements, and with clinical outcomes in a variety of diseases.

Metabolic Measurements

Measurement of energy expenditure and caloric requirements dates to the early 1900s. Basal metabolic rate (BMR) was measured by allowing subjects to rebreathe from a volume spirometer containing added oxygen. Plotting the rate at which oxygen was consumed derived an estimate of energy expenditure. Similar techniques are employed today, except that oxygen consumption and carbon dioxide production are monitored using exhaled gas analysis. **Resting energy expenditure (REE)** has replaced BMR as the primary variable related to metabolic needs. Although BMR was used to detect disorders that affected metabolism, REE is used to manage critically ill patients whose caloric requirements may be difficult to estimate.

INDICATIONS FOR PULMONARY FUNCTION TESTING

Each category of pulmonary function testing includes specific reasons why that test may be necessary. These reasons for testing are called *indications*. Some pulmonary function tests have well-defined indications. The same indications that apply to one type of test (e.g., spirometry) may apply to other categories as well.

Spirometry

Spirometry is the pulmonary function test performed most often because it is indicated in many situations (Box 1-2). Spirometry is often performed as a screening procedure. It may be the first test to indicate the presence of pulmonary disease. Spirometry is recommended as the "gold standard" for diagnosis of obstructive lung disease by the National Lung Health Education Program (NLHEP), the National Heart, Lung and Blood Institute (NHLBI),

BOX 1-2	Indications for Spirometry

Spirometry may be indicated to:
A. Diagnose the presence or absence of lung disease
  1. History of pulmonary symptoms
     a. Dyspnea, wheezing
     b. Cough, phlegm production
     c. Chest discomfort, orthopnea
  2. Physical indicators
     a. Decreased breath sounds
     b. Chest wall abnormalities
  3. Abnormal laboratory findings
     a. Chest x-ray or CT studies
     b. Blood gases or pulse oximetry
  4. Before beginning strenuous physical activities
B. Quantify the extent of known disease on lung function
  1. Pulmonary disease
     a. Chronic obstructive pulmonary disease
     b. Asthma
     c. Cystic fibrosis
     d. Interstitial diseases
  2. Cardiac disease (congestive heart failure)
  3. Neuromuscular disease (Guillain-Barré syndrome)
C. Measure effects of occupational or environmental exposure
  1. Smoking
  2. Working in hazardous or dusty environments
D. Determine beneficial or negative effects of therapy
  1. Bronchodilators or steroids
  2. Cardiac drugs (antiarrhythmics, diuretics)
  3. Lung resection, reduction, or transplant
  4. Pulmonary rehabilitation
E. Assess risk for surgical procedures
  1. Lung resection (lobectomy, pneumonectomy)
  2. Thoracic procedures (sternotomy)
  3. Upper abdominal procedures
F. Evaluate disability or impairment
  1. Social Security or other compensation programs
  2. Legal or insurance evaluations
  3. Cardiopulmonary rehabilitation assessment
G. Epidemiologic or clinical research involving lung health or disease

BOX 1-3	Indications for Lung Volume Determination

Lung volume determinations may be indicated to:
A. Diagnose or assess the severity of restrictive lung disease (reduced TLC)
B. Differentiate between obstructive and restrictive disease patterns
C. Assess response to therapeutic interventions
  1. Bronchodilators, steroids
  2. Lung transplantation, resection, reduction
  3. Radiation or chemotherapy
D. Make preoperative assessments of patients with compromised lung function
E. Determine the extent of hyperinflation
F. Assess gas trapping by comparison of plethysmographic lung volumes with gas dilution lung volumes
G. Standardize other lung function measures (e.g., specific conductance)

the World Health Organization (WHO), and numerous other organizations concerned with the diagnosis of lung diseases. However, spirometry alone may not be sufficient to completely define the extent of disease, response to therapy, preoperative risk, or level of impairment. Spirometry must be performed correctly because of the serious impact its results can have on the patient's life. Abnormal spirometric results can be the indication for more extensive tests, with increased risks and costs for the patient.

Lung Volumes

Lung volume determination usually includes the VC and its subdivisions, along with the FRC. From these two basic measurements, TLC and other lung volumes can be calculated (see Chapters 2 and 3). Lung volumes are almost always measured in conjunction with spirometry, although the indications for them are distinct (Box 1-3). The most common reason for measuring lung volumes is to identify restrictive lung disease. A reduced VC (or FVC) suggests restriction, particularly if airflow is normal. Measurement of FRC and determination of TLC are necessary to confirm restriction because a low FVC can be caused by either restriction or obstruction. If TLC is reduced below the 5th percentile of the predicted value, restriction is present. The severity of the restrictive process is determined by the extent of reduction of the TLC. TLC and its components can be determined by several methods. For patients with obstructive lung diseases (COPD, asthma), lung volumes measured by body plethysmography may be indicated (see Chapter 3) because multiple-breath or single-breath dilution techniques may underestimate TLC. In obstructive lung disease, lung volumes are necessary to determine whether air trapping or hyperinflation is present. The degree of hyperinflation, measured by indices such as the IC/TLC ratio, correlates with increased mortality in patients who have COPD.

Diffusing Capacity

Diffusing capacity is measured by having the patient inhale a low concentration of CO and a tracer gas to determine gas exchange within the lungs (DLCO). Several methods of evaluating the uptake of CO from the lungs are available, but the single-breath technique (DLCOsb) is most commonly used. This method is also called the breath-hold technique because CO transfer is measured during 10 seconds of breath holding. DLCO is usually measured in conjunction with spirometry and lung volumes. Although many pulmonary and cardiovascular diseases reduce DLCO (Box 1-4), it may be abnormally increased in some cases (see Chapter 5). DLCO testing is commonly used to monitor diseases caused by dust (pneumoconioses). These are conditions in which lung tissue is infiltrated by substances such as silica or asbestos that disrupt the normal structure of the gas exchange units. DLCO testing is also used to evaluate pulmonary involvement in systemic diseases such as rheumatoid arthritis. DLCO measurements are often included in the evaluation of patients with obstructive lung disease, particularly in emphysema. DLCO tests may be indicated to monitor changes in lung function (e.g., gas exchange) induced by drugs used to treat cardiac arrhythmias, as well as changes caused by chemotherapy and radiation therapy for lung cancer.

Blood Gases

Blood gas analysis is often done in conjunction with pulmonary function studies. Blood is drawn from a peripheral artery without being exposed to air (i.e., anaerobically). The radial artery is often used for a single arterial puncture or indwelling catheter. Blood gas analysis includes measurement

---

BOX 1-4	Indications for DLCO

Diffusing capacity (DLCO) measurements may be indicated to:
A. Evaluate or follow the progress of parenchymal lung diseases
  1. Dusts (asbestos, silica, metals)
  2. Organic agents (allergic alveolitis)
  3. Drugs (amiodarone, bleomycin)
B. Evaluate pulmonary involvement in systemic diseases
  1. Rheumatoid arthritis
  2. Sarcoidosis
  3. Systemic lupus erythematosus (SLE)
  4. Systemic sclerosis
  5. Mixed connective tissue disease
C. Evaluate obstructive lung disease
  1. Follow the progression of disease
    a. Emphysema
    b. Cystic fibrosis
  2. Differentiate types of obstruction
    a. Emphysema
    b. Chronic bronchitis
    c. Asthma
  3. Predict arterial desaturation during exercise in COPD
D. Evaluate cardiovascular diseases
  1. Primary pulmonary hypertension
  2. Acute or recurrent pulmonary thromboembolism
  3. Pulmonary edema and congestive heart failure
E. Quantify disability associated with interstitial lung disease
F. Evaluate pulmonary hemorrhage, polycythemia, or left-to-right shunts (increased DLCO)

---

of pH, along with PCO_2 and PO_2. Other calculated parameters (e.g., HCO_3^-, base excess) are often included in the standard blood gas report. The same specimen may be used for blood oximetry to measure total Hb, oxyhemoglobin saturation (O_2Hb), carboxyhemoglobin (COHb), and methemoglobin (MetHb).

Blood gas analysis is the ideal measure of pulmonary function because it assesses the two primary functions of the lung (oxygenation and CO_2 removal). Evaluation of many pulmonary disorders may include blood gas analysis. Specific indications for blood gas analysis are listed in Box 1-5. Blood gas analysis is most commonly used to determine the need for supplemental oxygen and to manage patients who require ventilatory support. Some pulmonary function measurements require blood

BOX 1-5	Indications for Blood Gas Analysis

Blood gas analysis and/or blood oximetry may be indicated to:
A. Evaluate adequacy of lung function
  1. Ventilation (Pa_{CO_2})
  2. Acid-base status
    a. pH
    b. Pa_{CO_2}
  3. Oxygenation and oxygen-carrying capacity
    a. Pa_{O_2}
    b. Total Hb, O_2Hb, COHb, MetHb
  4. Intrapulmonary shunt
  5. V_D/V_T ratio
B. Determine need for supplemental oxygen (for clinical or reimbursement purposes)
  1. Presence or severity of resting hypoxemia
  2. Exercise desaturation
  3. Nocturnal desaturation
  4. Adequacy of oxygen prescription
C. Monitor ventilatory support
  1. Assess or follow respiratory failure
  2. Adjust therapy to improve oxygenation (PEEP, CPAP, pressure support)
D. Document the severity or progression of known pulmonary disease
E. Provide data to correct or corroborate other pulmonary function measurements
  1. Correct D_{LCO} measurements (Hb and COHb)
  2. Determine accuracy of pulse oximetry, transcutaneous monitors, or indwelling blood gas devices

CPAP, Continuous positive airway pressure; *PEEP,* positive end-expiratory pressure.

BOX 1-6	Indications for Exercise Testing

Exercise testing may be indicated to:
A. Evaluation of exercise intolerance or level of fitness
B. Document or diagnose exercise limitation as a result of fatigue, dyspnea, or pain
  1. Cardiovascular diseases
    a. Myocardial ischemia or dyskinesis
    b. Cardiomyopathy
    c. Congestive heart failure
    d. Peripheral vascular disease
    e. Selection for heart transplantation
  2. Pulmonary diseases
    a. Airway obstruction (including cystic fibrosis) or hyperreactivity
    b. Interstitial lung disease
    c. Pulmonary vascular disease
  3. Mixed cardiovascular and pulmonary etiologies
  4. Unexplained dyspnea
C. Exercise evaluation for cardiac or pulmonary rehabilitation
  1. Exercise desaturation/hypoxemia
  2. Oxygen prescription
D. Assess preoperative risk, particularly lung resection or reduction
E. Assess disability, particularly related to occupational lung disease
F. Evaluate therapeutic interventions such as heart or lung transplantation

gas analysis as an integral part of the test (i.e., shunt or dead space studies). Blood gas analysis is invasive; noninvasive measurements of oxygenation or gas exchange are often preferred if they are safer or less costly. Many noninvasive techniques (e.g., pulse oximetry, transcutaneous monitoring, and capnography) rely on blood gas analysis to verify their validity (see Chapter 6).

Exercise Tests

Physical exercise stresses the heart, lungs, and the pulmonary and peripheral circulatory systems.

Exercise testing allows simultaneous evaluation of the cellular, cardiovascular, and ventilatory systems. Cardiopulmonary exercise tests can be used to determine the level of fitness or extent of dysfunction. Appropriately designed tests can determine the role of cardiac or pulmonary involvement. COPD, interstitial lung disease, pulmonary vascular disease, and exercise-induced bronchospasm are respiratory disorders that often require exercise evaluation. Understanding the physiologic basis for the patient's inability to exercise is an important aspect in prescribing effective therapy (i.e., cardiac or pulmonary rehabilitation). Exercise testing may also be required for determination of disability. Box 1-6 lists specific indications for exercise tests.

Equipment used to measure oxygen consumption and CO_2 production during exercise can also measure the REE. This allows estimates of caloric needs in patients who are critically ill. Indications for performing studies of REE are detailed in Chapter 9.

PATTERNS OF IMPAIRED PULMONARY FUNCTION

Patients are usually referred to the pulmonary function laboratory to evaluate signs or symptoms of lung disease. In some instances, the clinician may wish to exclude a specific diagnosis such as asthma. Indications for different categories of pulmonary function tests have been described previously. Sometimes, patients display patterns during testing that are consistent with a specific diagnosis. This section presents an overview of some commonly encountered forms of impaired pulmonary function.

Obstructive Airway Diseases

An obstructive airway disease is one in which airflow into or out of the lungs is reduced. This simple definition includes a variety of pathologic conditions. Some of these conditions are closely related regarding how they cause airway obstruction. For example, mucus hypersecretion is a component of chronic bronchitis, asthma, and cystic fibrosis (CF), although their causes are distinct.

Chronic Obstructive Pulmonary Disease

The term *COPD* is often used to describe long-standing airway obstruction caused by emphysema, chronic bronchitis, or asthma. These three conditions may be present alone or in combination (Figure 1-2). Bronchiectasis is sometimes considered a component of COPD. COPD is characterized by dyspnea at rest or with exertion, often accompanied by a productive cough. Delineation of the type of obstruction depends on the history, physical examination, and pulmonary function studies. Unfortunately, the term *COPD* is used to describe the clinical findings of dyspnea or cough without attention to the actual cause. This may lead to inap-

propriate therapy. Other similar terms include chronic obstructive lung disease (COLD) and chronic airway obstruction (CAO).

Emphysema. Emphysema means "air trapping" and is defined morphologically. The air spaces distal to the terminal bronchioles are abnormally increased in size. The walls of the alveoli undergo destructive changes. This destruction results in over-inflation of lung units. If the process mainly involves the respiratory bronchioles, the emphysema is termed *centrilobular*. If the alveoli are also involved, the term *panlobular* emphysema is used to describe the pattern. These distinctions require examination of lung tissue either by biopsy or at postmortem. Because this is often impractical, emphysema is suspected when there is airway obstruction with air trapping. Physical assessment, chest x-ray or CT studies, and pulmonary function studies are the primary diagnostic tools. Spirometry (FVC, FEV_1, and FEV_1/FVC) is used to determine the presence and extent of obstruction. Lung volumes (TLC, RV, IC, and RV/TLC) define the pattern of air trapping or hyperinflation caused by emphysema. D_{LCO} and blood gas analyses are useful in tracking the degree of gas exchange abnormality in emphysema. Exercise testing may be necessary if the emphysema patient is suspected of oxygen desaturation with exertion, or to plan pulmonary rehabilitation.

Emphysema is caused primarily by cigarette smoking. Repeated inflammation of the respiratory bronchioles results in tissue destruction. As the disease advances, more and more alveolar walls are destroyed. Loss of elastic tissue results in airway collapse, air trapping, and hyperinflation. Some emphysema is caused by the absence of a protective enzyme, α_1-antitrypsin. The lack of this enzyme is caused by a genetic defect. α_1-Antitrypsin inhibits proteases in the blood from attacking healthy tissue. Deficiency of α_1-antitrypsin causes gradual destruction of alveolar walls, resulting in panlobular emphysema. Chronic exposure to environmental pollutants can also contribute to the development of emphysema. The natural aging of the lung also causes some changes that resemble the disease entity. The natural decline of elastic recoil in the lung reduces maximal airflow and increases lung

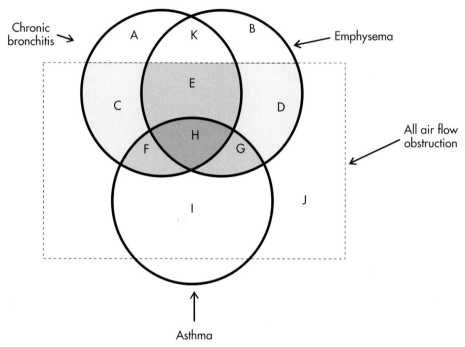

FIGURE 1-2   Nonproportional Diagram Depicting the Relationship Between Various Components of COPD. Emphysema, chronic bronchitis, and asthma overlap to varying degrees *(shaded areas)*. Chronic obstruction in small airways and all airway obstructive diseases *(large dashed square)* also overlap. **A,** Patients with chronic bronchitis but no airflow obstruction. **B,** Patients with anatomic changes related to emphysema, but no obstruction. **C,** Patients with chronic cough and airflow obstruction. **D,** Patients with emphysema and obstruction as demonstrated by spirometry. **E,** Combined chronic bronchitis and emphysema, commonly occurring in the same patient as a result of cigarette smoking. **F,** Combined chronic bronchitis and asthma. **G,** Combined emphysema and asthma. **H,** Combined asthma, chronic bronchitis, and emphysema. **I,** Patients with asthma manifested by reversible obstruction (spirometry or peak flow). **J,** Other forms of airway obstruction, including cystic fibrosis, bronchiolitis obliterans, or upper airway abnormalities (e.g., vocal cord dysfunction) are not considered part of COPD. **K,** Patients with cough and morphologic evidence of emphysema, but no obstruction. *(Modified from American Thoracic Society: Standards for the diagnosis and care of patients with chronic obstructive pulmonary disease, Am J Respir Crit Care Med 1995; 152:S77-S120.)*

volume as people age. Surgical removal of lung tissue sometimes causes the remaining lung to overinflate.

The main symptom of emphysema is breathlessness, either at rest or with exertion. Hypoxemia may contribute to this dyspnea, particularly in advanced emphysema. However, the destruction of alveolar walls also causes loss of the capillary bed. Ventilation-perfusion matching may be relatively well preserved in patients with emphysema. As a result, oxygen levels may be only slightly decreased, particularly at rest. This type of patient is sometimes called the "pink puffer." As the disease advances, the loss of alveolar surface causes a decreased ability to oxygenate mixed venous blood. DLCO is reduced. The patient becomes increasingly breathless, particularly with exertion. Muscle wasting seems to be common in emphysema, and patients are often below their ideal body weight. As noted, symptoms of chronic bronchitis and asthma may be present as well.

The chest x-ray film of a patient with emphysema shows flattened diaphragms and increased air spaces. The lung fields appear hyperlucent (dark) with little vascularity. The heart appears to be hanging from the great vessels. Computerized tomography (CT) scans, especially spiral CT scans, show a three-dimensional picture of enlarged air spaces and loss of supporting tissue. CT scans also delineate whether the emphysematous changes are localized or spread throughout the lungs.

The physical appearance of the chest confirms what is shown radiographically. The chest wall is immobile with the shoulders elevated. The diameter of the chest is increased in the anterior-posterior aspect (so-called barrel chest). There is little diaphragmatic excursion during inspiration. Intercostal retractions may be prominent. Accessory muscles (neck and shoulders) are used to lift the chest wall. Breath sounds are distant or absent. Patients may need to support the arms and shoulders to catch their breath. Breathing is often done through pursed lips in an attempt to alleviate the sensation of dyspnea.

Chronic Bronchitis. Chronic bronchitis is diagnosed by clinical findings. It is present when there is excessive mucus production, with a productive cough on most days, for at least 3 months for 2 years or more. The diagnosis is made by excluding other diseases that also result in excess mucus production. These include cystic fibrosis, tuberculosis, abscess, tumors, or bronchiectasis.

Chronic bronchitis, like emphysema, is caused primarily by cigarette smoking. It may also result from chronic exposure to environmental pollutants and secondhand smoke. Chronic bronchitis causes the mucus glands lining the airways to hypertrophy and increase in number. There is also chronic inflammation of the bronchial wall with infiltration of leukocytes and lymphocytes. The number of ciliated epithelial cells decreases. This causes impairment of mucus flow in the airways. Similar changes occur in respiratory bronchioles. Excessive mucus and poor clearance make the patient susceptible to repeated infections. Some patients who have chronic bronchitis caused by cigarette smoking experience a decrease in cough and mucus production after smoking cessation. Some airway changes, however, usually persist. Spirometry is useful in evaluating the extent of airway obstruction due to bronchitic changes. D_{LCO} may be helpful in distinguishing emphysema and chronic bronchitis; bronchitis patients may have

preserved D_{LCO}, while emphysema patients tend to have reduced D_{LCO}. However, D_{LCO} is usually not normal in chronic bronchitis because of mismatching of ventilation and perfusion caused by bronchial obstruction.

Chronic cough is the defining symptom of chronic bronchitis. Some patients do not consider cough abnormal and refer to it as "smoker's cough" or "morning cough." In addition to cough, chronic bronchitis may produce dyspnea, particularly with exertion. Blood gas abnormalities usually accompany chronic bronchitis. Ventilation-perfusion mismatching causes hypoxemia. If hypoxemia is significant and persists, the patient may develop secondary polycythemia. Cyanosis may be present due to the combination of arterial desaturation and increased Hb levels. Chronic hypoxemia may also lead to right-sided heart failure (cor pulmonale) with peripheral edema, particularly in the feet and ankles. Advanced chronic bronchitis is also often accompanied by CO_2 retention (**hypercapnia**).

Unlike the emphysema patient, the patient with chronic bronchitis may show few clinical signs of underlying disease. Body weight may be normal or increased with minimal changes to the chest wall. Patients with bronchitis may appear normal except for cough and dyspnea. The chest x-ray film in chronic bronchitis differs markedly from that in emphysema. The congested airways are easily visible. The heart may appear enlarged with the pulmonary vessels prominent. The diaphragms may appear normal or flattened, depending on the degree of air trapping present. If there is right-sided heart failure, swelling (**edema**) of the lower extremities is often present.

Pulmonary infections can seriously aggravate chronic bronchitis, and patients who have chronic bronchitis tend to have an increased number of chest infections. The appearance of the sputum produced can help predict worsening function. If it is normally white, a change to discolored sputum indicates the beginning of an infection. This may be accompanied by worsened hypoxemia and shortness of breath. Early treatment can potentially reverse an otherwise serious complication. Failure to manage the chest infection can result in severe hypoxemia and hypercapnia, with exacerbation of right-sided heart failure. Acute respiratory failure superimposed on chronic failure is a common cause of death in patients with COPD.

Bronchiectasis. Bronchiectasis is pathologic dilatation of the bronchi. It usually results from destruction of the bronchial walls by severe, repeated infections, but some individuals are born with it (congenital bronchiectasis). The terms *saccular, cystic,* and *tubular* are used to describe the appearance of the bronchi. Most bronchiectasis involves prolonged episodes of infection. Bronchiectasis is common in cystic fibrosis (CF), as well as following bronchial obstruction by a tumor or foreign body. When the entire bronchial tree is involved, it is assumed that the disease is inherited or caused by developmental abnormalities.

The main clinical feature of bronchiectasis is a very productive cough. The sputum is usually purulent and foul smelling. Hemoptysis is also common. Frequent bronchopulmonary infections lead to gas exchange abnormalities similar to those of chronic bronchitis. Right-sided heart failure follows advancement of the disease. Chest x-ray studies, bronchograms, and CT scans are used to identify the type and extent of the disease. As in chronic bronchitis, spirometry may be useful for assessing the degree of obstruction and response to therapy.

Treatment of bronchiectasis includes vigorous bronchial hygiene. Regular antibiotic therapy is used to manage the repeated infections. Bronchoscopy and surgical resection are sometimes required to manage localized areas of infection. Patients with recurrent hemoptysis may require resection of the offending lobe.

Management of Chronic Obstructive Pulmonary Disease. COPD is a leading cause of morbidity and mortality throughout the world. COPD often includes components of emphysema and chronic bronchitis (see Figure 1-2). This association most likely is due to the common risk factor of cigarette smoking. Hyperreactive airways disease (asthma) may also be present. Reversibility of obstruction, however, is usually less than in uncomplicated asthma. Bronchiectasis and bronchiolitis are also commonly found in patients with COPD.

An essential ingredient in COPD management is early diagnosis. The NLHEP and the WHO both recommend spirometry as a primary tool in early detection of chronic airflow limitation. Spirometry is recommended for all smokers over the age of 45 and for anyone with chronic cough, dyspnea on exertion, mucus hypersecretion, or wheezing.

Treatment of COPD begins with smoking cessation and avoiding irritants that inflame the airways. The rate of decline in lung function (FEV_1) in smokers is approximately twice that of nonsmokers. Smoking cessation decreases the accelerated decline in most, but not all, smokers. Other measures aimed at keeping the airways open are also important. Inhaled bronchodilators, especially β-agonists, are commonly used. Combinations of β-adrenergic and anticholinergic bronchodilators, together with inhaled corticosteroids, provide relief for many patients with COPD. This is often the case, even when there is little improvement in airflow assessed by spirometry. Some patients require oral steroids (e.g., prednisone) to manage chronic inflammation. Antibiotics are commonly used at the first sign of respiratory infections, and vaccination against viral and bacterial (pneumococcus) infection is recommended. Digitalis and diuretics are most often prescribed for the management of cor pulmonale.

Breathing retraining, bronchial hygiene measures, and physical reconditioning are important therapeutic modalities in addition to pharmacologic management. Breathing retraining is especially important for the patient with advanced COPD. Grossly altered pulmonary mechanics favor hyperinflation and use of accessory muscles. Training in the use of the diaphragm for slow, relaxed breathing can significantly improve gas exchange. Pulmonary rehabilitation, particularly physical reconditioning, permits many patients with otherwise debilitating disease to maintain their quality of life.

Supplemental O_2 therapy is indicated in COPD when the patient's oxygen tension at rest or during exercise is less than 55 mm Hg. Oxygen may also be prescribed when signs of cor pulmonale are present. Many patients desaturate only with exertion. Exercise testing is the only reliable method of detecting exertional desaturation. Low-flow O_2 therapy can be implemented by a number of methods, including portable systems. Chronic O_2 supplementation has been shown to improve survival in patients with COPD.

Single-lung transplantation has been used for patients with end-stage COPD who are younger than 60 years. Although lung transplantation causes immediate improvement in pulmonary function, it is expensive. The cost of hospitalization and follow-up care may be prohibitive. In addition, lack of donor organs means that many patients with COPD die while awaiting transplantation. The prognosis for those receiving lung transplants is generally good. In some transplant recipients, a severe form of airway obstruction (bronchiolitis obliterans) has been found to occur in the transplanted lung. The reason for this obstructive process is unclear, but the progression is rapid. Spirometry is used to monitor transplant recipients to detect early changes associated with bronchiolitis obliterans.

Lung volume reduction surgery (LVRS) has also been used to treat end-stage COPD. In this procedure, lung tissue that is poorly perfused is surgically removed. This allows the remaining lung units to expand with improved ventilation-perfusion matching. This technique works particularly well when there are well-defined areas of trapped gas with little perfusion (bullae). The procedure can be performed by sternotomy, or using a flexible thoracoscope. With both methods, lung volumes (TLC and RV) are reduced and spirometry and gas exchange improve. Spirometry, lung volume measurement, and blood gas analysis are used to monitor changes in these patients. Lung volume reduction is expensive, carries significant risk, and does not appear to benefit all patients who have air trapping.

Hyperreactive Airways Disease: Asthma

Asthma is characterized by reversible airway obstruction. Obstruction is caused by inflammation of the mucosal lining of the airways, bronchospasm, and increased airway secretions. Bronchospasm is usually reversed by inhalation of bronchodilators but may be persistent and severe in some patients. Inflammation is the essential element in the asthmatic response. Increased airway responsiveness is related to inhalation of antigens, viral infections, air pollution, occupational exposure, cold air, and exercise. Spirometry is the most useful tool for detecting reversible airway obstruction. Improvement in the FEV_1 or FVC (see Chapter 2) is the hallmark of reversibility. Airway resistance (Raw) and specific airway conductance (sGaw) are also useful in evaluation of reversible obstruction. Peak expiratory flow (PEF), measured using portable peak flow meters, can provide immediate information for a clinician or patient to modify therapy. Analysis of exhaled nitric oxide (eNO) can detect inflammatory changes in the airways even in the absence of spirometric or peak flow abnormalities.

Asthma can occur at any age but often begins during childhood. Even infants can have hyperreactive airways (see Chapter 8). Some asthmatic children outgrow the disease, but in others the disease continues into adulthood. In some individuals, asthma begins in adulthood, usually after age 40. There appears to be a hereditary component to asthma; many cases occur in patients who have a family history of asthma or allergic disorders.

Agents or events that cause an asthmatic episode are called *triggers* (Box 1-7). Antigens such as animal dander, pollens, and dusts are the most common triggers. Other common triggers include exposure to air pollutants, exercise in cold or dry air, occupational exposure to dusts or fumes, and viral upper respiratory infections. Aspirin or other drugs can also trigger asthma, as can food additives (e.g., metabisulfites) or emotional upset (e.g., crying, laughing). All of these triggers act on the hyperresponsive airway to produce the symptoms of asthma.

The most common presentation of asthma includes wheezing, cough, and shortness of breath. The severity of asthmatic episodes varies, even in the same individual at different times. In many patients, airway function is relatively normal between intermittent episodes or attacks. Some patients have only cough or chest tightness that subsides spontaneously. However, severe episodes may be life threatening. In its worst presentation,

---

BOX 1-7   Asthma Triggers

A. Allergic agents
  1. Pollens
  2. Animal dander (proteins)
  3. House dust mites
  4. Molds
B. Nonallergic agents
  1. Viral infections
  2. Exercise
  3. Cold air
  4. Air pollutants (sulfur, nitrogen dioxides)
  5. Cigarette smoke
  6. Drugs (aspirin, beta-blockers)
  7. Food additives
  8. Emotional upset
C. Occupational exposure
  1. Toluene 2,4-diisocyanate (TDI)
  2. Cotton, wood dusts
  3. Grain
  4. Metal salts
  5. Insecticides

---

asthma causes continuous chest tightness and wheezing that may not respond to the usual therapy. Dyspnea and cough can both be extreme, and if unresolved they can progress to respiratory failure.

During an attack there is usually wheezing, noisy breathing, and prolonged expiratory times. If the attack is severe, there may be significant air trapping, similar to the pattern seen in patients with emphysema. Accessory muscles of ventilation are used, and breathing may be labored. Spirometry or peak flows provide a simple means of tracking response to bronchodilators. Arterial blood gas testing may be necessary during severe asthmatic episodes. Hypoxemia is commonly present because of ventilation-perfusion mismatching. This usually results in a respiratory alkalosis, but evidence of respiratory acidosis suggests impending ventilatory failure.

Bronchial provocation tests using methacholine, histamine, exercise, or hyperventilation are often used to make the diagnosis of hyperreactive airways in patients who appear normal but have episodic symptoms. Skin testing is also used to demonstrate sensitivity to inhaled antigens. Elevated exhaled NO levels are also predictive of airway inflammation common in the asthmatic and usually correlate with hyperresponsiveness measured by conventional bronchial challenge tests.

Management of Asthma. The first step in asthma management is avoiding known triggers. In some instances this is easily accomplished. However, in the case of air pollution or occupational exposure, avoiding the offending substance may be expensive or impossible. Asthma education usually focuses on helping the affected individual identify and avoid triggers.

Pharmacologic management of asthma is usually based on a combination of bronchodilator, steroid, and anti-inflammatory therapy. For some patients with mild asthma, a β-adrenergic bronchodilator from a metered-dose inhaler (MDI) may be the only treatment required. A variety of β-agonists are available and these drugs are typically used as rescue medications. In moderate or severe asthma, long-acting β-adrenergic bronchodilators (such as salmeterol) are usually inhaled on a dosing schedule. Anticholinergic bronchodilators (such as ipratropium or tiotropium) have become widely prescribed for use in conjunction with β-agonists. Anticholinergic bronchodilators may be preferred in patients who experience tachycardia or tremor caused by adrenergic drugs. Although most β-agonists have a rapid onset of action (5–15 minutes), anticholinergic bronchodilators typically take 30–60 minutes for peak effect to occur, but with much longer lasting effects.

Inhaled corticosteroids (such as beclomethasone, fluticasone, budesonide, and mometasone) are the most effective treatment for mild, moderate, and severe asthma. Steroids act primarily as anti-inflammatory agents in the airways and may allow bronchodilators to work more effectively. Several different preparations are available in metered-dose or dry powder inhalers. Combinations of inhaled steroids and long-acting β-adrenergic bronchodilators seem to be effective at preventing asthma symptoms. Children and adolescents may not respond to inhaled steroids. Corticosteroids in general have a number of adverse side effects, including reduction in bone density and adrenal suppression. Inhaled steroids have relatively fewer side effects; fungal infection of the oral cavity is a common problem. Inhaled steroids decrease bone density, and their effect on growth in children is not completely understood.

Cromolyn sodium or nedocromil is used to prophylactically prevent bronchoconstriction by blocking the release of mediators from mast cells in the airways. They cannot be used for acute episodes but may decrease the amount of corticosteroids or bronchodilators necessary. Cromolyn derivatives are available as a nebulized solution, inhaled powder, or MDI.

Leukotriene receptor antagonists are also used to reduce airway inflammation in asthma. They block the release of leukotrienes, which potentiate inflammatory mediators. These drugs may be effective in cases in which inhaled steroids are not, and have been successfully used in conjunction with steroids. Some patients may better accept oral preparations of leukotriene inhibitors.

Some patients who have severe asthma caused by allergies may benefit from drugs that block immunoglobulin E (IgE)–mediated responses. Omalizumab blocks IgE from binding to mast cells and prevents activation that can lead to inflammation.

A significant tool in the management of asthma is the portable peak flow meter (see Chapters 2 and 10). This device allows simple monitoring of airway function by the patient at home, as well as by caregivers in a variety of settings. Measuring peak flow provides objective data to guide both the patient and physician in modifying bronchodilator therapy or seeking early treatment. Computerized peak flow meters that include symptom history (i.e., an electronic diary) allow asthma management to be tailored to the individual asthmatic's needs.

Cystic Fibrosis

Cystic fibrosis (CF) is a disease that primarily affects the mucus-producing apparatus of the lungs and pancreas. CF is an inherited disorder, transmitted as an autosomal recessive trait. In whites, it occurs in approximately 1 in 2000 live births; in African Americans CF is much less common, occurring in only 1 of 17,000 live births. A simple test, the sweat test, measures the chloride level in sweat, which is elevated in CF. Some states require a screening blood test for CF in newborns. CF was once considered a pediatric disease because affected individuals rarely lived to adulthood. Improved detection and aggressive treatment have increased the median survival age well into adulthood.

CF is characterized by malabsorption of food because of pancreatic insufficiency and progressive suppurative pulmonary disease. In infancy and early childhood, gastrointestinal manifestations seem to predominate. As the child gets older, respiratory complications related to the tenacious mucus production take over. Other organ systems may be involved as well. Children with CF tend to remain chronically infected with respiratory pathogens, such as *Staphylococcus aureus*, *Pseudomonas aeruginosa*, or *Burkholderia cepacia*.

Clinical manifestations of CF include chronic cough and sinusitis, bronchiectasis, and atelectasis. Hemoptysis and pneumothorax are common. Pulmonary function studies may be used to follow the progression of the disease. Spirometry (FEV_1) is frequently measured as an index of the need for lung transplantation. Chest x-ray studies show changes consistent with bronchiectasis and honeycombing. Atelectasis commonly affects entire lobes as a result of mucus impaction. Other complications center on gastrointestinal manifestations (e.g., bowel obstruction and vitamin deficiencies). Most individuals with CF are diagnosed in infancy or early childhood based on elevated sweat chloride levels. Occasionally, some young adults are not diagnosed until after age 15. In many instances, adolescents or even adults are misdiagnosed as having asthma or related pulmonary diseases. Misdiagnosis usually occurs in individuals who have mild CF with few complications.

Management of Cystic Fibrosis. Removal of the excess mucus produced in CF is the primary focus of management. This usually requires bronchial hygiene measures and pharmacologic intervention. Bronchodilators are used to reverse bronchospasm that commonly accompanies chronic inflammation. A genetically engineered enzyme is now used to reduce mucus viscosity in CF patients. This enzyme (rhDNase) is administered via an aerosol. This reduces the viscosity of secretions and improves airflow. Corticosteroids are used to combat both pulmonary inflammation and bronchial hyperreactivity. Continuous or intermittent antibiotics are also a mainstay of care in the patient with CF. Proper nutrition is similarly important in managing CF. Pancreatic insufficiency increases the patient's metabolic rate, even though nutrients are poorly absorbed in the intestine. Pancreatic enzyme supplements and vitamins are required, particularly in children with CF. For individuals with severe CF, lung transplantation has become a life-saving treatment. Pulmonary function studies are routinely used to assess lung function following transplantation.

Upper or Large Airway Obstruction

Many obstructive diseases involve the medium or small airways. Sometimes airway obstruction occurs in the upper airways (nose, mouth, or pharynx) or in the large thoracic airways (trachea, main stem bronchi). Obstruction can also occur where the upper and lower airways meet at the vocal cords. When obstruction occurs below the vocal cords, the degree of obstruction may vary with changes in thoracic pressure. This occurs because the airways themselves change size as thoracic pressure rises or falls. Obstructive processes above the vocal cords are not influenced by thoracic pressures but may still vary with airflow, depending on the type of lesion involved. Regardless of the location of the problem, large airway obstruction results in increased work of breathing. Extrathoracic or intrathoracic airway obstruction is frequently diagnosed using the flow-volume loop or measurements of airway resistance (see Chapter 2).

Vocal cord dysfunction or damage can result in significant airway obstruction. The vocal cords are normally held open or abducted during inspiration. When damaged, the vocal cords move toward the midline, narrowing the airway opening. This type of obstruction limits flow primarily during inspiration. In some cases, expiratory flow may be reduced as well, but inspiratory flow is typically lower. Common causes of vocal cord dysfunction (VCD) include laryngeal muscle weakness or mechanical damage as sometimes occurs during intubation of the trachea. Severe infections

involving the larynx can leave scar tissue on the vocal cords or supporting structures. Vocal cord dysfunction often mimics asthma. It may become noticeably worse when ventilation is increased, as happens during exercise. Neuromuscular disorders can cause paralysis of the vocal cords, also resulting in variable extrathoracic airway obstruction (see Chapter 2).

Tumors are a common cause of large airway obstruction. Lesions that invade the trachea or main stem bronchi can significantly diminish airflow. The decrease in flow is directly related to the decrease in cross-sectional area of the airway. If the airway lumen (i.e., the part not obstructed) varies in cross-sectional area with inspiration and expiration, the obstruction is described as variable. During inspiration, thoracic pressure decreases and large airways increase their cross-sectional area. During expiration, the opposite occurs. If the airway is partially obstructed by a tumor, airflow will be decreased during inspiration and expiration, but more so during expiration. If the tumor reduces the cross-sectional area of the airway but does not cause it to change with the phase of breathing, the obstruction is fixed. In this instance both inspiratory and expiratory flows are reduced approximately equally (see Chapter 2). Tumors involving the upper airway may cause variable or fixed obstruction. If an extrathoracic tumor causes the airway cross section to vary with breathing, inspiratory flow is usually reduced.

Neuromuscular disorders that affect the muscles of the upper airway can also affect airway patency. When the muscles of the pharynx or larynx are relaxed (reduced muscle tone), airway collapse may occur during the inspiratory phase of breathing. Any disorder that affects innervation of pharyngeal muscles can cause similar obstructive patterns. Abnormal airflow patterns are sometimes seen in patients who have obstructive sleep apnea (OSA), although flow measurements cannot predict sleep apnea. Myasthenia gravis affects the muscles of respiration, including the muscles of the upper airway. Generalized weakness of these muscles can result in variable extrathoracic obstruction.

Both extrathoracic and intrathoracic large airway obstruction commonly result from trauma to the airways. This can occur as the result of motor vehicle accidents or falls. Scarring or stenosis of the trachea may also occur after prolonged endotracheal intubation or tracheostomy. The typical pattern is one of fixed obstruction, although some lesions do vary with the phase of breathing. Granulomatous disease, such as sarcoidosis or tuberculosis, can occasionally cause upper airway obstruction. Extrinsic airway compression can also reduce airflow. Goiters or mediastinal masses are the most common culprits that compress the airways in this way.

Management of Upper or Large Airway Obstruction. Treatment of extrathoracic or intrathoracic large airway obstruction is aimed at reversing the process produced by the offending lesions. For vocal cord dysfunction, stopping inappropriate therapy (e.g., steroids) is the first step. Speech therapy and breathing retraining have been demonstrated to reduce inspiratory obstruction. In severe cases, a mixture of helium and oxygen (80% He – 20% O_2) may be needed to alleviate dyspnea and interrupt the episode. Treatment of neuromuscular disease, such as myasthenia gravis, often reverses the associated airway obstruction. Tumors usually require resection. Some neoplasms can be managed only by radiation or chemotherapy. In either case, spirometry with flow-volume curves (see Chapter 2) is used to assess airway obstruction. Surgical repair of trauma to the upper or large airways directly relieves airway obstruction and reduces the work of breathing.

Restrictive Lung Disease

Restrictive lung disease is characterized by reduction of lung volumes. The VC and TLC are both reduced below the lower limit of normal (LLN). Any process that interferes with the bellows action of the lungs or chest wall can cause restriction. Restriction is often associated with the following:

- Interstitial lung diseases, including idiopathic fibrosis, pneumoconioses, and sarcoidosis
- Disease of the chest wall and pleura
- Neuromuscular disorders
- Congestive heart failure (CHF)

- Obesity
- Lung resection
- Scarring (fibrosis) caused by radiation or chemotherapy
- Transient problems such as pleural effusions, abdominal ascites, or pregnancy.

Pulmonary Fibrosis

Pulmonary fibrosis involves scarring of the lung with involvement at the alveolar level. Multiple causes have been identified, including environmental pollutants, smoking, radiation, and connective tissue diseases. Patients who have pulmonary fibrosis present with dyspnea that increase with exertion and a dry, nonproductive cough.

Pulmonary fibrosis often follows the use of medications such as bleomycin, cyclophosphamide, methotrexate, or amiodarone. It is also associated with a number of autoimmune diseases. Rheumatoid arthritis, systemic lupus erythematosus (SLE), and scleroderma all produce alveolar wall inflammation and fibrotic changes. As each disease progresses, lung volumes are reduced. These reductions in VC and TLC occur as fibrosis causes the lungs to become stiff. Measurement of pulmonary compliance (see Chapter 2) is sometimes helpful in quantifying the effects of the fibrosis. DLCO (see Chapter 5) is often reduced because of loss of lung volume and ventilation-perfusion mismatching. The same processes also cause hypoxemia at rest that worsens with exertion.

When other causes of pulmonary fibrosis have been ruled out, this condition is called idiopathic pulmonary fibrosis (IPF). IPF is a chronic progressive interstitial lung disease of unknown etiology, characterized by alveolar wall inflammation resulting in fibrosis. Vascular changes are usually associated with pulmonary hypertension. These patients also have increasing exertional dyspnea, usually with a nonproductive cough. Clubbing of the fingers and expiratory rales are common physical findings. On the chest x-ray film, infiltrates are visible and advanced IPF shows a honeycombing pattern.

Management of pulmonary fibrosis relies primarily on corticosteroids (prednisone). Long-term therapy is usually indicated with large initial doses, followed by tapering and then maintenance. Immunosuppressive agents are sometimes used in conjunction with steroids in difficult cases. In the most severe presentations, lung transplantation may be required. Spirometry, lung volume measurements, and DLCO are routinely used to monitor the patient's progress and response to therapeutic interventions. Blood gases and exercise tests may be needed to gauge the degree of oxygen desaturation that is known to occur.

Pneumoconioses

Pneumoconiosis is lung impairment caused by inhalation of dusts. Specific types of dust exposures have been shown to result in pneumoconioses (Table 1-1). Dust particles in the size range between 0.5 and 5.0 microns are considered most dangerous because they are deposited throughout the lung. A carefully taken history of the patient's exposure, including work history, is essential. (See Pulmonary History in the Preliminaries to Patient Testing section.) Most pneumoconioses are characterized by pulmonary fibrosis and chest x-ray abnormalities. Pulmonary function studies typically reveal a restrictive pattern with reduction in DLCO.

Silicosis, caused by inhalation of silica dust, is common. Silica is found in sand, slate, granite and other ores; sandblasting, mining, and ceramic work are a few of the occupations commonly exposed to silica. Silica is deposited in the lung and ingested by macrophages. This results in the formation of nodules around bronchioles and blood vessels. As the silicosis advances, fibrosis occurs. The patient usually has cough and dyspnea, especially on exertion. In addition to restriction shown by pulmonary function studies, some airways may also be obstructed. As nodules increase in size to more than 1 cm, the condition is labeled progressive massive fibrosis (PMF). PMF is usually accompanied by hypoxemia and pulmonary hypertension. Treatment of silicosis is directed at relieving hypoxemia and managing right-sided heart failure.

Asbestosis results from inhalation of asbestos fibers. Asbestos has been commonly used in the manufacture of insulating materials, brake linings, roofing materials, and fire-resistant materials. As with most pneumoconioses, the risk of developing asbestosis is related to the intensity and duration of exposure. The onset of symptoms is usually delayed for 20 years. Cigarette smoking has been shown to shorten the period between exposure and onset of symptoms. Inhaled asbestos fibers are engulfed by alveolar macrophages. Fibrosis in alveolar walls and around bronchioles develops. The visceral pleura may also show fibrous deposits. Plaques, made up of collagenous connective tissue, are often found on the parietal pleura. The patient experiences dyspnea on exertion. Pulmonary function tests show restriction and impaired diffusion (DLCO). The chest x-ray film may show irregular densities in the lower lung fields, fibrotic changes (honeycombing), and diaphragmatic calcifications.

TABLE 1-1

Common Pneumoconioses

Dust	Pneumoconiosis	Occupation
Iron	Siderosis	Welder, miner
Tin	Stannosis	Metal worker
Barium	Baritosis	Miner, metallurgist, ceramics worker
Silica	Silicosis	Sandblaster, brick maker, coal miner
Asbestos	Asbestosis	Brake/clutch manufacturer, shipbuilder, steam fitter, insulator
Talc	Talcosis	Ceramics worker, cosmetics maker
Beryllium	Berylliosis	Alloy maker, electronic tube maker, metal worker
Coal	Coal worker's pneumoconiosis	Coal miner

COPD and lung cancer are also common in patients with asbestosis and are related to cigarette smoking. Treatment consists of assessment with pulmonary function tests (especially diffusing capacity) and relief of symptoms.

Coal worker's pneumoconiosis (CWP) is caused by an accumulation of coal dust (carbon particles) in the lungs. It should not be confused with black lung, which is a legal term used to describe any chronic respiratory disease in a coal miner. Some coal contains silica, but CWP begins with a reaction to an accumulation of dust, called a *coal macule*. These macules are usually found in the upper lobes. The black coal pigment is deposited around the respiratory bronchioles. Diagnosis of CWP is made by history and chest x-ray film interpretation. Onset of symptoms caused by CWP usually occurs in advanced cases. Coal workers often have respiratory symptoms and physiologic findings consistent with COPD. These symptoms may be related more to cigarette smoking than to coal dust exposure. CWP causes fibrosis, restriction on pulmonary function tests, hypoxemia, and pulmonary hypertension. As in the case of other pneumoconioses, treatment is aimed at relief of the symptoms.

Sarcoidosis

Sarcoidosis is a granulomatous disease that affects multiple organ systems. The lungs are often involved. The disease appears most often in the second through fourth decades. In the United States, it seems to occur more commonly in African Americans, especially in women. The granulomas found in sarcoidosis are composed of macrophages, epithelioid cells, and other inflammatory cells. Sarcoidosis has an active phase and a nonactive phase. In the active phase, granulomas form and increase in size. These granulomatous lesions may resolve with little or no structural change or may develop fibrosis in the target organ. In the nonactive phase, inflammation subsides but scar tissue usually remains.

Symptoms of sarcoidosis include fatigue, muscle weakness, fever, and weight loss. Other symptoms involve the specific organ system in which the granulomatous changes occur. The lungs and lymph nodes of the mediastinum are frequently involved in patients who have sarcoidosis. Dyspnea and a dry, nonproductive cough are the most common presenting symptoms. Chest x-ray films usually show enlargement of the hilar and mediastinal lymph nodes. Interstitial infiltrates may also be present. Other systems commonly involved in sarcoidosis include the skin, eyes, musculoskeletal system, heart, and central nervous system.

Pulmonary function tests show a pattern of restriction, with relatively normal flows. It is not unusual for sarcoidosis in the early stages to show completely normal lung function. Diffusing capacity may not be reduced, except when there is advanced fibrosis of lung tissue. Arterial blood gas measurements may be normal, or there may be hypoxemia. Cardiopulmonary exercise testing may show worsened gas exchange. Diagnosis of sarcoidosis is sometimes made via clinical findings and chest x-ray examination, but biopsy of affected tissue is often necessary. This may involve mediastinoscopy or fiberoptic bronchoscopy.

Management of sarcoidosis includes medications to treat symptoms such as fever, skin lesions, or arthralgia. Serious complications involving worsening pulmonary function are usually treated with corticosteroids.

Diseases of the Chest Wall and Pleura

Several disorders involving the chest wall or pleura of the lungs result in restrictive patterns on pulmonary function studies. Conditions affecting the thorax include kyphoscoliosis, pectus excavatum, and obesity. Pleural diseases include pleurisy, pleural effusions, and pneumothorax.

Kyphoscoliosis is a condition that involves abnormal curvature of the spine both anteriorly (kyphosis) and laterally (scoliosis). The degree of curvature is usually determined by x-rays, with curvature greater than 40 degrees requiring surgery. Patients who have kyphoscoliosis show rib cage distortion that can lead to recurrent infections as well as blood gas abnormalities. Depending on the degree of spinal curvature, the patient may have normal lung function or restriction. Ventilation may be normal. Lung compression usually causes ventilation-perfusion mismatching and hypoxemia. In severe cases, there may be hypercapnia and respiratory acidosis. Treatment of the disorder involves prevention of infections and relief of hypoxemia, if present. Surgical correction is necessary in many cases, and pulmonary function studies are used to evaluate patients both preoperatively and postoperatively.

Pectus excavatum (sunken chest) is a congenital abnormality affecting development of the sternum and ribs of the anterior chest. It is found more frequently in boys than in girls (approximately 3:1) and occurs in about 1 in 300–400 births, making it the most common congenital abnormality of the chest. The caved-in chest is usually obvious in infants, but often does not cause significant limitations until adolescence. Pectus excavatum varies in severity, but typically results in a restrictive pattern on pulmonary function tests. Exercise testing, or other tests of cardiac performance, may be indicated to assess functional limitations in severe cases. Pulmonary function and exercise tests may also be used to assess improvements following corrective surgery.

Obesity restricts ventilation, especially when the obesity is severe. Obesity is usually categorized using the body mass index (BMI). BMI equals body weight in kilogram divided by height in meters squared (BMI = kg/m^2). A BMI of 18.5–24.9 is normal; 25–29.9 is considered overweight, and 30 or greater is considered obese. A BMI of 40 or greater is sometimes referred to as morbid obesity. Increased mass of the thorax and abdomen interferes with the bellows action of the chest wall, as well as excursion of the diaphragm. Total lung capacity (TLC) and vital capacity (VC) are usually preserved in obese individuals, but FRC (functional residual capacity) and expiratory reserve volume (ERV) are characteristically reduced. Obesity is also sometimes associated with asthma-like symptoms. It is not clear whether asthma is related to obesity or if the restriction caused by obesity contributes to airflow limitation that mimics asthma.

Obesity may also be associated with a more general syndrome that consists of hypercapnia and hypoxemia, sleep apnea, and decreased respiratory drive. The combination of these findings is sometimes called the obesity-hypoventilation syndrome. Chronic hypoxemia in this syndrome results in polycythemia, pulmonary hypertension, and cor pulmonale. Not all patients who are obese show the signs of obesity-hypoventilation syndrome. However, pulmonary function studies often show restriction in proportion to the excess weight. Weight reduction relieves many of the associated symptoms. Respiratory stimulants, tracheostomy, and continuous positive airway pressure (CPAP) are used to manage the obstructive sleep apnea component.

Pleurisy and pleural effusions can each result in restrictive ventilatory patterns. Pleurisy is characterized by deposition of a fibrous exudate on the pleural surface. It is associated with other pulmonary diseases such as pneumonia or lung cancer. Pleurisy is often accompanied by chest discomfort or pain and may precede the development of pleural effusions. Pleural effusion is an abnormal accumulation of fluid in the pleural space. This fluid may be either a transudate or an exudate. Transudates occur when there is an imbalance in the hydrostatic or oncotic pressures, as occurs in congestive heart failure (CHF). Exudates are associated with infections or with inflammation, as in lung carcinoma. Patients with pleural effusions usually have symptoms that relate to the extent of the effusion. Small effusions often go unnoticed. If the effusion is large, there may be atelectasis from compression of lung tissue, and associated blood gas changes. Pulmonary function tests show restriction as a result of volume loss. In some cases, there is restriction caused by splinting as a result of pain. Treatment of pleurisy and pleural effusions is directed toward the underlying cause. Large or unresolved pleural effusions often require thoracentesis or chest tube drainage. Patients with painful pleural involvement may have difficulty performing spirometry or breath holding as required for DLCO.

Pneumothorax is a condition in which air enters the pleural space. This air leak may be due to a perforation of the lung itself or of the chest wall (e.g., chest trauma). A small pneumothorax may not cause any symptoms. A large pneumothorax results in severe dyspnea and chest pain. Physical examination of the patient reveals decreased chest movement on the affected side. Breath sounds are usually absent. A chest x-ray study shows a shift of the mediastinum away from the pneumothorax. Small pneumothoraces usually resolve without treatment as gas is reabsorbed from the pleural space. Large air leaks usually require a chest tube with appropriate drainage to allow lung re-expansion.

Pulmonary function tests are usually contraindicated in the presence of pneumothorax. However, undiagnosed pneumothorax may present a risk if pulmonary function studies are performed. Maneuvers that generate high intrathoracic pressures (i.e., FVC, MVV, MIP/MEP) can aggravate an untreated pneumothorax. The potential for development of a tension pneumothorax exists when these maneuvers are performed. In a tension pneumothorax, air enters the pleural space but cannot escape. Increasing pressure compresses the opposite lung, as well as the heart and great vessels. Compression of the mediastinum interferes with venous return to the heart and can cause a rapid drop in blood pressure. A tension pneumothorax can be fatal if not treated immediately. *Patients referred for pulmonary function studies who have a known or suspected pneumothorax should be tested very carefully, or not at all.* In many instances, the information obtained may not justify the risk to the patient.

Neuromuscular Disorders

Diseases that affect the spinal cord, peripheral nerves, neuromuscular junctions, and the respiratory muscles can all cause a restrictive pattern of pulmonary function. Most of these disorders result in an inability to generate normal respiratory pressures. The VC and TLC are often reduced, while the residual volume (RV) may be preserved. Some chronic neuromuscular disorders are associated with decreased lung compliance. Blood gas abnormalities, particularly hypoxemia, may result if the degree of involvement is severe. Stiff lungs and rapid respiratory rates often result in respiratory

alkalosis (**hyperventilation**). Progressive muscle weakness results in **hypoventilation** and respiratory failure.

Paralysis of the diaphragm may be bilateral or unilateral. Bilateral paralysis may be the end stage of various disorders. The most prominent finding is orthopnea, or shortness of breath in the supine position. In the upright position, the patient has a marked increase in VC and improvement in gas exchange. Simple spirometry in the supine and sitting positions can demonstrate the functional impairment. Unilateral paralysis often results from damage to one of the phrenic nerves (e.g., trauma, surgery, or tumor). As with bilateral paralysis, there is a marked change in VC from supine to sitting position. Diagnosis of which side is involved may require chest x-ray, or examination under fluoroscopy. Reduced inspiratory pressures (see Maximal Inspiratory Pressure in Chapter 2) may suggest diaphragmatic involvement.

Amyotrophic lateral sclerosis (ALS, or Lou Gehrig's disease) affects the anterior horn cells of the spinal cord (motor neurons). Progressive muscle weakness results in a gradual decrease in VC and TLC, which is invariably fatal. Pulmonary function studies may be done serially to assess the progression of the disease.

Guillain-Barré syndrome is a progressive disease in which the body's immune system attacks the peripheral nerves. Lower extremity weakness ascends to the upper extremities and face. There may be marked respiratory muscle weakness along with weakness of the pharyngeal and laryngeal muscles. Many patients eventually require mechanical support of ventilation. Serial measurements of the VC, MIP, and MEP are used to follow the disease progression.

Myasthenia gravis is chronic autoimmune disease affecting neuromuscular transmission. In myasthenia gravis, antibodies produced by the body's immune system block or destroy the receptors for acetylcholine at the neuromuscular junction, which prevents the muscle contraction from occurring. It particularly affects muscles innervated by the bulbar nuclei (i.e., face, lips, throat, and neck). The patient with myasthenia gravis has pronounced fatigability of the muscles. Speech and swallowing difficulties can occur with prolonged exercise of the associated muscles. Administration of edrophonium chloride (Tensilon) is sometimes used to confirm the diagnosis of myasthenia gravis; the drug blocks acetylcholinesterase and temporarily increases muscle strength in patients who have myasthenia gravis. When the ventilatory muscles become involved, a myasthenic crisis occurs. Progression of a myasthenic crisis can be assessed using VC and respiratory pressures. Analysis of the flow-volume curve (see Chapter 2) may be helpful in detecting upper airway obstruction brought on by muscular weakness.

Congestive Heart Failure

Congestive heart failure (CHF) is often used synonymously with left ventricular failure. Failure of the left ventricle may be caused by systemic hypertension, coronary artery disease, or aortic insufficiency. CHF may also be associated with cardiomyopathy, congenital heart defects, and left-to-right shunts. In each case, fluid backs up in the lungs. The pulmonary venous system becomes engorged. Fluid may spill into the alveolar spaces (pulmonary edema) or the pleural space (effusion).

The patient who has CHF usually has shortness of breath on exertion, cough, and fatigue. If coronary artery disease is the cause of CHF, there may be chest pain (angina) as well. Exertional dyspnea is related to pulmonary venous congestion. The fluid overload in the lungs reduces lung volume and makes the lungs stiff (decreased compliance). Dyspnea is usually worse when the patient is supine (i.e., orthopnea). This orthopnea results from increased pulmonary vascular congestion with increased venous return. Dyspnea brought on by CHF may be difficult to distinguish from other causes (e.g., chronic pulmonary disease), hence patients are often referred for pulmonary function studies. The chest x-ray film usually shows increased pulmonary congestion. The heart (left ventricle) may appear enlarged, particularly if systemic hypertension is the cause.

Treatment of CHF is directed at the underlying cause. Relief of systemic hypertension can reduce the myocardial workload. This is usually accomplished by vasodilator therapy. Reducing fluid retention is also important in managing CHF. Diuretics such as furosemide (Lasix) are commonly used to reduce the afterload on the ventricle. Oxygen therapy may also help reduce myocardial workload, especially if there is hypoxemia. If the cause of CHF is an arrhythmia, antiarrhythmic agents are typically used. Pulmonary function tests, particularly lung volumes and DLCO, may be used to monitor the effects of treatment.

Lung Transplantation

Lung transplantation has evolved as an effective treatment for end-stage lung disease. Lung transplantation has been used for patients with CF, primary pulmonary hypertension, and COPD (Table 1-2). Double-lung transplants are usually performed in patients who have CF, generalized bronchiectasis, or in some types of COPD. Heart-lung transplants have been used for Eisenmenger's syndrome, pulmonary hypertension with cor pulmonale, and end-stage lung disease coexisting with severe heart disease. Single-lung transplantation has been used effectively in patients with COPD who are younger than approximately 60 years old. Single-lung transplantation offers the benefit that two recipients can share a single donor's organs. Survival rates for lung transplant recipients have steadily improved. Longer survival is mainly due to more potent antirejection drugs (e.g., cyclosporine) and better adjunctive therapy. Pulmonary function tests are used to both assess potential transplant candidates and follow them postoperatively.

Preoperative evaluation consists of documentation of the severity of the specific disease process. Spirometry, lung volumes, DLCO, and blood gas analysis are all used to rank the level of dysfunction. The same tests are also used to detect sudden worsening of lung function that might necessitate rapid intervention. Cardiopulmonary exercise testing may be indicated to determine the extent of the physiologic abnormality. For example, a patient

TABLE 1-2	
Indications for Lung Transplantation	
Transplant Type	Disease State
Heart-lung	Eisenmenger's syndrome, severe cardiac defect
	Pulmonary hypertension, cor pulmonale
	End-stage lung disease, coexisting severe cardiac disease
Double-lung	Cystic fibrosis
	Generalized bronchiectasis
	COPD with severe chronic bronchitis or extensive bullae
Single-lung	Restrictive fibrotic lung disease
	Eisenmenger's syndrome (less severe cardiac anomalies)
	COPD
	Primary pulmonary hypertension

Modified from American Thoracic Society: Lung transplantation, *Am Rev Respir Dis* 1993; 147:772–776.

with borderline pulmonary hypertension at rest may develop severe hypertension during even mild exertion.

Most transplantation programs list patients as prospective candidates when their pulmonary disease has advanced beyond predefined limits. An extended wait for lung transplantation is a direct result of the shortage of donor organs. Patients are often referred for transplant evaluation when a major decline in their condition is observed. The term *transplant window* has been used to describe the time period during which the patient is sick enough to require transplantation, but healthy enough to have a reasonable chance of survival.

Posttransplant follow-up relies heavily on pulmonary function tests. Spirometry has been used extensively to monitor improvements resulting from transplantation. Recipients of double-lung transplants often show lung function values approaching those of normal patients within a few months. Blood gas changes usually occur immediately after surgery. Single-lung transplant (SLT) recipients show similar gains. However, because SLT patients retain a native lung, improvement in pulmonary function is usually less than when both lungs are replaced. Interpretation of spirometry, lung volumes, and blood gases in SLT patients is often complicated by the presence of the native lung along with the transplanted lung.

Besides monitoring improved lung function, pulmonary function tests are used to detect rejection and the development of bronchiolitis obliterans (BO). Rejection may be difficult to distinguish from other pulmonary complications (e.g., pneumonia) in patients who are immunosuppressed. There is some evidence that changes in spirometry (FVC, FEV_1, $FEF_{25\%-75\%}$) or distribution of gas (as measured by the single-breath technique) may signal episodes of acute rejection. Chronic rejection is thought to be associated with the development of BO. This pattern is characterized by the development of severe airflow limitation in the transplanted lung. Spirometry, particularly indices of small airway function such as $FEF_{25\%-75\%}$, may provide the earliest signs of bronchiolitis obliterans.

PRELIMINARIES TO PATIENT TESTING

Several preliminary steps precede any pulmonary function study. These include patient preparation, physical measurements and assessment, brief pulmonary history, and instructions to the patient in the performance of specific test maneuvers. In addition, pulmonary function tests are usually done in an ordered sequence. The testing sequence may be determined by laboratory policy, or it may be adapted for specific needs using a predefined protocol.

Patient Preparation

Patient preparation for pulmonary function studies consists mainly of instructions given to the patient in advance of the actual test session. These instructions focus on taking or withholding specific medications, refraining from smoking or eating, and other guidelines related to specific tests (e.g., exercise tests, blood gases).

Withholding Medications

Patients referred for evaluation of airflow limitation are often already taking bronchodilators or related drugs. If response to a bronchodilator is to be assessed, bronchodilators should be withheld before testing. The exact length of time to withhold a bronchodilator is dictated by the onset of action and how long it takes for the drug to be metabolized and/or excreted. Guidelines for withholding specific bronchodilators before simple spirometry are presented in detail in Chapter 2. Recommendations for withholding medications before bronchial challenge tests (e.g., methacholine, exercise, hyperventilation) are found in Chapter 9. Some patients may have difficulty withholding bronchodilators. In the case of simple spirometry, the test may be performed, if necessary, with a technologist comment describing the use of bronchodilators before testing. The patient should be instructed to take the bronchodilator when breathing problems require it. Patients scheduled for bronchial challenge who inadvertently take their bronchodilators may need to be rescheduled because bronchodilators can significantly alter airway response and lead to false-negative results.

Care should be taken when instructing outpatients about withholding medications. Some patients may be unable to correctly identify all of their medications; therefore it may be difficult for them to correctly withhold only bronchodilators. Some patients incorrectly withhold all medications.

This may cause serious problems for patients who rely on insulin (diabetic patients), antiarrhythmics, or antihypertensives used for high blood pressure. If the patient is uncertain, it may be preferable to not withhold any medications.

Smoking Cessation

Patients referred for pulmonary function tests should be asked to refrain from smoking for 24 hours before the test. Smoking cessation is especially important if D_{LCO} tests or arterial blood gas tests are ordered. Smoking has been shown to directly reduce diffusing capacity. Smoking also raises the level of CO in the blood, which also interferes with the measurement of diffusing capacity (CO back pressure in blood). Increased CO in the blood (COHb) also makes it difficult to interpret O_2 saturation measured by conventional pulse oximetry (see Chapter 6). Smoking has been shown to reduce the levels of exhaled nitric oxide (eNO), which may artifactually reduce the level of NO in patients who have airway inflammation.

Other Patient Preparation Issues

Patients referred for pulmonary function tests should refrain from eating a large meal immediately before their appointment. Two to four hours of fasting is usually sufficient to avoid vomiting or gastric distress during routine testing. The same is true if the patient will be exercising as part of the evaluation. Patients scheduled for a bronchial challenge test (see Chapter 9) should not drink beverages that contain caffeine or cola (theobromines) or eat chocolate. Outpatients scheduled for metabolic studies may need to fast for 8 hours before testing to ensure a stable baseline. Patients should refrain from alcohol consumption for at least 4 hours before testing.

Patients should refrain from vigorous exercise immediately before testing and should be relaxed and comfortable during the test session. Tight-fitting clothing (e.g., neckties) may need to be loosened during testing. Dentures should be left in place; many patients find it easier to hold the mouthpiece using their dentures. However, if the dentures are loose they may obstruct the mouthpiece, particularly during forced expiratory maneuvers.

Some patients may require special accommodations for pulmonary function tests to be performed safely and accurately. Patients, or those referring patients, should understand the requirements of the tests requested. Patients who are unable to sit or stand may require additional time or equipment for testing to be completed. Patients who have a permanent tracheostomy may also require special devices to allow connection to standard pulmonary function circuits. Patients who do not speak the primary language used in the laboratory may require an interpreter to be present during testing. Asking appropriate questions before the patient's appointment can identify each of these special needs.

Anthropometric Measurements

Various physical measurements are required for estimating each patient's expected level of pulmonary function. Age, height, and weight are usually recorded in addition to the patient's sex. Race or ethnic origin should also be recorded. Basic physical assessment of the patient's respiratory status may be needed before and during testing.

The patient's age should be recorded as of the last birthday. Some computerized pulmonary function systems store the patient's birth date and calculate the age. This approach is helpful, especially when the patient returns periodically for serial testing. Care should be used when entering specially formatted data (such as dates) into a computerized system. Data entry errors can result in gross overestimation or underestimation of the patient's expected values.

Standing height, in either inches or centimeters (to the nearest $1/4$ inch or 0.5 cm), should be recorded with the patient barefoot or in stocking feet. A wall-mounted ruler (stadiometer) allows the patient to stand with the back against the wall and the head close to the ruler. If the patient is unable to stand upright, the arm-span method should be used. Patients who have a history of kyphosis, scoliosis, or related problems should also have height estimated using their arm span. Arm span may be measured using a ruler or tape measure. The patient should extend the arms horizontally on both sides, and the distance between the tips of the middle fingers measured. Alternately, the distance from the tip of the middle finger to the center of the vertebrum at the level of the scapula is measured on each side, and then summed. Height may then be estimated as arm span/1.06 or may be estimated using regression equations that account for race, sex, and age in addition to arm span.

PF TIP

Always measure the patient's height (without shoes) and weight. Height should be measured to the nearest $1/4$ inch or $1/2$ centimeter. Self-reported heights and weights are usually inaccurate. Arm span may be used to estimate standing height for patients who are unable to stand, or who have significant spinal deformities.

The patient's weight in pounds or kilograms should be measured with an accurate scale. Because obesity may be related to restrictive lung disease, measurement of weight and calculation of body mass index (BMI) may be helpful for interpretation of reduced lung volumes (e.g., FRC, ERV). Body weight is used to calculate some reference values (see Appendix B). When weight is used to predict an expected value, the patient's ideal body weight should be used unless noted otherwise. Using actual weight in patients who are obese may overestimate expected values if the reference set is based on subjects with normal weights. Weight is also used to express oxygen consumption (i.e., ml/min/kg) for exercise and metabolic measurements. The patient's weight may also be required when lung volumes are determined with the body plethysmograph. Weight is used to estimate body volume in the plethysmograph (see Chapter 3).

Physical Assessment

Physical assessment of patients referred for pulmonary function studies may be needed to determine whether the individual can perform the test. Documentation concerning physical assessment of the patient can also assist with interpretation of test results. Physical assessment should focus on breathing pattern, breath sounds (if necessary), and respiratory symptoms (Box 1-8). These can be observed simply and noted as necessary. Commentary regarding the patient's signs or symptoms at the time of the test is a useful adjunct, especially if test performance is less than optimal.

Pulmonary History

Accurate interpretation of pulmonary function studies—from simple screening spirometry to com-

---

BOX 1-8	Physical Assessment During Pulmonary Function Testing

- Breathing pattern
  - Is the respiratory rate excessive?
  - Are there any complaints of chest tightness or chest discomfort?
  - Are accessory muscles being used for breathing?
  - Is the patient using pursed lips?
- Breath sounds (with and without auscultation)
  - Are there audible breath sounds? Are breath sounds distant or absent?
  - Is there any wheezing? Over which lung fields?
  - Is there stridor, especially on inspiration?
  - Are there any other unusual breath sounds (e.g., crackles, rubs)?
- Respiratory symptoms
  - Is there obvious shortness of breath (mild, moderate, severe)?
  - Is the patient coughing? If so, is the cough productive?
  - Is there any cyanosis?
  - Is the patient receiving supplemental oxygen? If so, how much?
  - What is the patient's oxygen saturation (pulse oximetry reading)?

---

plete cardiopulmonary evaluation—requires clinical information related to possible pulmonary disease. An ordered array of questions that can be easily answered by the patient provides the most useful history. The interpreter of pulmonary function studies may have little clinical information other than that obtained at the time of testing. A pulmonary history should be taken routinely before pulmonary function testing and should include the following:

1. Age, sex, standing height, weight, race
2. Current diagnosis or reason for test
3. Family history: Did anyone in the patient's immediate family (mother, father, brother, or sister) ever have the following:
   - Tuberculosis
   - Emphysema
   - Chronic bronchitis
   - Asthma
   - Hay fever or allergies
   - Lung cancer
   - Other lung disorders
4. Personal history: Have you ever had, or been told that you had, the following:
   - Tuberculosis
   - Emphysema
   - Chronic bronchitis
   - Asthma
   - Recurrent lung infections
   - Pneumonia or pleurisy
   - Allergies or hay fever
   - Chest injury (if so, what kind?)
   - Chest surgery (if so, what kind?)
5. Occupational/environmental exposure:
   - What is, or was, your occupation?
   - Have you ever been exposed to gases, dusts or fumes that caused breathing problems? If so, what were they?
   - Do you have hobbies or other activities that cause breathing problems? If so, what are they?
6. Smoking habits: Have you ever smoked the following:
   - Cigarettes (how many packs per day?)
   - Cigars (how many per day?)
   - Pipe (how many bowls per day?)
   - How long? How many years

- Do you still smoke? Y/N   If no, how long ago did you stop? How many years?
- Do you live with a smoker? Y/N

7. Cough:
   - On most days, do you have a cough? Y/N
   - How long have you had this cough?
   - Is the cough productive or nonproductive?

8. Dyspnea: Do you get short of breath at the following times:
   - At rest?   Y/N
   - On exertion? If so, what causes it?
   - At night?   Y/N

9. Current medications (for heart, lung, blood pressure, other). Last taken?

Most of these questions can be answered by Yes or No or by circling an appropriate response. Space should be provided so that the patient or history taker can enter comments. Computerized pulmonary function systems often allow history data to be stored in a database along with the patient's test results. This is a useful feature, but may limit the extent of the history that can be stored. In instances in which the physician performs the test, such history may be redundant if a medical history is available.

PF TIP

A brief pulmonary history can add significantly to the data provided by pulmonary function testing. Technologists who are familiar with pulmonary pathophysiology can implement protocols that are appropriate for the purpose of the test.

Interpretation of pulmonary function tests is best made if the clinical question asked of the test is considered. The clinician requesting the test should indicate the reason for the test. Examples of clinical questions asked of pulmonary function studies include "Does the patient have airway obstruction?" or "Does the patient have hyperreactive airways?" The pulmonary history, including the reason for the test, should be used to decide what is normal or abnormal. Clinical information

as provided by the history is especially important when the patient's pulmonary function tests are near the lower or upper limits of normal. For example, an FEV_1 that is near the lower limit of normal (LLN) would be interpreted differently in a healthy patient tested as part of a routine physical than it would be in a smoker who complained of increasing dyspnea.

TEST PERFORMANCE AND SEQUENCE

Pulmonary function laboratories should have written policies and procedures defining how each test is performed (see Chapter 11). Indications for performing a specific test should be related to the clinical question to be answered or to the patient's diagnosis. Testing protocols that can be modified for individual patients are usually the most cost-effective means of obtaining the required data. When the required tests have been determined, the exact sequence of tests can be selected. The sequence in which tests are performed may vary according to patient need and the test method used. For example, a patient with severe obstructive lung disease may not be able to perform an acceptable DLCO maneuver until a bronchodilator has been administered.

Technologist-Adapted Protocols

As described previously, the basis for deciding which pulmonary function tests are needed is related to the clinical question being asked. The clinical question is often inappropriately stated as a diagnosis. In fact, many patients are referred for pulmonary function studies to establish a diagnosis. For example, a patient may be referred with a diagnosis listed as "asthma." The clinical question is "Does the patient have asthma?" Pulmonary function studies may be able to help answer this question, but the exact tests to be performed may not be defined. In this example, spirometry is indi-

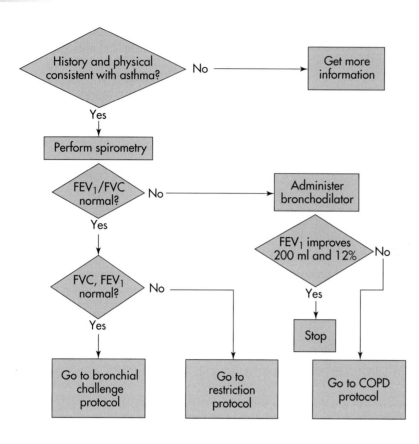

FIGURE 1-3 Protocol-decision diagram used by a pulmonary function technologist to select appropriate testing. A patient with possible asthma is referred for evaluation. The diagram shows routes to appropriate tests based on the results of simple spirometry. Note that if the patient history and physical assessment suggest diagnoses other than hyperreactive airways, more information may be needed.

cated. Using an adaptive protocol, spirometry can be performed and, based on the results, appropriate additional tests selected (Figure 1-3). Bronchial challenge tests may be performed if spirometry results are normal. Alternatively, additional tests such as lung volumes or DLCO may be necessary.

The correct sequence (and timing) for performing tests is important. Many laboratories use a fixed order for component pulmonary function tests. This may include spirometry, followed by lung volumes and DLCO. In some instances, the order of tests may need to be altered. The methodology used for some tests has definite effects on the results of subsequent procedures. For example, the multiple-breath N_2 washout test to determine FRC has the patient inhale 100% O_2 for several minutes. If this test is performed immediately before a DLCO test, the elevated O_2 level in the lungs (as well as in the blood and tissues) may reduce the measured DLCO. Similarly, before repetition of the DLCO maneuver or FRC determination by gas dilution techniques,

sufficient time must be allowed to wash out residual test gas.

Patient Instruction

Many pulmonary function tests are effort dependent. To obtain valid data, patients must be instructed and coached for each maneuver. Instruction and coaching are particularly important for the FVC maneuver. Instruction should include a description of what the patient is expected to do, such as "You will take a deep breath in, and then blow out as hard and as fast as possible." In addition to a description of the test, the maneuver should be demonstrated. During the actual test, vocal encouragement should be given so that the patient knows what is expected and continues for an appropriate interval. Any problems that occur with the first few efforts should be explained before the patient attempts the test again. For example,

"That was a very good effort, but you stopped before blowing out for 6 seconds. Let's try that again, and keep blowing out until I signal you to relax." This type of feedback is important because patients may be uncertain of what is required. Patients should be instructed that some maneuvers will be repeated so that their best effort can be obtained. They should be assured that repeating some tests is required and does not necessarily reflect a problem on their part.

PF TIP

The most effective way to get good patient effort is to demonstrate each maneuver. For spirometry, this can be accomplished by using a mouthpiece and simulating the maneuver expected of the patient. Be sure to show what is meant by a maximal effort and how long the effort should last.

Patients should also be carefully instructed for tests that require quiet breathing, such as lung volume determinations. Instructions about maintaining a good seal on the mouthpiece and continuing normal breathing can help reduce leaks or interrupted tests. Some maneuvers are complicated and may be difficult to describe to the patient. The DLCO maneuver and panting in the body plethysmograph each consist of several steps. For these tests, a combination of demonstration and practice may be the most efficient means of instructing the patient.

Even after adequate instruction and demonstration, some patients may be unable to perform certain tests. This may be caused by lack of coordination related to illness, pain due to their condition, or inability to follow instructions. For example, a patient may experience uncontrollable coughing when asked to inspire deeply for an FVC maneuver. If the coughing prevents obtaining valid spirometry results, the fact should be noted in the technologist's comments (see Chapter 11). Suboptimal effort by the patient can usually be detected as poorly repeatable results on effort-dependent tests (e.g., the FVC). Care should be taken that adequate instructions are given and a sufficient number of efforts recorded before deciding that the patient

did not give a maximal effort. If the patient cannot continue or refuses to continue a test, the exact reason should be documented in the technologist's comments.

SUMMARY

- This chapter serves as an introduction to pulmonary function testing. Categories of common pulmonary function tests are listed. This listing should acquaint the reader with the names of various tests, as well as their relationships to one another. Tests are categorized as airway function tests (spirometry), lung volume tests, diffusing capacity tests (DLCO), blood gases and gas exchange tests, cardiopulmonary exercise tests, and other specialized tests. Within each of these groups are a wide variety of tests and techniques.

- Indications for the various categories of tests are also listed. Indications are extremely important because they help the practitioner select appropriate tests. The clinical question asked of the test must be related to a valid indication for the test.

- This chapter also outlines patterns of impaired pulmonary function commonly encountered in the laboratory. This discussion assumes a basic knowledge of respiratory anatomy and physiology. The material presented aims to summarize the underlying pathology involved in common pulmonary diseases. The role of pulmonary function testing is discussed as it relates to diagnosis and assessment of these disease processes.

- Patient preparation for pulmonary function studies is covered in general terms. More detailed information for specific tests is presented in subsequent chapters. Many of the physical measurements and assessments, as well as the pulmonary history, are similar regardless of the tests being performed. Technologist-adapted protocols are described. Algorithms for selecting only appropriate tests are becoming increasingly popular. Such tools improve the sensitivity of the tests to answer the clinical question, as well as make tests more cost-effective.

CASE 1-1

Case Studies

 **Reason for test**: Does the patient have asthma? (This case should be evaluated in conjunction with the protocol described in Figure 1-3.)

HISTORY

J.C. is a 22-year-old physical therapy student referred by the student health center at her college. She complains of cough and shortness of breath after vigorous exercise such as playing soccer. She describes a history of "sinus problems" and allergies. No one in her family has a history of pulmonary disease. She has never smoked and has no history of unusual environmental exposure.

PULMONARY FUNCTION TESTING

Personal Data

Sex: Female
Age: 22
Height: 69 in (175 cm)
Weight: 122 lb (55 kg)

Spirometry							
	BEFORE DRUG				**AFTER DRUG**		
	Pred	LLN*	Actual	%	Actual	%	%Chg
FVC (L)	4.42	3.62	3.98	90	4.21	95	6
FEV$_1$ (L)	3.79	3.11	2.71	72	3.12	82	15
FEV$_1$%	86	76	68		74		
FEF$_{25\%-75\%}$ (L/sec)	4.00	2.56	1.71	43	2.55	64	49

*Lower limit of normal

TECHNOLOGIST'S COMMENTS

All efforts met ATS/ERS criteria for acceptable spirometry. Patient had some coughing during prebronchodilator efforts.

QUESTIONS

1. What is the interpretation of:
   • Prebronchodilator spirometry?
   • Response to bronchodilator?
2. What is the cause of the patient's symptoms?
3. What other tests might be indicated?
4. What treatment might be recommended based on these findings?

DISCUSSION

Interpretation

All spirometric efforts were performed acceptably. Prebronchodilator spirometry reveals mild obstruction. There is a significant improvement following inhaled bronchodilator.

Impression: Reversible airway obstruction with significant response to bronchodilator.

Cause of Symptoms

This patient's chief complaints of cough and shortness of breath following exertion are consistent with exercise-induced bronchospasm. The patient's FVC was above the lower limit of normal while her FEV$_1$ and FEV$_1$% were both below the LLN. These finding are diagnostic of obstruction that is relatively mild. Four puffs of a β-adrenergic bronchodilator produced a 0.41 L (15%) increase in her FEV$_1$. This was a significant improvement in airflow. (The American Thoracic Society/European Respiratory Society recommends a 12% *and* 200 ml improvement as evidence of significant response to bronchodilator.)

Other Tests

Using the sample protocol in Figure 1-3, no additional tests are necessary to support the diagnosis of reversible airway obstruction. Bronchial challenge is not needed to document reversible obstruction.

Treatment

The patient was treated with a combination of inhaled corticosteroid plus long-acting β-adrenergic bronchodilator, which alleviated most of her symptoms. She was also given a short-acting bronchodilator for premedication before vigorous exercise.

SELF-ASSESSMENT QUESTIONS

Entry-level

1. Measurement of airway resistance using the body plethysmograph was first described by
   a. Otis & McKerrow
   b. Meneely & Kaltreider
   c. Dubois & Comroe
   d. August & Marie Krogh

2. Indications for spirometry include which of the following?
   I. Preoperative evaluation for pneumonectomy
   II. Measurement of exercise capacity
   III. Determine the beneficial effects of a bronchodilator
   IV. Measure the effects of working in a dusty environment
   a. I, II, and III
   b. I, III, and IV
   c. II, III, and IV
   d. II and IV only

3. Measurement of lung volumes (TLC) is indicated
   a. To assess response to exercise training
   b. Whenever simple spirometry is performed
   c. To diagnose restrictive lung disease
   d. When hypoxemia is suspected

4. Arterial blood gases would be indicated in which of the following patients?
   a. An adult with exercise induced bronchospasm
   b. An adult with a suspected shunt
   c. An adolescent with myasthenia gravis
   d. An obese child

5. A 60-year-old male complains of dyspnea on exertion and when lying in bed; his FEV_1 and FVC are within normal limits. These symptoms are most consistent with which of the following?
   a. Emphysema
   b. Congestive heart failure
   c. Sarcoidosis
   d. Interstitial pulmonary fibrosis

6. Which of the following diseases often result in an obstructive pattern when spirometry is performed?
   I. Asthma
   II. Emphysema
   III. Bronchiolitis obliterans
   IV. Silicosis

   a. I, II, and III
   b. I, III, and IV
   c. II, III, and IV
   d. II and IV only

7. The most effective treatment for mild or moderate asthma is
   a. Beta-adrenergic bronchodilators
   b. Leukotriene receptor antagonists
   c. Inhaled corticosteroids
   d. IgE blockers

8. Which of the following should a pulmonary function technologist do before performing spirometry?
   a. Administer an anticholinergic bronchodilator
   b. Measure the patient's arm span
   c. Demonstrate how to correctly perform the test maneuver
   d. Explain the exact number of efforts that will be required for the test

Advanced

9. Which of the following would be indicated for a patient who complains of dyspnea on exertion and chest tightness?
   a. Diffusing capacity (D_{LCO})
   b. Cardiopulmonary exercise test
   c. Metabolic study
   d. Exhaled nitric oxide (FE_{NO})

10. Which of the following diseases is characterized by granulomatous changes and fibrosis in the lungs?
   a. Asthma
   b. Cystic fibrosis
   c. Emphysema
   d. Sarcoidosis

11. Pulmonary function testing is usually contraindicated in which of the following conditions?
   a. Amyotropic lateral sclerosis (ALS)
   b. Eisenmenger's syndrome
   c. Myasthenia gravis
   d. Untreated pneumothorax

12. Which of the following describe an appropriate physical measurement taken before pulmonary function testing?
   a. Actual body weight should be measured to calculate predicted values
   b. Standing height without shoes should be measured to the nearest cm

c. Arm span instead of height should be measured in children under 12

d. Sitting height x 1.32 may be used for patients who cannot stand

13. A 25-year-old patient with suspected asthma performs spirometry. Her FVC is 3.2 L and her FEV_1 is 2.2 L. Which of the following should the pulmonary function technologist do next?

a. Administer a bronchodilator

b. Evaluate for possible restrictive disorder

c. Perform a bronchial challenge test

d. Check oxygen saturation by pulse oximetry

14. A patient with COPD who is also a current smoker states that he has smoked within 1 hour before his scheduled pulmonary function test. Which of the following tests might produce inaccurate results because of this?

I. FRC by He dilution

II. D_{LCO}

III. Pulse oximetry

IV. MIP and MEP

   a. I, II and III

   b. II and III only

   c. II and IV only

   d. III and IV only

Selected Bibliography

GENERAL REFERENCES

Crapo RO: Pulmonary function testing, *N Engl J Med* 1994; 331:25-30.

Hess D: History of pulmonary function testing, *Respir Care* 1989; 34:427-445.

Spriggs EA: The history of spirometry, *Br J Dis Chest* 1978; 72:165-180.

INDICATIONS FOR PULMONARY FUNCTION TESTING

American Association for Respiratory Care: Clinical practice guidelines: body plethysmography: 2001 revision and update, *Respir Care* 2001; 46(5):506-513.

American Association for Respiratory Care: Clinical practice guidelines: single-breath carbon monoxide diffusing capacity: 1999 update, *Respir Care* 1999; 44(5):539-546.

American Association for Respiratory Care: Clinical practice guidelines: spirometry: 1996 update, *Respir Care* 1996; 41(7):629-636.

American Association for Respiratory Care: Clinical practice guidelines: static lung volumes: 2001 revision and update, *Respir Care* 2001; 46(5):531-539.

MacIntyre N, Crapo RO, Viegi G et al: Standardisation of the single-breath determination of carbon monoxide uptake in the lung, *Eur Resp J* 2005; 26:720-735.

Miller MR, Hankinson J, Brusasco V, et al: Standardisation of spirometry, *Eur Resp J* 2005; 26:319-338.

Pauwels RA, Buist SA, Calverley PMA, et al: GOLD Scientific Committee: Global strategy for the diagnosis, management, and prevention of chronic obstructive pulmonary disease, *Am J Resp Crit Care Med* 2001; 163:1256-1276.

Raffin TA: Indications for arterial blood gas analysis, *Ann Intern Med* 1986; 105:390-398.

Wanger J, Clausen JL, Coates A et al: Standardisation of the measurement of lung volumes, *Eur Resp J* 2005; 26:511-522.

Wasserman K, Hansen JE, Sue DY et al: *Principles of exercise testing and interpretation*, ed 3, Philadelphia, 1999, Lippincott, Williams & Wilkins.

Zibrak JD, O'Donnell CR, Marton K: Indications for pulmonary function testing, *Ann Intern Med* 1990; 112:763-771.

PATTERNS OF IMPAIRED PULMONARY FUNCTION

Aboussouan LS: Respiratory disorders in neurologic diseases, *Cleve Clin J Med* 2005; 72(6):511-520.

American Society for Transplant Physicians/American Thoracic Society/European Respiratory Society: International guidelines for the selection of lung transplant candidates, *Am J Respir Crit Care Med* 1998; 158:335-339.

American Thoracic Society/European Respiratory Society: Idiopathic pulmonary fibrosis: diagnosis and treatment, *Am J Respir Crit Care Med* 2000; 161:646-664.

Celli BR, MacNee W, ATS/ERS Task Force: Standards for the diagnosis and treatment of patients with COPD: a summary of the ATS/ERS position paper, *Eur Respir J* 2004; 23:932-946.

Davis PB, Drumm M, Konstan MW: Cystic fibrosis, *Am J Respir Crit Care Med* 1996; 154:1229-1256.

Dundas I, Mckenzie S: Spirometry in the diagnosis of asthma in children, *Curr Opin Pulm Med* 2006; 12(1):28-33.

Enright PL: The diagnosis of asthma in older patients, *Exp Lung Res* 2005; 31 Suppl 1:15-21.

Estenne M, Kotloff RM: Update in transplantation 2005, *Am J Respir Crit Care Med* 2006; 173(6):593-598.

Grissom LE, Harcke HT: Thoracic deformities and the growing lung, *Semin Roentgenol* 1998; 33(2):199-208.

National Asthma Education and Prevention Program: *Expert panel report 2: guidelines for the diagnosis and management of asthma*, Bethesda, Md, 1997, Department of Health and Human Services (NIH Publication No. 97-4051).

Putnam MT, Wise RA: Myasthenia gravis and upper airway obstruction, *Chest* 1996; 109:400-404.

Smith AD, Cowan JO, Filsell S, et al: Diagnosing asthma: comparisons between exhaled nitric oxide measurements and conventional tests, *Am J Respir Crit Care Med* 2004; 169(4):473-478.

Spurzem JR, Rennard SI: Pathogenesis of COPD, *Semin Respir Crit Care Med* 2005; 26(2):142-153.

PRELIMINARIES TO PATIENT TESTING

American Thoracic Society: *Pulmonary function laboratory management and procedure manual*, ed 2, Chapter 3: Quality system essentials for general operational issues, New York, 2005, American Thoracic Society.

Miller MR, Crapo R, Hankinson J, et al: General considerations for lung function testing, *Eur Resp J* 2005; 26:153-161.

NCCLS: A quality system model for health care. NCCLS document GP26-A, 1997, Wayne, Pa.

Social Security Administration: *Guide to pulmonary function studies under the Social Security Disability Program*, U.S. Department of Health and Human Services, http://www.ssa.gov/disability/professionals/pfs-pub055.htm. Updated: March 29, 2006. Accessed: October 1, 2006.

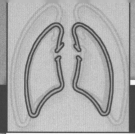

Chapter 2

Spirometry and Related Tests

DAVID A. KAMINSKY

CHAPTER OUTLINE

OBJECTIVES

After studying this chapter you will be able to:

Entry-level
1. Determine whether spirometry is acceptable and repeatable
2. Identify airway obstruction using vital capacity (VC) and forced expiratory volume in 1 second (FEV_1)
3. Differentiate between obstruction and restriction as causes of reduced VC
4. Determine whether there is a significant response to bronchodilators

Advanced
1. Select the appropriate VC and FEV_1 for reporting from a series of spirometry maneuvers
2. Identify at least two pathophysiologic conditions in which maximal inspiratory or expiratory pressures might be abnormal
3. Recognize abnormal values for airway resistance and specific conductance
4. Describe the technique for measuring pulmonary compliance

KEY TERMS

airway resistance (Raw)
body temperature, pressure, and
  saturation (BTPS)
expiratory reserve volume (ERV)
$FEF_{25\%-75\%}$
FEV_1/VC
forced expiratory volume (FEV_1)
forced vital capacity (FVC)

inspiratory capacity (IC)
isovolume correction
maximal expiratory flow volume
  (MEFV)
maximal expiratory pressure
  (MEP)
maximal inspiratory flow volume
  (MIFV)

maximal inspiratory pressure
  (MIP)
maximal voluntary ventilation (MVV)
peak expiratory flow (PEF)
peak flow meter
pulmonary compliance (C_L)
start-of-test
transpulmonary pressure (Ptp)

This chapter begins with measurement of the vital capacity (VC) using simple spirometry. Then the most widely used pulmonary function tests, those based on the forced vital capacity (FVC) maneuver, are described. Special emphasis is placed on the performance of each test. Criteria for judging the acceptability and repeatability of test data are provided, based on the most recent guidelines published by the American Thoracic Society/European Respiratory Society (ATS/ERS) Task Force on Standardization of Lung Function Testing. Volume-time and flow-volume curves are described as the two most common presentations of spirometric data. Bronchodilator studies to determine reversibility of airway obstruction are also presented. Other tests described include peak expiratory flow (PEF) and maximal voluntary ventilation (MVV). In addition, tests related to factors determining airflow are described, including maximal inspiratory pressure (MIP), maximal expiratory pressure (MEP), airway resistance (Raw) and its derivatives, and lung compliance (C_L). For each of these areas, interpretive strategies are suggested using questions that examiners might ask.

VITAL CAPACITY

Description

The vital capacity (VC) is the volume of gas measured from a slow, complete expiration after a maximal inspiration, without forced or rapid effort (Figure 2-1). Alternately, VC may be recorded as a maximal inspiration following a complete expiration. VC is normally recorded in either liters (L) or milliliters (ml), and reported at **body temperature, pressure, and saturation (BTPS).** VC is sometimes referred to as the slow vital capacity (SVC), distinguishing it from forced vital capacity (FVC). **Inspiratory capacity (IC)** and **expiratory reserve volume (ERV)** are subdivisions of the VC. IC is the largest volume of gas that can be inspired from the resting expiratory level (see Figure 2-1). IC is sometimes further divided into the tidal volume (V_T) and inspiratory reserve volume (IRV). ERV is the largest volume of gas that can be expired from the resting end-expiratory level (see Figure 2-1). Both the IC and ERV are recorded in liters or milliliters, corrected to BTPS.

Technique

VC is measured by having the patient inspire maximally and then exhale completely into a spirometer. (See Chapter 10 for a complete discussion of spirometers.) The patient is instructed to perform the maneuver slowly and completely. VC can also be measured from maximal expiration to maximal inspiration. The spirometer does not need to produce a graphic display if only VC is to be measured. However, if IC and ERV are to be determined (see Figure 2-1), some means of recording volume change is required. The graphic display may be a computer screen or a recording device (see Chapter 10). A graphic display allows the technologist to determine that the test is performed correctly

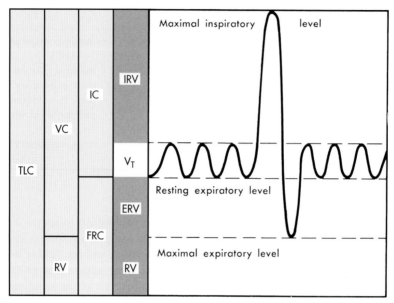

FIGURE 2-1 **Lung Volumes and Capacities.** Diagrammatic representation of lung volumes and capacities based on a simple spirogram. Relationships between the subdivisions and relative sizes as compared with TLC are shown *(shaded areas)*. Resting expiratory level is used as a starting point for FRC determinations because it remains more stable than other identifiable points during repeated measurements. ERV, expiratory reserve volume; FRC, functional residual capacity; IC, inspiratory capacity; IRV, inspiratory reserve volume; RV, residual volume; TLC, total lung capacity; VC, vital capacity; V_T, tidal volume. *(Modified from Comroe JH Jr, Forster RE, Dubois AB, et al: The lung: clinical physiology and pulmonary function tests, ed 2, St Louis, 1962, Mosby.)*

(Spirometry 2-1). A graphic display is also usually required for reimbursement purposes.

Obtaining a valid slow VC is important. The subdivisions of the VC (IC and ERV) are used in the calculation of residual volume (RV) and total lung capacity (TLC). An excessively large tidal volume or an irregular breathing pattern during the VC maneuver may alter ERV or IC. If either ERV or IC is erroneously recorded, other lung volumes may be incorrectly estimated (see Chapter 3).

IC is measured by having the patient breathe normally for three or four breaths and then inhale maximally. The volume inspired from the resting expiratory level is measured by the computer or from a spirogram. This is usually done as part of a slow VC maneuver. IC may also be calculated by subtracting the ERV from the VC. ERV is measured by having the patient breathe normally for three or four breaths and then exhale maximally. The change in volume from the end-expiratory level to the maximal expiratory level is the ERV. ERV may also

---

SPIROMETRY 2-1

CRITERIA FOR ACCEPTABILITY

Vital Capacity

1. End-expiratory volume varies by less than 100 ml for three preceding breaths.
2. Volume plateau observed at maximal inspiration and expiration.
3. Two acceptable VC maneuvers should be obtained; volumes within 150 ml.

---

be calculated by subtracting the IC from the VC. IC and ERV are usually measured from the same VC maneuver. IC and ERV should be reported as the average of at least three acceptable maneuvers, whereas VC is reported as the largest of at least three acceptable maneuvers.

The accuracy of the IC and ERV measurements depends on the stability of the end-expiratory level, which should vary by less than 100 ml. Three or more tidal breaths should be recorded before the

BOX 2-1   Contraindications to Spirometry

- Myocardial infarction within the last month
- Recent stroke, eye surgery, thoracic/abdominal surgery
- Uncontrolled hypertension
- Known thoracic, aortic, cerebral aneurysm
- Recent pneumothorax
- Relative contraindications: chest, abdominal, facial pain; headache; stress incontinence; dementia; confusion

Modified from AARC clinical practice guideline. Spirometry, 1996 update, *Respir Care* 1996; 41:629-636.

In adults, VC varies directly with height and inversely with age; tall patients have larger VCs than short patients. VC increases up to approximately age 20 and then decreases each year thereafter, with an average decrease of about 25 – 30 ml/year. It is usually smaller in women than in men because of differences in body size. Recent evidence indicates that lung volumes may differ significantly according to ethnic origin. VC also varies in individuals depending on body position or time of day. Interpretation of lung function should consider the key factors of age, sex, height, and race (see Appendix B).

VC maneuver is performed. If the end-expiratory volume is not consistent, IC and/or ERV may be measured incorrectly (e.g., too large or too small). Even if the end-expiratory level is constant, the V_T usually increases when the patient breathes through a mouthpiece with a nose clip in place. This increase in V_T may change the IC or ERV, depending on the patient's breathing pattern. Erroneous estimates of ERV may affect the calculation of RV, as described in Chapter 3.

Significance and Pathophysiology

Spirometry is indicated in a variety of situations (see Chapter 1). There are few contraindications to spirometry (Box 2-1), which basically relate to the high thoracic pressure developed during the test or to issues related to technique.

Normal VC may vary as much as 20% above or below the predicted value in healthy individuals, but must be above the bottom fifth percentile (lower limit of normal, see Appendix B) to be considered normal. The ATS/ERS guidelines recommend the use of the NHANES III reference equations (see Appendix B) for patients in the United States aged 8 – 80 years. For children younger than 8 years, the guidelines recommend the equations of Wang and colleagues.*

*Wang X, Dockery DW, Wypij D et al: Pulmonary function between 6 and 18 years of age, *Pediatr Pulmonol* 1993; 15:75-88.

PF TIP

Normal values for lung function parameters are obtained by studying healthy subjects. The predicted or reference value for VC is computed using an equation like:

$$VC = x\text{Height} - y\text{Age} - z$$

where:
x, y, and z are constants
Predicted values may be read from special diagrams called nomograms but are usually calculated by computer (see Appendix B.) The lower limit of normal, representing the lower 5th percentile of the normal distribution curve, is recommended as the cut-off to judge normality.

There are numerous causes of a decreased VC (Box 2-2). In general, these fall into the categories of loss of distensible lung tissue, obstructive lung disease, and reduced chest wall expansion.

When the VC is reduced, additional pulmonary function measurements may be indicated. Forced expiratory maneuvers (see the section on forced vital capacity) can reveal whether the reduced VC is caused by obstruction. Reduced VC without slowing of expiratory flow is a nonspecific finding. Measurement of other lung volumes (see Chapter 3) may be indicated to determine whether a restrictive defect is present. Measurement of muscle pressures (later) may help determine whether there is a problem with neuromuscular weakness.

BOX 2-2	Causes of Reduced Vital Capacity

Loss of distensible lung tissue
- Lung cancer
- Pulmonary vascular congestion, pulmonary edema
- Pneumonia
- Atelectasis
- Pulmonary fibrosis (e.g., from dust, drug toxicity, radiation, or idiopathic)
- Pleural effusion or pleural scarring
- Pneumothorax
- Surgical removal (e.g., lobectomy)

Obstructive lung disease (due to gas trapping, resulting in elevated RV but normal TLC)

Reduced chest wall excursion
- Neuromuscular weakness (e.g., myasthenia gravis)
- Chest wall deformity (e.g., kyphoscoliosis)
- Obesity, pregnancy, ascites
- Suboptimal patient effort (e.g., due to pain, motivation)

SPIROMETRY 2-2

INTERPRETIVE STRATEGIES

Vital Capacity

1. Was the test performed acceptably? Is it reproducible?
2. Are reference values correct? Age? Sex? Height? Race?
3. Is VC less than predicted? If so, to what extent? Is it less than the lower limit of normal?
4. How does VC relate to the clinical question to be answered? Is VC correlated to the history and physical findings?
5. Are additional tests indicated? Lung volumes? FVC?

In adults, VC less than the 95% confidence limit (see Appendix B) may be considered abnormal. Interpretation of the measured VC in relation to the reference value should consider the clinical question to be answered (Spirometry 2-2). The clinical question is often revealed in the history and physical findings of the patient (see Chapter 1). The terms mild, moderate, and severe may be used to qualify the extent of reduction of the VC in a manner similar to that described for FEV_1 (see FEV_1 section).

Artificially low estimates of the VC may result from poor patient effort. Similarly, inadequate patient instruction may affect performance of the test maneuver. These errors may be eliminated by applying appropriate criteria (see Spirometry 2-1). Values for at least two maneuvers should be reproducible within 150 ml (see Chapter 11).

IC and ERV are approximately 75% and 25% of the VC, respectively. Changes in IC or ERV usually parallel increases or decreases in the VC. Increased V_T caused by exertion or acid-base disorders (e.g., metabolic acidosis, respiratory alkalosis) may reduce IRV or ERV. This occurs because end-inspiratory and end-expiratory levels (see Figure 2-1) are altered. A similar pattern is commonly seen when patients breathe into a spirometer through a mouthpiece with nose clips in place. Changes in IC or ERV are of minimal diagnostic significance when considered alone. Reduction of IC or ERV is consistent with restrictive defects. Obese patients typically show a decrease in ERV, usually resulting in a low VC. A reduced ERV is one of the earliest lung function changes in obese patients.

FORCED VITAL CAPACITY, FORCED EXPIRATORY VOLUME, AND FORCED EXPIRATORY FLOW

Description

Forced vital capacity (FVC) is the maximum volume of gas that can be expired when the patient exhales as forcefully and rapidly as possible after a maximal inspiration. This procedure is often referred to as the FVC maneuver. A similar maneuver, beginning at maximal expiration and inspiring as forcefully as possible, is called forced inspiratory vital capacity (FIVC). The FVC and FIVC maneuvers are often performed in sequence to provide a continuous flow-volume loop (see the section on flow-volume curve).

The forced expiratory volume (FEV_T) is the volume of gas expired over a given time interval (T) from the beginning of the FVC maneuver. The time interval is stated as a subscript of FEV. The FEV_1 measurement is the most widely used. Other intervals in common use are $FEV_{0.5}$, FEV_3, and FEV_6. The FVC and FEV_T are both reported in liters corrected to BTPS. $FEV_{T\%}$ is the ratio of FEV_T to FVC expressed as a percentage, where T is the interval from the start of the FVC. The $FEV_{1\%}$ (FEV_1/FVC × 100) is by far the most widely used of the various $FEV_{T\%}$ parameters. VC (slow vital capacity) may be used in place of FVC if the VC is significantly larger. Because a low value for the ratio of FEV_1 to FVC is used to detect obstruction, using the largest value obtained for vital capacity (either VC or FVC) for the denominator may be helpful, and is currently recommended by the ATS/ERS guidelines.

Flows over specific intervals or at specific points in the FVC are expressed as FEF_X. The subscript X describes the point or interval in relation to the FVC maneuver. The **$FEF_{25\%-75\%}$** is the average flow during the middle half (from the 25%–75% points) of an FVC maneuver. FEF_X values are usually recorded in liters per second, BTPS. $FEF_{25\%-75\%}$ was formerly designated the maximum midexpiratory flow rate (MMFR). Other measures of average flow include the $FEF_{200-1200}$ (200–1200 ml portion of the FVC), and the $FEF_{75\%-85\%}$. FEF_X is also used to denote instantaneous flow at specific points in the FVC maneuver. Commonly reported flows are the $FEF_{25\%}$, $FEF_{50\%}$, and $FEF_{75\%}$. The subscript refers to the percentage of FVC that has been expired.

Technique

FVC is measured by having the patient, after inspiring maximally, expire as forcefully and rapidly as possible into a spirometer (see Chapter 11). The patient should inspire completely. The inhalation should be rapid but not forced. There should be little if any pause (less than 1–2 seconds) at maximal inspiration; a prolonged pause (4–6 seconds) may decrease flow during the subsequent expiration.

The volume expired may be read directly from a volume-time recording (Figure 2-2). This method is used by some small portable spirometers. More

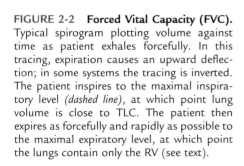

FIGURE 2-2 **Forced Vital Capacity (FVC).** Typical spirogram plotting volume against time as patient exhales forcefully. In this tracing, expiration causes an upward deflection; in some systems the tracing is inverted. The patient inspires to the maximal inspiratory level *(dashed line)*, at which point lung volume is close to TLC. The patient then expires as forcefully and rapidly as possible to the maximal expiratory level, at which point the lungs contain only the RV (see text).

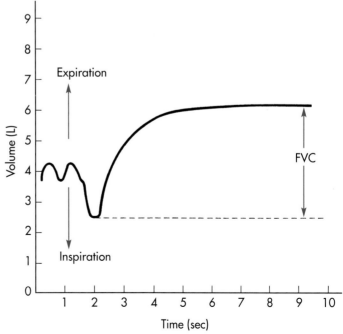

commonly, the maneuver is displayed on a computer monitor or liquid crystal display screen. The computer analyzes the signal from the spirometer, then calculates and displays the FVC. A spirometer that produces a graphical tracing (either volume-time or flow-volume) is essential for clinical laboratory purposes to allow visual inspection of the maneuver (Figure 2-3), and is also necessary for reimbursement purposes. Devices providing only numerical data may be helpful for simple screening. Whether used for diagnosis or monitoring, all spirometers should meet the criteria proposed by the ATS/ERS (see Chapter 11). The FVC maneuver depends on patient effort. Not all patients may be able to perform it acceptably (Spirometry 2-3).

FEV$_1$ (and other FEV$_T$ values) may be measured by timing the FVC maneuver over the described intervals. Historically this was done by recording the FVC spirogram on graph paper moving at a fixed speed. The FEV for any interval could then be

SPIROMETRY 2-3

CRITERIA FOR ACCEPTABILITY

FVC Maneuver

1. Maximal effort; no cough or glottic closure during the first second; no leaks or obstruction of the mouthpiece.
2. Good start-of-test; back-extrapolated volume less than 5% of FVC or 150 ml, whichever is greater.
3. Tracing shows 6 seconds of exhalation (3 seconds for children) or an obvious plateau; no early termination or cutoff; or subject cannot or should not continue to exhale.
4. Three acceptable spirograms obtained; two largest FVC values within 150 ml; two largest FEV$_1$ values within 150 ml.
5. Report the highest FVC and highest FEV$_1$, even if they come from separate maneuvers. The FEV$_1$/FVC ratio is derived from these values.

From ATS/ERS Task Force, 2005.

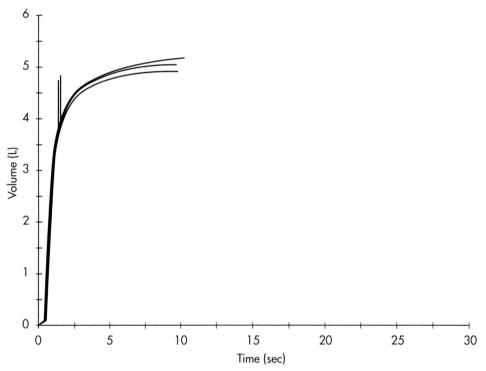

FIGURE 2-3 **Volume-Time Tracings of FVC Maneuvers from a Healthy Patient.** Tracings show the forced expiratory portion of the FVC maneuver. Three FVC efforts are superimposed, showing acceptable reproducibility of the maneuvers (see text). Tick marks indicate FEV$_1$.

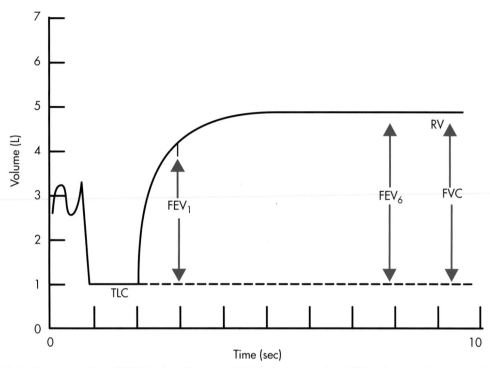

FIGURE 2-4   Determination of FEV_T Values from an FVC Maneuver. Various FEV_T values can be measured from the volume-time display of an FVC effort. FEV at intervals of 1 and 6 seconds, along with the FVC, are shown *(arrows)*. FEV_1 is the most commonly used index of airflow. FEV_6 is sometimes used as a surrogate for FVC in patients with airway obstruction. Precise timing and acceptable start-of-test are required to determine FEV_T values accurately (see Spirometry 2-3). FEV_1, forced expiratory volume in 1 second; FEV_6, forced expiratory volume in 6 seconds; FVC, forced vital capacity; RV, residual volume; TLC, total lung capacity.

read from the graph as shown in Figure 2-4. Most modern spirometers time the FVC maneuver with a computer. The computer then calculates and displays the FEV_1 or other FEV_T intervals. The spirometer should provide a volume-time display of each maneuver (Figure 2-5). A graphic representation allows monitoring of patient effort at the beginning of the test. Accurate measurement of FEV_1 (and other FEV_T intervals) depends on determination of the **start-of-test** (Figure 2-6). Computerized spirometers detect the start-of-test as a change in flow or volume above a certain threshold. The computer then stores volume and flow data points in memory and calculates the FEV_1.

Some spirometers allow tidal breathing and record both inspiratory and expiratory flows, whereas others record forced expiratory flow only. If only the expiratory spirogram is presented, assessing the start-of-test may be difficult. Inaccurate FEV_T values may result if the patient begins the FVC maneuver slowly, coughs, hesitates, or leaks at the mouthpiece. Most computerized spirometers correct for a slow start-of-test by back-extrapolation (see Figure 2-6). Visualization of the volume-time spirogram is the best means of identifying poor initial effort. Some portable spirometers report FEV_1 without a spirogram. Such measurements should be used with caution because it may be difficult to determine whether the maneuver was performed acceptably.

The ratio of the FEV_1 to FVC is expressed as follows:

$$FEV_{1\%} = \frac{FEV_1}{FVC} \times 100$$

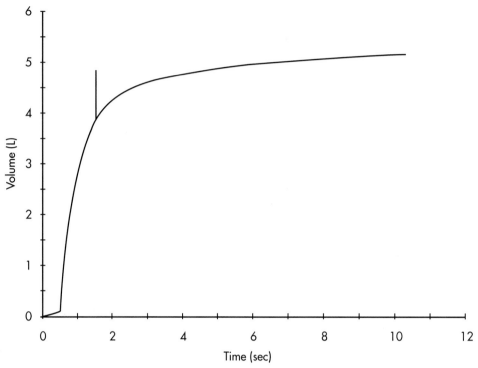

FIGURE 2-5 **Volume-Time Tracing from a Healthy Patient.** The graph shows an FVC tracing from a normal adult. The computer superimposes a tick mark on the curve to assist in identification of FEV_1.

$FEV_{1\%}$ is also commonly written as FEV_1/FVC. Both ratios are expressed as percentages, and this percentage is then related to normative values as a percentage of the predicted value. FEV_1 and FVC should be reported as the maximal values obtained from at least three acceptable FVC maneuvers. The FEV_1/FVC ratio based on these values may be different from the ratio obtained from any single maneuver. If both VC and FVC maneuvers have been performed, it is preferable to use the largest VC in the calculation. Some computerized spirometers calculate only the ratio obtained from FVC maneuvers.

The $FEF_{25\%-75\%}$ is measured from an FVC maneuver. The $FEF_{25\%-75\%}$ is the average flow during the middle half (from 25%–75%) of the VC. A computerized measurement of the $FEF_{25\%-75\%}$ requires storage of flow and volume data points for the entire maneuver. Calculation of the average flow over the middle portion of the exhalation is simply 50% of the volume expired divided by the time

required to get from the 25% point to the 75% point. To calculate the $FEF_{25\%-75\%}$ manually, a volume-time spirogram is used. The points at which 25% and 75% of the vital capacity have been expired are marked on the curve (Figure 2-7). A straight line connecting these points can be extended to intersect two timelines 1 second apart. The flow (in liters per second) can then be read directly as the vertical distance between the points of intersection. Instantaneous flows, such as the $FEF_{50\%}$ or $FEF_{75\%}$, cannot be read directly from a volume-time display, but can be measured using a flow-volume curve (see the section on flow-volume curve).

The $FEF_{25\%-75\%}$ depends on the FVC. Large $FEF_{25\%-75\%}$ values may be derived from maneuvers that produce small FVC measurements because the "middle half" of the volume is actually gas expired at the beginning of expiration. This effect may be particularly evident if the patient terminates the FVC maneuver before exhaling completely. When the $FEF_{25\%-75\%}$ is used for assessing the response to

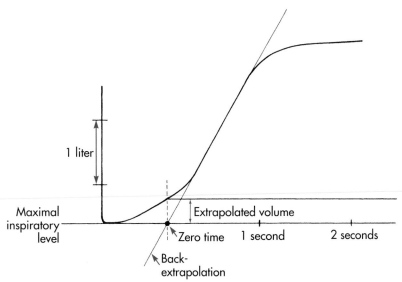

FIGURE 2-6   Back-Extrapolation of a Volume-Time Spirogram. Back-extrapolation is a method for correcting measurements made from a spirogram that does not show a sharp deflection from the maximal inspiratory level. This occurs when a patient does not begin forced exhalation rapidly enough or hesitates at the start-of-test. A straight line drawn through the steepest part of a volume-time tracing is extended to cross the volume baseline (maximum inspiration). The point of intersection is the back-extrapolated *time zero*. To accurately determine the new time zero, the display should include at least 0.25 second and preferably at least 1 second before the start of the exhalation. Timed volumes, such as FEV_1, are measured from this point rather than from the initial deflection from the baseline or from the point of maximal flow. The perpendicular distance from maximal inspiration to the volume-time tracing at time zero defines the back-extrapolated volume. To accurately determine FEV_1, the back-extrapolated volume should be less than 5% of the FVC or less than 150 ml, whichever is greater. FVC efforts with larger extrapolated volumes should be considered unacceptable. These measurements are commonly performed by computer.

FIGURE 2-7 $FEF_{25\%-75\%}$. Short horizontal lines on an FVC spirogram show points at which 25% and 75% of the FVC have been expired; these points may be determined by multiplying the FVC by 0.25 and 0.75, respectively. The slope of the line connecting the 25% and 75% points can be determined by dividing one half of the FVC by the time interval between the points. This slope is the average flow over the middle half of the FVC maneuver. Alternatively, a line connecting these points may be drawn to intersect two timelines 1 second apart (points A and B). The flow in liters per second can be read as the vertical distance between the points of intersection *(AC)*—in this case, approximately 2 L/sec. These measurements are usually calculated by computer.

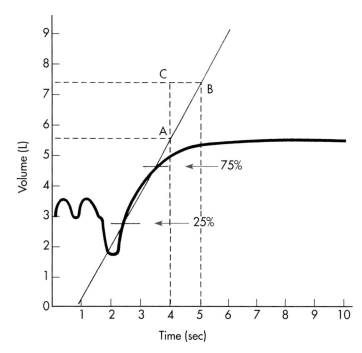

bronchodilator or bronchial challenge, the effect of changes in the absolute lung volumes must be considered. Measuring the $FEF_{25\%-75\%}$ at the same lung volumes in the comparison tests is called the isovolume technique. **Isovolume corrections** are usually applied when the FVC changes by more than 10% (indicating a change in TLC or RV). This technique requires that lung volumes (see Chapter 3) be measured in conjunction with flows. The isovolume technique may also be used with other flow measurements that are dependent on FVC.

The largest $FEF_{25\%-75\%}$ is not necessarily the value reported. The $FEF_{25\%-75\%}$ is recorded from the maneuver with the largest sum of FVC and FEV_1. Flows must be corrected to BTPS.

Criteria used to judge the acceptability of test results from the FVC maneuver include the following:

1. The volume-time tracing should show maximal effort with a smooth curve. There should be no coughing or hesitation during the first second. The tracing should show at least 6 seconds of forced effort. An obvious plateau with no volume change (25 ml or less) for at least 1 second should be achieved. Children, adolescents, and some restricted patients may plateau in less than 6 seconds (children younger than 10 years must exhale at least 3 seconds). Patients with severe obstruction may continue exhalation well past 15 seconds; therefore 6 seconds is simply a minimum. In severe obstruction, very low flows may be observed at the end of expiration. Continuation of the maneuver in these patients will not appreciably change the test results. The FVC maneuver may be stopped if the patient cannot continue for clinical reasons such as excessive coughing or dizziness. Multiple prolonged (longer than 6 seconds) exhalations are seldom necessary.

2. The start-of-test should be abrupt and unhesitating. Each maneuver should have the back-extrapolated volume calculated. FEV_1, and all other flows must be measured after back-extrapolation (see Figure 2-6). The ATS/ERS guidelines recommend that the volume-time tracing must begin at least 0.25 second before the beginning of the exhalation to be able to measure the back-extrapolated volume. If the volume of back-extrapolation is greater than 5% of the FVC or 150 ml (whichever is greater), the maneuver is unacceptable and should be repeated. The patient should be shown the correct technique for performing the maneuver. Demonstration by the technologist is often helpful.

3. A minimum of three acceptable efforts should be obtained. The test may be repeated multiple times, but if repeatable values cannot be obtained after eight attempts, testing may be discontinued. The only criterion for eliminating a test session completely is failure to obtain two acceptable maneuvers after at least eight attempts.

4. The two largest values for both FVC and FEV_1 should be within 150 ml (or within 100 ml if the FVC is 1 L or less). The second largest value is simply subtracted from the largest value for both FVC and FEV_1 to determine repeatability. Some clinicians prefer to use 5% as the repeatability criterion. This may be more appropriate than an absolute volume of 150 ml, particularly in children or those with large FVC values. However, the 150-ml absolute volume criterion has less variance than the 5% criterion, making it less dependent on individual characteristics and therefore more widely applicable to patients of different age, sex, and baseline lung function. If the two largest FVC or FEV_1 values are not within 150 ml (or 5%, if that criterion is applied), the maneuver should be repeated up to a maximum of eight times or until the patient cannot or will not continue. The repeatability criteria should be applied only after the maneuver has been judged acceptable. Individual spirometric maneuvers should not be rejected solely because they are not repeatable. Bronchospasm or fatigue often affects repeatability. Interpretation of the test should include comments regarding repeatability or lack of it. As a minimum, three acceptable satisfactory maneuvers should be saved for evaluation.

Data from all acceptable maneuvers should be examined. The largest FVC and the largest FEV_1 should be reported, even if the two values are from different test maneuvers. The reported FEV_1/FVC

ratio is taken from these values. Flows that depend on the FVC (e.g., the $FEF_{25\%-75\%}$) should be taken from the single best test maneuver, which is the maneuver with the largest sum of FVC and FEV_1 (Table 2-1). The reported flow-volume curve is also taken from the single best test maneuver.

A common problem may occur when using these criteria to produce a spirometry report. If a single volume-time or flow-volume tracing is included in the final report, it may not contain the FVC or FEV_1 that appears in the tabular data. It is advisable to maintain recordings, or raw data, for all acceptable maneuvers. Other methods of selecting the best test have been suggested and are sometimes used. PEF may be used to assess patient effort for an FVC maneuver. Selecting the effort with the largest PEF may cause errors if FVC and FEV_1 are not also evaluated.

Spirometry may be performed in either the sitting or standing position for adults and children, although the sitting position is recommended for safety, especially in adults. There is some evidence that FEV_1 may be larger in the standing position in adults and in children younger than 12 years. The position used for testing should be indicated on the final report. The patient should keep the head slightly elevated and should keep false teeth in if they fit well. The use of nose clips is recommended for spirometric measurements that require rebreathing, even if just for a few breaths. Spirometers that record only expiratory flow may require the patient to place the mouthpiece into the mouth after maximal inspiration. If this is the case, nose clips are usually unnecessary. Care should be taken, however, that the patient places the mouthpiece into the mouth before beginning a forced expiration. Failure to do so may result in an undetectable loss of volume. It may be impossible to calculate the volume of back-extrapolation from a tracing that displays only expiratory flow. Spirometers that use mechanical recorders should have pen or paper moving at recording speed when the forced expiration begins. Recorders that trigger pen or paper movement with exhalation may be unable to accurately record the start-of-test. Such spirometers often underestimate the FEV_1. Most spirometers use computer-generated graphics, avoiding the problems associated with mechanical recorders.

PF TIP

The largest FVC and FEV_1 are reported, even if they come from different efforts, as long as the efforts are acceptable. Peak flow (PEF) is always the largest value from an acceptable effort. All the other flows (e.g., $FEF_{25\%-75\%}$) are taken from the acceptable effort with the largest sum of FVC and FEV_1, as is the flow-volume loop.

TABLE 2-1				
Comparison of Spirometry Efforts				
Test	Trial 1	Trial 2	Trial 3	Best Test Reported
FVC (L)	5.20	5.30	5.35*	5.35
FEV_1 (L)	4.41*	4.35	4.36*	4.41
FEV_1/FVC (%)	85	82	82	82
$FEF_{25\%-75\%}$ (L/sec)	3.87	3.92	3.94	3.94
$FEF_{50\%}$ (L/sec)	3.99	3.95	3.41	3.41
$FEF_{25\%}$ (L/sec)	1.97	1.95	1.89	1.89
PEF (L/sec)	8.39	9.44	9.89	9.89

*These values are keys to selecting the best test results. The FEV_1 is taken from trial 1 and the FVC from trial 3, even though the largest sum of FVC and FEV_1 occurs in trial 3. All FVC-dependent flows (average and instantaneous flows) come from trial 3. The maximal expiratory flow-volume curve, if reported, would be the curve from trial 3 as well. It should be noted that the $FEV_{1\%}$ (FEV_1/FVC) is calculated from the FEV_1 of trial 1 and the FVC of trial 3.

Significance and Pathophysiology

Forced Vital Capacity

See Spirometry 2-4 for interpretive strategies. FVC usually equals VC in healthy individuals. In patients without obstruction, FVC and VC should be within 150 ml of each other. FVC and VC may differ if the patient's effort is variable or if significant airway obstruction is present (i.e., FEV_1/FVC less than 0.70). FVC is often lower than VC in patients with obstructive diseases if forced expiration causes airway collapse. This pattern is often seen in emphysema because of loss of tethering support of the airways. Large pressure gradients across the walls of the airways during forced expiration collapse the terminal portions of the airways. Gas is trapped in the alveoli and cannot be expired. This causes the

FVC to appear smaller than the VC. The FVC can appear larger than the VC if the patient exerts greater effort on the forced maneuver.

FVC can be reduced by mucus plugging and bronchiolar narrowing, as is common in chronic bronchitis, chronic or acute asthma, bronchiectasis, and cystic fibrosis. Reduced FVC is also present in patients whose trachea or mainstem bronchi are obstructed. Tumors or diseases affecting the patency of the large airways can produce this result.

Some obstructed patients have a relatively normal FVC in relation to their predicted values. However, the time required to expire their FVC (forced expiratory time or FET) is usually prolonged. Healthy adults can expire their FVC within 4–6 seconds. Healthy children and adolescents may exhale their FVC in less than 4 seconds. Patients with severe obstruction (e.g., those with emphysema) may require 15 seconds or more to exhale completely (Figure 2-8). Accurate measurement of FVC in such individuals may be limited by how long the spirometer can collect exhaled volume. Some spirometers allow only 15 seconds of volume recording. This is usually long enough to diagnose airway obstruction. However, the FVC and $FEV_{1\%}$ may be inaccurate if the patient continues to exhale for a longer time. The ATS/ERS recommends that spirometers measure FVC for at least 15 seconds (see Chapter 11).

An alternative to measuring FVC in severely obstructed patients is to use FEV_6. Because normal patients can exhale their FVC in 6 seconds, substituting FEV_6 for FVC allows the FEV_1/FEV_6 to be used as an index of obstruction. Using FEV_6 in place of FVC eliminates the necessity of having the patient try to exhale for a long interval. Predicted values for FEV_6 and FEV_1/FEV_6 may be calculated using coefficients in Appendix B. Because FEV_6 may underestimate FVC, use of FEV_1/FEV_6 instead of FEV_1/FVC may reduce the sensitivity of spirometry to detect airway obstruction, especially in older patients and those with mild obstruction.

Decreased FVC is seen in the same circumstances as described for reduced VC, which was discussed earlier. However, the reduction in FVC may be more evident than that of the slow VC in diseases that affect the bellows function of the chest, which is a

---

SPIROMETRY 2-4

INTERPRETIVE STRATEGIES

FVC Maneuver

1. Were at least three acceptable spirograms obtained? Are FVC and FEV_1 repeatable (within 150 ml)?
2. Are reference values appropriate? Age? Sex? Height? Race?
3. Is $FEV_{1\%}$ less than predicted? If so, obstruction is present.
   a. Is FVC also reduced? If so, is it caused by obstruction or restriction?
   b. If FVC is less than 80%, lung volumes may be indicated.
   c. Is the obstruction reversible? Bronchodilators may be indicated.
4. Is $FEV_{1\%}$ equal to or greater than expected?
   a. Are both FVC and FEV_1 reduced proportionately? If so, restriction may be present; lung volumes and/or muscle pressures may be indicated.
   b. Are FVC and FEV_1 within normal limits? If so, spirometry is likely normal.
5. Are the spirometric findings consistent with the patient history and physical findings? Is bronchial challenge indicated to reveal obstruction?

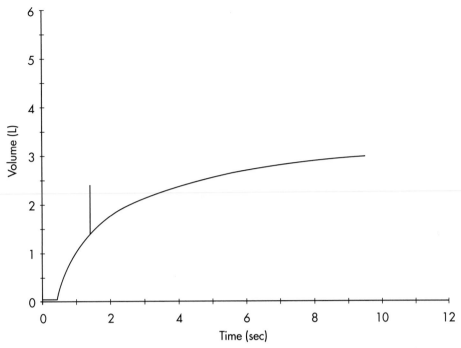

FIGURE 2-8   FVC Tracing from a Patient with Severe Airway Obstruction. A tick mark notes the point at which the patient exhaled his FEV_1. A significant volume is exhaled after the first second, and the tracing does not show an obvious plateau.

key determinant of the force generation involved in the FVC compared with the VC maneuver. Such diseases include neuromuscular disorders and chest wall mechanical abnormalities, such as kyphoscoliosis and obesity. A reduction in FVC when going from sitting to supine has been shown to be a good indicator of diaphragmatic weakness.

Reduced FVC (or VC) is a nonspecific finding. Values below the fifth percentile are considered abnormal (see Appendix B). Low FVC may be caused by either obstruction or restriction (see Box 2-2). Interpretation of the FVC in obstructive diseases requires correlation with flows. An FVC that is significantly lower than VC suggests airway collapse. In restrictive patterns, low FVC may indicate the need to assess other lung volumes, particularly total lung capacity (TLC, see Chapter 3). Interpretation of FVC values close to the lower limit of normal depends on the clinical question to be answered. An FVC at the fifth percentile would be interpreted differently in a healthy patient with no symptoms than in a patient with a history of cough or wheezing. An FVC much lower than expected is often accompanied by the complaint of exertional dyspnea.

A low value for FVC may also occur if the patient's effort is suboptimal. Patients who stop exhaling before achieving an obvious plateau (on a volume-time display) typically have an underestimated FVC. These patients should be encouraged to exhale longer and continue testing until three acceptable maneuvers are obtained. Premature termination of the FVC effort may cause the $FEV_{1\%}$ to be overestimated, masking the presence of obstruction.

An important quality issue to recognize is that a large FVC (and its derived parameters) derived from a flow sensor may result from improper zeroing or contamination of the sensor by condensation or mucus. This problem can usually be recognized by poor repeatability of measurements, characterized by progressively increasing test results within a single testing session.

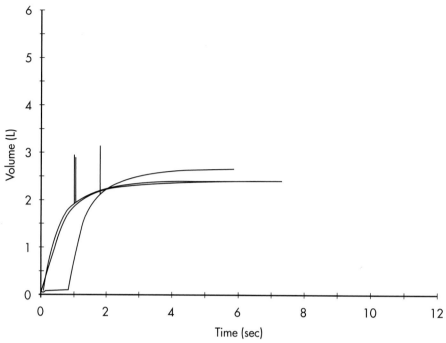

FIGURE 2-9 **Three FVC Maneuvers from a Patient with Moderately Severe Restriction.** All three maneuvers show relatively normal flows; most of the FVC is expired in the first second. However, the FVC is much lower than the expected value of 3.5 L for this patient. Notice the delayed start to the effort with the highest FVC, for which determination of back-extrapolated volume is necessary.

Forced Expiratory Volume (FEV₁)

Forced expiratory volume (FEV₁) measures the volume expired over the first second of an FVC maneuver. FEV_1 is reported as a volume, although it measures flow over a specific interval. FEV_1, like FVC, may be reduced in either obstructive or restrictive patterns (see Figures 2-8 and 2-9). FEV_1 values may also be reduced because of poor effort or cooperation by the patient.

An obstructive ventilatory defect is characterized by reduction of maximal airflow at all lung volumes. Flow is limited by airway narrowing during forced expiration. Airway obstruction may be caused by mucus secretion, bronchospasm, and inflammation such as in asthma or bronchitis. Airflow limitation may also result from loss of elastic support for the airways themselves, as in emphysema. The earliest changes in obstructive patterns may occur in the small airways (i.e., those less than 2 mm), which may or may not be detected by changes in FEV_1.

FEV_1 may also be decreased in large airway obstruction (trachea and bronchi). Tumors or foreign bodies that limit airflow cause the FEV_1 to be reduced. These defects can be identified by flow reductions across the entire forced expiration (see the section on flow-volume curve).

FEV_1 and **FEV_1/VC** are the most standardized indices of obstructive disease. An obstructive defect is defined best by a reduced FEV_1/VC ratio. The severity of obstructive disease may be gauged by the extent to which FEV_1 is reduced. The ability to work and function in daily life is related to FEV_1 and VC. Mortality (likelihood of dying) caused by respiratory disease is similarly related to the degree of obstruction as measured by FEV_1. Patients with markedly reduced FEV_1 values are much more likely to die from chronic obstructive pulmonary disease (COPD), lung cancer, and even cardiovascular disease, including myocardial infarction and stroke. Although FEV_1 correlates with prognosis and severity of symptoms in obstructive lung disease, outcomes for individual patients cannot be accurately predicted.

While the ratio of FEV_1/VC defines obstruction, the severity of obstruction is defined by the degree to which the FEV_1 is reduced. The ATS/ERS Task Force suggests the following classifications of severity:

Mild	$FEV_1 > 70\%$ predicted
Moderate	$FEV_1 = 60\% - 69\%$ predicted
Moderately severe	$FEV_1 = 50\% - 59\%$ predicted
Severe	$FEV_1 = 35\% - 49\%$ predicted
Very severe	$FEV_1 < 35\%$ predicted

The concept of grading severity based on FEV_1 applies best when the VC is in the normal range. Once the VC is below normal, a concomitant restrictive defect may also be present, and this can be determined only by further measurement of lung volumes, in particular TLC. Because the FEV_1 in restriction is reduced, in part, by the restrictive process itself, the decrement in FEV_1 due to the obstructive component of disease can no longer be assumed to reflect the severity of obstruction only. Thus the severity of obstruction in a combined restrictive and obstructive defect is typically overestimated when basing severity solely on the reduction in FEV_1.

Restrictive processes such as fibrosis, edema, space-occupying lesions, neuromuscular disorders, obesity, and chest wall deformities may all cause FEV_1 to be decreased. Reduction in FEV_1 occurs in much the same way as reduction in VC. Unlike the pattern seen in obstructive disease, in which VC is preserved and FEV_1 reduced, in restriction VC and FEV_1 values are proportionately decreased. Some patients with moderate or severe restriction have an FEV_1 nearly equal to the VC. The entire VC, because it is reduced, is exhaled almost completely in the first second. To distinguish between obstructive and restrictive causes of reduced FEV_1 values, the FEV_1/VC ratio ($FEV_{1\%}$) and other flow measurements are useful. Further definition of obstruction versus restriction may require measurement of lung volumes (e.g., functional residual capacity, or FRC, and TLC). However, studies have shown that when the FVC and FEV_1/VC ratio are both normal, restriction, as defined by a low TLC, is very unlikely.

FEV_1 is the most widely used spirometric parameter, particularly for assessment of airway obstruction. FEV_1 is used in conjunction with VC for simple screening, assessment of response to bronchodilators, inhalation challenge studies, and detection of exercise-induced bronchospasm (see Chapters 7 and 9). FEV_1 is the most robust pulmonary function test, making it the measurement of choice in evaluating lung function in general. In fact, the motto of the National Lung Health Education Program (NLHEP) is "Test your lungs. Know your numbers," and these numbers are the FEV_1 and FVC (or FEV_6). The NLHEP advocates the widespread use of simple office spirometry to increase the awareness and detection of COPD as well as other respiratory disorders. In particular, the NLHEP recommends that all smokers aged 45 years and older have spirometry done to detect airflow obstruction, even before the onset of clinical symptoms.

Forced Expiratory Volume Ratio ($FEV_{T\%}$)

Normal $FEV_{T\%}$ ratios for healthy adults are as follows:

$FEV_{0.5\%} = 50\% - 60\%$
$FEV_{1\%} = 75\% - 85\%$
$FEV_{2\%} = 90\% - 95\%$
$FEV_{3\%} = 95\% - 98\%$
$FEV_{6\%} = 98\% - 100\%$

These ratios may be derived by dividing predicted FEV_T by predicted VC. Some studies of healthy patients derive equations for the ratio itself. The reported FEV_1/VC ratio is calculated from the highest FEV_1 and the highest FVC. The FEV_1/VC ratio decreases with increasing age, presumably because of gradual loss of lung elasticity. For example, older healthy adults may have FEV_1/VC ratios in the $65\% - 70\%$ range. Thus the fifth percentile should be taken as the lower limit of normal when interpreting the FEV_1/VC, just as with FEV_1 and VC separately.

Patients with unobstructed airflow can usually exhale their entire FVC within 4 seconds. Conversely, patients with obstructive disease have reduced $FEV_{T\%}$

for each interval (e.g., 1 second, 2 seconds). The FEV_1/VC ratio is the most important measurement for distinguishing an obstructive impairment. A decreased FEV_1/VC ratio is the hallmark of obstructive disease. As already mentioned, the ratio decreases with age, so care should be taken in interpreting the FEV_1/VC ratio in absolute terms. The Global Initiative for Chronic Obstructive Lung Disease (GOLD) and ATS/ERS guidelines on COPD consider 70% as the absolute cutoff between normal airflow and airflow obstruction in defining COPD. However, this value may actually underestimate the presence of obstruction in younger adults, and overestimate it in older individuals (see Appendix B for predicted values).

Diagnosis of an obstructive pattern based on spirometry should focus on three primary variables: VC, FEV_1, and FEV_1/VC. Measurements such as $FEF_{25\%-75\%}$ should be considered only after the presence and severity of obstruction has been determined using the primary variables. If the FEV_1/VC is borderline abnormal, additional flow measurements may suggest the presence of an obstructive pattern. Care should be taken when interpreting the FEV_1/VC ratio in patients who have VC and FEV_1 values greater than predicted. The FEV_1/VC ratio may appear to indicate an obstructive pattern because of the variability of the greater than normal VC and FEV_1 values.

Although a low FEV_1/VC ratio is the key to defining obstruction, the ATS/ERS guidelines also define obstruction in the subset of patients who have a normal FEV_1/VC ratio but a low VC and a normal TLC. This pattern has been hypothesized to be due to small airways disease with resulting small airways closure and gas trapping.

PF TIP

Look at the FEV_1/FVC ratio first if obstruction is suspected. If the FEV_1/FVC ratio is lower than expected (the lower limit of normal), obstruction is present. If the ratio is normal or elevated, check the percent predicted for FVC and FEV_1. If FVC and FEV_1 are both reduced compared with the expected values, and FEV_1/FVC is normal or high, restriction or muscle weakness may be present.

Patients who have restrictive disease (e.g., pulmonary fibrosis) often have normal or increased $FEV_{T\%}$ values. Because airflow may be minimally affected in restrictive diseases, FEV_1 and VC are usually reduced in equal proportion. If the restriction is severe, FEV_1 may approach the VC value. In addition, the increased elastic recoil of fibrotic lungs may enhance expiratory airflow. As a result, $FEV_{1\%}$ appears to be higher than normal. The FEV_1/VC ratio may be 100% if the VC is severely reduced. The presence of a restrictive disorder may be suggested by a reduced VC and a normal or increased FEV_1/VC ratio. Further studies (e.g., measurement of TLC) should be used to confirm the diagnosis of restriction.

Forced Expiratory Flow$_{25\%-75\%}$

$FEF_{25\%-75\%}$ is measured from a segment of the FVC that includes flow from medium and small airways. Typical values for healthy young adults average 4 to 5 L/sec. These values decrease with age. $FEF_{25\%-75\%}$ is variable even in healthy patients, with one standard deviation (SD) equal to approximately 1 L/sec. Values as low as 50% of the predicted may be statistically within normal limits. This variability requires guarded interpretation of the $FEF_{25\%-75\%}$.

The $FEF_{25\%-75\%}$ may be indicative of the status of the medium to small airways. Decreased flows are common in the early stages of obstructive disease. Abnormalities in these measurements, however, are not specific for small airways disease. Although $FEF_{25\%-75\%}$ may suggest changes in the small airways, it should not be used to diagnose small airways disease in individual patients. In the presence of a borderline value for FEV_1/VC, a low $FEF_{25\%-75\%}$ may help confirm airway obstruction. Assessment of $FEF_{25\%-75\%}$ after bronchodilator must consider changes in FVC as well. If FVC increases markedly, $FEF_{25\%-75\%}$ may actually decrease. Likewise, if the FVC decreases, the $FEF_{25\%-75\%}$ may increase. Isovolume correction (as described previously) can be used to compare $FEF_{25\%-75\%}$ before and after bronchodilator therapy. However, the inherent variability of $FEF_{25\%-75\%}$ and its dependence on FVC make it less useful than the FEV_1 for assessing bronchodilator response.

Reduced $FEF_{25\%-75\%}$ values are sometimes seen in cases of moderate or severe restrictive patterns. This is assumed to be caused by a decrease in the cross-sectional area of the small airways. $FEF_{25\%-75\%}$ depends somewhat on patient effort because it depends on the FVC exhaled. Patients who perform the FVC maneuver inadequately often show widely varying midexpiratory flow rates.

The $FEF_{25\%-75\%}$/FVC ratio is thought to reflect relative airway size to lung size, and, as such, has been found to be significantly associated with airways hyperresponsiveness. The clinical importance of this finding is unknown.

Validity of FVC maneuvers depends largely on patient effort and cooperation. Equally important is the instruction and coaching supplied by the technologist. Many patients need several attempts before performing the maneuver acceptably. Demonstration of proper technique by the technologist helps the patient give maximal effort. Placement of the mouthpiece behind the teeth and lips, maximal inspiration, little if any pause, and maximal expiration should all be demonstrated. Emphasis should be placed on the initial burst of air and on continuing expiration for at least 6 seconds. Acceptability of each FVC maneuver should be evaluated according to specific criteria (see Spirometry 2-3). The final report should include comments on the quality of the data obtained (see Chapter 11). These comments may be provided by the technologist, physician, or both.

Validity of the FEV_1 also depends on cooperation and effort. Adequate instruction and demonstration of the maneuver by the technologist is essential. Repeatability of FEV_1 should be within 150 ml for the two best of at least three acceptable maneuvers. Accurate measurement of FEV_1 requires an acceptable spirometer (see Chapter 11), preferably one that allows inspection of the volume-time curve and back-extrapolation.

Validity of the $FEV_{1\%}$ also depends on patient effort and cooperation. Because the values used to derive the ratio may be taken from separate maneuvers, both FEV_1 and FVC should be reproducible. Poor effort on an FVC test may result in an overestimate of $FEV_{T\%}$. If the patient stops prematurely, the FVC (i.e., denominator of the ratio) will appear smaller than it actually is. The $FEV_{1\%}$ will then appear larger than it actually is. Some clinicians prefer to use the VC to calculate the $FEV_{1\%}$. This may be useful if the VC is significantly larger than FVC because of airway compression.

Patients who have moderate or severe obstruction may require longer than 10 seconds to completely exhale. Although continuing to exhale increases measured FVC, the diagnosis of obstruction can be made with less than complete expiration. The FEV_6 may be a useful surrogate measurement in obstructed patients who have difficulty with prolonged exhalation. In some cases, prolonged effort may be difficult for the patient. The large transpulmonary pressure generated by a forced expiratory maneuver often reduces cardiac output. Patients may complain of dizziness, seeing "spots," ringing in the ears, or numbness of extremities. A patient may occasionally faint as a result of decreased cerebral blood flow. This complication may be serious if it causes the patient to fall from a standing or sitting position. Because of these issues, the NLHEP recommends use of the FEV_6 rather than the FVC for ease of performance and safety in office spirometry.

FLOW-VOLUME CURVE

Description

The FVC graphs the flow generated during an FVC maneuver against volume change. The FVC may be followed by an FIVC maneuver, plotted similarly. Flow is usually recorded in liters per second, and the volume is recorded in liters, BTPS. The **maximal expiratory flow-volume (MEFV)** curve shows flow as the patient exhales from maximal inspiration (TLC) to maximal expiration (RV). The **maximal inspiratory flow volume (MIFV)** curve displays inspiratory flow plotted from RV to TLC. When MEFV and MIFV curves are plotted together, the resulting figure is called a flow-volume (F-V) loop (Figure 2-10). The reported F-V loop is taken from the single best test maneuver (highest sum of FEV_1 and FVC).

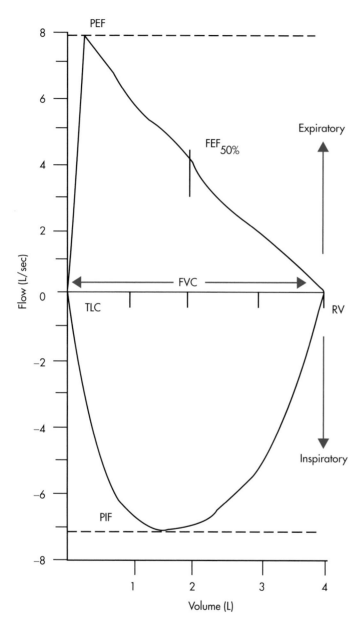

FIGURE 2-10 **Flow-Volume Loop.** A flow-volume recording in which an FVC and an FIVC maneuver are recorded in succession. Flow in liters per second is plotted on the vertical axis and volume, in liters, on the horizontal axis. By convention, expiratory flow is plotted upward (positive), and inspiratory flow is plotted downward (negative). The maximal exhalation begins with the patient at total lung capacity (TLC) and continues until residual volume (RV) is reached; a maximal inspiration then returns to TLC. The forced vital capacity (FVC) can be read from the tracing as the maximal horizontal deflection along the zero flow line. Peak flows for expiration and inspiration (PEF and PIF) can be read directly from the tracing as the maximal deflections on the flow axis (positive and negative). The instantaneous flow (FEF) at any point in the FVC can also be measured directly. Abnormalities, such as small or large airway obstruction, may show up as characteristic changes in the maximal flow rates. The flow-volume loop is a graphic display of the MEFV and MIFV curves combined.

Technique

The patient performs an FVC maneuver, inspiring fully and then exhaling as rapidly as possible. To complete the loop, the patient inspires as rapidly as possible from the maximal expiratory level back to maximal inspiration. Volume is plotted on the horizontal x-axis, and flow is plotted on the vertical y-axis. The F-V loop is usually displayed on a computer screen. It can also be printed or plotted. Expiratory flow is plotted upward. Expired volume is usually plotted from left to right. Sometimes, when concomitant lung volumes have also been measured, an absolute lung volume scale is used, usually with

TLC on the left and RV on the right. Airflow should be recorded at 2 L/sec/unit distance on the y-axis. Volume should be recorded at 1 L/unit distance on the volume axis. Scale factors should be at least 5 mm/L/sec for flow and 10 mm/L for volume. These factors are required so that manual measurements can be made from a printed copy of the maneuver.

FVC, as well as PEF and peak inspiratory flow (PIF), can be read directly from the F-V loop. Instantaneous flow at any lung volume can be measured directly from the F-V loop. Maximal flow at 75%, 50%, and 25% of the FVC are commonly reported as the $\dot{V}max_{75}$, $\dot{V}max_{50}$, and $\dot{V}max_{25}$. The subscript in these terms refers to the portion of the FVC remaining. The same flows are also reported as the $FEF_{25\%}$, $FEF_{50\%}$, and $FEF_{75\%}$, with the subscripts referring to the percentage of FVC exhaled. This latter terminology is now preferred by the ATS/ERS guidelines. Most computerized spirometers superimpose timing marks (ticks) on the MEFV curve (Figure 2-11). These marks allow FEV_1 (or other FEV_T) values to be read from the F-V loop.

F-V loop data, stored in computer memory, can be easily manipulated. Multiple loops can be compared by superimposing them with contrasting colors. Bronchodilator or inhalation challenge F-V loops can be presented in a similar manner. A predicted MEFV curve can be plotted using points for PEF and maximal flows at 75%, 50%, and 25% of the FVC. A patient's flow-volume curve can then be superimposed directly over the expected values (see Figure 2-11). Superimposing multiple FVC maneuvers as F-V loops can be used to assess reproducibility of the patient's effort. Positioning loops side by side or superimposing can also help detect decreasing flows with repeated efforts. This pattern may be seen because FVC maneuvers can induce bronchospasm. Storing tests in the order performed is recommended. This allows review of the test session and detection of bronchospasm or fatigue.

Reproducible MEFV curves, particularly the PEF, are good indicators of adequate patient effort (Spirometry 2-5). Assessing the start-of-test and determining whether exhalation lasted at least 6 seconds may be difficult if only the F-V loop is displayed. Simultaneous display of flow-volume and

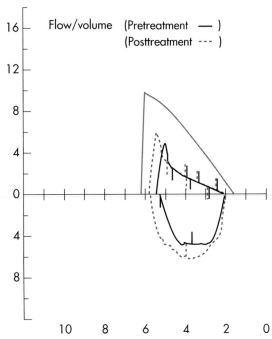

FIGURE 2-11 Superimposed Flow-Volume Loops on an Absolute Volume Scale. Flow-volume curves from a patient with combined obstruction and restriction. Multiple F-V loops (in this case before and after bronchodilator therapy) are superimposed by the computer at RV. *Upward ticks* on the expiratory limb represent $FEV_{0.5}$, FEV_1, and FEV_3, respectively. *Downward ticks* on the expiratory curve represent the $FEF_{25\%}$, $FEF_{50\%}$, and $FEF_{75\%}$, respectively. *Upward ticks* on the inspiratory loop represent the $FIF_{50\%}$. The large gray expiratory curve is a computer-generated plot of the patient's predicted MEFV. As can be seen from the curves, expiratory flow is decreased at all lung volumes. The patient's FVC *(horizontal axis)* is also lower than predicted.

volume-time curves is useful (Figure 2-12). Although computerized systems calculate back-extrapolated volume, a volume-time tracing may be necessary to perform back-extrapolation manually (see Figure 2-6). Common technical problems with volume-time tracings and F-V loops are shown in Figure 2-13.

Significance and Pathophysiology

See Spirometry 2-6 for interpretive strategies. Maximal flow at any lung volume during forced expiration or forced inspiration can be easily measured from the F-V loop (see Figure 2-10). Significant decreases in flow or volume are easily detected from a single graphic display. Many clinicians prefer to include the F-V loop or MEFV curve as part of the patient's medical record.

SPIROMETRY 2-5

CRITERIA FOR ACCEPTABILITY

Flow-Volume Loop

1. Rapid rise from maximal inspiration to PEF.
2. Maximal effort until flow returns to zero baseline; no glottic closure or abrupt end of flow.
3. Maximal inspiratory effort with return of volume to point of maximal inspiration (Failure to close loop indicates that effort was not started from maximal inspiration, inspiratory effort was submaximal, or spirometer error).
4. At least three acceptable loops recorded; superimposed or side-by-side loops should be reproducible, unless bronchospasm occurs.
5. Report the F-V loop from the single best test maneuver (highest sum of FEV_1 and FVC).

The shape of an MEFV curve from approximately 75% of FVC to maximal expiration is largely independent of patient effort. Flow over this segment is determined by two properties of the lung: elastic recoil and flow resistance. The lung is stretched by maximal inspiration. Elastic recoil determines the pressure applied to gas in the lung during a forced expiration. This pressure is determined by the recoil of the lung and chest wall. Resistance to flow in the airways is the second factor affecting the shape of the flow-volume curve. Flow limitation occurs in the large and medium airways during the early part of a forced expiration. The site of flow limitation migrates "upstream" rapidly during forced expiration. Resistance to flow in small (less than 2 mm) airways is determined primarily by the cross-sectional area. This cross-sectional area can be affected by a number of factors. Destruction of alveolar walls, as in emphysema, reduces support of the small airways. Bronchoconstriction and inflammation directly reduce the lumen of the small airways.

In healthy patients, flow ($\dot{V}max$) over the effort-independent segment decreases linearly as lung volume decreases. Pressures around airways are

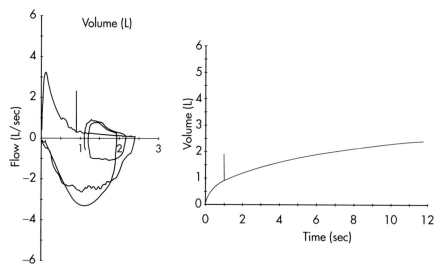

FIGURE 2-12   MEFV and Volume-Time Tracings from a Patient with Severe Obstruction. The expiratory flow-volume curve shows severely reduced flows at all lung volumes; inspiratory flows are also markedly reduced. Note that the tidal breathing loop (recorded immediately before the forced effort) shows higher flows than the MEFV curve. This is consistent with dynamic airway compression during forced exhalation. The expiratory volume-time tracing reveals reduced flow with no obvious plateau even after 12 seconds of exhalation.

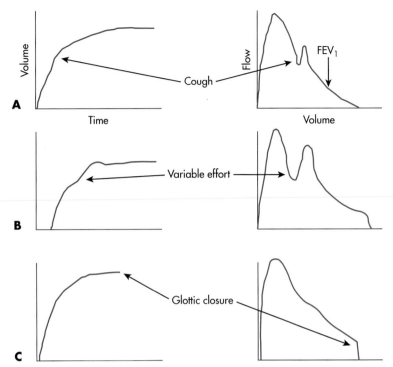

FIGURE 2-13 **Common Technical Problems with Flow-Volume Loops. A,** Cough during the first second of exhalation will interfere with proper measurement of forced expiratory volume in 1 second; (FEV₁). **B,** Variable efforts will result in poorly reproducible loops. **C,** Glottic closure results in abrupt termination of expiration and will affect accurate measurement of FVC.

SPIROMETRY 2-6

INTERPRETIVE STRATEGIES

Flow-Volume Loop

1. Were at least three acceptable F-V loops obtained? Does the beginning of the expiratory curve show a sharp rise to PEF? If not, suspect patient effort or large airway obstruction.
2. Are the PEF and PIF values consistent? Does PEF or other expiratory flows fall with repeated efforts? If so, suspect hyperreactive airways.
3. Does the expiratory curve from PEF to maximal exhalation appear concave? If so, suspect intrathoracic airway obstruction.
4. Do either the expiratory or inspiratory portions of the curve show a "squared off" pattern? If so, suspect large airway obstruction. If both, suspect a fixed obstruction.
5. Is the inspiratory curve repeatable? If not, suspect variable extrathoracic obstruction or suboptimal effort or fatigue.
6. Does the F-V loop show any other unusual patterns (sudden changes in flow that are reproducible, or "sawtooth" pattern)?

balanced by gas pressures in the airways so that flow is limited at an "equal pressure point." As the lung empties, the equal pressure point moves upstream into increasingly smaller airways and continues until small airways begin to close, trapping some gas in the alveoli (the RV). This pattern of airflow limitation in healthy lungs causes the MEFV curve to have a linear or slightly concave appearance (see Figure 2-10). This degree of concavity increases with age, presumably due to reduced flows secondary to loss of elastic recoil with aging.

Flow-Volume Loops in Small Airway Obstruction

Maximal flow is decreased in patients who have obstruction in small airways, particularly at low lung volumes. The effort-independent segment of the MEFV curve appears more concave or "scooped out" (see Figure 2-12). Values for $\dot{V}max_{50}$ and $\dot{V}max_{25}$ are characteristically decreased. Decreases in $\dot{V}max_{50}$ correlate well with the reduction in $FEF_{25\%-75\%}$ in patients with small airway obstructive disease.

Because elastic recoil *and* resistance in small airways determine the shape of the MEFV tracing, different lung diseases can cause similar F-V patterns. Emphysema destroys alveoli with loss of elastic tissue and support for small airways. Flow through small airways decreases because of collapse of the unsupported walls. In contrast, bronchitis, asthma, and similar inflammatory processes increase resistance in the small airways. Increased resistance is caused by edema, mucus production, and smooth muscle constriction. Reduction in the cross-sectional area of the small airways reduces flow. Emphysema and chronic bronchitis are often found in the same

individual because of their common cause—cigarette smoking. The MEFV curve thus presents a picture of the extent of obstruction without identifying its cause.

Flow-Volume Loops in Large Airway Obstruction

Obstruction of the upper airway, trachea, or mainstem bronchi also shows characteristic patterns. Both expiratory and inspiratory flow may be limited. The F-V loop is extremely useful in diagnosing these large airway abnormalities (Figure 2-14).

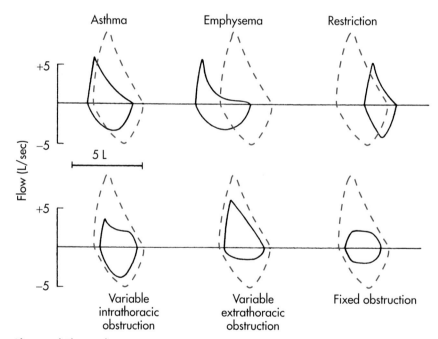

FIGURE 2-14 **Abnormal Flow-Volume Loops Patterns.** Six curves are shown plotting flow in liters per second against the FVC on an absolute volume scale, with higher lung volumes on the left. In each example, the expected curve is shown *(dashed lines)*, while the curve illustrating the particular disease pattern is superimposed. In patients who have asthma and emphysema, the portion of the expiratory curve from the peak flow to residual volume (RV) is characteristically concave. Both the TLC and RV points are displaced toward higher lung volumes (to the left of the expected curves). These patterns are indicative of hyperinflation and/or air trapping. In restrictive patterns, the shape of the loop is preserved but the FVC is decreased. The TLC and RV displaced toward lower lung volume (to the right of the expected curves). The bottom three examples depict types of large airway obstruction. Variable intrathoracic obstruction shows reduced flows on expiration despite near-normal flows on inspiration resulting from flow limitation in the large airways during a forced expiration. Variable extrathoracic obstruction shows an opposite pattern. Inspiratory flow is reduced, while expiratory flow is relatively normal. Fixed large airway obstruction is characterized by equally reduced inspiratory and expiratory flows. Comparison of the $FEF_{50\%}$ with the $FIF_{50\%}$ may be helpful in differentiating large airway obstructive processes. However, because the magnitude of inspiratory flow is highly effort dependent, low inspiratory flows should be carefully evaluated.

Comparison of expiratory and inspiratory flows at 50% of the FVC ($FEF_{50\%}$ and $FIF_{50\%}$, respectively) may help determine the site of obstruction. In healthy patients, the ratio of $FEF_{50\%}$ to $FIF_{50\%}$ is approximately 1.0 or slightly less. Fixed large airway obstruction causes equally reduced flows at 50% of the VC during inspiration and expiration (Figure 2-15). Obstructive lesions that vary with the phase of breathing also produce characteristic patterns. Variable extrathoracic obstruction usually shows normal expiratory flow but diminished inspiratory flow. The $FEF_{50\%}/FIF_{50\%}$ is often greater than 1.0. Because the obstructive process is outside of the thorax, the MEFV portion of the curve appears as it would in a healthy individual, but the inspiratory portion of the loop is flattened. Inspiratory flow depends on how much obstruction is present. A common cause of variable extrathoracic obstruction, resulting in truncated inspiratory flow, is paradoxical vocal cord closure during inspiration, also known as vocal cord dysfunction. In variable intrathoracic obstruction, PEF is reduced. Expiratory flow remains constant until the site of flow limitation reaches the smaller airways. This gives the expiratory limb a "squared-off" appearance (see Figure 2-14). The inspiratory portion of the loop may be completely normal. The $FEF_{50\%}/FIF_{50\%}$ will be typically much less than 1.0, depending on the severity of obstruction.

PF TIP

Reduced peak expiratory flow (PEF) and/or peak inspiratory flow (PIF) as seen on the F-V loop may be due to disease or poor patient effort. Be sure to look at *all* maneuvers performed. If peak expiratory or peak inspiratory flows are uniformly reduced in all efforts, large airway obstruction may be present. An F-V loop performed with poor effort may mimic large airway obstruction.

Airway obstruction associated with abnormality of the muscular control of the posterior pharynx and larynx sometimes produces a "sawtooth" pattern visible on the inspiratory and expiratory limbs of the MEFV curve. This pattern is sometimes observed in patients suspected of having sleep apnea.

Peak inspiratory flow and the pattern of flow during inspiration are largely effort dependent. Poor patient effort may result in inspiratory flow patterns similar to variable extrathoracic obstruction. Instruction by the technologist should emphasize maximal effort during inspiration as well as expiration. If repeated efforts produce reduced inspiratory flows, an obstructive process should be suspected.

Restrictive disease processes may show normal or greater than normal peak flows with linear decreases in flow versus volume. The lung volume displayed on the x-axis is decreased. Moderate or severe restriction demonstrates equally reduced flows at all lung volumes. Reduced flows are primarily caused by the decreased cross-sectional area of the small airways at low lung volumes. Simple restriction causes the F-V loop to appear as a miniature of the normal curve (see Figure 2-14), often with supranormal flow as seen by elevated FEV_1/VC.

Before- and after-bronchodilator F-V loops can be superimposed to measure changes in flow at specific lung volumes. The curves are usually positioned by superimposing at maximal inspiration. This method assumes that any increase in FVC occurs while TLC remains constant. If postbronchodilator lung volume tests are performed, the curves may be superimposed on an absolute volume scale (i.e., isovolume correction). This method shows bronchodilator-induced changes in lung volumes as well as flows. Sometimes, lung volumes will change after bronchodilator without any change in FEV_1. Inhalation challenge studies (see Chapter 9) can be displayed similarly to assess the reduction in flows at specific lung volumes.

Tidal breathing curves or MVV curves can also be superimposed on the F-V loop. The patient's ventilatory reserve can be assessed by comparing the areas enclosed under each of the curves. Patients who have obstructive lung disease may generate F-V loops only slightly larger than their tidal breathing curves. In severe obstruction, flow during tidal breathing may actually exceed flow during a forced expiration. Dynamic compression of small airways

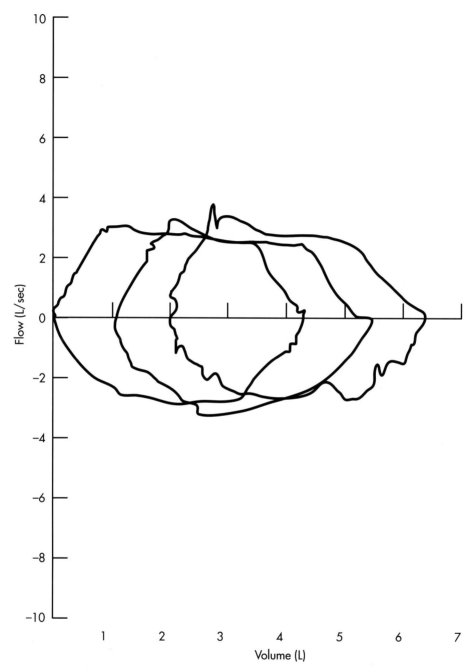

FIGURE 2-15   MEFV Tracings from a Patient with a Fixed Upper Airway Obstruction. Three flow-volume loops are displayed with the starting point (TLC) offset by 1 L. On each curve, the expiratory and inspiratory limbs show flattening consistent with a fixed obstruction. Note that maximal flow on both limbs is about 3 L/sec, much less than expected in a healthy patient.

during forced expiration causes airway collapse, while tidal breathing may not. These patients have limited ventilatory reserve and shortness of breath with exertion.

F-V loops may also be measured during exercise (see Chapter 7). By superimposing a flow-volume curve during exercise over the maximal F-V loop, specific patterns of ventilatory response can be assessed. Patients who have airflow limitation are typically unable to increase ventilation during exercise when expiratory flow equals maximal flow. Exercise F-V curves can be used to demonstrate this phenomenon.

PEAK EXPIRATORY FLOW

Description

Peak expiratory flow (PEF) is the maximum flow attained during an FVC maneuver. When reported in conjunction with other spirometric variables, PEF is expressed in liters per second, BTPS. When performed alone using a **peak flow meter**, PEF is usually reported in liters per minute, BTPS.

Technique

PEF can be easily measured from a flow-volume curve (MEFV). PEF may also be measured by using devices that sense flow directly (see Chapter 10) or by using volume displacement spirometers and deriving the rate of volume change. Many portable devices (e.g., peak flow meters) are available to measure maximal flow during forced expiration. Most sense flow as movement of air against a turbine or through an orifice. PEF done in conjunction with spirometry is performed as described for F-V loops.

Measuring PEF with a peak flow meter may be done at the bedside, in the emergency department, in the clinic setting, or at home. In each setting, the individual performing the measurement must know how to operate the specific peak flow meter. The maneuver should be demonstrated to the patient. A return demonstration is essential when the patient is being trained to use the peak flow meter at home.

The peak flow meter should be set or zeroed, as required. When performed at home with a portable device as part of ambulatory monitoring, the standing position is usually recommended. (If performed as part of a spirometry maneuver in the office or hospital setting, the patient should be sitting.) The patient should inhale maximally; the inhalation should be rapid but not forced. The patient then exhales with maximal effort as soon as the teeth and lips are placed around the mouthpiece. The neck should be in a neutral position to avoid tracheal compression with neck flexion or extension, because this will reduce PEF. As in the FVC maneuver, a long pause (4–6 seconds) at maximal inspiration may decrease the PEF; there should be no more than 1-second hesitation. The expiratory effort only needs to be 1–2 seconds to record PEF.

At least three maneuvers should be performed and recorded, along with the order in which the values were obtained. All readings are recorded to detect effort-induced bronchospasm. The largest PEF obtained should be reported. The PEF is effort dependent and variable. It may be particularly variable in patients with hyperreactive airways (Spirometry 2-7). Up to five attempts should be made to achieve adequate repeatability, defined as no more than 0.67 L/sec (40 L/min) difference between the largest of two out of three acceptable efforts.

When PEF is used to monitor asthmatic patients, it is important to establish each person's best PEF (i.e., the largest PEF achieved). Best values can be obtained over 2–3 weeks. PEF should be measured twice daily (morning and evening). The personal best is usually observed in the evening after a period of maximum therapy. Daily measurements are then compared with the personal best. The personal best PEF should be reevaluated annually. This allows PEF to be adjusted for growth in children or for progression of disease. PEF should be periodically compared with regular spirometry results (FEV_1).

Portable peak flow meters need to be precise (low variability in the same instrument). *Precision* is more important than accuracy for detecting changes from serial measurements. Peak flow meters should

---

SPIROMETRY 2-7

CRITERIA FOR ACCEPTABILITY

Peak Flow

1. Patient was standing or sitting up straight.
2. Patient inhaled maximally (rapid, but not forced) and exhaled maximally without holding his or her breath.
3. At least three efforts were performed and recorded in order.
4. The largest two out of three efforts were reproducible within 0.67 L/sec (40 L/min)
5. Largest PEF obtained is reported.

From ATS/ERS Task Force, 2005.

SPIROMETRY 2-8

INTERPRETIVE STRATEGIES

Peak Flow

1. What is the patient's personal best PEF?
2. Is the current PEF the best of three trials? Was it obtained in the morning or evening? Was it obtained before or after inhaled bronchodilator therapy?
3. Zone system*:

   Green   80%–100% of personal best
           Routine treatment can be continued; consider reducing medications.

   Yellow 50%–80% of personal best
           Acute exacerbation may be present; temporary increase in medication may be indicated; maintenance therapy may need to be increased.

   Red   < 50% of personal best
           Bronchodilators should be taken immediately; begin oral steroids; clinician should be notified if PEF fails to return to yellow or green within 2–4 hours.

* From National Asthma Education Program, NIH, 1991.

---

have ranges of 60–400 L/min for children and 100 to 850 L/min for adults. Standards for peak flow monitoring devices have been published by the ATS/ERS (see Chapters 10 and 11).

Significance and Pathophysiology

See Spirometry 2-8 for interpretive strategies. The PEF attainable by healthy young adults may exceed 10 L/sec or 600 L/min, BTPS. Even when an accurate pneumotachometer is used, the value of PEF measurements may be limited. Peak flow is effort dependent. It primarily measures large airway function and muscular effort. Decreased PEF values should be evaluated for consistent patient effort. PEF values for patients without hyperreactive airways are usually similar with repeated efforts. Asthmatic patients often have a pattern of decreasing PEF with repeated trials. Widely varying peak flows without a pattern of induced bronchospasm suggest poor effort or cooperation. However, PEF measurements alone are not sufficient to make a diagnosis of asthma. Spirometry, lung volumes, diffusing capacity, and airway resistance measurements may be required to evaluate fully the associated physiologic impairment.

Effort dependence of PEF makes it a good indicator of patient effort during spirometry. Maximal transpulmonary pressures correlate well with maximal PEF. Patients who exert variable effort during FVC maneuvers are seldom able to reproduce their PEF. Some clinicians use PEF in addition to the FVC and FEV_1 to gauge maximal effort during spirometry. PEF measurements, when performed with a good effort, correlate well with the FEV_1 as measured by spirometry.

Patients with early small airway obstruction may initially have high flows during an FVC maneuver. Despite obstruction, these individuals show relatively normal PEF values. When small airway obstruction becomes severe, PEF also decreases. Reduction in PEF is often less than the decrease in $FEF_{50\%}$ or $FEF_{75\%}$ in patients with severe obstruction.

PEF measurements are particularly useful for monitoring asthma patients at home. Daily monitoring of PEF can provide early detection of asthmatic episodes. It can be used to detect day-night patterns (circadian rhythms) related to airway reactivity. PEF monitoring provides objective criteria for treatment. It can help determine specific triggers (e.g., allergens) or workplace exposures that cause symptoms. Daily morning and evening readings are recommended. For patients taking inhaled bronchodilators, PEF may be measured before and after treatment. Significant variation from their personal best or from one reading to the next should be emphasized.

The National Asthma Education and Prevention Program suggests a "zone" system, based on the individual's personal best or predicted PEF (see Spirometry 2-8). The zone system uses green, yellow, and red as indicators for maintaining or altering therapy. Green (80%–100% of the personal best PEF) indicates continuation of routine therapy. Yellow (50%–80% of the personal best PEF) indicates that an acute episode may be starting. Increased medication may be necessary. Red (less than 50% of the personal best PEF) indicates that an acute change has occurred. Immediate treatment is required, and the clinician should be notified. This approach dramatically improves the patient's ability to communicate symptomatic changes to the clinician.

Uniformly decreased PEF is often associated with upper airway obstruction but is nonspecific. PEF assessed from F-V loops (along with PIF) helps define both the severity and site of large airway obstruction.

MAXIMUM VOLUNTARY VENTILATION

Description

Maximum voluntary ventilation (MVV) is the volume of air exhaled in a specific interval during rapid, forced breathing. The maneuver should last at least 12 seconds. It is recorded in liters per minute, BTPS, by extrapolating the volume to 1 minute.

Technique

MVV is measured by having the patient breathe deeply and rapidly for a 12-second interval. Patients should set the rate, but breathe rapidly and deeply.

The volume breathed should be greater than their V_T but less than their VC. Instruct the patient to move as much air as possible into and out of the spirometer. The technologist should encourage the patient throughout the maneuver. An ideal rate is 90–110 breaths per minute, and an ideal tidal volume is approximately 50% of the VC.

MVV is continued for at least 12 seconds but no more than 15 seconds. The patient is hyperventilating. Efforts longer than 15 seconds exaggerate the sensation of lightheadedness. Even the 12-second interval may produce dizziness or syncope. The test may be performed with the patient in either a sitting or standing position. If done while standing, a chair should be available in case of dizziness. Some automated spirometers allow MVV to be terminated before 12 seconds. This accommodates patients who cannot continue because of coughing or lightheadedness. If MVV does not last 12 seconds, it should be noted in the technologist's comments (see Chapter 11). At least two MVV maneuvers should be performed. The two largest should be within 20% of each other. The largest value is reported (Spirometry 2-9).

PF TIP

You can quickly check the validity of the MVV by comparing it with the patient's FEV_1 multiplied by 40. If the MVV is significantly lower than $FEV_1 \times 40$, patient effort may be the cause. Neuromuscular disease may also cause a reduced MVV in relation to FEV_1.

SPIROMETRY 2-9

CRITERIA FOR ACCEPTABILITY

MVV

1. Volume-time tracing shows continuous, rhythmic effort for at least 12 seconds.
2. Volume is approximately 50% of VC and rate is 90–110 breaths per minute.
3. Two acceptable maneuvers are obtained; MVV values are within 20%.
4. Report the highest acceptable MVV and breathing rate.

From ATS/ERS Task Force, 2005.

The volume expired is measured by a spirometer. The spirometer must have adequate frequency response over a wide range of flows (see Chapters 10 and 11). Historically, the volume of each breath was read from a volume-time spirogram or from a recording of accumulated volume (Figure 2-16). Now volume data from each breath are summed by computer for the interval measured. The MVV (for a 12-second test) is calculated as flow in liters per minute, as follows:

$$MVV = Vol_{12} \times \frac{60}{12}$$

where:
Vol_{12} = volume in liters expired in 12 seconds
60 = factor for extrapolation from seconds to minutes

For other intervals, the MVV is calculated similarly. The MVV must be corrected to BTPS.

Significance and Pathophysiology

See Spirometry 2-10 for interpretive strategies. MVV tests the overall function of the respiratory system. It is influenced by airway resistance, respiratory muscles, compliance of the lung and/or chest

SPIROMETRY 2-10

INTERPRETIVE STRATEGIES

MVV

1. Was MVV test performed acceptably? At least 12 seconds?
2. Does MVV approximate $FEV_1 \times 40$? If not, suspect suboptimal effort or neuromuscular weakness.
3. Is MVV less than 75% of predicted? If so, correlate with obstruction ($FEV_1\%$).
4. If no obstruction, look for clinical correlation for reduced MVV. Consider testing maximal respiratory pressures, compliance.

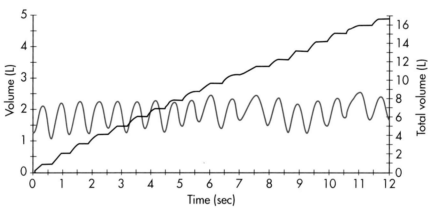

FIGURE 2-16 Maximum Voluntary Ventilation (MVV). A composite MVV spirogram on which breath-by-breath volume change and accumulated volume are plotted against time. The undulating line shows the tidal volume (approximately 1 L in this test) moved during each breath over a 12-second interval. The stair-step tracing depicts the accumulated (total) volume, in liters, exhaled during the 12-second maneuver. In this example, the volume is approximately 17 L, as read from the scale on the right. To calculate MVV, the volumes of individual breaths can be added and multiplied by a factor of 5 (i.e., 60 seconds/12 seconds = 5). Alternatively, the accumulated volume can be multiplied by 5. Because the MVV is reported in liters per minute, values for 12 seconds must be extrapolated to 1 minute. Healthy patients can maintain the same MVV flow throughout the maneuver. Patients who have pulmonary disease will show decreased absolute values. The MVV may decrease significantly as the maneuver progresses because of respiratory muscle fatigue, increased work of breathing, or air trapping.

wall, and ventilatory control mechanisms. Values in healthy young men average between 150 and 200 L/min. Values are slightly lower in healthy women. MVV decreases with age in both men and women and varies considerably in healthy patients. Only large reductions in MVV (25% or more) are considered significant.

MVV is decreased in patients with moderate or severe obstructive disease. This may be the result of the increased airway resistance caused by bronchospasm or mucus secretion. Reduction of MVV may also occur because of airway collapse and hyperinflation, as in emphysema. The MVV maneuver exaggerates air trapping and airflow limitation. Volume-time MVV tracings may show a shift if gas trapping occurs during the test. A slight shift is usually noted during the first few breaths even in healthy patients. The patient adjusts to a lung volume that allows maximal airflow. These first few breaths are usually excluded from the MVV calculation.

The MVV maneuver also places a load on the respiratory muscles. Both inspiratory and expiratory muscles are used in the MVV maneuver. Weakness or decreased endurance of either system may result in low MVV values. Poor coordination of the respiratory muscles caused by a neurologic deficit may also cause a low MVV. Disorders such as paralysis or nerve damage reduce MVV as well.

A markedly reduced MVV correlates with postoperative risk for patients having abdominal or thoracic surgery. Patients who have low preoperative MVV values show an increased incidence of complications. Reduced strength or endurance of the respiratory muscles may be the factor that allows MVV to predict postoperative problems.

The MVV value may be helpful in estimating ventilation during exercise. Note, however, that the MVV maneuver does not mimic the true respiratory pattern during maximal exercise, and thus is only an estimate of maximal breathing capacity during exercise (see Chapter 7). Airway-obstructed patients who have an MVV less than 50 L/min often have a ventilatory limitation to exercise. Maximal exercise ventilation in healthy patients is usually less than 70% of their MVV. In airway-obstructed patients, maximal ventilation during

exercise approaches or even exceeds their MVV. This pattern occurs partly because the MVV itself is reduced in obstruction. Highly conditioned healthy patients may also reach their MVV during maximal exercise (see Chapter 7).

MVV may be normal in patients who have restrictive pulmonary disease. Diseases that limit lung or chest wall expansion may not interfere significantly with airflow. Patients who have restrictive disease can compensate by performing the MVV maneuver with low V_T and high breathing rates.

The MVV maneuver depends on patient effort and cooperation. Low MVV values may indicate obstruction, muscular weakness, defective ventilatory control, or poor patient performance. Patient effort during the MVV maneuver may be estimated by multiplying their FEV_1 by 40. For example, a patient with an FEV_1 of 2.0 L might be expected to ventilate approximately 80 L/min (40×2.0 L) during the MVV test. If the measured MVV is less than 80% of ($FEV_1 \times 40$), poor patient effort or neuromuscular weakness may be suspected. If the MVV exceeds ($FEV_1 \times 40$) by a large volume, the FEV_1 may be erroneous.

BEFORE- AND AFTER-BRONCHODILATOR STUDIES

Description

Spirometry can be performed before and after bronchodilator administration to determine the reversibility of airway obstruction. An $FEV_1\%$ less than predicted is a good indication for bronchodilator studies. Patients whose FEV_1 and VC are within normal limits may have a low $FEV_{1\%}$. This happens when the VC is greater than 100% of predicted while the FEV_1 is slightly reduced. Even if the FEV_1 and $FEV_{1\%}$ are normal, one may still test for a bronchodilator response in patients for whom there is a high clinical suspicion of airflow obstruction because the normal range is defined for a population, not for any one individual. In addition, airflow obstruction may not be reflected in the FEV_1 and $FEV_{1\%}$. Although any pulmonary function parameter may be measured before and after bronchodilator therapy, FEV_1 and specific airway conductance (sGaw) are usually evaluated.

Technique

The patient may take an array of tests, including spirometry, lung volumes, and diffusing capacity (DLCO). Lung volumes should be recorded before bronchodilator administration. This provides a baseline for comparing lung volume changes after bronchodilator therapy. Even though indices of flow (FEV_1, $FEF_{25\%-75\%}$, and sGaw) usually show the greatest change, lung volumes and DLCO may also respond to bronchodilator therapy.

Patients referred for spirometry testing should withhold routine bronchodilator therapy before the procedure (Table 2-2). Some patients may be unable to manage their symptoms if bronchodilators are withheld. These patients should be instructed to take their bronchodilator medication as needed. In these instances, the time when the medication was last taken should be noted. Some patients who use bronchodilators shortly before testing (within 4 hours) still show significant improvement after a repeated dose.

Inhaled bronchodilators can be administered by a metered-dose inhaler (MDI) or a small-volume nebulizer. An MDI provides a reproducible means of administering the bronchodilator. Some patients are unable to coordinate activation of the MDI with slow, deep inspiration. For these patients, use of an aerosol reservoir, or spacer, may provide a more consistent delivery of medication. If the patient is unfamiliar with the MDI, the technologist may need to activate the device (Spirometry 2-11). Small-volume, jet-powered nebulizers may be used to administer more bronchodilator over a longer interval. Nebulizers, if reused, must be carefully disinfected between patients.

β_2-Adrenergic aerosols, such as albuterol, are most commonly used. Each of these drugs has a rapid onset of action, usually within 5 minutes. Maximum bronchodilatation usually takes longer. An interval of 10-15 minutes between administration and repeat testing is recommended for short-acting β-agonists, and an interval of 30 minutes for ipratropium bromide.

The ATS/ERS guidelines recommend a relatively high dose of bronchodilator be used to ensure that a bronchodilator response will be seen if it exists. Thus the recommended dose of albuterol is 400 mcg delivered as 4 inhalations of 100 mcg each by MDI, separated by 30-second intervals. For ipratropium bromide, the recommended dose is 160 mcg delivered as 4 inhalations of 40 mcg each by MDI.

TABLE 2-2

Withholding Medications

Medication	Time to Withhold*
Short-acting β-agonists	4 hours
Short-acting anticholinergic	4 hours
Long-acting β-agonists	12 hours
Long-acting anticholinergic	24 hours
Methylxanthines (theophyllines)	12 hours
Slow-release methylxanthines	24 hours
Cromolyn sodium	8-12 hours
Leukotriene modifiers	24 hours
Inhaled steroids	Maintain dosage

Modified from Miller MR, Hankinson J, Brusasco et al; ATS/ERS Task Force: Standardisation of spirometry, *Eur Respir J* 2005; 26:319-338.
*Approximate times; may be adjusted for individual patients.

SPIROMETRY 2-11

USING AN MDI

- Shake the MDI; activate once to prime and check contents. If empty, replace.
- Hold the MDI mouthpiece slightly away from the patient's open mouth; or, if a spacer is used, place the spacer mouthpiece between the lips, per manufacturer's instructions.
- As the patient inspires slowly from the resting expiratory level, activate the MDI.
- Have the patient continue slowly inhaling to maximal inspiration.
- Have patient hold the breath for 5-10 seconds, followed by a slow exhalation.
- Repeat inhalations as indicated (see text). Inhalations can be repeated at 30-second intervals.

Bronchodilator administration often causes side effects. The most common side effect of β-agonist use is tachycardia. Increased blood pressure, flushing, dizziness, or lightheadedness is not unusual. Monitoring pulse rate and blood pressure is recommended for susceptible patients. This includes patients with known cardiac arrhythmias or elevated blood pressure. Marked changes in heart rate, rhythm, or blood pressure, or symptoms such as chest pain indicate a need to stabilize the patient. The referring physician or laboratory medical director should be notified immediately. Management of the patient's symptoms and continuation of testing are the decision of the physician.

Measurements of FEV_1, FVC, $FEF_{25\%-75\%}$, PEF, and sGaw are commonly made before and after bronchodilator administration. In each case, the percentage of change is calculated as follows:

$$\% \, \text{Change} = \frac{\text{Postdrug} - \text{Predrug}}{\text{Predrug}} \times 100$$

where:
Postdrug = test parameter after administration
Predrug = test parameter before administration

If the test value improves, the percentage of change will be positive. If the parameter worsens, a negative percentage results. Small prebronchodilator values (e.g., an FEV_1 of 0.5 L) may show large changes even though the improvement is minimal.

FEV_1 is the most commonly used test for quantifying bronchodilator response. If $FEF_{25\%-75\%}$ or flows such as $Vmax_{50}$ are used, they should be isovolume-corrected for changes in the FVC. If FVC increases more than FEV_1 after bronchodilator therapy, $FEV_{1\%}$ may actually decrease. $FEV_{1\%}$ should not be used to judge bronchodilator response. sGaw may show a marked increase after bronchodilator therapy. Improved conductance may occur despite minimal change in FEV_1 or conventional measures of flow. Spirometry or plethysmography after bronchodilator therapy should meet the usual criteria for acceptability and reproducibility.

SPIROMETRY 2-12

INTERPRETIVE STRATEGIES
Bronchodilator Studies

1. Are the prebronchodilator and postbronchodilator measurements acceptable? Reproducible within 150 ml? If not, postbronchodilator changes may be erroneous.
2. Is there a 12% or greater improvement in FEV_1 or FVC? Is there also a 200-ml increase? If so, there is a significant improvement.
3. Is there an increase in sGaw (if done) greater than 30%–40%? If so, there is a significant improvement.
4. No significant improvement observed? Trial of bronchodilator therapy still may be recommended, if clinically indicated.

PF TIP

Patients who have a normal FEV_1/FVC ratio may be candidates for a bronchodilator study, even if they have taken their own medication within 4 hours. Many patients with a history of asthma or COPD may show a significant improvement if they have been using their MDI incorrectly (see Spirometry 2-11). Alternatively, some patients may have a bronchodilator response even with a normal baseline FEV_1 or FEV_1/FVC ratio.

Significance and Pathophysiology

See Spirometry 2-12 for interpretive strategies. Reversibility of airway obstruction is considered significant for increases of greater than 12% *and* 200 ml for either the FEV_1 or FVC (Table 2-3). If the sGaw is assessed, an increase of 30%–40% is usually considered significant. Some patients may show little or no improvement in FEV_1 but have a significant improvement in sGaw. Changes in $FEF_{25\%-75\%}$ of 20%–30% are sometimes considered significant. However, flows that depend on the FVC should be volume-corrected (see Case 2-2). If not corrected, $FEF_{25\%-75\%}$ may appear to decrease although FEV_1

TABLE 2-3			
Illustration of Bronchodilator Response			
Test	Prebronchodilator	Postbronchodilator	Absolute (%) Change
FVC (L)	2.80	3.25	+ 0.45 (16)
FEV$_1$ (L)	1.82	2.07	+ 0.25 (14)

and FVC improve. Likewise, the FEF$_{25\%-75\%}$ may appear to increase even though there is no change in FEV$_1$. This tends to occur when the postbronchodilator FVC falls from the baseline value, often because of suboptimal technique or effort.

Diseases involving the bronchial (and bronchiolar) smooth muscle usually improve most from "before" to "after." Increases greater than 50% in the FEV$_1$ may occur in patients with asthma. Patients with chronic obstructive diseases may show little improvement in flows. Poor bronchodilator response may be related to inadequate deposition of the inhaled drug because of poor inspiratory effort. Failure to show a significant improvement after inhaled bronchodilator therapy does not exclude a response. This is especially true if only the FEV$_1$ is being monitored. Changes in lung volumes, in particular, may occur without substantial change in FEV$_1$, but this may not be evident during spirometry. Such changes may still result in significant symptomatic improvement. Some patients have a significant response to one drug but little or no response to another. Efficacy of a specific drug may require repeat testing after a trial on the medication. Long-acting bronchodilators or inhaled corticosteroids may significantly improve a patient's lung function, even if there is no acute response to an inhaled β-agonist.

Some patients show a paradoxical response to bronchodilator therapy. In these individuals, flows may actually decrease after the bronchodilator therapy. Decreased flows after bronchodilator therapy may also be related to fatigue from multiple FVC efforts. Changes of less than 8% or 150 ml are within the variability of measurement of FEV$_1$. Such small changes may occur just with testing and are unlikely to be significant.

MAXIMAL INSPIRATORY PRESSURE AND MAXIMAL EXPIRATORY PRESSURE

Description

Forced maneuvers during spirometry require the patient to give a maximal effort, as well as to have normal muscle function. Muscle function is best assessed by measurement of maximal inspiratory and expiratory pressures. **Maximal inspiratory pressure (MIP)** is the lowest pressure developed during a forceful inspiration against an occluded airway. It is usually measured at maximal expiration (near RV). It is recorded as a negative number in either cm H$_2$O or mm Hg. **Maximal expiratory pressure (MEP)** is the highest pressure that can be developed during a forceful expiratory effort against an occluded airway. It is usually measured at maximal inspiration (near TLC) and reported as a positive number in either cm H$_2$O or mm Hg. MIP and MEP are sometimes measured at the resting end-expiratory level (FRC). If so, this volume must be specified.

Technique

The patient is connected to a valve or shutter apparatus, with a flanged mouthpiece and nose clip in place. The mouthpiece can be placed in the mouth with teeth resting on bite blocks, or the lips pressed against the mouthpiece opening, as would be done with a bugle. With either technique, there should be a tight fit so that the patient can exert maximal pressure. The airway is occluded by blocking a port in the valve or by closing a shutter. In either system, a small, fixed leak is introduced between the occlusion and the patient's mouth. The leak can be created using a large-bore needle or similar small opening (~2 mm inner diameter and 20–30 mm in length). The leak eliminates pressures generated by the cheek muscles during the MEP maneuver by allowing a small amount of gas to enter the oral cavity. Likewise, the leak prevents glottic closure during the MIP maneuver. The incorporation of this small leak does not significantly change lung volume or the pressure measurement.

Pressure may be measured using a manometer, an aneroid-type gauge, or a pressure transducer. The pressure-monitoring device should be linear over its range. It should be able to record pressures from −200 to approximately +200 cm H_2O. If a pressure transducer is used, its signal can be directed to a recorder or computer display. If a manometer or aneroid gauge is used, the technologist observes the pressure and records it. Devices that use a "trip" indicator can be misleading. The highest pressure recorded may be a transient pressure that occurs at the very beginning of the maneuver (Figure 2-17). The technologist should record the plateau pressure that the patient can maintain for 1–3 seconds.

For the MIP test, the patient is instructed to expire maximally. Monitoring expiratory flow or having the patient signal helps determine when maximal expiration has been achieved. Then the airway is occluded as described. The patient inspires maximally and maintains the inspiration for 1–3 seconds. The first portion of each maneuver is disregarded because it may include transient pressure changes that occur initially (see Figure 2-17). The most negative value from at least three efforts that vary less than 20% is recorded.

MEP is recorded similarly. The patient inhales as much as possible, then exhales maximally against the occluded airway for 1–3 seconds. Longer efforts should be avoided. Cardiac output can be reduced by the high thoracic pressures (e.g., Valsalva maneuvers) that are sometimes developed. MEP is usually larger than MIP in healthy patients. The pressure-monitoring device should be able to withstand the higher pressure without damage. The best of at least three MEP efforts is reported. As for MIP, initial pressure transients during the MEP are disregarded. Both MIP and MEP require patient cooperation and effort (Spirometry 2-13). Low values may reflect lack of understanding or insufficient effort.

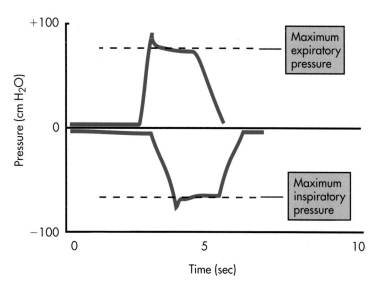

FIGURE 2-17 **Maximal Inspiratory Pressure (MIP) and Maximal Expiratory Pressure (MEP).** These tracings plot the respective pressures recorded in cm H_2O against time on a single graph. Maximal inspiratory pressure shows a downward or negative deflection. Maximal expiratory pressure shows a positive or upward deflection. Each maneuver is conducted with the airway occluded (see text). The occlusion is maintained for a short interval (1–3 seconds), and any initial transient tracings are discarded.

Significance and Pathophysiology

MIP primarily measures inspiratory muscle strength. Healthy adults can generate inspiratory pressures greater than −50 cm H_2O in women, and −75 cm H_2O in men. Decreased MIP is seen in patients with neuromuscular disease or diseases involving the diaphragm, intercostals, or accessory muscles. MIP may also be decreased in patients with hyperinflation, as in emphysema. The diaphragm is flattened by the increased volume of trapped gas in the lungs. The intercostals and accessory muscles may also be compromised by injury to or diseases of the chest wall. Patients with chest wall or spinal deformities (e.g., kyphoscoliosis) may also have reduced inspiratory pressures. MIP is sometimes used to assess patient response to strength training of respiratory muscles. MIP is often used in the assessment of respiratory muscle function in patients who need ventilatory support.

MEP measures the pressure generated during maximal expiration. It depends on the function of the abdominal muscles and accessory muscles of respiration and the elastic recoil of the lungs and thorax. Healthy adults can generate MEP values greater than 80 cm H_2O in women, and greater than 100 cm H_2O in men. MEP may be decreased in neuromuscular disorders, particularly those resulting in generalized muscle weakness. Another common disorder that results in reduction of MEP is high cervical spine fracture. Damage to nerves control-

ling abdominal and accessory muscles of expiration can dramatically reduce MEP. However, MIP may be preserved in these patients.

Reduced MEP often accompanies increased RV, as seen in emphysema. A low MEP is associated with inability to cough effectively. Inability to generate an adequate cough may complicate chronic bronchitis, cystic fibrosis, or other diseases that result in excessive mucus secretion.

Accurate measurement of MIP and MEP depends largely on patient effort. The technologist should carefully instruct the patient how to do the maneuver. Low values may result if the patient fails to inhale or exhale completely before the airway is occluded. At least three maximal efforts should be recorded. Some patients may show increased MIP or MEP with repeated efforts (training effect). Others may demonstrate decreasing pressures with repeated efforts (muscle fatigue). The best efforts should be reproducible within 20% or 10 cm H_2O, whichever is greater. Widely varying pressures for either MIP or MEP should be assessed carefully before interpretation.

AIRWAY RESISTANCE AND CONDUCTANCE

Description

The forces governing maximal airflow are the elastic recoil pressure of the lung and airway resistance upstream from the equal pressure point. This section addresses measurement of airway resistance.

Airway resistance (Raw) is the pressure difference per unit flow as gas flows into or out of the lungs. Raw is the difference between mouth pressure and alveolar pressure, divided by flow at the mouth. This pressure difference is caused primarily by the friction of gas molecules in contact with the airways. Raw is recorded in centimeters of water per liter per second (cm H_2O/L/sec).

Airway conductance (Gaw) is the flow generated per unit of pressure drop across the airways. It is the reciprocal of Raw (1/Raw) and is recorded in liters per second per centimeter of water (L/sec/cm

H$_2$O). Gaw is not commonly reported because it changes with lung volume. Instead, specific airway conductance (sGaw), which is Gaw divided by the lung volume (in liters) at which the measurement was made, is usually reported. It is reported in liters per second per centimeter of water per liter of lung volume (L/sec/cm H$_2$O/L).

Technique

Raw can be measured as the ratio of alveolar pressure (P$_A$) to airflow (V̇). Gas flow at the mouth is measured with a pneumotachometer (see Chapter 10). P$_A$ is measured in the body plethysmograph (Figure 2-18, A). For gas to flow into the lungs during inspiration, P$_A$ must fall below atmospheric pressure (mouth pressure). During expiration, P$_A$ rises above atmospheric pressure. Changes in V̇ are plotted against plethysmograph pressure changes. Changes in plethysmograph pressure are proportional to alveolar volume changes. The patient pants with a small V$_T$ at a rate of about 1.5–2.5 breaths/sec (1.5–2.5 Hz). Shallow, rapid breathing produces an S-shaped pressure-flow curve (see Figure 2-18, B). A tangent (the slope) is measured from this curve. The tangent passes through zero flow and connects the +0.5 L/sec and –0.5 L/sec flow points. The slope of this line is the ratio of V̇/ P$_{BOX}$.

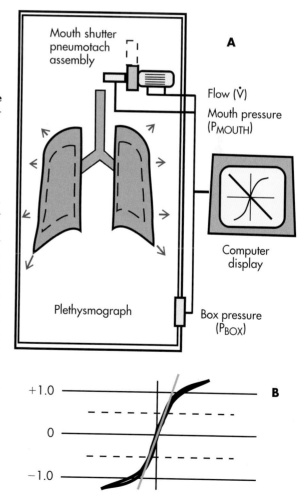

FIGURE 2-18 Measurement of Airway Resistance (Raw) Using the Body Plethysmograph. A, Diagrammatic representation of airway resistance measurement:

$$Raw = \frac{\text{Atmospheric pressure} - \text{alveolar pressure}}{\text{Flow}}$$

Flow (V̇) is measured directly by means of the pneumotachometer. As the patient pants with the shutter open, flow is plotted against box pressure (V̇/P$_{BOX}$) as an S-shaped curve on the computer display. A shutter occludes the airway momentarily, usually at end-expiration, and a sloping line representing the ratio of mouth pressure to box pressure (P$_{MOUTH}$/P$_{BOX}$) is recorded in a manner similar to that used for measurement of V$_{TG}$ (see Chapter 3). In this example, the flow tracing (shutter open) and volume tracing (shutter closed) are superimposed on the computer display. The P$_{MOUTH}$/P$_{BOX}$ tangent is measured as for the V$_{TG}$. **B,** The flow tangent is measured from the steep portion of the flow tracing, from –0.5 to +0.5 L/sec. Airway resistance is then calculated as the ratio of these two tangents using appropriate calibration factors (see text and Appendix F).

$\dot{V}$ is flow at the mouth, and P_{BOX} is plethysmograph pressure.

Problems with the open-shutter panting technique are illustrated by the loops seen in Figure 2-19. The most common problems are thermal drift, or panting at too high or low a frequency or volume.

Immediately after the open-shutter panting measurement, a shutter at the mouthpiece is closed, and the patient continues panting. The optimal rate for closed-shutter panting is about 1 Hz, slightly slower than open-shutter panting. Changes in P_{BOX} are then plotted against airway pressure at the mouth (P_{MOUTH}). Because there is no flow into or out of the lungs, P_{MOUTH} equals P_A. A second tangent is measured from this curve. The slope of this line is P_A/P_{BOX}, where P_A equals alveolar pressure. Computerized plethysmographs usually calculate a "best fit" line to measure the open-shutter and closed-shutter tangents. The technologist should visually inspect all computer-fitted lines. The system should allow the technologist to adjust computer-generated tangents manually. Problems with the closed-shutter panting technique are similar to those that plague the open-shutter panting measurement, and also include leak around the mouth or nose.

Raw is then calculated by taking the ratio of these two slopes, as follows:

$$Raw = \frac{P_A/P_{BOX}}{\dot{V}/P_{BOX}} \times \frac{Mouth\ cal}{Flow\ cal}$$

where:

$\dot{V}$	=	airflow
P_A	=	alveolar pressure
P_{BOX}	=	plethysmographic pressure, measured with the shutter open and closed
Mouth cal	=	calibration factor for the mouth pressure transducer
Flow cal	=	calibration factor for the pneumotachometer

This formula shows how Raw is calculated from the ratio of PA and $\dot{V}$, as P_{BOX} cancels out. Calibration factors for the flow and mouth pressure transducers are included in the previous equation. (See sample calculations in Appendix F.)

Panting eliminates a number of artifacts from the tracing. Small, rapid breaths (1.5-2.5 per second) reduce thermal drift, both in the box and in the pneumotachometer. Panting helps keep the glottis open, allowing measurement of alveolar pressure. Panting also allows measurements to be made near FRC. The resistances of the mouthpiece and pneumotachometer are subtracted from the patient's Raw.

Airway conductance (Gaw) can be calculated as the reciprocal of Raw. Specific conductance is calculated by dividing Gaw by the lung volume at which it was measured. Lung volume is measured at the same time, using the plethysmographic method (see Chapter 3). sGaw should be calculated separately for each maneuver because the lung volume at which measurements are made influences Raw and Gaw. After three to five acceptable trials are obtained, calculated Raw and sGaw are averaged. Individual values should be within approximately 10% of the mean (Spirometry 2-14).

Computerized plethysmographs permit thoracic gas volume (V_{TG}), Raw, and sGaw to be measured from a combined maneuver. The patient breathes through the pneumotachometer with the plethysmograph sealed. Tidal breathing is recorded with the patient breathing near FRC. The computer stores this end-expiratory volume as a reference

---

SPIROMETRY 2-14

CRITERIA FOR ACCEPTABILITY

Raw and sGaw

1. Pressure-flow loops should be closed; pressure and flow should be within the calibrated range of the respective transducers.
2. Thermal equilibrium should be established; no drift during recording.
3. Panting frequency should be 1.0-1.5 Hz for each maneuver.
4. Raw and sGaw should be calculated for each maneuver; do not average tangents.
5. Mean of three or more acceptable efforts should be reported; individual values should be within 10% of mean.

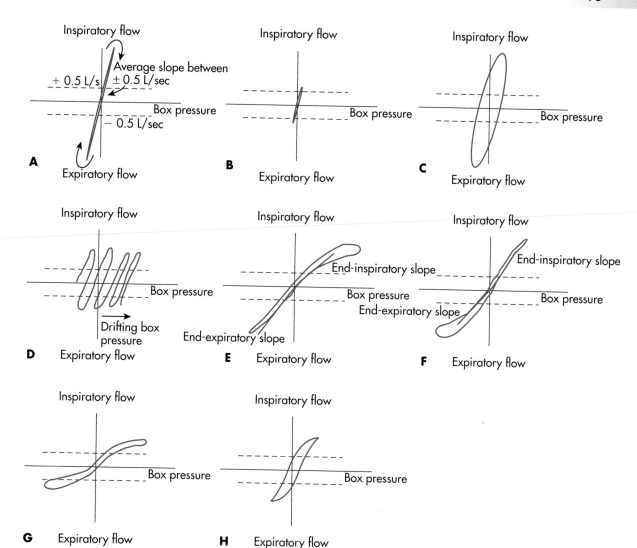

FIGURE 2-19   **Normal and Abnormal Open Shutter Tracings. A,** Normal tracing, showing narrow loop and consistent slope on both inspiration and expiration. **B,** Small, narrow loop due to panting frequency that is too high or panting volume that is too small. **C,** Wide, large loop (hysteresis) due to panting frequency that is too low or panting volume that is too large. **D,** Thermal drift, due to failure of body plethysmograph to come to a steady temperature prior to obtaining panting loops. **E,** High inspiratory resistance, causing hysteresis and flattening of inspiratory portion of panting loop. Notice that separate inspiratory and expiratory tangents (slopes) can be obtained. **F,** High expiratory resistance, causing hysteresis and flattening of expiratory portion of panting loop. **G,** High inspiratory and expiratory resistance due to fixed airway obstruction, causing flattening of both inspiratory and expiratory portions of panting loops. **H,** Typical loop seen in asthma, with slight widening and flattening of loop, indicative of overall increased resistance.

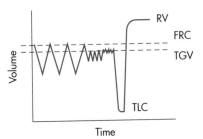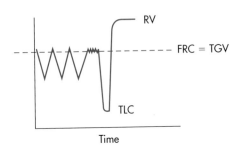

FIGURE 2-20 **Difference in TGV and FRC Measured in a Combined Maneuver.** On the left, a combined open-followed by closed-shutter maneuver was performed to obtain both Raw and TGV. Inhalation is down and exhalation is up. Because TGV drifted above FRC (downward in the tracing) during the open-panting maneuver, TGV is higher than FRC. TGV in this case is still necessary to calculate sGaw, but it is a poor approximation of FRC. On the right, only a closed-shutter maneuver was performed to measure TGV, which closely approximates FRC. In this case, a separate open-shutter maneuver is needed to measure Raw, followed by closed-shutter maneuver to calculate sGaw. FRC, functional residual capacity; RV, residual volume; TGV, thoracic gas volume; TLC, total lung capacity.

point. Then the patient pants, and the open-shutter slope of $\dot{V}/P_{BOX}$ is recorded. The mouth shutter is then closed and P_{MOUTH}/P_{BOX} is recorded as described previously. The V_{TG} in this maneuver does not equal the FRC because the shutter is closed at a volume different from the FRC. However, the change in volume from the tidal breathing level was stored at the beginning of the maneuver. This volume can be added to or subtracted from the V_{TG} to determine FRC. Most patients pant above their FRC, so the V_{TG} in this combined method is usually slightly greater (Figure 2-20). Because of this issue, a separate test to measure FRC for use in calculating absolute lung volumes may need to be done.

Raw and Gaw may be expressed per liter of lung volume as specific airway resistance and specific airway conductance (sRaw and sGaw, respectively). Expressing Raw and Gaw in this way allows comparisons to be made between patients with different lung volumes or in the same patient when lung volume changes.

Significance and Pathophysiology

See Spirometry 2-15 for interpretive strategies. Normal values of Raw in adults range from 0.6 to 2.4 cm H_2O/L/sec. Gaw in healthy adults is between 0.42 and 1.67 L/sec/cm H_2O. sGaw varies in a manner similar to Gaw. sGaw values less than 0.15

to 0.20 L/sec/cm H_2O/L are consistent with airway obstruction. Measurements are standardized at flow rates of ±0.5 L/sec, as described previously.

Raw in healthy adults is divided across the airway as follows:

Nose, mouth, upper airway = 50%
Trachea and bronchi   = 30%
Small airways   = 20%.

Small airways (less than 2 mm in diameter) contribute only approximately one fifth of the total resistance to flow. Significant obstruction can develop in the small airways with little increase in Raw or decrease in sGaw. Early or mild obstructive processes are not usually identified by abnormal Raw or sGaw. Raw may be increased in an acute asthmatic episode by as much as three times the normal values. Inflammation, mucus secretion, and bronchospasm all increase Raw in the small and medium airways. Raw is increased in advanced emphysema because of airway narrowing and collapse, especially in the bronchioles. Other obstructive diseases (e.g., bronchitis) may cause increases in Raw proportionate to the degree of obstruction in medium and small airways.

PF TIP

sGaw measurements are easy to evaluate in adult patients. Healthy subjects have an sGaw of 0.15 L/sec/cm H$_2$O/L or greater. Values much lower than 0.15 L/sec/cm H$_2$O/L are usually associated with increased airway resistance and are commonly found in patients who have obstructive lung disease.

Lesions obstructing the larger airways (e.g., tumors, traumatic injuries, or foreign bodies) may also cause a significant increase in Raw. Large airway obstruction is often accompanied by increased work of breathing and dyspnea on exertion. Airflow in the trachea and mainstem bronchi is predominately turbulent. Any large airway obstruction can exaggerate this turbulent flow. For this reason, Raw and sGaw may be more sensitive to elevations in central airway resistance than FEV$_1$. Breathing low-density gas mixtures (e.g., helium + oxygen) reduces Raw and hence the work of breathing. The shapes of the open panting loops may give clues as to the underlying pathophysiology, as seen in Figure 2-19.

Raw is decreased at increased lung volume. The airways (particularly large and medium airways) are distended slightly, and their cross-sectional area increases. For this reason, the V$_{TG}$ is always obtained with Raw measurements. Raw and Gaw are often expressed per liter of lung volume. This allows comparison of values in different patients or in the same patient after treatment. sGaw is particularly useful for assessing changes in airway caliber after bronchodilator therapy or inhalation challenge. sGaw may change significantly after bronchodilator or inhalation challenge, even though other measures of flow (i.e., FEV$_1$) vary only slightly. The primary site of airway obstruction (i.e., large versus small airways) may determine which parameters reflect changes in airway caliber.

Raw and sGaw measurements are not influenced by the degree of patient effort. Raw and sGaw measurements may be useful for determining airway status in patients who are unable or unwilling to exert maximum effort. Acceptable panting maneuvers in the plethysmograph require a certain degree of patient coordination. Not all patients may be able to perform these maneuvers. Patients with severe obstruction may produce pressure-flow curves during panting that are difficult to measure. Such curves may be flat (see Figure 2-19) or show widening (hysteresis). Inspiratory and expiratory flows may produce different resistances, causing the curve to appear as a loop (see Figure 2-19). In these cases, inspiratory flow resistance is usually reported.

In addition to resistance caused by flow through conducting airways, some frictional resistance is caused by the displacement of the lungs, rib cage, and diaphragm. In healthy patients, this tissue resistance is only approximately one fifth of the total resistance, and therefore total pulmonary resistance is approximately 20% greater than the measured Raw.

In addition to measuring Raw by use of the body plethysmograph, measurement of Raw by means of the forced oscillation technique is becoming increasingly common. For further discussion, see Chapter 9.

PULMONARY COMPLIANCE

Description

The other major factor determining maximal airflow is elastic recoil, or its reciprocal, pulmonary compliance. **Pulmonary compliance (C$_L$)** is volume change per unit of pressure change for the lungs. Lung compliance is recorded in liters (or milliliters) per cm H_2O. Elastic recoil pressure of the lungs is the **transpulmonary pressure (Ptp),** or pressure across the lung from alveoli to pleural space. Ptp is reported in centimeters of water.

Technique

Determination of C_L requires measurement of Ptp, which itself requires measurement of alveolar pressure and pleural pressure. Ptp equals alveolar pressure minus pleural pressure. Alveolar pressure is estimated by mouth pressure during a brief period of no flow, because no flow between mouth and alveoli imposes equalization of pressure between the two regions. Pleural pressure is estimated by esophageal pressure. To measure esophageal pressure, the patient is asked to swallow an esophageal catheter that has a 10-cm-long balloon at its tip and is connected to a pressure transducer. The catheter is inserted through the nose, and then advanced to a position approximately 10 cm above the lower esophageal sphincter, placing it in the lower to midthorax. Proper positioning of the catheter is verified by noting negative pressure deflections on inspiration. If the catheter is advanced too far, the balloon may enter the stomach. This causes positive pressure changes with inspiration. If the balloon is positioned at the level of the heart, cardiac action may cause an unwanted artifact (Spirometry 2-16).

The pressure transducer is set at zero with a small volume (0.5 – 1.0 ml) of air in the balloon. Pressures are then recorded at different lung volumes. These pressures are plotted to produce a compliance curve (Figure 2-21). The patient inhales maximally before the test to standardize the measurements. C_L increases slightly after a full inspiration. Then the patient inhales again to TLC, and slowly and gently allows the air to be exhaled. Pressure and volume are measured during the exhalation. To approximate alveolar pressure, pressure measurements must be made at zero flow. To do this, the patient may hold his or her breath periodically with the glottis open, or, more commonly, flow may be interrupted periodically with a shutter. Flow interruption usually occurs every 1 – 2 seconds to allow 6 – 8 data points to be collected. Esophageal pressure is subtracted from mouth pressure to obtain the recoil pressure of the lungs (Ptp) at each point of shutter closure. A pneumotachometer is used to measure lung volumes (V). A curve is then fit to the pressure-volume data, usually of the form $V = A - Be^{-kPtp}$, where V is volume, A is the curve's volume asymptote, B is the volume intercept, and k is a variable known as the shape factor that describes the curve's shape. There are no standardized measures of repeatability, but at least three to five efforts should be obtained and examined for consistency.

C_L is conventionally measured from the expiratory curve developed as the patient expires slowly from TLC to FRC. Static C_L is the slope of the line defined by:

$$\frac{\Delta V \text{ (Liters)}}{\Delta Ptp \text{ (cm } H_2O)}$$

C_L is usually recorded as the slope of the pressure-volume curve from FRC to FRC + 0.5 L (see Figure 2-21). Because the deep inspiration increases compliance, measurements are usually recorded from the exhalation curve. Maximum static elastic recoil pressure (Ptp-max) is the highest Ptp recorded at maximal inspiration. Another way of describing the maximal point of the compliance curve is to calculate the coefficient of retraction (Coeff R), which equals the Ptp-max divided by TLC. The

---

SPIROMETRY 2-16

CRITERIA FOR ACCEPTABILITY

Lung Compliance

1. Catheter is positioned properly; negative deflection on inspiration; minimal cardiac artifact.
2. At least three inspiratory and expiratory maneuvers are obtained.
3. Compliance and maximal recoil values are reproducible within 10% of their mean.
4. Report the mean compliance of three or more acceptable maneuvers.

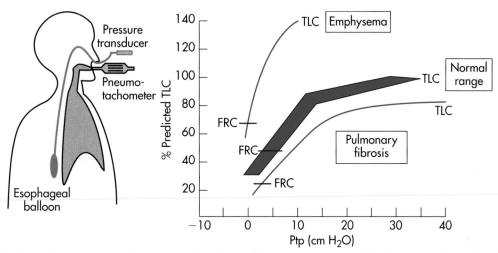

FIGURE 2-21   Measurement of Pulmonary Compliance (C_L) Using Esophageal Balloon Technique. On the left is shown a depiction of the placement of the esophageal balloon catheter to record esophageal pressure, an estimate of pleural pressure, and the pneumotach to record mouth pressure and flow, to estimate alveolar pressure (at zero flow) and lung volume, respectively. On the right is a graph of the expiratory pressure-volume curve. Ptp is plotted on the x-axis, and percentage of predicted TLC on the y-axis. The normal range is represented by the *shaded area*. Two examples of abnormal pressure-volume curves are shown. The curve up and to the left of the normal range is from a patient with emphysema, and reveals the increased compliance (reduced stiffness) of the lungs in that disease. Compliance is conventionally measured as the slope of the curve at FRC, estimated by the slope of the line from FRC to FRC + 0.5 L. Notice that the peak pressure is reduced and the TLC increased compared to the normal curve, resulting in a low coefficient of retraction. The curve down and to the right of the normal range is from a patient with pulmonary fibrosis, and reveals the reduced compliance (increased stiffness) of the lungs in that disease. Here, the coefficient of retraction is increased. FRC, functional residual capacity; Ptp, transpulmonary pressure; TLC, total lung capacity.

normal range for Coeff R = 2 – 8 cm H_2O, with lower values seen in diseases with loss of elastic recoil, such as emphysema, and higher values seen in diseases of increased elastic recoil, such as interstitial lung disease. The optimal method of presenting compliance data is to plot the entire pressure curve (inflation and deflation) versus lung volume. The C_L curve can then be plotted along with normal ranges.

Compliance is sometimes measured in patients supported by positive pressure mechanical ventilation. The ventilator inflates the lungs-thorax system with a fixed volume. By recording pressure when flow is zero (by occlusion of the exhalation valve), a compliance measurement can be obtained. Pressure may be measured from the ventilator circuit. This compliance measure differs slightly from true C_L. It measures the distensibility of the chest wall as well as the lungs. This technique may be influenced by the patient's position or by any contribu-

tion from the respiratory muscles. A more sophisticated technique uses an esophageal balloon like the laboratory method, which therefore isolates lung compliance from that of the chest wall. In each case, the volume of gas compressed in the patient's lungs is divided by the observed pressure.

Significance and Pathophysiology

See Spirometry 2-17 for interpretive strategies. C_L measures the distensibility of the lungs. The average C_L in a healthy adult is approximately 0.2 L/cm H_2O. The lungs are distended in series with the chest wall. The compliance of the thorax (C_T) is also approximately 0.2 L/cm H_2O in healthy patients. In series, the total compliance (C_{LT}) is calculated using the following equation:

$$\frac{1}{C_{LT}} = \frac{1}{C_T} + \frac{1}{C_L}$$

SPIROMETRY 2-17

INTERPRETIVE STRATEGIES

Lung Compliance

1. Were the data obtained reproducible? C_L? Pst?
2. Is C_L less than the lower limit of normal? If so, check for clinical correlation. Are lung volumes also reduced?
3. Is C_L greater than the upper limit of normal? Check for findings consistent with obstruction (e.g., $FEV_{1\%}$). Is maximal static recoil decreased?

---

or substituting the normal values:

$$\frac{1}{C_{LT}} = \frac{1}{0.2} + \frac{1}{0.2} = 10\,cm\,H_2O/L$$

or:

$$C_{LT} = 0.1\,L/cm\,H_2O$$

It should be noted that C_{LT} is less than (approximately half) C_L or C_T alone. The elastic forces act in series, counterbalancing the lung tissue and the chest wall. C_L varies with the lung volume at the end-expiratory level (i.e., FRC). To compare the C_L of diseased and normal lungs, the FRC in each case should be known. Plotting the entire C_L curve against lung volume helps relate the two factors. The volume axis is usually depicted as percentage of predicted TLC so that the influence of lung volume can also be seen.

Lung compliance is decreased in diseases such as pulmonary edema. Congestion of the pulmonary blood vessels makes the lung stiff. The same is true for diseases in which airways become filled with fluid. Such disorders include atelectasis, pneumonia, or loss of surfactant. Diseases that alter elasticity of lung tissue also lower compliance. Examples include pulmonary fibrosis resulting from silicosis, asbestosis, or sarcoidosis (see Figure 2-21). Decreased C_L may also result when lung volume is reduced as a result of space-occupying lesions such as tumors. When C_L is severely reduced from any cause, symptoms such as dyspnea on exertion are usually present. C_L increases with age, presumably because of changes in the connective tissues of the lung. This loss of elastic recoil likely accounts for the reduction in FEV_1 that occurs with aging.

Emphysema is often accompanied by an increase in C_L (see Figure 2-21). Emphysema destroys alveolar septa with loss of elastic tissue. As a result, the balance between the lungs and chest wall is upset. The chest wall tends to spring outward. The highly compliant lungs exert less pressure to cause recoil. Hyperinflation results as thoracic volume increases. Patients with severe air trapping typically have abnormal breathing patterns and markedly increased work of breathing.

Measurement of C_L requires cooperation by the patient. Some patients may be unable to swallow the esophageal balloon easily. If a mouth shutter is not used to interrupt flow, the patient must hold his or her breath with the glottis open. The C_L and elastic recoil pressure measurements are largely independent of effort, provided the patient is cooperative.

SUMMARY

- This chapter describes spirometry—the most commonly performed pulmonary function study.
- Techniques for performing the tests and criteria for acceptability are enumerated.
- Simple spirometry, F-V loops, and bronchodilator studies are discussed.
- Obstructive and restrictive disorders are differentiated by explaining the pathophysiologic conditions involved.
- Other tests of respiratory mechanics related to airflow are also discussed.
- Maximum voluntary ventilation, maximal respiratory pressures, airway resistance and conductance, and pulmonary compliance are related to diagnosis of various lung diseases.
- Interpretive strategies, in the form of questions, provide a systematic approach to understanding the implications of the test results.
- Case studies, with representative data and graphics, are included to help relate the tests to real pulmonary disorders.
- Multiple-choice self-assessment questions and selected references follow.

CASE 2-1

Case Studies

 HISTORY
L.L. is a 21-year-old male in good health who plays college football. His chief complaint is shortness of breath after wind sprints and similar vigorous exercises. L.L. denies any other symptoms, including cough or sputum production. He has never smoked. His grandfather had lung problems, but there is no other history of pulmonary disease involving the family. He states that his brothers and sisters have hay fever. There is no history of exposure to environmental pollutants.

PULMONARY FUNCTION TESTING

Personal Data

Sex:	Male
Age:	21 yr
Height:	73 in (185 cm)
Weight:	180 lb (81.6 kg)

Spirometry and Airway Resistance

	Predrug	Pred*	LNN†	% Pred	Postdrug	% Pred	% Change
FVC (L)	6.85	6.04	5.07	113	6.73	111	−2
FEV$_1$ (L)	4.65	5.03	4.18	92	5.45	108	17
FEV$_{1\%}$ (%)	68	84	74	—	81	—	—
FEF$_{25\%-75\%}$ (L/sec)	3.9	5.0	3.46	78	4.88	97	25
MVV (L/min)	218	166	—	131	215	130	−1
Raw (cm H$_2$O/L/sec)	2.1	0.6–2.4	—	—	1.6	—	−24
sGaw (L/sec/cm H$_2$O/L)	0.14	0.2	—	—	0.22	—	57

*Predicted value, based on NHANES III (Appendix B).
†Lower limit of normal, based on NHANES III (Appendix B).

TECHNOLOGIST'S COMMENTS
All FVC efforts performed acceptably. All tests meet ATS/ERS criteria. Body plethysmograph efforts were reproducible.

QUESTIONS
1. What is the interpretation of:
   - Prebronchodilator spirometry?
   - Response to bronchodilator?
   - Airway resistance and conductance?
2. What is the cause of the patient's symptoms?
3. What other tests might be indicated?
4. What treatment might be recommended based on these findings?

DISCUSSION

Interpretation

All spirometry efforts before and after bronchodilator therapy were performed acceptably. All body-box maneuvers were acceptable. Spirometry results are within normal limits except for a decrease in the FEV$_{1\%}$. There is a significant increase in the FEV$_1$ after administration of the bronchodilator. MVV is normal, as are Raw and sGaw. Raw and sGaw also show significant improvement after bronchodilator therapy.

Impression: Mild obstructive defect with significant response to bronchodilator. Evaluation for exercise-induced bronchospasm may be indicated.

Cause of Symptoms

This patient has normal or slightly above average values for most of his lung function parameters. The exception is his FEV$_{1\%}$. It is below the expected value, consistent with mild obstruction. Simply evaluating FVC and FEV$_1$ compared with predicted values might give the impression that he is normal. The FEV$_{1\%}$ indicates that the patient, whose FVC is slightly larger than normal, expired a disproportionately small FEV$_1$. This pattern of supranormal volumes with lower than normal FEV$_{1\%}$ is sometimes seen in healthy young adults. Although the FEF$_{25\%-75\%}$ also appears low, the variable and poorly reproducible nature of this number make it less reliable in diagnosing airway obstruction. Obstruction is already evident in the low FEV$_{1\%}$. There is a 17% increase (0.8 L) in FEV$_1$ after administration of a bronchodilator (Figure 2-22). This response is signifi-

continued

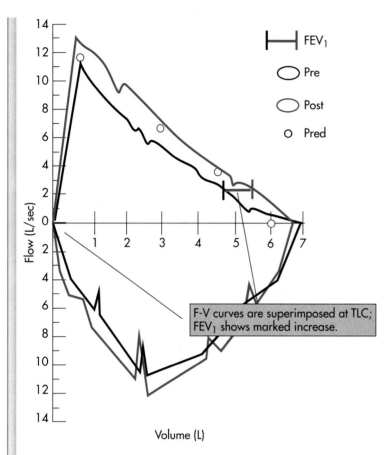

FIGURE 2-22   Flow-volume loops superimposed at total lung capacity (TLC).

F-V curves are superimposed at TLC; FEV$_1$ shows marked increase.

cant in view of the patient's complaint of shortness of breath after exercise. He appears to have reversible airway obstruction triggered by exercise.

Other Tests

Further evaluation of L.L. included an exercise test to demonstrate exercise-induced asthma (EIA). He jogged for 6 minutes on a treadmill at 85% of his predicted maximal heart rate. After he completed the exercise, L.L.'s FEV$_1$ began to decrease. Five minutes after stopping the test, his FEV$_1$ decreased to 3.81 L, a fall of 18% from the baseline value of 4.65 L. This extent of change (10%–15% or greater fall in FEV$_1$)

after exercise is diagnostic of exercise-induced bronchospasm. Scattered wheezes were heard on auscultation. The obstruction was readily reversed by inhaled bronchodilator. Inhalation-challenge testing was deferred because the obstructive defect was obvious after the exercise test.

Treatment

The patient was given a regimen of inhaled short-acting β-agonist. He was given a portable peak flow meter to monitor his lung function. He reported marked decrease in symptoms by pretreating himself with the inhaled medication 15 min before athletic activities.

CASE 2-2

Case Studies

 HISTORY

R.Z. is a 47-year-old carpenter whose chief complaint is shortness of breath on exertion. His dyspnea, although worse recently, has been present for several years. He smoked $1^1/_2$ packs of cigarettes per day for 32 years (48 pack years). He has a cough in the morning. He says that he produces a "small amount of grayish sputum." R.Z.'s father had tuberculosis. A sister had asthma as a child and now as an adult. He denies any extraordinary exposure to environmental dusts or fumes.

PULMONARY FUNCTION TESTING

Personal Data

Sex:	Male
Age:	47 yr
Height:	70 in (178 cm)
Weight:	190 lb (86.4 kg)

Spirometry and Airway Resistance

	Predrug	Pred*	LLN†	% Pred	Postdrug	% Pred	% Change
FVC (L)	4.01	5.15	4.22	78	4.49	87	12
FEV$_1$ (L)	2.05	4.03	3.26	51	2.20	55	7
FEV$_{1\%}$ (%)	51	78	69	—	49	—	−4
FEF$_{25\%-75\%}$ (L/sec)	1.2	3.69	2.03	33	1.3	35	8
V̇max$_{50}$ (L/sec)	1.35	5.54		24	2.67	30	98
V̇max$_{25}$ (L/sec)	0.55	2.58		21	1.02	40	85
MVV (L/min)	81	146		55	97	67	20
Raw (cm H$_2$O/L/sec)	3.1	0.6–2.4		—	2.9	—	−6
sGaw (L/sec/cm H$_2$O/L)	0.07	0.20		—	0.11	—	57

*Predicted value, based on NHANES III (Appendix B).
†Lower limit of normal, based on NHANES III (Appendix B).

TECHNOLOGIST'S COMMENTS

All tests met ATS/ERS criteria. All body plethysmograph efforts were performed acceptably.

QUESTIONS

1. What is the interpretation of:
   - Prebronchodilator spirometry?
   - Response to bronchodilator?
   - Airway resistance and conductance?
2. What is the cause of the patient's symptoms?
3. What other tests might be indicated?
4. What treatment might be recommended based on these findings?

DISCUSSION

Interpretation

All spirometry efforts were acceptable. All body-box efforts were reproducible. The patient has a reduced FEV$_1$, and his FVC appears only slightly decreased based on the percentage of the predicted value. How-

ever, the FVC is below the LLN, revealing a significant reduction in the FVC. FEF$_{25\%-75\%}$ is decreased, as are V̇max$_{50}$ and V̇max$_{25}$. MVV is reduced in proportion to the patient's FEV$_1$. Raw is greater than the reference value, and sGaw is below the LLN. Little or no change occurs in FEV$_1$ after inhaled bronchodilator therapy. FVC does improve significantly. sGaw is significantly better after bronchodilator.

Impression: Moderately severe airway obstruction with significant improvement in vital capacity and airway conductance after inhaled bronchodilator.

Cause of Symptoms

R.Z. is a smoker who has developed moderate airway obstruction. His spirometry results reveal the extent of the obstruction: FEV$_1$, 51% of predicted; FEF$_{25\%-75\%}$, 33% of predicted; and MVV, 55% of predicted. The FVC is also decreased, but it increases significantly after bronchodilator. The FEF$_{25\%-75\%}$ must always be interpreted cautiously because it is variable even in

continued

normal patients. The 95% confidence limits for this patient include values from 1.45 – 5.93 L/sec. (See Appendix B for predicted values and the standard error of estimate.) His $FEF_{25\%-75\%}$ is well below the lower limit. MVV is reduced as might be expected, almost exactly 40 times his FEV_1. This indicates that the patient made a consistent effort on both the FEV_1 and MVV.

Raw is above the upper normal limit of 2.4 cm H_2O/L/sec. This is consistent with moderate airway obstruction. Specific conductance is quite low, consistent with increased Raw.

FEV_1 does not improve significantly after bronchodilator therapy. The $FEV_{1\%}$ actually decreases as a result of the greater increase in FVC. This pattern is not unusual in patients with obstructive airway disease. The improvement in FVC makes obstruction with air trapping the most likely cause of his reduced FVC at baseline because a reduced FVC from other causes, such as restriction or weakness, would not be expected to improve after bronchodilator. Airway resistance falls slightly with inhaled bronchodilator therapy. Most notably, sGaw improves by 57%. The large increase in conductance with only marginal change in

flow suggests a shift in lung volumes, with a reduction in thoracic gas volume (TGV) (less hyperinflation). Figure 2-23 shows F-V curves plotted at absolute lung volumes (measured in the body-box). Improvement in flow is evident by noting the curves at any particular lung volume.

Other postbronchodilator changes are also important. MVV improves by 20%. This may be related to a change in lung volume. The $FEF_{25\%-75\%}$ is hardly changed after bronchodilator therapy. This pattern is often seen when the FVC improves. A larger FVC means the time required to exhale the middle half of the breath may be longer. Because the $FEF_{25\%-75\%}$ depends on the FVC, the calculated flow may not improve; it may even go down. Once again, this illustrates the limited utility of interpreting obstructive airway disease based on using the $FEF_{25\%-75\%}$.

Other Tests

The lung function of this patient is common in both emphysema and chronic bronchitis. Air trapping is consistent with emphysematous changes but may also be present in bronchitis and asthma. Further evaluation of R.Z. included measurement of lung volumes,

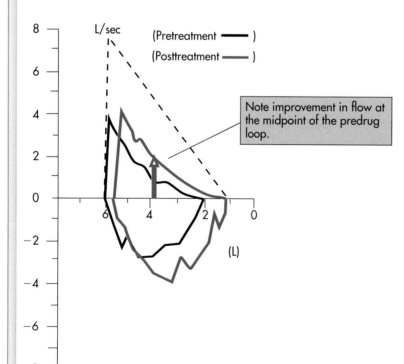

FIGURE 2-23 Isovolume flow-volume loops. Each loop is plotted at the absolute lung volume at which it was measured. The increase in $FEF_{50\%}$ accurately describes the degree of bronchodilator response. Notice that expiratory flow is increased after bronchodilator for every matched absolute lung volume.

DLCO, and blood gas analysis. The findings from each of these additional tests were consistent with the results of his spirometry. He had some air trapping (elevated RV/TLC), which would explain the improved FVC after bronchodilator therapy. Blood gases and diffusing capacity were relatively normal, the latter finding making chronic bronchitis, and not emphysema, the likely diagnosis.

Treatment

A combination of bronchodilators and inhaled steroids was prescribed. The patient was also referred to a counselor for smoking cessation and successfully quit smoking. His cough gradually subsided during a 6-month period. The patient noted a marked improvement in his dyspnea.

CASE 2-3

Case Studies

HISTORY

P.W. is a 27-year-old auto mechanic referred to the pulmonary function laboratory by his private physician. His chief complaint is "breathing problems." He describes breathlessness that occurs suddenly and then subsides. He has no other symptoms and no history of lung disease. None of his immediate family has any lung disease. He has smoked one pack of cigarettes per day for the past 10 years (10 pack years). He has no unusual environmental exposure. He claims that gasoline fumes sometimes bring on the episodes of shortness of breath.

PULMONARY FUNCTION TESTING

Personal Data

Sex: Male
Age: 27 yr
Height: 68 in (173 cm)
Weight: 150 lb (68.2 kg)

Spirometry	Before Drug	Predicted	LLN*	% Predicted
FVC (L)	3.80	5.21	4.32	73
FEV$_1$ (L)	3.70	4.30	3.55	86
FEV$_{1\%}$ (%)	97	83	73	—
FEF$_{25-75\%}$ (L/sec)	4.62	4.49	2.94	103
FEF$_{50\%}$ (L/sec)	4.81	6.01	—	80
FEF$_{75\%}$ (L/sec)	3.12	3.33	—	94
MVV (L/min)	77	146	—	53

*Lower limit of normal, based on NHANES III (Appendix B).

Respiratory Pressures	Before Drug	Predicted	% Predicted
MIP (cm H$_2$O)	118	128	92
MEP (cm H$_2$O)	57	240	24

TECHNOLOGIST'S COMMENTS

None of the FVC maneuvers were acceptable; they did not last 6 seconds or show an obvious plateau. Best FVC values were not within 150 ml. Inspiratory efforts were variable. A total of eight maneuvers were attempted. Respiratory pressure measurements were variable. The patient had difficulty completing all maneuvers.

QUESTIONS

1. What is the interpretation of:
   - Spirometry
   - Low value for MEP
   - Variability of the patient's efforts
2. What is the cause of the patient's symptoms?
3. What other tests might be indicated?
4. What treatment might be recommended based on these findings?

DISCUSSION

Interpretation

All spirometry maneuvers and respiratory pressures are unacceptable because of poor patient effort or technical errors. The patient's best effort shows a reduced FVC. The FEV$_1$ is normal, and the FEV$_{1\%}$ is above the expected range. All other flows and the MVV are within normal limits. MIP is normal, but MEP is reduced.

continued

Impression: Spirometry results are inconsistent. The FVC and FEV_1 are not reproducible. Expiratory muscle pressure is reduced. Overall, inadequate patient effort or technical errors are present.

Cause of Symptoms

This test shows poor reproducibility, especially for effort-dependent measurements. Figure 2-24 shows the variability for three FVC maneuvers. The tracings show incomplete exhalations, as well as variability.

The low FVC seems to be consistent with a mild restrictive process. The FEV_1, however, is close to normal. If simple restriction were present, both FVC and FEV_1 should be reduced similarly. The patient's other flows are normal. Flows that depend on the FVC (e.g., the $FEF_{25\%-75\%}$) might also be in error if the FVC is incorrect. The FEV_1 and MVV do not depend on the FVC. The MVV is much less than 40 times the FEV_1, so the MVV is probably not accurate.

Because of the low MVV, respiratory pressures were measured. MIP appears to be normal but was variable. MEP was also performed variably. The best effort was only 24% of expected. Both MEP and MIP depend largely on patient effort.

Examination of the volume-time spirograms reveals that the patient terminated each FVC maneuver after approximately 2 seconds. The FVC values all varied by more than 150 ml, confirming poor patient cooperation. However, lack of repeatability of the FVC maneuvers is not sufficient reason for discarding the test results. This patient's FVC maneuvers lasted only 2 seconds, despite repeated coaching by the technologist. The efforts did not meet the criteria of continuing for at least 6 seconds or showing an obvious plateau. Failure to exhale completely is one of the most common errors in spirometry. This error may be caused by lack of cooperation on the part of the patient or inability to continue exhalation due to cough. It may also occur if the technologist does not adequately explain or demonstrate the maneuver.

The technologist performing this test repeated the FVC maneuver eight times. Only the three best efforts were recorded. Appropriate comments were added at the end of the test data. The poor quality of the data makes it impossible to determine whether the patient's symptoms are real. The patient appears to be malingering; that is, not giving maximal effort on tests that are effort dependent. Poor reproducibility in a patient who is free of symptoms at the time of the test suggests poor effort or lack of cooperation.

Other Tests

Alternative tests for this patient should be independent of patient effort. A simple blood gas analysis was performed. The results indicated normal oxygenation and acid-base status. Testing of lung volumes and diffusing capacity was postponed because both of these depend on patient effort and cooperation. A *bronchial challenge* test (see Chapter 9) might have been indicated because the patient had asthma-like symptoms.

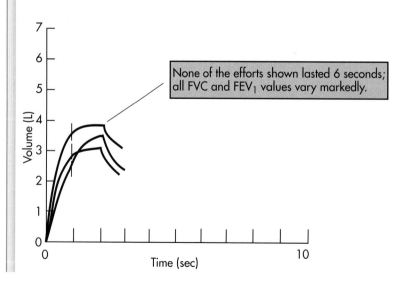

None of the efforts shown lasted 6 seconds; all FVC and FEV_1 values vary markedly.

FIGURE 2-24 Multiple forced vital capacity (FVC) maneuvers are superimposed. None of the recorded efforts are acceptable.

However, bronchial challenge tests use spirometry, which this patient was unable or unwilling to perform acceptably.

Treatment

Before suggesting any treatment, the referring physician contacted the patient's employer to ask about possible environmental hazards that might cause the symptoms. He learned that the patient was facing possible termination for excessive absence from work. The patient's supervisor revealed that the patient claimed to have asthma, which caused his excessive absenteeism.

SELF-ASSESSMENT QUESTIONS

Entry-level

1. A patient performs three FVC maneuvers using a computerized spirometer. The spirometer reports that all maneuvers had a back-extrapolated volume of less than 5% and 150 ml. The maneuvers met all other criteria for acceptability and repeatability. The technologist should:
   a. Repeat all maneuvers
   b. Correct the FEV_1 and all other flows by the amount of the back-extrapolated volume
   c. Perform at least one more maneuver
   d. Report the average of the three FVC values

2. A 58-year-old man who complains of increased shortness of breath with exercise has the following spirometry results:

	Measured	Predicted	LLN*	% Predicted
FVC (L BTPS)	5.11	4.93	4.19	104
FEV_1 (L BTPS)	2.57	3.95	3.38	65

*Lower limit of normal, based on NHANES III (Appendix B).

These results are consistent with which of the following?
   a. Normal lung function
   b. Restrictive lung disease
   c. Obstructive lung disease
   d. Incorrect predicted values

3. An 81-year-old man performs three acceptable spirometry efforts and records these results:

	Measured	Predicted	LLN*	% Predicted
FVC (L BTPS)	2.17	3.82	3.25	57
FEV_1 (L BTPS)	1.71	2.41	2.05	71

*Lower limit of normal, based on NHANES III (Appendix B).

Which of the following do these values suggest?
   a. Normal spirometry for an elderly man
   b. Obstructive lung disease
   c. Restrictive lung disease
   d. Erroneously measured FEV_1

4. Which of the following best describes the flow-volume curve shown?

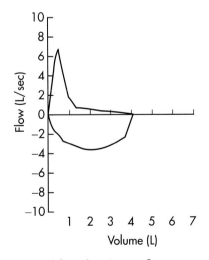

   a. Normal forced expiratory flow pattern
   b. Variable intrathoracic obstruction
   c. Variable extrathoracic obstruction
   d. Fixed large airway obstruction

continued

5. A 20-year old man complains of shortness of breath with exercise. The following results of spirometry are obtained:

	Measured	Predicted	LLN*	% Predicted	After Bronchodilator	% Change
FVC (L BTPS)	4.98	5.83	4.96	85	5.98	20
FEV$_1$ (L BTPS)	3.18	4.68	3.98	68	3.5	10

*Lower limit of normal, based on NHANES III (Appendix B).

Which of the following statements best describes these findings?
a. Normal spirometry
b. There is moderate obstruction with significant response to bronchodilators
c. There is moderate obstruction without significant response to bronchodilators
d. Results are inconsistent and must be repeated

6. A 33-year-old woman complains with increasing shortness of breath with exertion. Her spirometry results are as follows:

	Measured	Predicted	LLN*	% Predicted
FVC (L BTPS)	2.25	3.09	2.62	73
FEV$_1$ (L BTPS)	1.84	2.62	2.23	70
PEF (L/s)	2.77	6.17	5.24	45
MVV (L/min)	45	104	—	43

*Lower limit of normal, based on NHANES III (Appendix B).

Which of the following is most consistent with these results?
a. Moderate obstructive lung disease
b. Normal spirometry
c. Severe lung volume restriction
d. Muscle weakness or poor effort

7. How long should the pulmonary function technologist wait after giving inhaled β-agonist before conducting post-bronchodilator testing?
a. 5 minutes
b. 15 minutes
c. 30 minutes
d. 45 minutes

Advanced

8. A 14-year-old male with cystic fibrosis performs three spirometry trials:

	Trial 1	Trial 2	Trial 3
FVC (L BTPS)	3.01	2.99	3.12
FEV$_1$ (L BTPS)	1.99	2.01	1.95

The reported flow-volume loop should come from which data?
a. Trial 1
b. Trial 2
c. Trial 3
d. Average of all 3 trials

9. In which of the following conditions would an abnormal MIP and MEP be expected?
I. Measurements starting at FRC
II. Myasthenia gravis
III. Poor effort
IV. Kyphoscoliosis
   a. II and III only
   b. I, II, III, and IV
   c. II only
   d. I, II, III only

10. An open-shutter panting loop that is flattened at the midpoint of both inspiration and expiration is most compatible with which diagnosis?
a. Asthma
b. Emphysema
c. Tracheal stenosis
d. Pneumonia

11. A patient with pulmonary fibrosis has a compliance study performed. Which set of findings is most likely?
a. Low compliance, low coefficient of retraction, curve down and to the right
b. High compliance, high coefficient of retraction, curve down and to the right
c. High compliance, high coefficient of retraction, curve up and to the left
d. Low compliance, high coefficient of retraction, curve down and to the right

12. A patient with severe emphysema has airway resistance measured in a body plethysmograph. The Raw = 3.25 cm H_2O/L/sec and the sGaw = 0.05 cm H_2O/L/sec/L. The patient's TGV for this maneuver was which of the following?
   a. 4.25 L
   b. 5.35 L
   c. 6.15 L
   d. 6.50 L

13. A healthy, physically fit patient performs spirometry, and the following values are recorded:

	Trial 1	Trial 2	Trial 3	Trial 4
FVC (L BTPS)	6.52	6.23	6.17	6.37
FEV$_1$ (L BTPS)	5.01	5.22	5.13	5.19

   Which values of FVC, FEV$_1$, and FEV$_{1\%}$ should be reported for this patient?
   a. FVC = 6.52 L, FEV$_1$ = 5.22 L, FEV$_{1\%}$ = 80%
   b. FVC = 6.23 L, FEV$_1$ = 5.22 L, FEV$_{1\%}$ = 84%
   c. FVC = 6.52 L, FEV$_1$ = 5.01 L, FEV$_{1\%}$ = 77%
   d. FVC = 6.52 L, FEV$_1$ = 5.22 L, FEV$_{1\%}$ = 82%

14. A patient, whose chief complaints are cough and hoarseness, performs a series of FVC efforts, and flow-volume curves are recorded as shown in the following figure. Which of the following diagnoses seems most likely?
   a. Fixed airway obstruction
   b. Variable intrathoracic obstruction
   c. Variable extrathoracic obstruction
   d. The patient was malingering

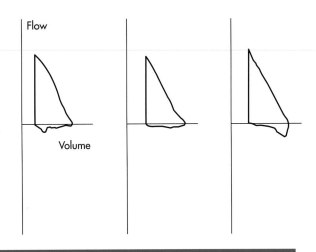

Selected Bibliography

GENERAL REFERENCES

Clausen JL: *Pulmonary function testing guidelines and controversies*, New York, 1982, Grune & Stratton.

Crapo RO: Pulmonary function testing, *N Engl J Med* 1994; 331:25-30.

Ferguson GT, Enright PL, Buist SA, et al: Office spirometry for lung health assessment in adults: a consensus statement from the National Lung Health Education Program, *Chest* 2000; 117:1146-1161.

Forster RE: *The lung: clinical physiology and pulmonary function tests*, ed 3, St Louis, 1986, Mosby.

West JB: *Pulmonary physiology and pathophysiology: an integrated, case-based approach*, Baltimore, 2001, Lippincott, Williams & Wilkins.

SPIROMETRY

Aaron SD, Dales RE, Cardinal P: How accurate is spirometry at predicting restrictive pulmonary impairment? *Chest* 1999; 115:869-873.

Balfe DL, Lewis M, Mohsenifar Z: Grading the severity of obstruction in the presence of a restrictive ventilatory defect, *Chest* 2002; 122:1365-1369.

Dillard TA, Hnatiuk OW, McCumber TR: Maximum voluntary ventilation: spirometric determinants in chronic obstructive pulmonary disease patients and normal subjects, *Am Rev Respir Dis* 1993; 147:870-875.

Eaton T, Withy S, Garrett JE et al: Spirometry in primary care practice: the importance of quality assurance and the impact of spirometry workshops, *Chest* 1999; 116:416-423.

Enright PL, Linn WS, Avol EL et al: Quality of spirometry test performance in children and adolescents: experience in a large field study, *Chest* 2000; 118:665-671.

Hansen JE, Sun X-G, Wasserman K: Should forced expiratory volume in six seconds replace forced vital capacity to detect airway obstruction? *Eur Respir J* 2006; 27:1244-1250.

Knudson RJ, Lebowitz MD: Maximal mid-expiratory flow (FEF$_{25\%-75\%}$): normal limits and assessment of sensitivity, *Am Rev Respir Dis* 1978; 117:609.

Krowka MJ, Enright PL, Rodarte JR et al: Effect of effort on measurement of forced expiratory volume in one second, *Am Rev Respir Dis* 1987; 136:829.

Leuallen EC, Fowler WS: Maximal midexpiratory flow, *Am Rev Tuberculosis* 1955; 72:783.

Litonjua, AA, Sparrow D, Weiss ST: The FEF $_{25-75}$/FVC ratio is associated with methacholine airway responsiveness. The Normative Aging Study, *Am J Respir Crit Care Med* 1999; 159:1574-1579.

Roberts SD, Farber MO, Knox KD et al: FEV1/FVC ratio of 70% misclassifies patients with obstruction at the extremes of age, *Chest* 2006; 130:200-206.

Swanney MP, Beckert LE, Frampton CM et al: Validity of American Thoracic Society and other spirometric algorithms using FVC and forced expiratory volume at 6 s for predicting a reduced total lung capacity, *Chest* 2004; 126:1861-1866.

Townsend MC, Hankinson JL, Lindesmith LA et al: Is my lung function really that good? Flow-type spirometer problems that elevate test results, *Chest* 2004; 125:1902-1909.

PEAK EXPIRATORY FLOW

Godfrey S: Monitoring asthma severity and response to treatment, *Respiration* 2001; 68:637-648.

Hankinson JL: Beyond the peak flow meter: newer technologies for determining and documenting changes in lung function in the workplace, *Occup Med* 2000; 15:411-420.

Kennedy DT: Selection of peak flowmeters in ambulatory asthma patients: a review of the literature, *Chest* 1998; 114:587-592.

Lebowitz MD: The use of peak expiratory flow rate measurements in respiratory disease, *Pediatr Pulmonol* 1991; 11:166-174.

BEFORE- AND AFTER-BRONCHODILATOR STUDIES

Brocklebank D, Ram F, Wright J et al: Comparison of the effectiveness of inhaler devices in asthma and chronic obstructive airways disease: a systematic review of the literature, *Health Technol Assess* 2001; 5:1-149.

Casaburi R, Adame D, Hong CK: Comparison of albuterol to isoproterenol as a bronchodilator for use in pulmonary function testing, *Chest* 1991; 100:1597-1600.

Dales RE, Spitzer WO, Tousignant P et al: Clinical interpretation of airway response to a bronchodilator: epidemiologic considerations, *Am Rev Respir Dis* 1988; 138:317.

Guyatt GH, Townsend M, Nogradi S et al: Acute response to bronchodilator, an imperfect guide for bronchodilator therapy in chronic airflow limitation, *Arch Intern Med* 1988; 148:1949.

Light RW, Conrad SA, George RB: The one best test for evaluating the effects of bronchodilator therapy, *Chest* 1977; 72:512.

Smith HR, Irvin CG, Cherniack RM: The utility of spirometry in the diagnosis of reversible airways obstruction, *Chest* 1992; 101:1577-1581.

FLOW-VOLUME CURVES

Acres J, Kryger M: Clinical significance of pulmonary function tests: upper airway obstruction, *Chest* 1981; 80:207.

Bass H: The flow volume loop: normal standards and abnormalities in chronic obstructive pulmonary disease, *Chest* 1973; 63:171.

Chan ED, Irvin CG: The detection of collapsible airways contributing to airflow limitation, *Chest* 1995; 107:856-859.

Haponik EF, Blecker ER, Allen RP et al: Abnormal inspiratory flow-volume curves in patients with sleep disordered breathing, *Am Rev Respir Dis* 1981; 124:571.

Hyatt RE, Black LF: The flow volume curve, *Am Rev Respir Dis* 1973; 107:191.

Knudson RJ, Lebowitz MD, Holberg CJ et al: Changes in the normal maximal expiratory flow-volume curve with growth and aging, *Am Rev Respir Dis* 1983; 127:725.

Knudson RJ, Slatin RC, Lebowitz MD et al: The maximal expiratory flow-volume curve: normal standards, variability and effects of age, *Am Rev Respir Dis* 113:587, 1976.

Lunn WW, Sheller JR: Flow volume loops in the evaluation of upper airway obstruction, *Otolaryngol Clin North Am* 1995; 28:721-729.

Miller RD, Hyatt RE: Evaluation of obstructing lesions of the trachea and larynx by flow volume loops, *Am Rev Respir Dis* 1973; 108:475.

MAXIMAL RESPIRATORY PRESSURES

Aldrick TK, Spiro P: Maximal inspiratory pressure: does reproducibility indicate full effort? *Thorax* 1995; 50:40-43.

Black LF, Hyatt RE: Maximal static respiratory pressure in generalized neuromuscular disease, *Am Rev Respir Dis* 1971; 103:641.

Karvonen J, Soarelainen S, Nieminen MM: Measurement of respiratory muscle forces based on maximal inspiratory and expiratory pressures, *Respiration* 1994; 61:28-31.

Vincken GH, Cosio MG: Maximal static respiratory pressures in adults: normal values and their relationship to determinants of respiratory function, *Bull Eur Physiopathol Respir* 1987; 23:435.

COMPLIANCE AND AIRWAY RESISTANCE

Baydur A, Behrakis PK, Zin WA, et al: A simple method for assessing the validity of the esophageal balloon technique, *Am Rev Respir Dis* 1982; 126:788.

Behrakis PK, Baydur A, Jaeger MJ et al: Lung mechanics in sitting and horizontal body positions, *Chest* 1983; 83:643.

Dubois AB, Bothello SV, Comroe JH: A new method for measuring airway resistance in man using a body plethysmograph: values in normal subjects and in patients with respiratory disease, *J Clin Invest* 1956; 35:327.

National Heart and Lung Institute, Division of Lung Diseases: *Procedures for standardized measurements of lung mechanics: principles of body plethysmography,* Bethesda, Md, 1974, National Heart and Lung Institute, pp 1-21.

Wagers SS, Bouder TG, Kaminsky DA, Irvin CG: The invaluable pressure-volume curve, *Chest* 2000; 117:578-583.

STANDARDS AND GUIDELINES

American Association for Respiratory Care: Clinical practice guidelines: assessing response to bronchodilator therapy at the point of care, *Respir Care* 1995; 40:1300-1307.

American Association for Respiratory Care: Clinical practice guidelines: body plethysmography, *Respir Care* 2001; 46:506-513.

American Association for Respiratory Care: Clinical practice guidelines: spirometry, *Respir Care* 1996; 41:629-636.

American Association for Respiratory Care: Clinical practice guidelines: static lung volumes, *Respir Care* 2001; 46:531-539.

American Thoracic Society: Lung function testing: selection of reference values and interpretative strategies, *Am Rev Respir Dis* 1991; 144:1202.

American Thoracic Society: Standardization of spirometry: 1994 update, *Am J Respir Crit Care Med* 1995; 152:1107-1136.

American Thoracic Society/European Respiratory Society: Statement on respiratory muscle testing, *Am J Respir Crit Care Med* 2002; 166:518-624.

American Thoracic Society/European Respiratory Society Task Force: Standardization of lung function testing. Number 1: general considerations for lung function testing, *Eur Respir J* 2005; 26:153-161.

American Thoracic Society/European Respiratory Society Task Force: Standardization of lung function testing. Number 2: standardization of spirometry, *Eur Respir J* 2005; 26:319-338.

American Thoracic Society/European Respiratory Society Task Force: Standardization of lung function testing. Number 5: interpretative strategies for lung function tests, *Eur Respir J* 2005; 26:948-968.

British Thoracic Society and the Association of Respiratory Technicians and Physiologists: Guidelines for the measurement of respiratory function, *Respir Med* 1994; 88:165-194.

National Asthma Education Program: *Expert panel report 2: guidelines for the diagnosis and management of asthma,* Bethesda, Md, 1979, Department of Health and Human Services (NIH Publication No. 97-4051).

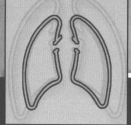

Chapter 3

Lung Volumes and Gas Distribution Tests

JACK WANGER

CHAPTER OUTLINE

Lung Volumes: Functional Residual Capacity, Residual Volume, Total Lung Capacity, and Residual Volume/Total Lung Capacity Ratio
Description
Technique
Significance and Pathophysiology

Gas Distribution Tests: Single-Breath Nitrogen Washout, Closing Volume, and Closing Capacity
Description
Technique
Significance and Pathophysiology

OBJECTIVES

After studying this chapter you will be able to:

Entry-level
1. Describe the measurement of lung volumes using gas dilution/washout methods
2. Explain two advantages of measuring lung volumes using the body plethysmograph
3. Calculate residual volume and total lung capacity from FRC and the subdivisions of VC
4. Identify a restricted disease process from measured lung volumes

Advanced
1. Calculate FRC using helium dilution and nitrogen washout methods
2. Describe the correct technique for measuring thoracic gas volume
3. Identify air trapping and hyperinflation using measured lung volumes
4. Identify uneven distribution of gas in the lungs by either single- or multiple-breath techniques

KEY TERMS

Boyle's law
closed-circuit multiple-breath helium dilution (FRC_{He})
closing capacity (CC)

dilutional lung volumes
distribution of ventilation
end-expiratory level
FRC_{pleth}

functional residual capacity (FRC)
hyperinflation
lung volume reduction surgery (LVRS)

open-circuit multiple-breath
   nitrogen washout technique
   (FRC_{N2})
residual volume (RV)

RV/TLC ratio
single-breath nitrogen washout
   test (SBN_2)
slope of phase III

"switch-in" error
total lung capacity (TLC)
thoracic gas volume (V_{TG})

This chapter introduces the measurement of absolute lung volumes beyond the inspired and expired lung volumes measured by spirometry. The gas volume remaining in the lungs after the vital capacity (VC) has been exhaled must be measured indirectly. Several methods can accomplish this. Each method has its own advantages and disadvantages. Two methods—helium (He) dilution and nitrogen (N_2) washout—involve having the patient breathe gases or gas concentrations not normally present in the lungs: He or 100% oxygen (O_2). These techniques are sometimes referred to as **dilutional lung volumes.** A third method uses the body plethysmograph to measure the volume of thoracic gas (V_{TG}). The gas dilution techniques can also provide information about the distribution of gas in the lungs. Conventional radiographs, nuclear medicine imaging of the lungs, computerized tomography (CT), and magnetic resonance imaging (MRI) all provide an estimate of lung volumes, especially in patients with limited ability to cooperate. However, submaximal lung inflation leads to underestimation of true lung volume in these imaging techniques, and comparisons with lung volume determined by physiologic methods are not recommended.

LUNG VOLUMES: FUNCTIONAL RESIDUAL CAPACITY, RESIDUAL VOLUME, TOTAL LUNG CAPACITY, AND RESIDUAL VOLUME/TOTAL LUNG CAPACITY RATIO

Description

Functional residual capacity (FRC) is the volume of gas remaining in the lungs at the end of a quiet breath. On a simple spirogram, this point is termed the **end-expiratory level** (see Figure 2-1). **Residual volume (RV)** is the volume of gas remaining in the lungs at the end of a maximal expiration regardless of the lung volume at which exhalation was started (see Figure 2-1). **Total lung capacity (TLC)** is the volume of gas contained in the lungs after maximal inspiration. FRC, TLC, and RV are reported in liters (L) or milliliters (ml), corrected to BTPS. The **RV/TLC ratio** defines the fraction of TLC that cannot be exhaled (RV), expressed as a percentage.

Thoracic gas volume (V_{TG}) is the absolute volume of gas in the thorax at any point in time and any level of alveolar pressure. V_{TG} is usually measured at the end-expiratory level and is then equal to FRC. It also may be measured at other lung volumes and corrected to relate to FRC. The V_{TG} is reported in liters or milliliters, BTPS.

Technique

There are a variety of methods for measuring absolute lung volumes (Table 3-1). FRC is measured directly with the open-circuit multiple-breath N_2 washout, closed-circuit multiple-breath He dilution, and body plethysmographic techniques. Once FRC and VC have been measured, RV and TLC can be calculated. TLC can be estimated directly with the single-breath N_2 washout, and single-breath He dilution as part of the diffusing capacity (DLCO) test, and chest radiography. RV can only be measured indirectly once FRC or TLC has been determined.

Open-Circuit Multiple-Breath Nitrogen Washout

Determination of FRC with the **open-circuit multiple-breath nitrogen washout technique (FRC_{N2})** is based on washing out the N_2 from the

TABLE 3-1		
Methods for Measurement of Lung Volumes		
Method	Lung Volume	Advantages/Disadvantages
Multiple-breath He dilution	FRC	Simple, relatively inexpensive; affected by distribution of ventilation in moderate or severe obstruction; multiple-breath; requires IC, ERV to calculate other lung volumes
Multiple-breath N_2 washout	FRC	Simple, relatively inexpensive; affected by distribution of ventilation in moderate or severe obstruction; multiple-breath; requires IC, ERV to calculate other lung volumes
Single-breath N_2 washout	TLC	Calculated from single-breath N_2 distribution test; may underestimate lung volume in the presence of obstruction
Single-breath He dilution	TLC	Calculated as part of D_{LCO} (V_A); may underestimate lung volume in the presence of obstruction
Plethysmography	V_{TG} (FRC)	Plethysmographic method somewhat complex; not affected by degree of airway obstruction
Chest radiograph	TLC	Requires posterior-anterior and lateral chest x-ray films; not accurate in the presence of diffuse, space-occupying diseases

D_{LCO}, Diffusing capacity; IC, inspiratory capacity; N_2, nitrogen; V_A, alveolar volume.

lungs while the patient breathes 100% O_2 for several minutes. At the start of the test the N_2 concentration in the lungs is approximately 75%–80%. As the patient breathes 100% O_2, the N_2 in the lungs is gradually washed out. At the end of the test the N_2 concentration in the lungs is approximately 1%. The initial N_2 concentration, amount of N_2 washed out, and final N_2 concentration are measured and can then be used to calculate the volume of air in the lungs at the start of the test (FRC) using the following formula:

$$FRC = \frac{F_E N_{2final} \times Expired\ Volume - N_{2tissue}}{F_A N_{2alveolar1} - F_A N_{2alveolar2}}$$

where:

$F_E N_{2final}$ = fraction of N_2 in volume expired
$F_A N_{2alveolar1}$ = fraction of N_2 in alveolar gas initially
$F_A N_{2alveolar2}$ = fraction of N_2 in alveolar gas at end (from an alveolar sample)
$N_{2tissue}$ = volume of N_2 washed out of blood/tissues

A correction must be made for N_2 washed out of the blood and tissue. For each minute of O_2 breathing, approximately 30–40 ml of N_2 is removed from blood and tissue. $N_{2tissue} = 0.04$ times T (where T is

time of the test). This value is subtracted from the total volume of N_2 washed out.

The original N_2 washout technique lasted 7 minutes. However, not all of the N_2 in the lungs may be washed out, even after 7 minutes of 100% O_2 breathing. The $F_A N_{2alveolar2}$ is measured at the end of the test and subtracted from the initial N_2 concentration. Correction for the **"switch-in" error** should also be made. The final FRC is then corrected to BTPS, and volume of the equipment dead space (including filters) must be subtracted (see Appendix F for a sample calculation).

To obtain RV, the ERV measured immediately after the acquisition of FRC as a "linked" maneuver (i.e., without the patient coming off the mouthpiece), is subtracted from the FRC:

$$RV = FRC - ERV$$

To obtain TLC, the calculated value for RV is added to the "linked" inspiratory vital capacity (IVC).

Some available commercial systems use a rapid N_2 analyzer in combination with a spirometer to provide a "breath-by-breath" analysis of expired N_2 (Figure 3-1, A). An alternative approach is to use fast-response O_2 and carbon dioxide (CO_2) analyz-

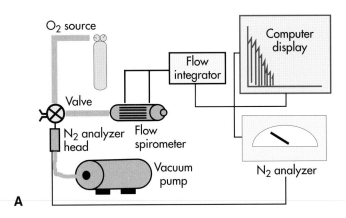

FIGURE 3-1   Open-Circuit and Closed-Circuit FRC Systems. A, Open-circuit equipment used for N_2 washout determination of FRC. The patient inspires O_2 from a regulated source and exhales past a rapidly responding N_2 analyzer into a pneumotachometer. Flow and gas concentration are integrated and displayed on a computer screen. FRC is calculated from the total volume of N_2 exhaled and the change in alveolar N_2 from the beginning to the end of the test (Figure 3-2 and Open-Circuit Method). **B,** Closed-circuit equipment used for He dilution FRC determination includes a volume-based spirometer with He analyzer, CO_2 absorber, and a directional breathing circuit. A fan or blower promotes gas mixing within the rebreathing system. A breathing valve near the mouth allows the patient to be "switched in" to the system after He has been added and the system volume determined. The O_2 source allows the addition of O_2 during the test to replenish that taken up by the patient and to maintain a constant system volume. The CO_2 absorber permits rebreathing without accumulation of CO_2. Water vapor is removed by a chemical absorber before the gas is sampled by the He analyzer. Tidal breathing and the He dilution curve are displayed on the computer.

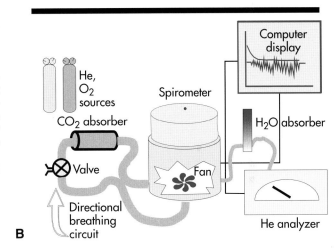

ers to calculate the concentration of N_2 in expired gas during the washout:

$$N_2 = 1 - F_EO_2 - F_ECO_2$$

where:
F_EO_2 = fraction of O_2 in expired gas (dry)
F_ECO_2 = fraction of CO_2 in expired gas (dry)

The patient, wearing a nose clip, breathes through a mouthpiece-valve system. Precisely at end-expiration, a valve is opened to allow 100% O_2 breathing to begin. Each breath of 100% O_2 washes out some of the residual N_2 in the lungs. Analog signals proportional to N_2 concentration and volume (or flow) are integrated to derive the volume of

N_2 exhaled for each breath. Values for each breath are summed to provide a total volume of N_2 washed out (Figure 3-2). The test is continued until the N_2 in alveolar gas has been reduced to approximately 1% (Lung Volumes 3-1). Some older systems terminate the test at 7 minutes. However, the O_2 breathing should be continued until alveolar N_2 falls to less than 1.5% for at least three consecutive breaths. A change in inspired N_2 concentration of greater than 1% or sudden large increases in expiratory N_2 concentrations indicate a leak, in which case the test should be stopped and repeated.

At least one technically satisfactory FRC_{N2} determination should be made. If additional washouts are performed, a waiting period of at least 15

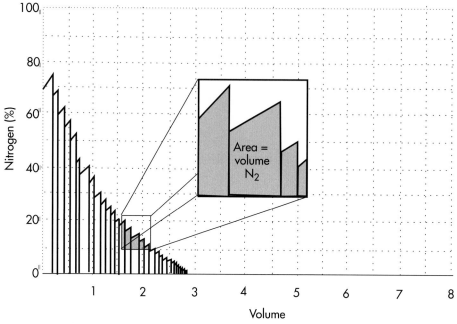

FIGURE 3-2   **Open-Circuit (N$_2$ Washout) Determination of FRC.** The concentration (or log concentration) of N$_2$ is plotted against time or against the volume expired as the patient breathes through a circuit (Figure 3-1, *A*). The volume of N$_2$ expired with each breath is measured by integrating flow and N$_2$ concentration to determine the area under each curve (see inset). The volume of N$_2$ expired for each breath is summed. The test continues until most of the N$_2$ in the lung has been washed out (usually 1.5% or less). FRC is determined by dividing the volume of N$_2$ expired by the change in alveolar N$_2$ from the beginning to the end of the test, with corrections, as described in the text.

LUNG VOLUMES 3-1

CRITERIA FOR ACCEPTABILITY

N$_2$ Washout FRC

1. The washout tracing or display should indicate a continually falling concentration of alveolar N$_2$.
2. The test should be continued until the N$_2$ concentration falls to 1.5%.
3. Washout times should be appropriate for the type of subject tested. Healthy subjects should wash out N$_2$ completely within 3 – 4 minutes.
4. The washout time should be reported. Failure to wash out N$_2$ within 7 minutes should be noted.
5. Multiple measurements should agree within 10%; the average FRC from acceptable trials should be used to calculate lung volumes. At least 15 minutes of room-air breathing should elapse between repeated trials.

minutes is recommended to allow normal concentrations of N$_2$ to be reestablished in the lungs, blood, and tissues. If more than one FRC measurement is obtained, the mean of the technically acceptable results that agree within 10% should be reported.

Some pulmonary function systems use pneumotachometers that may be sensitive to the composition of expired gas. These devices correct for changes in the viscosity of the gas as O$_2$ replaces N$_2$ in the expirate. Such corrections are easily accomplished by software or electronic correction of the analyzer output.

Closed-Circuit Multiple-Breath Helium Dilution

FRC can also be determined by equilibrating the gas in the lungs with a known volume of gas containing He (**closed-circuit multiple-breath helium dilution [FRC$_{He}$]**). A spirometer is filled with a known volume of air, and then a volume of He is added so that a concentration of approximately 10% is achieved (see Figure 3-1, *B*). The exact concentration of He and spirometer volume are measured and recorded before the test is begun. The patient breathes through a valve that allows connection to a rebreathing system. The valve is opened at the end of a quiet breath (i.e., the end-expiratory level). Then the patient rebreathes the gas in the spirometer, with a CO_2 absorber in place, until the concentration of He falls to a stable level (Figure 3-3). A fan or blower mixes the gas within the spirometer system. O_2 is added to the spirome-

ter system to maintain the FIO_2 near or above 0.21 and to keep system volume relatively constant.

An older method (i.e., the bolus method) added a large volume of O_2 to the spirometer at the beginning of the test. The patient then rebreathed and gradually consumed the O_2. Because of the possibility of equilibrium not being attained before the added O_2 was depleted, this method is no longer used.

Equilibration between normal lungs and the rebreathing system takes place in approximately 3 minutes when a 10% He mixture in a system volume of 6–8 L is used (Figure 3-4). The final concentration of He is then recorded. The system volume is computed first. System volume is the volume of the

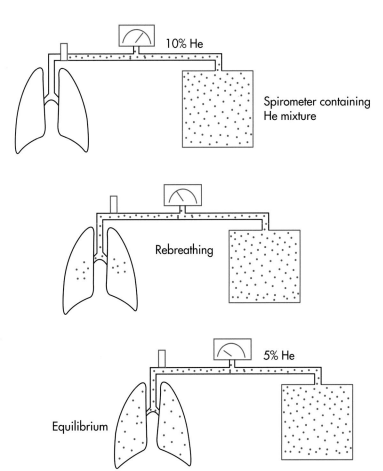

FIGURE 3-3 Closed-Circuit (He Dilution) Determination of FRC. At the beginning of the test, the patient's lungs contain no He. The spirometer contains a known concentration of He in a known volume (see text). The patient then rebreathes the He mixture from this system (Figure 3-1, *B*). He is diluted until equilibrium is reached. At the end of the test, the known volume of He has been diluted in the rebreathing system and the lungs. FRC is calculated from the change in He concentration and the known system volume. The patient must be switched from breathing air to the He mixture at the end-expiratory level for accurate measurement of FRC. RV is derived by subtracting the ERV. *(Modified from Comroe JH Jr, Forster RE, Dubois AB, et al: The lung: clinical physiology and pulmonary function tests, ed 2, St Louis, 1962, Mosby.)*

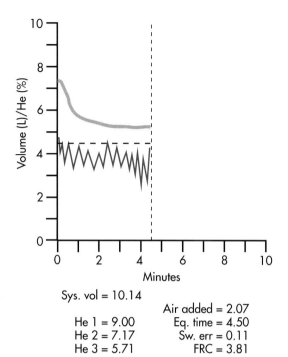

Sys. vol = 10.14

He 1 = 9.00	Air added = 2.07
He 2 = 7.17	Eq. time = 4.50
He 3 = 5.71	Sw. err = 0.11
	FRC = 3.81

FIGURE 3-4   Computer-Generated Recording of Closed-Circuit Multiple-Breath FRC Determination in a Healthy Patient. Graph shows He concentration from the beginning of rebreathing until equilibrium is achieved *(upper line)*. System volume of the spirometer and the patient's tidal breathing is also shown *(lower line)*. A CO_2 absorber removes carbon dioxide produced by the patient. A computerized valve system replaces O_2 to keep the system volume constant. Measurements of He concentrations and system variables are also displayed.

LUNG VOLUMES 3-2

CRITERIA FOR ACCEPTABILITY

He Dilution FRC

1. A tracing or display of spirometer volume should indicate that no leaks are present (system baseline flat). He concentration should be stable before testing.
2. The rebreathing pattern should be regular. If recorded, successive tidal breaths should show a gradually falling end-tidal level as O_2 is consumed. Addition of O_2 should return breathing to close to the system baseline.
3. The test should be continued until the He readings change by less than 0.02% in 30 seconds or until 10 minutes has elapsed.
4. Addition of O_2 should be appropriate for quiet tidal breathing (i.e., 200–400 ml/min).
5. The He equilibration curve, if plotted or displayed, should show a smooth and regular fall of He concentration until equilibrium is achieved.
6. Multiple measurements of FRC should agree within 10%; the average of acceptable multiple measurements should be reported.

spirometer, breathing circuitry, and valves before the patient is connected. It can be calculated as follows:

$$\text{System volume (L)} = \frac{\text{He}_{added}(L)}{F_{He\ initial}}$$

where:

He_{added} = volume of He placed in the spirometer in liters (L)

$F_{He\ initial}$ = %He converted to a fraction (%He/100)

When the system volume is known, FRC can be computed as follows:

$$\text{FRC} = \frac{(\%He_{initial} - \%He_{final})}{\%He_{final}} \times \text{System volume}$$

Either percent or fractional concentration of He may be used because the term is a ratio.

Some automated systems use a similar method to calculate the system volume; a small amount of He is added to the closed system, followed by a known volume of air. The change in He concentration after the addition of the air is used to determine the system volume. Rebreathing is continued until the He concentration changes by no more than 0.02% in 30 seconds (Lung Volumes 3-2).

At least one technically satisfactory measurement should be obtained. If additional dilutions are performed, a waiting period of at least 5 minutes is recommended between repeated tests. If more than one measurement of FRC_{He} is obtained, it is recommended that the mean of the technically acceptable results that agree within 10% should be reported.

Although a small volume of He dissolves in the blood during the test, it results in a negligible increase in FRC, and it is recommended that no correction be made. The volume of the equipment dead space (including filters) must also be subtracted from the measured FRC.

Most manufacturers provide "switch-in" error correction when the patient begins the test at a point either above or below the actual end-expiratory level (FRC). Depending on the patient's breathing pattern, a volume difference of several hundred milliliters may result. The effect of the switch-in error may be insignificant, especially with the closed-circuit method. Equilibrium does not occur instantaneously at switch-in. The total volume of spirometer and lungs is constantly changing with tidal breathing, removal of CO_2, and addition of O_2. If the switch-in error is large or the end-expiratory level appears to change during the maneuver, the test may need to be repeated.

Additional Comments on FRC by Gas Dilution Techniques

In the gas dilution techniques, RV is measured indirectly as a subdivision of the FRC. This method is preferred because the resting end-expiratory level depends less on patient effort than on maximal inspiration or expiration. The end-expiratory level (and the ERV) must be accurately measured. If tidal breathing is irregular, ERV may be overestimated or underestimated. Subtraction of an ERV value that is too large from the FRC will cause the RV to appear smaller than it actually is. Similarly, a small ERV will produce a larger than actual RV. The patient's tidal breathing pattern must be carefully monitored during the VC measurement.

The accuracy of the gas dilution techniques depends on all parts of the lung being well ventilated. In patients who have obstructive disease, some lung units are poorly ventilated. In these patients, it is often difficult to wash N_2 out or mix He to a stable level in poorly ventilated parts of the lungs. Thus FRC, RV, and TLC may all be underestimated, usually in proportion to the degree of obstruction. Extending the time of these tests improves their accuracy. However, prolonging the

test may not measure completely trapped gas, as found in bullous emphysema.

The graphic method of displaying breath-by-breath N_2 washout provides a means of quantifying the evenness of ventilation. Some systems plot the logarithm of the N_2 concentration against time or volume exhaled. The slope of the washout curve is determined by the FRC, tidal volume, dead space volume, and frequency of breathing. If N_2 is washed out of the lungs evenly, the log N_2 plot appears as a straight line. Because the lung is not perfectly symmetrical, the washout curve is slightly concave. The deviation from the expected curve indicates the extent to which ventilation is uneven. Washout should be complete within 3–4 minutes in healthy patients. The time to reach He equilibrium during the closed-circuit FRC determination can also be used as an index of **distribution of ventilation.** By simply recording the time to reach equilibrium and plotting the dilution curve, an estimate of the evenness of ventilation is obtained. In healthy patients, either type of gas dilution should be complete in 3–4 minutes. Use of gas dilution techniques to assess distribution has been replaced by ventilation scans using radioisotopes, as well as by CT scanning.

PF TIP

The gas dilution techniques of measuring lung volumes usually *underestimate* lung volumes in the presence of moderate or severe obstruction. Both methods (N_2 washout and He dilution) are also subject to leaks in their respective breathing circuits. Leaks usually cause the measured lung volume to be *overestimated*.

In either of the gas dilution techniques, a leak will cause erroneous estimates of FRC. Leaks may occur in breathing valves or circuitry, or at the patient connection. Some patients have difficulty maintaining an adequate seal at the mouthpiece throughout the test. Failure to properly apply nose clips can also result in a leak. Leaks usually result in an overestimate of lung volume. A leak in the open-circuit N_2 washout system allows room air to enter, increasing the volume of N_2 washed out. A leak in the closed-circuit He dilution system allows air to dilute the He concentration or He to escape. Each situation causes the test gas concentration to change more than it should. Leaks during the N_2 washout can usually be identified by inspection of

A

B

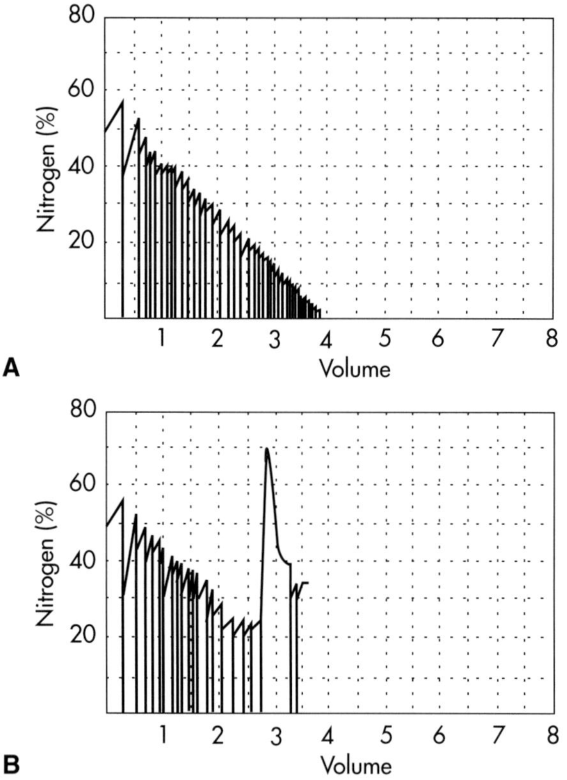

FIGURE 3-5   Open-Circuit Multiple-Breath N_2 Washout Tracings. A, A computer-generated recording of a nitrogen (N_2) washout test in a healthy patient. The tracings show a continuous decrease in end-tidal N_2 concentration with successive breaths. The test is continued until the N_2 concentration falls to less than 1%. **B,** A similar plot of N_2 washout from a healthy patient, but in this instance a leak occurs during the test. Leaks may occur if the patient does not maintain a tight seal at the mouthpiece. Leaks are usually easy to detect because room air enters the system and indicates an abrupt increase in N_2 concentration.

the graphic display or recording (Figure 3-5). Inaccuracy or malfunction of the gas analyzers in either method often causes errors. Leaks or analyzer problems should be considered whenever FRC values are inconsistent with spirometry results.

Body Plethysmography

FRC measured with the body plethysmograph (**FRC$_{pleth}$**) (Figure 3-6) refers to the volume of intrathorax gas measured when airflow occlusion occurs at FRC. The technique is based on **Boyle's law** relating pressure to volume. A volume of gas varies in inverse proportion to the pressure to which it is subjected if the temperature remains constant (isothermal). The patient has an unknown volume of gas in the thorax at the end of a normal expiration (i.e., the FRC). The airway is occluded momentarily at or near FRC; the patient is asked to gently pant at a frequency between 0.5 and 1.0 Hz (0.5 – 1.5 cycles per second), allowing the air in the chest to be compressed and decompressed. This causes a change in volume and pressure. The changes in pressure are easily measured at the mouth (P_{MOUTH}) with a pressure transducer. Mouth pressure theoretically equals alveolar pressure when there is no airflow. Changes in pulmonary gas volume are estimated by measuring pressure changes in the plethysmograph. The pressure in the plethysmograph is measured by a sensitive transducer. This transducer is calibrated by introducing a small, known volume of gas into the sealed box and relating the pressure change to the known volume (P_{BOX}). The calibration factor is then applied to measurements made on human patients.

The display of the panting maneuver is a graph with P_{MOUTH} and P_{BOX}. P_{MOUTH} is plotted on the vertical axis, and P_{BOX} is plotted on the horizontal axis (Figure 3-7). The resulting figure appears as a sloping line equal to $\Delta P/\Delta V$, where ΔP equals change in alveolar pressure and ΔV equals change in alveolar volume. Change in alveolar volume is measured indirectly by noting the reciprocal change in plethysmograph volume.

The V_{TG} can then be obtained from the slope of the tracing by applying a derivation of Boyle's law:

FIGURE 3-6 Components of the Body Plethysmograph Used to Measure Thoracic Gas Volume (V_{TG}). Boyle's law states that volume varies inversely with pressure if temperature is held constant. A pressure-type (constant volume) plethysmograph, with pressure transducers for measurements of box pressure and mouth (alveolar) pressure, is shown. A pneumotachometer measures flow to track lung volumes. The mouth shutter occludes the airway momentarily so alveolar pressure can be estimated. The patient pants gently against the closed shutter. Gas in the lungs is alternately compressed and decompressed. Changes in lung volume are reflected by changes in box pressure. These changes are displayed as a sloping line on a computer display. When the original pressure (P), the new pressure (P′), and the new volume (V′ or V + ΔV) are known, the original volume (V or V_{TG}) can be computed from Boyle's law (see the section on the technique of thoracic gas volume and Appendix E).

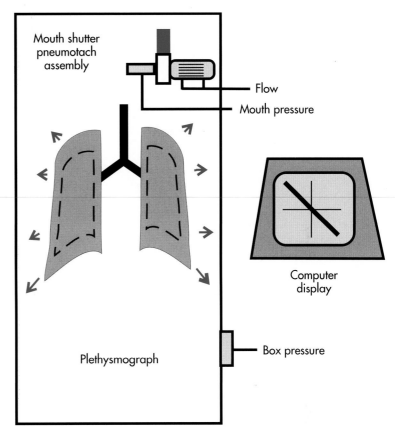

$$V_{TG} = \frac{P_B}{\lambda V_{TG}} \times \frac{P_{BOX}cal}{P_{MOUTH}cal} \times K$$

where:

V_{TG}	= thoracic gas volume
P_B	= barometric pressure minus water vapor pressure
λV_{TG}	= slope of the displayed line equal to $\Delta P / \Delta V$
$P_{BOX}cal$	= box pressure transducer calibration factor
$P_{MOUTH}cal$	= mouth pressure transducer calibration factor
K	= correction factor for volume displaced by the patient

For the complete derivation of the equation and sample calculations, see Appendixes E and F.

Computerized plethysmograph systems permit monitoring of tidal breathing in conjunction with the V_{TG} maneuver. Instantaneous changes in lung volume can be monitored by continuously integrating the flow through the plethysmograph's pneumotachometer. The end-expiratory level can be determined from tidal breathing. The patient then pants with the mouth shutter open. The computer records the change in lung volume above or below the resting level (FRC). When asked to pant, most patients do so slightly above FRC. The shutter then closes automatically, the patient continues panting, and V_{TG} is measured as described. The computer then adds or subtracts the change in volume from the end-expiratory level (before panting began) to calculate the true FRC. This computerized technique allows the patient to pant at the correct frequency and depth before the shutter is closed. It also eliminates the necessity of closing the shutter precisely at end-expiration. Airway resistance (Raw) and specific airway conductance (sGaw) can also be

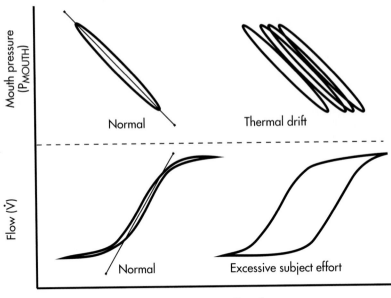

FIGURE 3-7 **Normal and Abnormal Plethysmograph Recordings.** *Top left,* Normal closed-shutter maneuver in which mouth pressure is plotted against box pressure. The loop should be closed, or nearly so. If thermal equilibrium has not been achieved, the loop (shown on the *top right*) tends to be open and to drift across the screen. *Bottom left,* Normal open-shutter measurement in which flow is plotted against box pressure. If the patient pants near FRC, the loop takes on a nearly closed S-shaped appearance. If the patient pants too rapidly or too deeply, the tracing becomes open and flattened (shown on the *bottom right*). Thermal drift can also cause the open-shutter tracing to resemble excessive patient effort.

measured simultaneously during the open-shutter panting (see Chapter 2). It should be noted that the correct panting frequencies for measuring Raw and V_{TG} are slightly different. Raw measurements should be made with the patient panting at about 1.5–2.5 Hz (1.5–2.5 cycles per second, or 90–150 breaths/min), whereas V_{TG} should be measured with the patient panting at a slower rate of 0.5–1 Hz. Many computerized systems display the panting frequency so the technologist can coach the patient to achieve the correct rate.

A VC maneuver along with its subdivisions (ERV and IC) should be performed immediately after the acquisition of FRC_{pleth}. Most plethysmograph systems allow these measurements using the built-in pneumotachometer. The same standards for accuracy should be applied to a slow VC measured in the plethysmograph as for any other spirometer. When FRC_{pleth} has been determined, the remaining

lung volumes can be calculated as described for the gas dilution techniques.

Measurement of FRC_{pleth} is a complex procedure. Each patient must be carefully instructed in the required maneuvers. Allowing the patient to sit in the box with the door open is helpful. A few patients may experience claustrophobia in the plethysmograph. The panting maneuver should be demonstrated by the technologist and then practiced by the patient. The patient should be instructed to place both hands against the cheeks. This prevents unwanted pressure changes in the mouth when the patient pants against the closed shutter. If practical, the shutter may be closed so that the patient knows what to expect during the test. The door of the plethysmograph can then be closed. The patient should understand that the plethysmograph can be opened if he or she becomes uncomfortable. Most systems allow the patient to open the door from within the box. If the plethysmograph is equipped with a communication device, it should be adjusted so the patient can hear instructions.

Depending on the construction of the plethysmograph, venting to the atmosphere is usually required to establish thermal equilibrium. Equilibrium can be presumed when the flow-volume recording stabilizes (i.e., does not drift). The patient is then instructed to pant. When the correct panting frequency and depth have been established, the shutter may be closed. Some plethysmograph systems require tidal breathing before shutter closure to establish the patient's end-expiratory level. In either type of system, the patient should pant against the closed shutter until a stable tracing is produced. Two to four pants are usually sufficient. If the patient pants too hard, the tracing may drift or appear as an "open" loop (see Figure 3-7). The recorded pressure changes should be within the range over which the transducers were calibrated. The entire tracing should be visible on the display. If the tracing goes offscreen, the pressure changes probably exceed the calibration ranges. Three or more technically satisfactory maneuvers should be recorded, each followed by ERV and IVC maneuvers (Lung Volumes 3-3). At least 3 FRC_{pleth} values that agree within 5% should be obtained and the mean value reported. The technologist's comments should note the acceptability of the maneuvers. Most computerized plethysmographs automatically measure the slope of the $\Delta P/\Delta V$ tracings. This is done by using the least-squares method to calculate a "best-fit" line through the recorded data points. The technologist may need to correct computer-generated tangents, depending on data quality from the panting maneuvers.

Additional Comments on FRC by Plethysmography

The plethysmographic method is a quick and accurate means of measuring lung volumes. It can be used in combination with simple spirometry to derive all lung volume compartments. The plethysmograph's primary advantage is that it measures all gas in the thorax, whether in ventilatory communication with the atmosphere or not. The plethysmographic measurement of FRC is often larger than that measured by He dilution or N_2 washout. This is the case in emphysema and other diseases characterized by air trapping, as well as in the presence of uneven distribution of ventilation. When gas dilution tests are continued for more than 7 minutes, the results for FRC determinations approach the V_{TG} value. Lung Volumes 3-4 lists interpretive strategies.

LUNG VOLUMES 3-3

CRITERIA FOR ACCEPTABILITY

FRC_{pleth}

1. The panting maneuver shows a closed loop without drift or other artifact.
2. Pressure changes are within calibration ranges; the tracing does not go offscreen.
3. Panting frequency should be between 0.5 and 1.0 Hz.
4. A series of three to five technically satisfactory panting maneuvers should be recorded.
5. At least three FRC_{pleth} values that agree within 5% should be obtained.
6. Reported FRC_{pleth} is averaged from the three acceptable and repeatable panting maneuvers.

PF TIP

Plethysmography offers several advantages over other methods of measuring lung volumes. V_{TG} is not affected by the distribution of ventilation. Multiple measurements can be made quickly and averaged. It provides a more accurate estimate of lung volumes in patients who have airway obstruction. In addition, Raw and sGaw can be measured in the same testing session.

It is often useful to compare FRC values obtained by plethysmography with values obtained by gas dilution methods, particularly in patients with obstructive disease. The ratio of FRC_{pleth}/FRC_{N2} or FRC_{pleth}/FRC_{He} can be used as an index of gas trapping. This ratio is usually near 1.0 in patients with

---

LUNG VOLUMES 3-4

INTERPRETIVE STRATEGIES

FRC_{pleth}

1. Were the panting maneuvers performed acceptably? Was the panting frequency appropriate (0.5–1.0 Hz)? If not, interpret results cautiously.
2. Were at least three maneuvers averaged to obtain FRC? Were individual values repeatable (within 5%)? If not, interpret cautiously.
3. Are reference values appropriate? Age, height, weight, race? Were they obtained plethysmographically?
4. Were other lung volumes (TLC) calculated appropriately? Were VC, ERV, and IC acceptable? If not, evaluate only FRC.
5. If the TLC is less than the lower limit of normal, suspect restriction.
6. If the TLC is greater than the upper limit of normal, suspect hyperinflation.
7. Are lung volumes consistent with spirometric findings? If not, evaluate carefully for combined obstruction and restriction.

---

panting rates aggravate this inaccuracy. Care should be taken that patients with spirometric evidence of obstruction pant at a rate of 0.5–1 Hz.

Spirometry (e.g., FVC, FEV_1, and VC) may be performed with the patient in the plethysmograph. The pneumotachometer must be capable of accurately measuring the entire range of gas flows required (i.e., up to 12 L/sec).

Two varieties of body boxes are commonly used: constant-volume and flow-based (see Chapter 10). For constant-volume plethysmographs, spirometry is done with the door open. Flow-based plethysmographs have the advantage of allowing forced spirometry with the door closed. Flow boxes also allow a slightly different type of flow-volume curve to be recorded. Normal spirometry plots airflow at the mouth against volume at the mouth (as detected by the spirometer). With the patient in a flow box, flow at the mouth can be plotted against actual lung volume changes as detected by the box. This may be particularly useful in patients with severe airway obstruction. It is possible to detect a significant compression volume during forced expiration and plot it against the flow generated. Spirometry, lung volumes, and airway resistance can all be obtained in a single sitting with either type of plethysmograph.

normal lungs, or even those with a restrictive lung disorder. Values greater than 1.0 indicate gas volumes detectable by the plethysmograph but hidden to the gas dilution techniques. Care must be taken that lung volumes determined by the two separate methods are reliable before the values can be expressed as a ratio. This ratio has been used to evaluate candidates for **lung volume reduction surgery (LVRS).** In LVRS removal of unperfused and diseased lung tissure will directly reduce gas trapping. Patients with severe bullous emphysema may have a difference in TLC of more than 1 L between FRC_{pleth} and the gas dilutional methods of measuring FRC.

Some evidence suggests that in severe airway obstruction, FRC may actually be overestimated when the plethysmographic technique is used. This occurs primarily because P_{MOUTH} (measured when the shutter is closed) may not equal alveolar pressure if the airways are severely obstructed. Rapid

Total Lung Capacity and Residual Volume/Total Lung Capacity Ratio

TLC is calculated combining other lung volume measurements. The two most common are as follows:

$$TLC = RV + VC$$

$$TLC = FRC + IC$$

Each method requires accurate measurement of the subdivisions of the VC. TLC can also be calculated with single-breath techniques (i.e., single-breath He dilution or single-breath N_2 washout). Single-breath measurements of lung volumes are usually done as part of other tests, such as the diffusing capacity (DLCO) test (see Chapter 5). Single-breath lung volumes correlate well with multiple-breath techniques in healthy patients. However, single-breath lung volumes tend to underestimate true values in moderate to severe obstruction. TLC can also be measured from standard chest x-ray films, as well as from CT scans of the thorax.

The RV/TLC ratio is calculated by dividing the RV by the TLC. This ratio is expressed as a percentage. Either ATPS (ambient temperature, pressure, saturation) or BTPS values may be used in the ratio, but both RV and TLC must be expressed in the same units.

The FRC, RV, and TLC should be reported in liters or milliliters, BTPS. Barrier filters may be used during lung volume determinations, particularly in rebreathing systems. If a filter is used, its volume must be subtracted from the lung volume measured.

Significance and Pathophysiology

FRC varies with body size, with change in body position, and with time of day (i.e., diurnal variation). As with other lung volumes, normal FRC may be affected by racial or ethnic background (Lung Volumes 3-5). Equations for calculating predicted FRC are found in Appendix B.

Increased FRC is considered pathologic. FRC values greater than approximately 120% of predicted values represent air trapping. Air trapping may result from emphysematous changes or from obstruction caused by asthma or bronchitis. Compensation for surgical removal of lung tissue or thoracic deformity can also cause increased FRC. Elevated FRC usually results in muscular and mechanical inefficiency of the respiratory apparatus. As lung volume increases, the chest wall and lungs themselves become "stiffer." This causes an increase in the work of breathing. FRC can increase dynamically; patients with airway obstruction may increase their end-expiratory lung volume (EELV) during exercise. This change in lung volume with increased ventilatory demand often results in a sensation of breathlessness.

The RV is the volume left in the lungs after the VC is exhaled. An increased RV indicates that, despite maximal expiratory effort, the lungs contain

---

LUNG VOLUMES 3-5

INTERPRETIVE STRATEGIES

Dilutional Lung Volumes

1. Was the FRC determination performed acceptably? Were multiple trials performed? If so, were they within 10%?
2. Was the VC maneuver acceptable? Were the ERV and IC measurements within 5% or 60 ml?
3. Were other lung volumes calculated appropriately (TLC, RV)?
4. Are the reference values appropriate? Age, height, sex, race?
5. Is the TLC less than the lower limit of normal? If so, restriction is present. Are other lung volumes (FRC, RV) reduced in similar proportion?
6. Is the TLC greater than the upper limit of normal? If so, suspect hyperinflation.
7. Is the RV/TLC ratio greater than predicted (approximately 35%)? Is the TLC normal or increased? If both are true, suspect air trapping.
8. Are lung volumes consistent with spirometric findings in regard to obstruction or restriction? Are they consistent with the history and physical findings?
9. Are additional tests indicated (plethysmographic lung volumes)?

---

a larger volume of gas than normal. Increased RV often results in an equivalent decrease in VC (Figure 3-8). Elevated RV may occur during an acute asthmatic episode but is usually reversible. Increased RV is characteristic of emphysema and bronchial obstruction; both may cause chronic air trapping. RV and FRC usually increase together. As RV becomes larger, increased ventilation is needed to adequately exchange O_2 and CO_2 in the lung. This requires an increase in tidal volume, respiratory rate, or both. Because of altered pressure-volume characteristics of the lung, work of breathing is also increased. Patients with increased RV often display gas exchange abnormalities such as hypoxemia or CO_2 retention.

FRC, RV, and TLC are typically decreased in restrictive diseases. Decreased lung volumes are

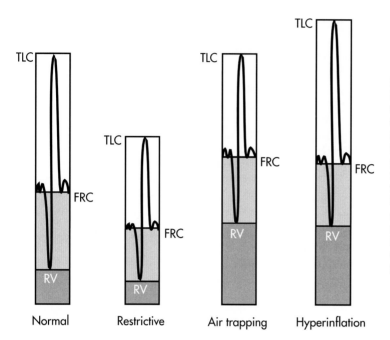

TLC

TLC

TLC

FRC

FRC

TLC

FRC

FRC

RV

RV

RV

RV

Normal   Restrictive   Air trapping   Hyperinflation

FIGURE 3-8   Lung Volumes in Normal, Restrictive, and Obstructive Patterns. A comparison of changes in lung volume compartments and VC *(superimposed)* shows the following: in restrictive patterns FRC, RV, and VC are all decreased proportionately, resulting in a decrease in the TLC, which defines restriction (see text). In obstruction (with air trapping) FRC and RV are both increased at the expense of the VC, and hence TLC remains relatively unchanged. Similar increases in RV and FRC may occur without reduction of VC, in which case the TLC increases (hyperinflation).

seen in interstitial diseases associated with extensive fibrosis (e.g., sarcoidosis, asbestosis, and complicated silicosis). Restrictive disorders affecting the chest wall include kyphoscoliosis, neuromuscular disorders, and obesity. Diseases that impair the diaphragm often result in reduced lung volumes, particularly TLC. Lung volumes may also be decreased in diseases that occlude many alveoli, such as pneumonia. Congestive heart failure causes pulmonary congestion, which can also reduce lung volume. Any disease process that occupies volume in the thorax can reduce lung volume. Examples include tumors and pleural effusions.

Table 3-2 lists comparative lung volumes for a healthy adult male and for patients with air trapping (as in emphysema), hyperinflation, and restriction (as in sarcoidosis). Restrictive processes usually cause lung volumes to be reduced equally. Proportional relationships between lung volume compartments, such as the RV/TLC ratio, may be relatively normal in restrictive diseases.

In obstruction, two different patterns may be observed. RV is usually increased. This increase may be at the expense of a reduction in VC (see Figure 3-6), with TLC remaining close to normal. In other cases, RV may increase while VC is preserved, so TLC is greater than predicted. The term *air trapping* is sometimes used to describe an increase in FRC and RV, and the term **hyperinflation** is used to describe the absolute increase in TLC. TLC may be either normal or increased in obstructive processes such as asthma, chronic bronchitis, bronchiectasis, cystic fibrosis, and emphysema. TLC does not appear to change dynamically, even though FRC may increase acutely during exercise.

PF TIP

Total lung capacity (TLC) is an important diagnostic tool in both obstructive and restrictive lung diseases. In restriction, the TLC is usually less than 80% of the predicted value, or below the lower limit of normal (LLN). In obstruction, the TLC is either normal or increased (hyperinflation).

Processes that occupy space in the lungs such as edema, atelectasis, neoplasms, or fibrotic lesions may decrease TLC. Other diseases that commonly result in decreased TLC include pulmonary congestion, pleural effusions, pneumothorax, or thoracic

TABLE 3-2

Comparative Lung Volumes for a Healthy Adult Male and Patients with Air Trapping, Hyperinflation, and Restriction

Value	Normal	Air Trapping	Hyperinflation	Restriction
VC (L)	4.80	3.00	4.80	3.00
FRC (L)	2.40	3.60	3.60	1.50
RV (L)	1.20	3.00	3.00	0.75
TLC (L)	6.00	6.00	7.80	3.75
RV/TLC (%)	20	50	38	20

deformities. Pure restrictive defects show proportional decreases in most lung compartments as described for FRC and RV. When the TLC value is less than 80% of predicted, or less than the 95% confidence limit, a restrictive process is present. Reduced VC, along with a normal or increased FEV_1/FVC ratio, is suggestive of restriction, but a measurement of TLC is needed to confirm the diagnosis of a restrictive defect.

The RV/TLC ratio describes the percentage of total lung volume that must be ventilated by tidal breathing. In healthy adults, the RV/TLC ratio may vary from 20% in young adults to 35% in older patients. Values greater than 35% may result from absolute increases of RV (as in emphysema) or from a decrease in TLC because of a loss of VC. A large RV/TLC in the presence of increased TLC is often indicative of hyperinflation. An increased RV/TLC with a normal TLC indicates that air trapping is present.

GAS DISTRIBUTION TESTS: SINGLE-BREATH NITROGEN WASHOUT, CLOSING VOLUME, AND CLOSING CAPACITY

Description

The **single-breath nitrogen washout test (SBN_2)** measures the distribution of ventilation. Distribution is analyzed by measuring the change in N_2 concentration during expiration of the VC after a single breath of 100% O_2. Evenness of distribution is assessed by two parameters: the change in per-centage of N_2 between the 750- and 1250-ml portion of the SBN_2 test ($\Delta\%N_{2\ 750-1250}$) and the **slope of phase III** of the expiratory tracing. Each of these indices is recorded as a percent. Closing volume (CV) is the portion of the VC that can be exhaled from the lungs after the onset of airway closure. CV is also measured from the SBN_2 maneuver and is usually expressed as a percentage of the VC. A related measurement, **closing capacity (CC),** is the sum of the CV and RV. CC is expressed as a percentage of the TLC.

Technique

The test is performed with equipment similar to that used for the open-circuit FRC_{N2} determination (see Figure 3-1, A). The patient exhales to RV, then inspires a VC breath of 100% O_2 from a reservoir or demand valve. The 100% O_2 dilutes the N_2 present in the lungs. Without holding the breath, the patient exhales slowly and evenly at a flow of 0.3–0.5 L/sec. The N_2 concentration is measured by an N_2 analyzer, while the exhaled volume is measured by the spirometer. Volume expired is plotted against N_2 concentration on a graph (Figure 3-9). This washout curve can be divided into four phases:

Phase I: upper airway gas from the anatomic dead space (V_{Danat}), consisting of 100% O_2

Phase II: mixed dead space gas in which the relative concentrations of O_2 and N_2 change abruptly as the V_{Danat} volume is expired

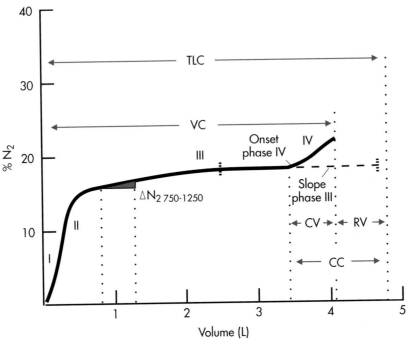

FIGURE 3-9   Single-Breath Nitrogen Elimination (SBN$_2$). A plot of increasing N$_2$ concentration on expiration after a single VC breath of 100% O$_2$. The curve is divided into four phases. Phase I is the extreme beginning of the expiration, when only O$_2$ is being exhaled. Phase II shows an abrupt rise in N$_2$ concentration as mixed bronchial and alveolar air is expired. Phase III is the alveolar gas plateau. N$_2$ concentration changes slowly as long as ventilation is uniformly distributed. Phase IV is an abrupt increase in N$_2$ concentration as basal airways close and a larger proportion of gas comes from the N$_2$-rich lung apices. Several useful parameters are derived from the SBN$_2$ tracing. The $\Delta N_2\,{}_{750-1250}$ and slope of phase III are indices of the evenness of ventilation distribution. CV can be read directly from the onset of phase IV until RV is reached; VC can also be read directly. RV, TLC, and CC can be calculated if the area under the curve is determined either by planimetry or electronic integration (see text).

Phase III: a plateau caused by the exhalation of alveolar gas in which relative O$_2$ and N$_2$ concentrations change slowly and evenly

Phase IV: an abrupt increase in the concentration of N$_2$ that continues until RV is reached

The initial 750 ml of expired gas contains dead space gas from phases I and II and is not used to assess distribution of ventilation. The difference in N$_2$ concentration between the 750-ml and 1250-ml points is called the delta N$_2$ ($\Delta\%N_2\,{}_{750-1250}$).

The slope of phase III is the change in N$_2$ concentration from the point at which 30% of the VC remains up to the onset of phase IV. It is recorded as $\Delta\%N_2$ per liter of lung volume.

The volume expired after the onset of phase IV is the CV. CV may be added to the RV, if the RV has been determined, and expressed as the CC. CV is reported as a percentage of VC:

$$\frac{CV}{VC}\times100$$

CC is recorded as a percentage of TLC:

$$\frac{CC}{TLC}\times100$$

TLC can be determined from the SBN$_2$ test by integrating the area of the washout curve. When the volume of N$_2$ is known, a dilution equation can be used to calculate RV. RV is then added to the measured VC to derive TLC. RV is calculated as follows:

$$RV = VC \times \frac{F_{\bar{E}}N_2}{F_A N_2 - F_{\bar{E}}N_2}$$

where:

$F_{\bar{E}}N_2$ = mean expired N_2 concentration determined by integration of the area under the curve

$F_A N_2$ = N_2 concentration in the lungs at the beginning of inspiration, approximately 0.75 – 0.79

This method is accurate only in patients who do not have significant obstruction or dead space–producing disease. CV and CC measurements may be in error if the patient does not perform an acceptable VC maneuver (Lung Volumes 3-6). The inspired and expired VC should be within 5%. The VC during the SBN_2 should match the FVC or VC within 5% or 200 ml. Expiratory flow should be maintained between 0.3 and 0.5 L/sec.

Significance and Pathophysiology

Lung Volumes 3-7 lists interpretive strategies.

Δ%N₂ 750-1250

The normal $\Delta\%N_{2\ 750-1250}$ is 1.5% or less for healthy young adults and slightly higher for healthy older adults (up to approximately 3%). Increased $\Delta\%N_{2\ 750-1250}$ is found in diseases characterized by

---

> ### LUNG VOLUMES 3-7
>
> #### INTERPRETIVE
>
> **SBN_2**
>
> 1. Was the test performed acceptably? VC reproducible within 5% or 200 ml? Expiratory flow appropriate?
> 2. Are reference values appropriate? Age, height, sex, race?
> 3. Is $\Delta\%N_{2\ 750-1250}$ greater than 1.5%? If so, suspect uneven distribution of ventilation.
> 4. Is slope of phase III greater than 1.0% – 1.5%? If so, there is uneven distribution of ventilation.
> 5. Is CV/VC% greater than 20% (or age-related expected value)? If so, suspect small airway abnormalities. Correlate with clinical findings.

uneven distribution of gas during inspiration or unequal emptying rates during expiration. In patients with severe emphysema, $\Delta\%N_{2\ 750-1250}$ may exceed 10%.

Slope of Phase III

A best-fit line is drawn through the phase III segment of the tracing from the point where 30% of the VC remains above RV to the onset of phase IV. The slope of this line is an index of gas distribution, similar to the $\Delta\%N_{2\ 750-1250}$. Values in healthy young adults range from 0.5% – 1.0% N_2/L of lung volume, with wide variability. Very slow expiratory flow rates may cause oscillations in the tracing of phase III, making the accurate measurement of $\Delta\%N_2$ difficult. These oscillations are attributed to changes in alveolar N_2 concentrations as blood pulses through the pulmonary capillaries during cardiac systole. Increasing the expiratory flow rate slightly eliminates this artifact. Patients who have small VC values may have difficulty exhaling enough gas to make the $\Delta\%N_2$ or slope of phase III meaningful.

Other gases, such as He or sulfur hexafluoride (SF_6), may also be used to assess the distribution of ventilation. The slope of the alveolar phase using these gases may be useful in detecting early changes in the small airways. Detecting these changes may

---

> ### LUNG VOLUMES 3-6
>
> #### CRITERIA FOR ACCEPTABILITY
>
> **SBN_2**
>
> 1. Inspired and expired VC should be within 5% or 200 ml.
> 2. The VC during SBN_2 should be within 200 ml of a previously determined VC.
> 3. Expiratory flow should be maintained between 0.3 and 0.5 L/sec.
> 4. The N_2 tracing should show minimal cardiac oscillations.

identify bronchiolitis obliterans in double–lung transplant recipients.

Closing Volume and Closing Capacity

After maximal expiration by an upright patient, more RV remains at the apices of the lungs than at the bases. Gravity causes this difference. When the test gas (O_2) is inspired, the apices receive the gas occupying the patient's dead space, which consists mostly of N_2. O_2 then goes preferentially to the bases of the lungs. Gas concentrations in the lungs become widely different. The apices contain RV gas plus dead space gas rich in N_2. The bases of the lungs contain a higher concentration of the test gas O_2. Compression of the airways during the subsequent expiration causes airways to narrow and then close, as lung volume approaches RV. Airways at the bases close first because of gravity and the weight of the lung in patients sitting upright. As airways at the bases close, proportionately more gas comes from the apices. This appears as an abrupt rise in the concentration of N_2—the onset of phase IV.

The onset of phase IV marks the lung volume at which airway closure begins. The point at which this occurs in the VC depends on the caliber of the small airways. In healthy young adults, airways begin closing after 80%–90% of the VC has been expired. This equates to a CC in healthy young adults of approximately 30% of the TLC, with wide variations. CV and CC may be increased, indicating earlier onset of airway closure in the following:

- Elderly patients
- Restrictive disease patterns in which the FRC becomes less than the CV
- Smokers and other patients with early obstructive disease of small airways
- Congestive heart failure when the caliber of the small airways is compromised by edema

Patients with moderate or severe obstructive disease may have no sharp inflection separating phases III and IV of the SBN_2. This lack of a clear point of airway closure is the result of grossly uneven distribution of gas in the lungs. Patients who have airway obstruction typically show greater than normal values for the $\Delta\%N_2{}_{750-1250}$ and slope of phase III.

In some patients with no pulmonary disease, the onset of phase IV cannot be accurately determined. Because of the variability in both the CV and CC, the mean of three tests is usually reported. Because of its poor reproducibility, the CV test is not widely used. Although it appears to be a sensitive indicator of abnormalities in the small airways, particularly in smokers, an increased CV/VC ratio is not highly predictive of which individuals will have chronic airway obstruction. To calculate normal values for CV/VC and CC/TLC according to age and sex, see Appendix B.

SUMMARY

- To measure TLC, the functional residual capacity (FRC) is measured first. FRC can be measured with N_2 washout (FRC_{N2}), He dilution (FRC_{He}), or body plethysmograph (FRC_{pleth}) techniques.
- TLC is calculated by adding the inspiratory capacity (IC, measured from simple spirometry) to the FRC.
- The expiratory reserve volume (ERV, also measured by simple spirometry) may be subtracted from FRC to derive RV.
- The addition of RV and VC (from spirometry) also provides an estimate of TLC.
- The plethysmographic technique is the preferred method because it is largely independent of gas distribution in the lungs.
- Gas dilution techniques may underestimate lung volumes in the presence of significant airway obstruction.
- Gas dilution techniques, along with analysis of N_2 after a single breath of oxygen (SBN_2), provide a qualitative means of assessing gas distribution in the lungs.

CASE 3-1

Case Studies

HISTORY

M.B. is a 27-year-old male high school teacher whose chief complaint is dyspnea on exertion. He states that his breathlessness has worsened over the past several months. He has smoked one pack of cigarettes per day for 10 years (10 pack years). He denies a cough or sputum production. No one in his family ever had emphysema, asthma, chronic bronchitis, carcinoma, or tuberculosis. There is no history of exposure to extraordinary environmental pollutants.

PULMONARY FUNCTION TESTING

Personal Data

Sex:	Male
Age:	27 yr
Height:	65 in
Weight:	297 lb
Body surface area (BSA):	2.28 m^2

Spirometry and Airway Resistance			
	Before Drug	Predicted	%
FVC (L)	2.9	4.7	62
FEV$_1$ (L)	2.47	3.86	64
FEV$_{1\%}$ (%)	85	82	—
FEF$_{25\%-75\%}$ (L/sec)	4.62	4.35	106
FEF$_{50\%}$ (L/sec)	4.94	5.82	85
MVV (L/min)	178	130	137
Raw (cm H$_2$O/L/sec)	2.33	0.6–2.4	—
sGaw (L/sec/cm H$_2$O/L)	0.23	0.12–0.50	—

Lung Volumes (by Plethysmograph)			
	Before Drug	Predicted	%
VC (L)	2.9	4.7	62
IC (L)	1.96	2.91	67
ERV (L)	0.94	1.8	59
FRC (L)	1.87	3.29	57
RV (L)	0.93	1.49	57
TLC (L)	3.83	6.2	62
RV/TLC (%)	25	24	—

TECHNOLOGIST'S COMMENTS

Spirometry results met all American Thoracic Society (ATS) acceptability and repeatability recommendations. Good patient cooperation and effort.

QUESTIONS

1. What is the interpretation of:
   - Spirometry?
   - Lung volumes?
   - Airway resistance?
2. What is the cause of the patient's symptoms?
3. What other tests might be indicated?
4. What treatment might be recommended based on these findings?

DISCUSSION

Interpretation

All data from spirometry and lung volumes are acceptable. Spirometry shows a decreased FVC and FEV$_1$. The FEV$_{1\%}$ is normal. Flows are within normal limits, as is the maximal voluntary ventilation (MVV). Raw is near the upper limit of normal, but sGaw is normal. Lung volumes are decreased, with the RV/TLC ratio preserved.

Impression: Moderate restrictive lung disease without evidence of obstruction. The restrictive pattern may be related to the patient's weight. Recommend arterial blood gas testing to evaluate gas exchange abnormalities.

Cause of Symptoms

This case is a good example of what might be considered a pure restrictive defect. A proportional decrease in all lung volumes, including FVC and FEV$_1$, is characteristic of a restrictive process. Flows such as FEF$_{25\%-75\%}$ or FEF$_{50\%}$ show little or no decrease (Figure 3-10). In addition, characteristic of simple restriction is the well-preserved ratio of FEV$_1$ to FVC. The volume expired in the first second was in correct proportion to the VC, despite decreases in their absolute volumes. The MVV demonstrates the patient's ability to move a normal maximal volume. This may be accomplished despite moderately severe restriction by an increase in the rate rather than the tidal volume.

The explanation for the restrictive pattern lies in the patient's weight of 297 pounds. His actual weight

continued

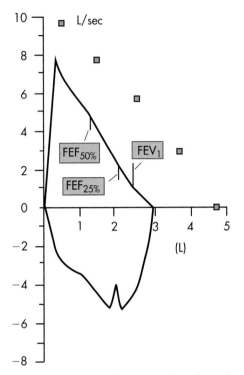

FIGURE 3-10   Flow-Volume Loop from the Patient.
Upward tick mark superimposed on the loop denotes the FEV$_1$, whereas downward tick marks show FEF$_{50\%}$ and FEF$_{25\%}$, respectively. Small, shaded boxes represent the patient's reference values.

is approximately 200% of his ideal weight. Obesity commonly causes restrictive patterns.

Other Tests

The patient returned for analysis of arterial blood gases, which revealed resting hypoxemia and slightly elevated PaCO$_2$. Blood gas measurements confirmed the degree of impairment caused by the moderately severe restrictive pattern. Other tests that might be considered include ventilatory response tests for hypoxemia or hypercapnia (see Chapter 4). Studies to diagnose sleep apnea might be indicated if the patient had symptoms of disordered breathing during sleep or excessive daytime sleepiness. This patient's border-line Raw suggests upper airway involvement, which might predispose him to obstructive sleep apnea.

Treatment

The patient was referred to a dietician for counseling in weight management.

CASE 3-2

Case Studies

HISTORY

R.B. is a 37-year-old pipe fitter whose chief complaint is shortness of breath at rest and with exertion. His dyspnea has worsened in the past 6 months, so much so that he is no longer able to work. Additional symptoms include a dry cough. He admits some sputum production when he has a chest cold. He has smoked one pack of cigarettes per day for 19 years (19 pack years). He quit smoking approximately 3 weeks before the tests. His father died of emphysema, and his mother of lung cancer. His brother is in good health. His occupational exposure includes working for the past 13 years in the assembly room of a boiler plant. He admits to seldom using the respirators provided at work despite a dusty environment.

PULMONARY FUNCTION TESTS

Personal Data

Sex:	Male
Age:	37 yr
Height:	69 in
Weight:	143 lb

Spirometry

	Before Drug	Predicted	%	After Drug	%
FVC (L)	3.04	5.05	60	3.1	61
FEV_1 (L)	2.03	3.90	52	2.26	58
$FEV_{1\%}$ (%)	67	77	—	73	—
$FEF_{25\%-75\%}$ (L/sec)	1.3	4.09	32	1.60	39
$FEF_{50\%}$ (L/sec)	2.12	5.78	37	2.42	42
$FEF_{25\%}$ (L/sec)	0.78	2.95	26	1.2	41
MVV (L/min)	83	141	59	91	65
Raw (cm H_2O)/L/sec)	2.51	0.6–2.4	—	2.47	—
sGaw (L/sec/cm H_2O/L)	0.14	0.11–0.44	—	0.15	—

Lung Volumes (by N_2 Washout)

	Before Drug	Predicted	%
VC (L)	3.04	5.05	60
IC (L)	1.62	3.18	51
ERV (L)	1.42	1.87	76
FRC (L)	2.75	3.81	72
RV (L)	0.33	1.94	69
TLC (L)	4.37	6.99	63
RV/TLC (%)	30	28	—

TECHNOLOGIST'S COMMENTS

Spirometry results met all American Thoracic Society (ATS) recommendations, prebronchodilator and postbronchodilator. Lung volumes by N_2 washout: all maneuvers were performed acceptably. Duplicate measurements were averaged. Raw and sGaw efforts were performed appropriately.

QUESTIONS

1. What is the interpretation of:
   - Prebronchodilator spirometry?
   - Response to bronchodilator?
   - Airway resistance and conductance?
   - Lung volumes?
2. What is the cause of the patient's symptoms?
3. What other tests might be indicated?
4. What treatment might be recommended based on these findings?

DISCUSSION

Interpretation

All data from spirometry and lung volumes are acceptable. Spirometry shows a reduced FVC and FEV_1. The $FEF_{25\%-75\%}$, $FEF_{50\%}$, and $FEF_{25\%}$ are all reduced. The MVV is low. Raw and sGaw are close to their respective limits of normal. Response to bronchodilators is borderline, with an increase in the FEV_1 of 230 ml (11%). The $FEF_{25\%}$ improved somewhat more than the other flows. The patient's lung volumes are all decreased. His RV/TLC ratio is normal.

Impression: There is moderate airway obstruction combined with a restrictive pattern. The response to inhaled bronchodilator medication is borderline. A trial of bronchodilators should be considered. Recommend arterial blood gas testing to evaluate possible hypoxemia.

Cause of Symptoms

R.B. typifies a patient who has combined obstructive and restrictive disease. His spirometry results indicate that a serious obstructive component is present, as revealed by his FEV_1 (52% of predicted) and the other flows. His $FEV_{1\%}$, however, is close to normal because his FVC is also reduced. Airway narrowing as a result of restriction is sometimes responsible for decreased flows. This is particularly evident when restriction is severe. R.B.'s symptoms of cough and sputum suggest a genuine obstructive process. His smoking and family history place him at risk. Because FVC can be reduced in either obstructive or restrictive processes, spirometry alone would not have adequately defined the patient's disease.

Lung volume measurements (Figure 3-11) confirm the presence of a restrictive component (see Figure 3-8). All lung volumes are reduced in similar proportions. The reduction in VC matches decreases in FRC, RV, and TLC. The patient's history and symptoms suggest the possibility of restrictive or obstructive disease or both. The obstructive component may be related to the patient's smoking history, but the etiology of the restrictive component is less clear. On further inquiry, it was learned that the patient's occupation

continued

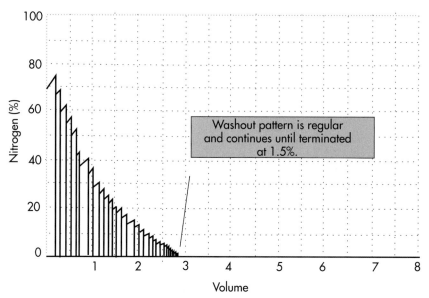

FIGURE 3-11   **Open-Circuit Multiple-Breath N₂ Washout Graph.** Tracing shows a normal pattern of washout with N₂ concentration plotted against lung volume (FRC). The test was terminated when N₂ concentration fell to less than 1.5%.

involved exposure to asbestos, which can cause fibrosis and/or carcinoma. Chest radiographs revealed linear calcifications of the diaphragmatic pleura and pleural thickening, as well as fibrotic changes. These findings are all consistent with asbestos exposure.

Other Tests

A sputum examination was performed, and asbestos bodies were identified from the patient's sputum. Open-lung biopsy was deferred because both the obstructive and restrictive components seemed to be appropriately identified. Measurement of pulmonary compliance (CL) could be used to document the severity of the fibrosis. Analysis of resting arterial blood gases is probably indicated because the patient has a significant degree of restriction. Diffusing capacity (DLCO) could also be used to identify possible gas exchange abnormalities.

Because of his dyspnea on exertion, the patient returned for an exercise evaluation. He walked on a treadmill with an arterial catheter in place. His PaO₂ fell from 65 mm Hg (rest) to 55 mm Hg after only 2 minutes of walking at 2 miles per hour. The desaturation was corrected when the patient breathed O₂ by nasal cannula at 1 L/min.

Treatment

The patient was given a trial of bronchodilators and reported significant symptomatic improvement. He began using supplemental O₂ via a portable system and was able to return to work in a position modified to accommodate his abilities.

CASE 3-3

Case Studies

HISTORY

J.A. is a 68-year white woman, whose chief complaint is worsening dyspnea, was seen by a pulmonologist in the office. She admitted to having been a heavy smoker (90 pack years), but recently quit. She has a productive cough and trouble sleeping at night. She had worked in the meat department of a grocery store for many years, and there was no history of exposure to extraordinary environmental pollutants. She is 62 inches tall and weighs 110 pounds. Her chest radiograph had an emphysematous appearance with increased diameters.

DOCTOR'S OFFICE PULMONARY FUNCTION TEST

Spirometry

	Before Drug	Predicted	%	After Drug	%
FVC (L)	2.18	3.63	60	2.38	66
FEV$_1$ (L)	1.09	2.57	42	1.19	46
FEV$_{1\%}$ (%)	50	71	—	50	—
FEF$_{25\%-75\%}$ (L/sec)	0.65	2.38	26	0.71	30

Lung Volumes (by N$_2$ Washout)

	Before Drug	Predicted	%
VC (L)	2.47	3.63	68
IC (L)	2.05	2.02	101
ERV (L)	0.50	0.89	56
FRC$_{N2}$ (L)	2.58	2.80	92
RV (L)	2.08	1.91	109
TLC (L)	4.63	4.82	96
RV/TLC (%)	45	40	—

After seeing the results of the office pulmonary function test, the doctor ordered another pulmonary function test at the area hospital.

HOSPITAL PULMONARY FUNCTION TEST

Spirometry and D$_{LCO}$

	Before Drug	Predicted	%	After Drug	%
FVC (L)	2.30	3.63	63	2.45	67
FEV$_1$ (L)	1.12	2.57	44	1.30	51
FEV$_{1\%}$ (%)	49	71	—	53	—
FEF$_{25\%-75\%}$ (L/sec)	0.59	2.38	25	0.83	35
Raw (cm H$_2$O/L/sec)	2.89	0.6–2.4	—		
sGaw (L/sec/ cm H$_2$O/L)	0.06	0.12–0.50	—		
D$_{LCO}$(ml/min/ mm Hg)	17.4	23.5	74		
D$_{LCO}$/V$_A$	3.66	4.88	75		

Lung Volumes (by Plethysmography)

	Before Drug	Predicted	%
VC (L)	2.50	3.63	69
IC (L)	1.80	2.02	89
ERV (L)	0.86	0.89	97
FRC$_{pleth}$ (L)	3.99	2.80	142
RV (L)	3.13	1.91	164
TLC (L)	5.79	4.82	120
RV/TLC (%)	54	40	—

QUESTIONS

1. What is the interpretation of the pulmonary function tests done in the doctor's office?
2. What concerns did the doctor have that prompted sending the patient for another test?
3. What is the interpretation of the pulmonary function tests done in the hospital laboratory?
4. Why is there such a difference?

DISCUSSION

Interpretation of Tests from Doctor's Office

Pulmonary function test data from the doctor's office reveal normal lung volumes (TLC, FRC, and RV) and a reduced SVC. The results also reveal severe airflow limitation with a small but clinically insignificant response to bronchodilator (9.2% and 100-ml improvement in FEV$_1$). The most likely interpretation of these data would state a mixed obstructive-restrictive disorder.

Concerns About Office Data

The main concern by the office physician was the low lung volumes and lack of hyperinflation that would be consistent with this degree of obstruction and the chest radiograph interpretation.

Interpretation of Tests from Hospital Laboratory

Pulmonary function data from the hospital pulmonary function laboratory, which used a body plethysmograph, reveal severe airflow limitation, decreased diffusing capacity, but markedly increased lung volumes. There is a better bronchodilator response (16.1% and 180-ml improvement in FEV$_1$). The interpretation of these data is that of severe airflow limitation. There is no evidence of a mixed obstructive-restrictive disorder.

Why the Difference?

The major difference between the two pulmonary function tests is the measurement of FRC. In the doctor's office, the FRC$_{N2}$ value was 2.58 L. In the hospital laboratory the body plethysmography was used in determining a FRC$_{pleth}$ of 3.99 L. The difference between these values can be explained by the presence of trapped gas or poorly communicating airways. In patients with significant airways obstruction, the gas dilutional methods (i.e., N$_2$ washout and He dilution) will likely underestimate true lung volume, and the body plethysmograph is a better instrument to use.

SELF-ASSESSMENT QUESTIONS

Entry-level

1. All of the following are techniques for determining FRC except:
   a. Single-breath nitrogen washout
   b. Open-circuit multiple-breath nitrogen washout
   c. Closed-circuit multiple-breath helium dilution
   d. Body plethysmography

2. In patients with obstructive lung disease, the gas dilution methods for FRC determination:
   a. Overestimate FRC
   b. Equal body plethysmography FRC
   c. Underestimate FRC
   d. Equal radiographic FRC

3. According to the 2005 ATS/ERS Guidelines for standardizing the measurement of lung volumes, the N_2 washout test is considered complete when the:
   a. N_2 concentration has decreased to less than 2.5% after 7 minutes
   b. N_2 concentration has decreased to less than 1.5% for at least 3 consecutive breaths
   c. N_2 concentration changes by less than 0.02% in 30 seconds
   d. N_2 concentration has reached equilibrium

4. A patient has the following results from a pulmonary function test:

VC	4.35 L
IC	3.15 L
ERV	1.20 L
FRC_{He}	3.40 L

   What is the patient's RV and RV/TLC ratio?
   a. 4.60 L and 70%
   b. 1.80 L and 27%
   c. 2.20 L and 34%
   d. 1.95 L and 26%

5. A patient has the following lung volumes measured using a body plethysmograph:

	Measured	Predicted	%Predicted
VC (L)	3.50	4.30	81
FRC_{pleth} (L)	3.80	3.00	127
RV (L)	3.00	2.00	150
TLC (L)	7.20	6.30	114

These values are most consistent with:
   a. Normal lung volumes
   b. A restrictive pattern as in pulmonary fibrosis
   c. An obstructive pattern such as emphysema
   d. A mixed obstructive and restrictive pattern

6. The calculation of FRC with the body plethysmograph is based on:
   a. Charles' law
   b. Poiseuille's law
   c. Boyle's law
   d. Dalton's law

Advanced

7. Which of the following are true about the measurement of lung volumes using the body plethysmograph?
   I. The plethysmograph measures all gas in the thorax.
   II. Gas in the thorax that does not communicate with the mouth is not measured by the plethysmograph.
   III. FRC_{pleth} is often larger than gas dilutional FRC determinations.
   IV. FRC_{pleth} can overestimate true FRC in severe airway obstruction.
   a. I, II, III, and IV
   b. I and II
   c. I, III, and IV
   d. II and III

8. A 53-year-old woman has the following measurements obtained during pulmonary function testing:

FVC	2.55 L
FEV_1	1.20 L
FEV_1/FVC	47%
FRC_{He}	2.32 L
FRC_{pleth}	3.59 L

   Which of the following best explains these findings?
   a. A leak during the FRC_{He} determination
   b. Normal pulmonary function
   c. Airflow obstruction with air trapping
   d. Poor patient effort

9. In measuring FRC by body plethysmography, which of the following is most correct?
   I. Patient should pant at a rate between 0.5 and 1 Hz

II. Patient should pant at about 90 breaths/min

III. The largest of three acceptable tests is reported

IV. The average of three acceptable tests that agree within 5% is reported

   a. I and III only
   b. II and IV only
   c. I and IV only
   d. I, II, and III

10. A 25-year-old patient performs an SBN_2 test and records a slope of phase III of 2.9%. This value is:

   a. Consistent with increased physiologic dead space
   b. Indicative of uneven distribution of gas within the lungs
   c. Within normal limits
   d. Consistent with a gas analyzer malfunction

11. A patient with alpha-1 antitrypsin deficiency and severe airway obstruction has lung volumes measured with the open-circuit N_2 washout method and by plethysmography with the following results:

FRC_{N2}	2.99 L
FRC_{pleth}	4.58 L
VC	2.77 L
IC	1.54 L
FRC predicted	3.67 L

The volume of trapped gas is:

   a. 0.91 L
   b. 3.04 L
   c. 1.81 L
   d. 1.59 L

12. A patient with an FEV_1 of 1.24 L and an FVC of 3.10 L performs the FRC_{He} test. The He concentration between 6 and 6.5 minutes changed by 0.1%, and between 7 and 7.5 minutes changed by 0.08%. The technician correctly concludes equilibration has not been reached. The most likely explanation is:

   a. The patient is malingering.
   b. The N_2 analyzer has malfunctioned.
   c. The CO_2 absorber is contaminated.
   d. This is consistent with severe airway obstruction.

Selected Bibliography

GENERAL REFERENCES

Crapo RO, Morris AH, Clayton PD et al: Lung volumes in healthy nonsmoking adults, *Bull Eur Physiopathol Respir* 1982; 18:419.

Forster RE: *The lung: clinical physiology and pulmonary function tests,* ed 3, St Louis, 1988, Mosby.

Goldman HI, Becklake MR: Respiratory function tests: normal values at median altitudes and the prediction of normal results, *Am Rev TB Pulm Dis* 1959; 79:457.

Hibbert ME, Lanigan A, Raven J et al: Relation of armspan to height and the prediction of lung function, *Thorax* 1988; 43:657.

Ries A: Measurement of lung volumes, *Clin Chest Med* 1989; 10:177-186.

THORACIC GAS VOLUME

Begin P, Peslin R: Influence of panting frequency on thoracic gas volume measurements in chronic obstructive pulmonary disease, *Am Rev Respir Dis* 1984; 130:121.

Dubois AB, Bothelo SY, Bedell GH et al: A rapid plethysmographic method for measuring thoracic gas volume: a comparison with a nitrogen washout method for measuring functional residual capacity, *J Clin Invest* 1956; 35:322.

Habib MP, Engel LA: Influence of the panting technique on the plethysmographic measurement of thoracic gas volume, *Am Rev Respir Dis* 1978; 117:265.

Lourenco RV, Chung SYK: Calibration of a body plethysmograph for measurement of lung volume, *Am Rev Respir Dis* 1967; 95:687.

Rodenstein DO, Stanescu DC, Francis C: Demonstration of failure of body plethysmography in airway obstruction, *J Appl Physiol* 1982; 52:949.

GAS DILUTION LUNG VOLUMES

Hathirat S, Renzetti AD, Mitchell M: Measurement of the total lung capacity by helium dilution in a constant volume system, *Am Rev Respir Dis* 1970; 102:760.

McMichael J: A rapid method of determining lung capacity, *Clin Sci* 1939; 4:167.

Meneely GR, Ball CO, Kory RC et al: A simplified closed-circuit helium dilution method for the determination of the residual volume of the lungs, *Am J Med* 1960; 28:824.

Rodenstein DO, Stanescu DC: Reassessment of lung volume measurements by helium dilution and by body plethysmography in chronic airflow obstruction, *Am Rev Respir Dis* 1982; 126:1040.

Schaaning CG, Gulsvik A: Accuracy and precision of helium dilution technique and body plethysmography in measuring lung volume, *Scand J Clin Invest* 1973; 32:271.

GAS DISTRIBUTION

Berend N, Glanville AR, Grunstein MM: Determinants of the slope of phase III of the single-breath nitrogen test, *Bull Eur Physiopathol Respir* 1984; 20:521.

Buist AS, Ross BB: Quantitative analysis of the alveolar plateau in the diagnosis of early airway obstruction, *Am Rev Respir Dis* 1973; 108:1078-1087.

Estenne M, Van Muylem A, Knoop C et al: Detection of obliterative bronchiolitis after lung transplantation by indexes of ventilation distribution, *Am J Respir Crit Care Med* 2000; 162:1047-1051.

Fowler WS: Lung function studies. III. Uneven pulmonary ventilation in normal subjects and in patients with pulmonary disease, *J Appl Physiol* 1949; 2:283.

Hathirat S, Renzetti AD, Mitchell M: Intrapulmonary gas distribution: a comparison of the helium mixing time and nitrogen single-breath test in normal and diseased subjects, *Am Rev Respir Dis* 1970; 102:750.

STANDARDS AND GUIDELINES

American Association for Respiratory Care: Clinical practice guidelines: body plethysmography: 2001 revision and update, *Respir Care* 2001; 46:506-513.

American Association for Respiratory Care: Clinical practice guidelines: static lung volumes: 2001 revision and update, *Respir Care* 2001; 46:531-539.

American Thoracic Society: Lung function testing: selection of reference values and interpretive strategies, *Am Rev Respir Dis* 1991; 144:1202.

British Thoracic Society and Association of Respiratory Technicians and Physiologists: guidelines for the measurement of respiratory function, *Respir Med* 1994; 88:165-194.

Martin R, Macklem PT: Suggested standardization procedures for closing volume determinations (nitrogen method), *DHD-NHLBI*, 1973.

Quanjer PH, Tammeling GJ, Cotes JE et al: Lung volumes and forced ventilatory flows. Report Working Party Standardization of Lung Function Tests, European Community for Steel and Coal. Official Statement of the European Respiratory Society, *Eur Respir J Suppl* 1993; 16:5-40.

Wanger J, Clausen JL, Coates A et al: Standardisation of the measurement of lung volumes. *Eur Respir J* 2006; 26:511-522.

Ventilation and Ventilatory Control Tests

OBJECTIVES

After studying this chapter you will be able to:

Entry-level
1. Describe the measurement of tidal volume and minute ventilation
2. Identify at least two causes of decreased minute ventilation
3. Calculate the V_D/V_T ratio using the modified Bohr equation

Advanced
1. Compare the calculation of V_D/V_T using $PaCO_2$ and $PETCO_2$
2. List at least two causes for an increased V_D/V_T ratio
3. Explain the function of a variable CO_2 scrubber in a circuit for measuring ventilatory response to hypoxia

KEY TERMS

alveolar dead space
alveolar ventilation ($\dot{V}_A$)
anatomic dead space
Bohr equation
end-tidal PCO_2

hypercapnia
hypoxemia
occlusion pressure (P_{100} or $P_{0.1}$)
recruitment
respiratory dead space (V_D)

respiratory exchange ratio (RER)
respiratory frequency (f_B)
tidal volume (V_T)
V_D/V_T ratio
ventilatory response

This chapter discusses the measurement of ventilation and its components: tidal volume (V_T), respiratory frequency (f), and minute ventilation ($\dot{V}_E$). Wasted or dead space ventilation is defined, and techniques for estimating dead space (V_D) and alveolar ventilation ($\dot{V}_A$) are described. Because a variety of diseases can increase dead space, measurements of V_D and the V_D/V_T ratio are used to evaluate many disorders. Ventilation and V_D measurements are used in several different clinical situations. These parameters may be measured in the critical care unit and in the pulmonary function or exercise laboratory.

Assessment of ventilatory responses is closely related to measurement of resting ventilation. The responses to two stimuli, carbon dioxide (CO_2) and oxygen (O_2), are commonly evaluated. **Ventilatory response** is usually assessed by measuring the change in ventilation that occurs with elevated CO_2 (**hypercapnia**) or decreased O_2 (**hypoxemia**). The output of the central respiratory centers is also sometimes measured as the pressure developed during the first tenth of a second when the airway is blocked (P_{100} or $P_{0.1}$).

TIDAL VOLUME, RATE, AND MINUTE VENTILATION

Description

Tidal volume (V_T) is the volume of gas inspired or expired during each respiratory cycle (see Figure 2-1). It is usually measured in liters or milliliters and corrected to BTPS. Conventionally, the volume expired is expressed as V_T. The respiratory rate is the number of breaths per minute (sometimes called breathing frequency or f_B). The total volume of gas expired per minute is $\dot{V}_E$, or minute ventilation. $\dot{V}_E$ includes alveolar and dead space ventilation and is recorded in liters per minute, BTPS.

Technique

V_T can be measured directly by simple spirometry (see Figure 2-1). The patient breathes into a volume-displacement or flow-sensing spirometer (see Chapter 10). Volume change may be measured directly from the excursions of a volume spirometer. V_T may also be measured from an integrated flow signal (see Chapter 10). A graphic representation of tidal breathing can be displayed on a computer screen. Because no two breaths are the same, inhaled or exhaled tidal breaths should be measured for at least 1 minute and then divided by the rate to determine an average volume:

$$V_T = \frac{\dot{V}}{f_B}$$

where:
$\dot{V}$ = volume expired or inspired per minute (usually the $\dot{V}_E$)
f_B = number of breaths for same interval (i.e., the respiratory rate)

The inspired minute volume ($\dot{V}_I$) and V_T are normally slightly greater than the $\dot{V}_E$ because at rest the body produces a slightly lower volume of CO_2 than the volume of O_2 consumed. This exchange difference is termed the **respiratory exchange ratio (RER).** It is calculated as the $\dot{V}CO_2/\dot{V}O_2$, where $\dot{V}CO_2$ is the volume of CO_2 produced and $\dot{V}O_2$ is the volume of O_2 consumed per minute. It is assumed that RER is approximately 0.8 in resting patients. For most clinical purposes, expired volume is measured to calculate V_T.

V_T may also be estimated by means of a respiratory inductive plethysmography (RIP). The RIP uses coils of wire as transducers that respond to changes in the cross-sectional area of the rib cage and abdominal compartments. With appropriate calibration, inductive plethysmography can be used to measure V_T. This method allows measurement of V_T and minute ventilation without direct connection to the patient's airway.

PF TIP

Not all spirometers allow bidirectional breathing (i.e., breathing in and out of the spirometer). For flow-based spirometers that do not measure flow in both directions, a one-way breathing circuit may be used. To measure ventilation with a volume-based spirometer, the subject rebreathes; CO_2 must be removed and O_2 added for prolonged measurements.

Respiratory frequency (f_B) may be determined by counting chest movements, noting the excursions of a volume displacement spirometer (Ventilation 4-1), or most commonly by measuring flow changes while the subject breathes through a flow-sensing spirometer. Counting the rate for several minutes and taking an average produces a more accurate value than shorter measurements. Prolonged measurement of V_T and rate with a volume-displacement spirometer requires a means of removing CO_2. This is called a rebreathing system and uses a chemical CO_2 absorber (see Figure 3-1, *B*). Sodium hydroxide crystals (Sodasorb) or barium hydroxide crystals (Baralyme) are commonly used to scrub CO_2 from rebreathing systems. Flow-sensing spirometers usually do not require a chemical absorber.

The $\dot{V}_E$ may be measured by allowing the patient to breathe into or out of a volume- displacement or flow-sensing spirometer for at least 1 minute. A shorter breathing interval can be used with minute volume extrapolated but may give a misleading estimate of ventilation if the patient's breathing rate is irregular. If a rebreathing system is used, a CO_2 absorber must be included, as well as a means of replenishing O_2. Measuring expired gas volume for several minutes and dividing by the time gives an average $\dot{V}_E$. $\dot{V}_E$, measured from expired gas, is usually slightly smaller than $\dot{V}_I$ because of the RER as described previously. For most clinical purposes, this difference is negligible. BTPS corrections should be made.

Significance and Pathophysiology

See Ventilation 4-2 for interpretive strategies. Average V_T for healthy adults at rest ranges between 400 and 700 ml, but there is considerable variation. Decreased V_T occurs in many types of pulmonary disorders, particularly those that cause severe restrictive patterns. Pulmonary fibrosis and neuro-muscular diseases (e.g., myasthenia gravis) often cause reduced V_T. Decreased tidal breathing usually accompanies changes in the mechanical properties of the lungs or chest wall (i.e., compliance and resistance). These changes usually produce an increased respiratory rate (f_B) required to maintain an adequate $\dot{V}_A$. Decreases in both V_T and respiratory rate are often associated with respiratory center depression because of drugs or pathologic conditions affecting the brain stem. Low V_T and rate usually result in alveolar hypoventilation.

Some patients who have pulmonary disease may exhibit increased V_T, particularly at rest. The V_T alone is not a good indicator of the adequacy of

---

VENTILATION 4-1

CRITERIA FOR ACCEPTABILITY

Tidal Volume, Rate, Minute Ventilation

1. V_T averaged from at least 60 seconds of ventilatory data; either accumulated volume divided by respiratory rate or multiple breaths summed and averaged.
2. $\dot{V}_E$ measured for at least 60 seconds; one-way breathing circuit or appropriate rebreathing system used. Repeated measurements should be within 10%.
3. Respiratory rate measured for at least 15 seconds; longer intervals may be necessary for patients with disordered breathing patterns.

VENTILATION 4-2

INTERPRETIVE STRATEGIES

Tidal Volume, Rate, Minute Ventilation

1. Were V_T, respiratory rate, and $\dot{V}_E$ measured appropriately? Was the data collection adequate? Did the ventilatory pattern (i.e., rate or tidal volume) change during the measurements? If so, suspect breathing circuit problems.
2. Is the pattern of ventilation consistent with the patient's clinical status?
3. Is V_T, respiratory rate, and/or $\dot{V}_E$ excessive? If so, suspect hyperventilation. Arterial blood gases (pH and $PaCO_2$) may be necessary to document respiratory alkalosis.
4. Is V_T, respiratory rate, and/or $\dot{V}_E$ decreased? If so, suspect hypoventilation. Arterial blood gases (pH and $PaCO_2$) may be necessary to document respiratory acidosis.

alveolar ventilation ($\dot{V}_A$). Tidal volume should always be considered in conjunction with respiratory rate and $\dot{V}_E$. Many healthy patients display increased V_T simply because of breathing into the pulmonary function apparatus with the nose occluded. Estimates of resting ventilation may be artifactually increased when measured during pulmonary function testing. Some subjects adopt unusual breathing strategies (e.g., large tidal volumes with slow respiratory rate or small tidal volumes with rapid breathing rates) during exercise or stress for nonphysiologic reasons.

The normal respiratory rate (f_B) ranges from 10–20 breaths/min in adults. Increased demand for ventilation, such as during exercise, usually results in increases in both the rate and depth of breathing (i.e., the tidal volume). Increases or decreases in the respiratory rate are indications of a change in the ventilatory status. Breathing frequency, when evaluated with the V_T, may be used as an index of ventilation. Hypoxia, hypercapnia, metabolic acidosis, decreased lung compliance, and exercise can all result in increased respiratory rate. Rapid breathing rates and small tidal volumes may suggest increased V_D or hypoventilation but must be correlated with arterial pH and PCO_2 values to confirm those conditions. Decreased breathing frequency is common in central nervous system depression and in CO_2 narcosis. Respiratory rate may be falsely elevated in patients connected to unfamiliar breathing circuits, with or without a nose clip.

Normal $\dot{V}_E$ ranges from 5–10 L/min in healthy adults with wide variations in normal patients. The $\dot{V}_E$, when used in conjunction with blood gas values, indicates the adequacy of ventilation. $\dot{V}_E$ is the sum of the $\dot{V}_D$ (dead space ventilation per minute) and $\dot{V}_A$. Because the relative proportions of these components can change, absolute values for $\dot{V}_E$ do not necessarily indicate either hypoventilation or hyperventilation. In other words, low minute ventilation does not necessarily indicate hypoventilation. Similarly, elevated $\dot{V}_E$ does not indicate hyperventilation. To make these diagnoses, arterial pH and PCO_2 must be measured.

A large $\dot{V}_E$ at rest (greater than 20 L/min) may result from an enlarged V_D because an increase in total ventilation is required to maintain adequate

$\dot{V}_A$. $\dot{V}_E$ increases in response to hypoxia, hypercapnia, metabolic acidosis, anxiety, and exercise. Hyperventilation is ventilation in excess of that needed to adequately remove CO_2, resulting in respiratory alkalosis.

Decreased ventilation may result from hypocapnia, metabolic alkalosis, respiratory center depression, or neuromuscular disorders that involve the ventilatory muscles. Hypoventilation is defined as inadequate ventilation to maintain a normal arterial PCO_2, with respiratory acidosis as the result. The diagnosis of either hyperventilation or hypoventilation requires blood gas analysis (see Chapter 6).

RESPIRATORY DEAD SPACE AND ALVEOLAR VENTILATION

Description

Respiratory dead space (V_D) is the lung volume that is ventilated but not perfused by pulmonary capillary blood flow. V_D can be divided into the conducting airways, or **anatomic dead space,** and the nonperfused alveoli, or **alveolar dead space.** The combination of alveolar and anatomic dead space is respiratory (or physiologic) dead space. V_D is recorded in milliliters or liters, BTPS.

$\dot{V}_A$ is the volume of gas that participates in gas exchange in the lungs. It can be expressed as:

$$\dot{V}_A = \dot{V}_E - \dot{V}_D$$

where:

$\dot{V}_A$ = alveolar ventilation
$\dot{V}_E$ = minute ventilation
$\dot{V}_D$ = dead space ventilation per minute

For a single breath, the V_A equals the V_T minus the V_D. $\dot{V}_A$ is usually expressed in liters per minute, BTPS.

Technique

Dead Space

Anatomic dead space is sometimes estimated from an individual's body size as 1 ml/lb of ideal body weight. The actual respiratory dead space, however, is of greater clinical importance. V_D can be calculated in two ways. The first uses the Enghoff modification of Bohr's equation defining V_D:

$$V_D = \frac{F_ACO_2 - F_{\bar{E}}CO_2}{F_ACO_2} \times V_T$$

where:
V_T = tidal volume
F_ACO_2 = fraction of CO_2 in alveolar gas
$F_{\bar{E}}CO_2$ = fraction of CO_2 in mixed expired gas

Because the fractional concentration of alveolar CO_2 is difficult to measure, partial pressure of CO_2 may be substituted and the equation written as follows:

$$V_D = \frac{(PaCO_2 - P_{\bar{E}}CO_2)}{PaCO_2} \times V_T$$

where:
$PaCO_2$ = arterial PCO_2
$P_{\bar{E}}CO_2$ = PCO_2 of mixed expired gas sample

Note that the $PaCO_2$ is substituted for the alveolar PCO_2. This substitution presumes perfect equilibration between alveoli and pulmonary capillaries. This may not be true in certain diseases. The test also assumes that little CO_2 is in the atmosphere. Therefore the PCO_2 in expired gas is inversely proportional to the V_D. Exhaled gas is collected over a short interval, and arterial blood is obtained simultaneously to measure $PaCO_2$. V_D is calculated by applying the previous equation. The estimate usually becomes more representative as more expired gas is collected. Accuracy depends on measurement of V_T (usually derived from $\dot{V}_E$ and f_B) and on the precision of the partial pressures of CO_2 measured in expired gas and arterial blood. The mixed expired gas sample is usually collected in a bag or balloon after filling and emptying it several times with expired gas to wash out room air from the valves, tubing, and bag itself. The volume of gas in the bag can be measured during collection by including a flow-sensing spirometer in the circuit. If $\dot{V}_E$ and respiratory rate are recorded, the volumes of V_D and V_T can be determined. If expired volume is not measured, only a dilution ratio can be determined; this is called the **V_D/V_T ratio.**

The V_D/V_T ratio can be calculated if arterial and mixed-expired PCO_2 values are known. It can also be estimated noninvasively. **End-tidal PCO_2** (see the section on capnography in Chapter 6) can be used to estimate $PaCO_2$. The main advantage of this method is that it is not necessary to obtain an arterial blood sample. This technique is often used in systems that monitor expired CO_2 continuously and in breath-by-breath metabolic measurement devices. V_D/V_T may be calculated as follows:

$$\frac{V_D}{V_T} = \frac{(PETCO_2 - P_{\bar{E}}CO_2)}{PETCO_2}$$

where:
$PETCO_2$ = end-tidal PCO_2
$P_{\bar{E}}CO_2$ = PCO_2 of mixed-expired gas sample

PF TIP

Dead space consists of anatomic and alveolar components. Anatomic dead space is usually estimated from body weight (1 ml/lb ideal body weight). Respiratory dead space, measured using mixed-expired and arterial CO_2, measures both components.

In some patients, particularly those with severe obstruction, $PETCO_2$ may not accurately reflect $PaCO_2$. Consequently, the V_D/V_T ratio may be estimated incorrectly. $PaCO_2$ should be used in the V_D calculation whenever possible.

Alveolar Ventilation

$\dot{V}_A$ can be calculated in two ways:

$$\dot{V}_A = f_B(V_T - V_D)$$

where:
V_T = tidal volume
V_D = respiratory dead space
f_B = respiratory rate

For convenience, V_D is often estimated as equal to anatomic dead space. This method is valid only when there is little or no alveolar dead space, as in individuals who do not have pulmonary disease.

Because atmospheric gas contains almost no CO_2, $\dot{V}_A$ can be calculated on the basis of CO_2 elimination from the lungs. A volume of expired gas may be collected in a bag, balloon, or spirometer and analyzed to determine the volume of CO_2 (see Chapter 7). The following equation can then be used:

$$\dot{V}_A = \frac{\dot{V}CO_2}{F_ACO_2}$$

where:

$\dot{V}CO_2$ = volume of CO_2 produced in liters per minute (STPD)

F_ACO_2 = fractional concentration of CO_2 in alveolar gas

If an end-tidal CO_2 monitor (i.e., a capnograph) is used, a close approximation of the concentration of alveolar CO_2 is easily obtained, and the equation is simplified as follows:

$$\dot{V}_A = \frac{\dot{V}CO_2}{\% \text{ alveolar } CO_2} \times 100$$

End-tidal CO_2 may not equal alveolar CO_2 in patients with grossly abnormal patterns of ventilation-perfusion (see Chapter 6).

The same equation can be used substituting $PaCO_2$ for the alveolar PCO_2 (i.e., P_ACO_2), again presuming that arterial blood and alveolar gas are in equilibrium. The equation is then as follows:

$$\dot{V}_A = \frac{\dot{V}CO_2}{PaCO_2} \times 0.863$$

where:

$\dot{V}CO_2$ = CO_2 production in ml/min (STPD)

$PaCO_2$ = partial pressure of arterial CO_2

0.863 = conversion factor (concentration to partial pressure, correcting $\dot{V}CO_2$ to BTPS)

Significance and Pathophysiology

See Ventilation 4-3 for interpretive strategies. Measurement of V_D yields important information regarding the ventilation-perfusion characteristics of the lungs. Anatomic dead space is larger in men than in women because of differences in body size.

VENTILATION 4-3

INTERPRETIVE STRATEGIES

V_D and $\dot{V}_A$

1. Was dead space determination based on $PaCO_2$? If not, interpret cautiously.
2. Was $\dot{V}_E$ or V_T measured? If not, then interpret only V_D/V_T.
3. Is the V_D/V_T ratio greater than 0.40? If so, elevated dead space is likely. Consider clinical correlation, especially pulmonary embolism or pulmonary hypertension.
4. Is the V_D/V_T ratio less than 0.20 with the patient at rest? Is there an elevated level of ventilation? Consider technical problems.
5. Is $\dot{V}_A$ (if measured) consistent with the patient's clinical signs and symptoms?

It increases along with the V_T during exercise, as well as in certain forms of pulmonary disease (e.g., bronchiectasis). It may be decreased in asthma or in diseases characterized by bronchial obstruction or mucus plugging. Because of the difficulty in measuring the anatomic dead space, estimates based on age, sex, functional residual capacity, or body size may be used. For clinical purposes, anatomic dead space in milliliters is sometimes considered equal to the patient's ideal body weight in pounds.

Of greater clinical significance is the measurement of respiratory dead space, which is accomplished reasonably well by applying the **Bohr equation.** The portion of ventilation wasted on the conducting airways and poorly perfused alveoli is usually expressed as the V_D/V_T ratio. The normal value for V_D/V_T in adults is about 0.3 (with a range of 0.2–0.4). V_D/V_T is also commonly expressed as a percentage, with a value of 30% considered normal. Expressing dead space in this way eliminates the need to measure the volume of expired gas in the Bohr equation. However, if V_T or $\dot{V}_E$ is known, dead space volume can be easily calculated. Physiologic dead space measurements are a good index of ventilation-blood flow ratios because all CO_2 in expired gas comes from perfused alveoli (see Chapter 6). If there were no dead space in the lung, arterial and mixed-expired CO_2 would be equal. As the difference between arterial and mixed-expired CO_2 increases, the volume of "wasted" ventilation rises.

The V_D/V_T ratio decreases in healthy subjects during exercise. As cardiac output increases, perfusion of alveoli at the lung apices also increases. This increased perfusion is referred to as **recruitment**. Alveoli at the apices are poorly perfused at rest, accounting for some of the normal resting dead space. Both V_D and V_T increase with exercise. In healthy individuals, the V_T increases more than V_D; thus the ratio decreases.

Increased dead space, and V_D/V_T ratio, may be observed in pulmonary embolism and in pulmonary hypertension. In pulmonary embolism, large numbers of arterioles may be blocked, resulting in little or no CO_2 removal in the associated alveoli. In pulmonary hypertension, increased pulmonary arterial pressure causes most alveoli to be perfused, so there is little or no recruitment of underperfused gas exchange units. This is most notable during exercise when the V_D/V_T ratio normally decreases. In both pulmonary embolism and hypertension, the patient may be very short of breath (i.e., dyspneic) because of the increased dead space.

The $\dot{V}_A$ at rest is approximately 4–5 L/min with wide variations in healthy adults. The adequacy of $\dot{V}_A$ can be determined only by arterial blood gas studies. Low $\dot{V}_A$ associated with acute respiratory acidosis ($PaCO_2$ greater than 45 and pH less than 7.35 in healthy patients) defines hypoventilation. Excessive $\dot{V}_A$ ($PaCO_2$ less than 35 and pH greater than 7.45 in healthy patients) defines hyperventilation. Chronic hypoventilation and hyperventilation are associated with abnormal $PaCO_2$ values but near-normal pH values (see Chapter 6). Decreased $\dot{V}_A$ can result from absolute increases in dead space and decreases in $\dot{V}_E$.

VENTILATORY RESPONSE TESTS FOR CARBON DIOXIDE AND OXYGEN

Description

Ventilatory response to CO_2 is a measurement of the increase or decrease in $\dot{V}_E$ caused by breathing various concentrations of CO_2 under normoxic conditions ($PaO_2 \approx 100$ mm Hg). It is recorded as L/min/mm Hg PCO_2.

Ventilatory response to O_2 is a measurement of the increase or decrease in $\dot{V}_E$ caused by breathing various concentrations of O_2 under isocapnic conditions ($PaCO_2 \approx 40$ mm Hg). The change in ventilation (in liters per minute) may be recorded in relation to changes in PaO_2 or saturation as monitored by oximetry.

Occlusion pressure (P_{100} or $P_{0.1}$) is the pressure generated at the mouth during the first 100 msec of an inspiratory effort against an occluded airway. Changes in P_{100} are related to changes in the ventilatory stimulant (hypercapnia or hypoxemia). P_{100} is usually measured in centimeters of water (cm H_2O).

Technique

The response to increasing levels of CO_2 (hypercapnia) can be measured in two ways:

1. *Open-circuit technique.* The patient breathes increasing concentrations (1%–7%) of CO_2 in air or O_2 from a demand valve or reservoir until a steady state is reached. Measurements of $PETCO_2$, $PaCO_2$, P_{100}, and $\dot{V}_E$ may be made at each concentration.

2. *Closed-circuit or rebreathing technique.* The patient rebreathes from a reservoir (usually an anesthesia bag) of 7% CO_2 in O_2. The breathing circuit usually includes ports for pressure monitoring (P_{100}), and for extracting gas samples ($PETCO_2$). A pneumotachometer is placed in the rebreathing circuit to record $\dot{V}_E$. Alternatively, the gas reservoir bag may be placed in a rigid container or box, and volume change measured by connecting a spirometer to the container (i.e., "bag-in-box" setup). The patient rebreathes until the concentration of $PETCO_2$ exceeds 9% or until 4 minutes have elapsed. The rebreathed gas may be analyzed to ensure that the FIO_2 remains above 0.21. The patient's SpO_2 may also be monitored by means of a pulse oximeter. Changes in $\dot{V}_E$ are monitored and plotted against $PETCO_2$ to obtain a response curve. A plot of $\dot{V}_E$ versus

$PETCO_2$ may be used to determine a slope or response curve. The CO_2 response curve may be extrapolated backward to determine the PCO_2 at which ventilation would be zero. This PCO_2 is termed the threshold and is sometimes used as a measure of sensitivity to the ventilatory stimulant.

Response to decreasing levels of O_2 (hypoxemia) can also be measured by either open-circuit or closed-circuit techniques:

1. *Open-circuit technique.* The patient breathes gas mixtures containing O_2 concentrations from 20%–12%, to which CO_2 is added to maintain

alveolar PCO_2 ($PaCO_2$) at a constant level. When a steady state is reached, PaO_2, $\dot{V}_E$, and P_{100} can be measured. This procedure, often called a step test, is repeated with decreasing O_2 concentrations to produce the response curve. Continuous monitoring of $PETCO_2$ is necessary to titrate addition of CO_2 to the system to maintain isocapnia (Figure 4-1). Pulse oximetry may be used to monitor changes in saturation. CO_2 response curves are sometimes measured at widely varying PaO_2 levels, and the subsequent difference in ventilation or P_{100} at any particular PCO_2 is attributed to the response to hypoxemia.

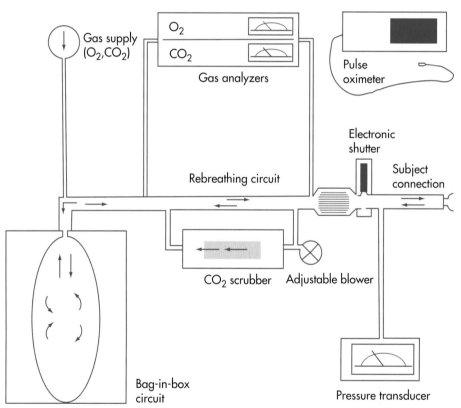

FIGURE 4-1   Closed-Circuit System for the Rebreathing O_2 Response Test. The circuit allows the patient to rebreathe from a bag to which CO_2 or O_2 can be added. Gas analyzers allow continuous monitoring of gas concentrations in the circuit during testing. Ventilation is measured by integrating flow from the pneumotachometer or attaching a spirometer to the bag-in-box setup. A pressure transducer and mouth shutter allow the measurement of P_{100}, and a pulse oximeter provides data on the patient's saturation. A CO_2 scrubber with an adjustable blower allows the level of CO_2 in the system to be maintained at baseline levels (isocapnia). Increases in ventilation caused by the gradual consumption of O_2 in the circuit can be measured by scrubbing just enough of the exhaled CO_2 to maintain a near-normal alveolar PCO_2. A similar circuit can be used to measure response to CO_2 by rebreathing. The bag is filled with 5%–7% CO_2 in O_2, and the scrubber is removed from the circuit.

2. *Closed-circuit technique (progressive hypoxemia)*. The patient rebreathes from a system similar to that used for the closed-circuit CO_2 response, but the system contains a CO_2 scrubber. CO_2 can be added to the inspired gas to maintain isocapnia, or an adjustable blower may be used to direct a portion of the rebreathed gas through the scrubber to maintain isocapnia (see Figure 4-1). Response to decreasing inspired PO_2 is monitored by recording $\dot{V}_E$ or P_{100}, and the PaO_2 or saturation is measured either directly by indwelling catheter or by pulse oximetry.

PF TIP

To measure response to hypoxemia, it is necessary to maintain a constant level of CO_2 (isocapnia). To measure response to hypercapnia, it is necessary to maintain normoxia (PaO_2 of 80–100 mm Hg).

VENTILATION 4-4

CRITERIA FOR ACCEPTABILITY

Ventilatory Response Tests

1. CO_2 response—Appropriate concentrations of CO_2 (i.e., 7% CO_2 in O_2 for rebreathing studies) must be used.
2. CO_2 response—Normoxia maintained; subject's SpO_2 should remain >95% during testing.
3. O_2 response—FIO_2 appropriate to induce hypoxic response; isocapnia demonstrated by monitoring $PETCO_2$.
4. P_{100}—Pressure transducer and monitor capable of recording up to 50 cm H_2O with a recorder speed of 50–100 mm/sec. Occlusion device should be hidden from the patient.
5. Ventilatory responses (O_2, CO_2) should be reproducible within 10%; average of two trials should be reported if clinically practical.
6. Reported P_{100} should be the average of three or more occlusions at each level of challenge.

P_{100} is measured with a system similar to that in Figure 4-1. A port at the mouth records pressure changes versus time, by means of a computer or high-speed recorder. A large-bore stopcock or electronic shutter mechanism is included in the inspiratory line so that inspiratory flow can be randomly occluded. The stopcock or shutter can be closed so that inspiration occurs against a complete occlusion near functional residual capacity. The entire apparatus is usually hidden so that the patient is unaware of the impending airway occlusion. A pressure-time curve is recorded. P_{100} is usually measured at varying $PETCO_2$ values or levels of desaturation to assess the effect of changing stimuli to ventilation. P_{100} and $\dot{V}_E$ are usually graphed against $PETCO_2$ (Figure 4-2) or versus O_2 saturation (for O_2 response tests). See Ventilation 4-4 for acceptability criteria for ventilatory response measurements.

Significance and Pathophysiology

See Ventilation 4-5 for interpretive strategies. The response to an increase in $PaCO_2$ in a normal individual is a linear increase in $\dot{V}_E$ of approximately

3 L/min/mm Hg (PCO_2). The normal range of response varies from 1–6 L/min/mm Hg PCO_2. Some variation is present in repeated testing of the same individual. The response to CO_2 in patients who have obstructive disease may be reduced. This is partially attributable to increased airway resistance, which has been shown to reduce ventilatory drive in healthy individuals. It is unclear why some patients who have obstructive disease increase ventilation to maintain a normal $PaCO_2$, whereas others tolerate an increased $PaCO_2$. Genetic variation in drive may explain some of the differences in blood gas tensions in patients with chronic obstructive pulmonary disease (COPD). Lesions in the central nervous system may also cause a decreased sensitivity to CO_2. Some individuals who have no respiratory muscle weakness, mechanical ventilatory problems, or neurologic disease have a decreased sensitivity to CO_2. This condition is described as primary alveolar hypoventilation. These patients can lower their PCO_2 by voluntary hyperventilation.

The normal response to a decrease in PaO_2 varies depending on the level of PCO_2 at which the measurement is made. There is little change in ventilation until the PaO_2 falls to less than 60 mm Hg. The

---

VENTILATION 4-5

INTERPRETIVE STRATEGIES

Ventilatory Response Tests

1. CO_2 response—Were appropriate levels of elevated CO_2 attained? If rebreathing was used, was test terminated at 4 minutes or an F_ECO_2 of 0.09 (9%)?
2. CO_2 response—Was normoxia maintained? Did SpO_2 demonstrate adequate saturation? If not, interpretation may be compromised.
3. O_2 response—Were appropriate low levels of FIO_2 attained? Was isocapnia maintained as demonstrated by $PETCO_2$? If not, interpretation may be compromised.
4. Were repeat tests reproducible? If not, interpret cautiously.
5. CO_2 response—Did ventilation increase by at least 1 L/mm Hg change in $PETCO_2$? If not, decreased ventilatory response to CO_2 is likely.
6. O_2 response—Did ventilation increase exponentially at SpO_2 levels less than 90%? If not, suspect decreased ventilatory response to hypoxia.
7. P_{100}—Was the occlusion pressure appropriate for the baseline $PaCO_2$ (1.5–5.0 cm H_2O at a $PaCO_2$ of 40 mm Hg)? Did P_{100} increase by at least 0.5 cm H_2O/mm Hg change in $PETCO_2$? If not, a decreased central ventilatory drive is likely.

response appears to be exponential once the PaO_2 has fallen to the range of 40–60 mm Hg, and it varies widely between individuals on a genetically determined basis. The hypoxic response is increased in the presence of hypercapnia and decreased in hypocapnia. Patients who have severe COPD with CO_2 retention receive their primary respiratory stimulus from the hypoxemic response. This group of patients may experience severe or even fatal respiratory depression if that response is obliterated by uncontrolled O_2 therapy.

Some patients with minimal intrinsic lung disease show markedly decreased response to hypoxemia or hypercapnia. These include patients with myxedema, obesity-hypoventilation syndrome, obstructive sleep apnea, and idiopathic hypoventilation. CO_2 and O_2 response measurements, along with tests of pulmonary mechanics, may be particularly valuable in the evaluation and treatment of these types of patients.

The P_{100} ($P_{0.1}$) has been suggested as a measurement of ventilatory drive independent of the mechanical properties of the lungs. Because no airflow occurs during occlusion of the airway, significant interference from mechanical abnormalities (e.g., increased resistance or decreased compliance) is omitted. Reflexes from the airways and chest wall are also of little influence during the first 100 msec of the occluded breath. Therefore the pressure generated can be viewed as proportional to the neural output of the medullary centers that drive the rate and depth of breathing. This proportionality may be influenced by other factors, however, such as body position and the contractile properties of the respiratory muscles.

Individuals with normal $PaCO_2$ values have P_{100} values in the range of 1.5–5 cm H_2O. P_{100} has been shown to increase in hypercapnia and hypoxia and appears to correlate well with the observed ventilatory responses. Increasing PCO_2, and thereby inducing hypercapnia, in healthy patients typically results in an increase in the occlusion pressure of 0.5–0.6 cm H_2O/mm Hg PCO_2, with as much as 20% variability. Healthy subjects increase their P_{100} when breathing through artificial resistance on challenge with high PCO_2 or low PO_2. Some patients who have chronic airway obstruction demonstrate no increase in P_{100} in response to increasing PCO_2, even with increased airway resistance. This failure to respond to increased resistance in the airways may predispose individuals with COPD to respiratory failure when lung infections occur. Similarly, patients supported by mechanical ventilation may be difficult to wean if their ventilatory drive is compromised, as demonstrated by failure to increase P_{100} when challenged with increased PCO_2. Determination of P_{100} may prove helpful in determining the effects of treatment in patients who have abnormal ventilatory responses.

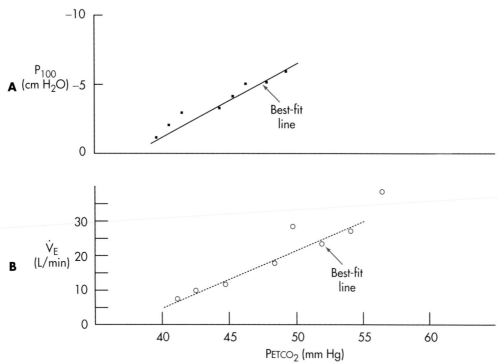

FIGURE 4-2   A, P_{100} plotted against end-tidal CO_2 ($PETCO_2$), as might be obtained during a CO_2 rebreathing study. **B,** Minute ventilation plotted against $PETCO_2$ during the same study. Individual points may be plotted and a "best-fit" line constructed by statistical methods. The slope of the best-fit line is the rate at which ventilation or occlusion pressure increases with increasing stimulation from the rebreathed CO_2.

SUMMARY

- This chapter discusses measurement of $\dot{V}_E$, V_T, respiratory rate, alveolar ventilation, dead space, and the ventilatory responses to hypercapnia and hypoxemia.
- Resting ventilatory measurements can be used in conjunction with blood gases to evaluate respiratory status.
- One of the most important parameters is the respiratory or physiologic dead space. An estimate of wasted ventilation can be made by comparing expired CO_2 with arterial PCO_2. Dead space and reduced $\dot{V}_A$ are common in many pulmonary disorders. When dead space

increases, ventilation must increase to maintain a normal acid-base status.
- Disorders of ventilatory control are also common to many diseases. Evaluation of responses to hypoxemia and hypercapnia are often useful in characterizing types of ventilatory response disorders. Different techniques of assessing responses have been described.
- The rebreathing techniques for O_2 and CO_2 are used most often. P_{100} can discriminate central ventilatory drive problems from other causes of abnormal responses.

CASE 4-1

Case Studies

HISTORY

T.J. is a 45-year-old man admitted to the hospital for acute shortness of breath. He has never smoked but has a family history of heart disease. His lungs are clear during auscultation. He becomes breathless just moving around his hospital room. He denies any recent respiratory infections. Because of his rapid respiratory rate, his attending physician requested an arterial blood gas test using room air and a V_D/V_T ratio determination.

PULMONARY FUNCTION STUDIES

Personal Data

Age:	45
Height:	67 in (170 cm)
Weight:	175 lb (80 kg)
Race:	White

Blood Gas Analysis

pH	7.49
P_{CO_2} (mm Hg)	29
P_{O_2} (mm Hg)	102
HCO_3^- (mEq/L)	21
Hb (g/dl)	14.2
Sa_{O_2} (%)	98

Exhaled Gas Analysis

$\dot{V}_E$ (L/min)	24.20
f_B (breaths/min)	20
$P_{\bar{E}CO_2}$ (mm Hg)	14

QUESTIONS

1. Determine the following for this patient:
   - V_T
   - V_D/V_T
   - $\dot{V}_A$
2. What is the interpretation of the patient's ventilation?
3. What other tests might be indicated?
4. What treatment might be indicated based on these findings?

DISCUSSION

Calculations

a.
$$V_T = \frac{\dot{V}_E}{f_B}$$
$$= \frac{24.2}{20}$$
$$V_T = 1.21 L$$

b.
$$\frac{V_D}{V_T} = \frac{(Pa_{CO_2} - P_{\bar{E}CO_2})}{Pa_{CO_2}}$$
$$= \frac{(29-14)}{29}$$
$$\frac{V_D}{V_T} = 0.517$$

c.
$$\dot{V}_A = f_B(V_T - V_D)$$

where:
$$V_D = \frac{V_D}{V_T}(V_T)$$
$$= 0.517(1.21)$$
$$V_D = 0.626$$

Substituting this value in the alveolar ventilation equation:

$$\dot{V}_A = 20(1.21 - 0.626)$$
$$= 20(0.584)$$
$$\dot{V}_A = 11.68$$

Ventilation

This patient has a rapid respiratory rate and a large V_T. The result of this is a large $\dot{V}_E$ (i.e., 24.2 L/min). The blood gas analysis shows hyperventilation (respiratory alkalosis) consistent with excessive ventilation. The V_D/V_T ratio is increased at 52% (0.517 as a fraction). Healthy patients have V_D/V_T ratios of 30%–40% at rest. In effect, this patient is wasting more than half of each breath. Calculation of the $\dot{V}_A$ similarly reveals that less than half of his $\dot{V}_E$ is actually available for gas exchange. To maintain a normal Pa_{CO_2} (or in this case, to hyperventilate), patients who have increased dead space must increase their total ventilation. Large increases in dead space can occur as a result of obstruction of pulmonary arterial vessels by blood clots or similar lesions. Congestion of pulmonary vessels (resulting from pulmonary hypertension) can also cause imbalances in ventilation-perfusion ratios, especially during exercise.

Other Tests

Other diagnostic procedures that might be indicated include perfusion or ventilation-perfusion scanning of the lungs. Perfusion scans can identify areas of the lung in which there is little or no blood flow. $\dot{V}/\dot{Q}$ scans can detect which areas of the lungs have decreased blood flow in relation to their ventilation. These imaging tests are often used when pulmonary emboli are suspected. Ventilation-perfusion scans of T.J. indicated multiple areas of decreased perfusion in both lower lobes, consistent with multiple pulmonary emboli.

Treatment

The patient had been given O_2 therapy after the blood gas test results were obtained. Because there was adequate oxygenation on room air, the O_2 therapy was inappropriate and was discontinued. After the lung scans, the patient was started on anticoagulant therapy (heparin). During the next week, the pattern of pulmonary embolization gradually resolved. His ventilation and V_D/V_T ratio returned to normal.

CASE 4-2

Case Studies

HISTORY

T.B. is a 37-year-old white male who is 69 inches tall and weighs 275 pounds (BMI = $40.6\,kg/m^2$). He was referred to the pulmonary function laboratory after an evaluation in the sleep laboratory revealed obstructive sleep apnea (OSA). He admits to daytime somnolence. Baseline pulmonary function studies revealed the following:

	Actual	% Predicted
FVC (L)	3.2	72
FEV₁ (L)	2.7	81
TLC (L)	4.1	71
RV/TLC	22%	

Baseline blood gas results were as follows:

pH	7.36
P_{CO_2} (mm Hg)	47
P_{O_2} (mm Hg)	77
HCO_3^- (mEq/L)	28
Sa_{O_2} (%)	93

A CO_2 response test (rebreathing method) was performed to assess the patient's respiratory drive. T.B. rebreathed a mixture of 7% CO_2 in O_2 for 4 minutes. Triplicate measurements of P_{100} were made at intervals throughout the test with a pneumatically operated occlusion valve. The following data were obtained:

P_{ETCO_2} (mm Hg)	$\dot{V}_E$ (L/min)	P_{100} (cm H_2O)
43	4.5	2.2
46	4.4	—
50	5.9	—
54	7.9	7.8
57	15.1	—
59	17.1	12.0

QUESTIONS

1. What is the interpretation of:
   a. Ventilatory response to CO_2 stimulation?
   b. Respiratory drive response to CO_2 stimulation?
2. What is the cause of the patient's daytime somnolence?
3. What treatment(s) might be indicated based on these findings?

DISCUSSION

Interpretation

All data obtained during the CO_2 rebreathing test were acceptable. The P_{ETCO_2} increased appropriately, and the test was terminated after 4 minutes of rebreathing. P_{100} was obtained at baseline, after 2 minutes, and near the end of the test. All pressures were repeatable, and the average values were reported. Ventilatory response was diminished at 0.8 L/mm Hg P_{CO_2}. P_{100} appeared to increase appropriately.

Impression: Markedly reduced ventilatory response to CO_2, with a normal occlusion pressure.

Cause of Symptoms

This patient, who has documented sleep apnea, also displays a reduced sensitivity to increasing levels of CO_2. His spirometry and total lung capacity show a restrictive pattern. His baseline blood gases indicate mild CO_2 retention. His slightly elevated HCO_3^- suggests that this is a chronic condition. The P_{O_2} is mildly reduced as a result of hypoventilation.

The CO_2 rebreathing test documents that the patient does not increase his ventilation appropriately in response to an increasing load of CO_2 (Figure 4-3). At the same time, the patient's P_{100} shows a relatively normal response to hypercapnia. This pattern suggests that the patient does not increase ventilation, although his respiratory center is signaling otherwise. These find-

continued

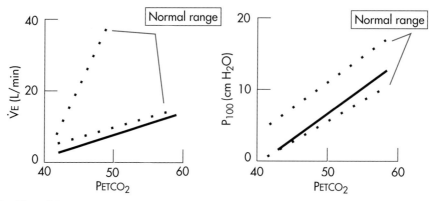

FIGURE 4-3   Plot of Data.

ings are consistent with his obstructive sleep apnea. Patients who retain CO_2 because of large airway or small airway obstruction often have reduced sensitivity to elevated CO_2. This patient might be suspected of having obesity-hypoventilation syndrome. However, patients with obesity-hypoventilation typically have a decreased central drive to ventilation along with their daytime hypercapnia. Obesity-hypoventilation is often associated with OSA or central apnea and usually involves severe hypoxemia and hypercapnia. T.B. has less severe blood gas abnormalities and a normal respiratory drive (P_{100}),

suggesting a different cause for the reduced ventilatory response to CO_2.

Treatment

This patient's treatment was nasal continuous positive airway pressure (CPAP) at night. Nasal CPAP alleviates much of the obstruction occurring in the upper airway. The patient reported a marked decrease in daytime hypersomnolence. He was also referred for weight-loss counseling because his increased weight and reduced ventilatory response placed him at increased risk for pulmonary and cardiac complications.

SELF-ASSESSMENT QUESTIONS

Entry-level

1. During a rebreathing test, a patient with COPD has his ventilation measured for 3 minutes with the following results:

   Total volume expired: 12.4 L (BTPS)
   Total breaths: 30

   This patient's VT is approximately _____?
   a. 0.10 L (BTPS)
   b. 0.41 L (BTPS)
   c. 1.24 L (BTPS)
   d. 4.13 L (BTPS)

2. Decreased minute ventilation might be expected in which of the following conditions?
   a. Hypercapnia with acidosis
   b. Mild hypoxemia
   c. Respiratory center depression
   d. Compensated metabolic acidosis

3. In order to calculate the V_D/V_T ratio, what else is needed in addition to the mixed expired CO_2 ($P_{\bar{E}CO_2}$)?

   I. V_T
   II. $\dot{V}_E$
   III. $PaCO_2$
   IV. $P_{ET}CO_2$
      a. I and II
      b. Either I or II
      c. Either III or IV
      d. I and IV

4. An outpatient has her V_D/V_T ratio measured as 0.48 (48%); this finding is
   a. Normal for an adult female
   b. Consistent with pulmonary hypertension
   c. Diagnostic of mild restrictive lung disease
   d. Expected after surgical removal of one lung

5. A healthy adult subject who weighs 150 pounds has a $\dot{V}_E$ of 9.0 L/min (BTPS) and a respiratory rate of 10/min. His $\dot{V}_A$ can be estimated as _____?
   a. 7.5 L (BTPS)
   b. 6.0 L (BTPS)

c. 4.5 L (BTPS)
d. 3.0 L (BTPS)

Advanced

Questions 6 and 7 refer to the same case.

6. The following data are recorded from a patient with suspected pulmonary embolism:

P_ECO_2:   20 mm Hg
pH: 7.39
$PaCO_2$:   40
PaO_2:   72

What is this patient's V_D/V_T ratio?
a. 0.15
b. 0.25
c. 0.33
d. 0.50

7. Based on the V_D/V_T ratio (question 6), what is the patient's alveolar ventilation ($\dot{V}_A$) if his minute ventilation ($\dot{V}_E$) is 16.0 L/min (BTPS)?
a. 13.6 L/min
b. 12.0 L/min
c. 10.7 L/min
d. 8.0 L/min

8. A patient has the following results after 4.0 minutes of a CO_2 rebreathing test:

	Time 0	4 Min
P_ETCO_2 (mm Hg)	38	62
$\dot{V}_E$ (L/min)	3.7	7.0

Which of the following diagnoses is most consistent with these findings?
a. Obesity-hypoventilation syndrome
b. COPD
c. Coal worker's pneumoconiosis
d. Normal lung function

9. The purpose of a variable speed blower in the closed-circuit rebreathing system used to measure the response to hypoxemia is to
a. Reduce the inspired FIO_2
b. Mix gas in the rebreathing circuit
c. Maintain isocapnia
d. Allow measurement of P_{100}

10. A patient has the following findings during a CO_2 rebreathing test:

	Time 0	3 Min
P_ETCO_2 (mm Hg)	41	51
$\dot{V}_E$ (L/min)	5.7	23.0
P_{100} (cm H_2O)	2.7	7.8

These data suggest
a. Normal ventilatory response to CO_2
b. Decreased output of the respiratory centers
c. Normal respiratory drive but decreased ventilatory response
d. Abnormally increased P_{100} with hypercapnia

Selected Bibliography

GENERAL REFERENCES

Levitzky MG: *Pulmonary physiology*, ed 6, Columbus OH, 2003, McGraw-Hill.

West JB: *Pulmonary pathophysiology: the essentials*, ed 6, Baltimore, 2003, Lippincott, Williams & Wilkins.

West JB: *Pulmonary physiology and pathophysiology: an integrated, case-based approach*, Baltimore, 2000, Lippincott, Williams & Wilkins.

VENTILATION

Hardman JG, Aitkenhead AR: Estimating alveolar dead space from the arterial to end-tidal CO(2) gradient: a modeling analysis, *Anesth Analg* 2003; 97:1846-1851.

Hedenstierna G, Sandhagen B: Assessing dead space. A meaningful variable? *Minerva Anestesiol* 2006; 72:521-528.

Kline JA, Israel EG, Michelson EA et al: Diagnostic accuracy of a bedside D-dimer assay and alveolar dead-space measurement for rapid exclusion of pulmonary embolism: a multicenter study, *JAMA* 2001; 285:761-768.

Koulouris NG, Latsi P, Dimitroulis J et al: Noninvasive measurement of mean alveolar carbon dioxide tension and Bohr's dead space during tidal breathing, *Eur Respir J* 2001; 17:1167-1174.

Riley RL, Cournand A: "Ideal" alveolar air and the analysis of ventilation-perfusion relationships in the lungs, *J Appl Physiol* 1949; 1:825.

Rodger MA, Jones G, Rasuli P et al: Steady-state end-tidal alveolar dead space fraction and D-dimer: bedside tests to exclude pulmonary embolism, *Chest* 2001; 120:115-119.

CONTROL OF VENTILATION

Benlloch E, Cordero P, Morales P et al: Ventilatory pattern at rest and response to hypercapnic stimulation in patients with obstructive sleep apnea, *Respiration* 1995; 62:4-9.

Caruana-Montaldo B, Gleeson K, Zwillich CW: The control of breathing in clinical practice, *Chest* 2000; 117:205-225.

Cherniack NS, Lederer DH, Altose MD et al: Occlusion pressure as technique in evaluating respiratory control, *Chest* 1976; 70 (suppl):137.

Howard LS, Robbins PA: Problems with determining the hypoxic response in humans using stepwise changes in end-tidal PO_2, *Respir Physiol* 1994; 98:241-249.

Marin JM, Montes de Oca M, Rassulo J et al: Ventilatory drive at rest and the perception of exertional dyspnea in severe COPD, *Chest* 1999; 115:1293-1300.

Misuri G, Lanini B, Gigliotti F et al: Mechanism of CO_2 retention in patients with neuromuscular disease, *Chest* 2000; 117:447-453.

Mohan RM, Amara CE, Cunningham DA et al: Measuring central-chemoreflex sensitivity in man: rebreathing and steady-state methods compared, *Respir Physiol* 1999; 115:23-33.

Read DJ: A clinical method for assessing the ventilatory response to carbon dioxide, *Australas Ann Med* 1967; 16:20-32.

Rebuck AS, Campbell EJM: A clinical method for assessing the ventilatory response to hypoxia, *Am Rev Respir Dis* 1974; 109:345-350.

Zhang S, Robbins PA: Methodological and physiological variability within the ventilatory response to hypoxia in humans, *J Appl Physiol* 2000; 88:1924-1932.

Chapter 5

Diffusing Capacity Tests

CHAPTER OUTLINE

Carbon Monoxide Diffusing Capacity
Description
Techniques
Significance and Pathophysiology

OBJECTIVES

After studying this chapter you will be able to:

Entry-level
1. Identify the steps for performing the single-breath DLCO
2. List at least two criteria for an acceptable single-breath DLCO test
3. Describe why DLCO is often reduced in emphysema

Advanced
1. Describe at least two nonpulmonary causes for reduced DLCO
2. Explain the significance of a reduced DL/V_A
3. Compare diffusion limitation due to membranes and pulmonary capillary blood volume

KEY TERMS

alveolar sample	Jones method	standard temperature, pressure,
alveolar volume	membrane resistance	dry (STPD)
alveolitis	Müller maneuver	three-equation method
breath hold	multigas analysis	tracer gas
DL/V_A	O_2 desaturation	transfer factor (DLCO)
DLCOsb	rebreathing method	Valsalva maneuver
intrabreath method		washout volume

This chapter describes measurement of diffusion in the lungs. Diffusing capacity (also referred to as **transfer factor**) is usually measured using small volumes of carbon monoxide (CO) and is referred to as DLCO or D_{CO}. DLCO is used to assess the gas-exchange ability of the lungs, specifically oxygenation of mixed venous blood. Various methods, all of which use CO, have been described. The most commonly used method is the single-breath, or breath-hold, technique. The single-breath method is also the most widely standardized. The techniques section focuses on the single-breath method

133

but also describes some of the other methods that are used for specific applications.

DLCO measurements are used in the diagnosis and management of most pulmonary disorders. The importance of standards and guidelines in the performance of DLCO tests and in the overall interpretation of results is highlighted. Interpretive strategies are presented in a format similar to those in previous chapters.

CARBON MONOXIDE DIFFUSING CAPACITY

Description

DLCO measures the transfer of a diffusion-limited gas (CO) across the alveolocapillary membranes. DLCO is reported in milliliters of CO/minute/millimeter of mercury at 0°C, 760 mm Hg, dry (i.e., **standard temperature, pressure, dry [STPD]**).

Techniques

CO combines with hemoglobin (Hb) approximately 210 times more readily than oxygen (O_2). In the presence of normal amounts of Hb and normal ventilatory function, the primary limiting factor to diffusion of CO is the status of the alveolocapillary membranes. This process of conductance across the membranes can be divided into two components: membrane conductance (D_M) and the chemical reaction between CO and Hb. D_M reflects the process of diffusion across the alveolocapillary membrane. Uptake of CO by Hb depends on the reaction rate (θ) and the pulmonary capillary blood volume (V_C). These two components occur in series, so the diffusion conductance can be expressed as:

$$\frac{1}{DLCO} = \frac{1}{D_M} + \frac{1}{\theta V_C}$$

Diffusing capacity can be affected by factors that change the membrane component, as well as by alterations in Hb and the capillary blood volume.

A small amount of CO in inspired gas produces measurable changes in the concentration of inspired versus expired gas. Because little or no CO is normally present in pulmonary capillary blood, the pressure gradient causing diffusion is basically the alveolar pressure (P_ACO). If the partial pressure of CO in the alveoli and the rate of uptake of the gas can be measured, the DLCO of the lung can be determined. There are several methods for determining DLCO (Table 5-1). All methods are based on the following equation:

$$DLCO = \frac{\dot{V}CO}{P_ACO - P_CCO}$$

where:

$\dot{V}CO$ = milliliters of CO transferred/minute (STPD)
P_ACO = mean alveolar partial pressure of CO
P_CCO = mean capillary partial pressure of CO, assumed to be 0

DLCO is expressed in milliliters of gas/minute/unit of driving pressure at STPD conditions.

Single Breath–Breath-Hold Technique (Modified Krogh Technique)

The patient exhales to RV and then inspires a vital capacity breath (referred to as the IVC or V_I) from a system such as that in Figure 5-1. A special diffusion gas mixture is delivered either from a spirometer, a reservoir bag, or by means of a demand valve. The diffusion mixture usually contains 0.3% CO, a "tracer" gas, 21% O_2, and the balance is N_2. The **tracer gas** is usually an insoluble, inert gas such as helium (He), methane (CH_4), or neon (Ne). The tracer used depends on the type of analyzer implemented to analyze the exhaled gas. The traditional method used He (usually about 10%) as the tracer gas. Rapidly responding infrared analyzers (see Chapter 10) have been used for continuous analysis of the small changes in CO. The same type of infrared analyzer can use CH_4 as the tracer gas, so that a single analyzer can rapidly detect changes in both CO and the tracer. Another method uses gas chromatography (see Chapter 10) to detect changes in CO with neon used as the tracer gas.

TABLE 5-1				
Advantages and Disadvantages of DLCO Testing Methods				
Method	Technique	Advantages	Disadvantages	Applications
DLCOsb (breath hold)	CO and tracer gas analysis relatively simple; 10-sec breath hold	Easy calculations, simple, fast; highly standardized and automated; minimal COHb back-pressure effect	Sensitive to distribution of ventilation and V/Q matching; "nonphysiologic"; not practical for exercise testing	Screening and clinical applicatons
DLCOrb (rebreathing)	Rapid analysis of CO and tracer gas required; rebreathing must be controlled	Less sensitive to V_A than DLCOsb; less sensitive to V/Q abnormalities; can be used with NO to measure DL_{NO}	Complex calculations (computerized); rapidly responding analyzers required; sensitive to COHb back-pressure	Clinical and research applications; provides most accurate DLCO
DLCOib (intrabreath)	Rapid analysis of CO and tracer gas during single controlled exhalation	Breath holding not required; can be used during exercise	Complex calculations (computerized); flow must be controlled; sensitive to uneven V/Q; not standardized	Screening and clinical applications; may be useful in patients who cannot hold their breath
1/Dm + 1/θVc (membrane diffusing capacity)	DLCOsb repeated at two different levels of alveolar PO_2	Differentiates membrane transfer resistance from red cell uptake	Complex calculations; estimates of alveolar PO_2 are critical	Research with limited clinical applications

After inspiring the VC breath, the patient holds the breath at total lung capacity (TLC) for approximately 10 seconds. The patient then exhales. After a suitable **washout volume** (750–1000 ml) has been discarded, a sample of alveolar gas is collected (Figure 5-2). The **alveolar sample** may be collected in a small bag (~500 ml or less) or by continually aspirating a sample of the exhaled gas.

The sample is analyzed to obtain the fractional CO and tracer gas concentrations in alveolar gas, F_ACO_T (where T is the time of the breath hold), and $F_A$tracer, respectively. The concentration of CO in the alveoli at the beginning of the **breath hold** (F_ACO_0) must be determined as well. It is calculated as follows:

$$F_ACO_0 = F_ICO \times \frac{F_A\text{tracer}}{F_I\text{tracer}}$$

where:

F_ACO_0 = fraction of CO in alveolar gas at beginning of breath hold (time = 0)

F_ICO = fraction of CO in reservoir (usually 0.003)

$F_A$tracer = fraction of tracer in alveolar gas sample

$F_I$tracer = fraction of tracer in inspired gas (varies with tracer gas used)

The change in tracer gas concentration reflects dilution of inspired gas by the gas remaining in the lungs (i.e., RV). This change is used to determine the CO concentration at the beginning of the breath hold, before diffusion from the alveoli into the

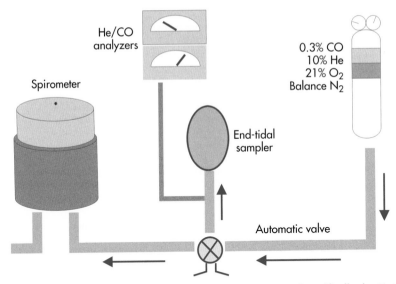

FIGURE 5-1   DLCO Apparatus. Basic equipment for performing a DLCO test (specifically the DLCOsb). The test gas contains 0.3% CO, 10% He, 21% O_2, and the balance N_2 (some systems use a tracer gas other than He). Gas is delivered to the automated valve from a reservoir bag (not shown), the spirometer, or a demand valve (not shown). The automated valve allows the patient to inhale the test gas rapidly. The valve then closes, assisting the breath-hold maneuver. After 10 seconds, the valve opens, allowing exhalation to the spirometer to measure dead space (washout). Exhaled gas is then directed to an alveolar sampling device. Gas analyzers for CO and the tracer gas then measure concentrations of gas from the alveolar sample. Some systems measure exhaled gas continuously with rapidly responding analyzers (see text). In these systems, gas is sampled directly at the mouth without an alveolar sample bag. A computer usually displays a volume-time tracing along with signals from the gas analyzer(s) (see Figures 5-2, 5-3, and 5-4). Timing of the maneuver is usually performed by the computer.

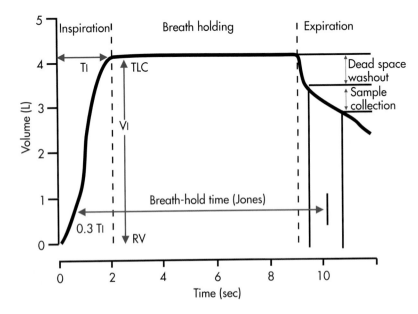

FIGURE 5-2   DLCOsb Maneuver Tracing. Tracing of a single-breath DLCO maneuver proceeding from left to right *(heavy line)*. Inspiration is up. After exhaling to RV (0 L on the volume axis), the patient rapidly inspires a vital capacity breath (V_I) of the test gas, then holds the breath at TLC for approximately 10 seconds. At the end of the breath hold, the patient exhales the dead space washout volume (usually 0.750 – 1.0 L). A sample of the alveolar gas is then collected (usually 0.5 – 1.0 L). Any remaining volume is discarded. The recommended timing method is illustrated. The Jones method measures from 0.3 of the inspiratory time (T_I) to the midpoint of the alveolar sample.

pulmonary capillaries. The **DLCOsb** (single-breath) is then calculated as follows:

$$DLCOsb = \frac{V_A \times 60}{(P_B - 47) \times (T)} \times Ln\frac{F_ACO_0}{F_ACO_T}$$

where:
V_A = alveolar volume, ml (STPD)
60 = correction from seconds to minutes
P_B = barometric pressure, mm Hg
47 = water vapor pressure at 37° C, mm Hg
T = breath-hold interval, seconds
Ln = natural logarithm
F_ACO_0 = fraction of CO in alveolar gas at beginning of breath hold
F_ACO_T = fraction of CO in alveolar gas at end of breath hold

V_A may be calculated from the single-breath dilution of the tracer gas:

$$V_A = (V_I - V_D) \times \frac{F_I tracer}{F_A tracer} \times STPD\ correction\ factor$$

where:
V_I = volume of test gas inspired, ml (see Figure 5-2)
V_D = dead space volume (anatomic and instrumental), ml
$F_A tracer$ = fraction of tracer in alveolar gas sample
$F_I tracer$ = fraction of tracer in inspired gas (depends on tracer used)

Note that the V_A, usually expressed in BTPS units, must be converted to STPD for the single-breath calculation. The dilution of tracer gas is used twice: to determine the CO concentration at the beginning of the breath hold and to determine the lung volume (i.e., V_A) at which the breath hold occurred.

A simplification of the single-breath method described earlier is widely used. The tracer gas and CO analyzers may be calibrated to read full scale (100% or 1.000) when sampling the diffusion mixture, and to read zero when sampling air (no tracer or CO). If the analyzers have a linear response to each other, the fractional concentration of the tracer gas in the alveolar sample is equal to the F_ACO_0. This technique assumes that both the tracer gas and CO are diluted equally during inspiration. Because no tracer gas leaves the lung during the

breath hold, its concentration in the alveolar sample approximates that of the CO before any diffusion occurred. The exponential rate of CO diffusion from the alveoli can then be expressed as follows:

$$Ln\left(\frac{F_A tracer}{F_ACO_T}\right)$$

where:
$F_A tracer$ = fraction of tracer in alveolar gas, equal to F_ACO_0
F_ACO_T = fraction of CO in alveolar gas at end of breath hold
Ln = natural logarithm of the ratio

This technique avoids the necessity of analyzing the absolute concentrations of the two gases. However, it requires that the analyzers be linear with respect to each other. Analysis of CO is often done using infrared analyzers (see Chapter 10), and their output is nonlinear. Care must be taken to ensure that corrected CO readings are used in the computation. These corrections are easily accomplished either electronically or via software in computerized systems. Systems that use the same detector for both CO and the tracer gas (e.g., infrared, gas chromatography) also need to provide linear output. The linearity of the system should be within 0.5% of full scale. This means that any drift or nonlinearity should cause no more than a 0.5% error when analyzing a known gas concentration. (See Chapter 11 for techniques to assess linearity of gas analyzers.)

DLCO gas analysis is commonly performed with either a rapidly responding multigas analyzer or gas chromatography. **Multigas analysis** uses specialized infrared analyzers capable of detecting several gases simultaneously. These systems use methane (CH_4) as a tracer gas. One advantage of multigas analysis is that CO and CH_4 are measured rapidly and continuously (Figure 5-3) so that the calculated DLCO is available as soon as the exhalation has been completed. Gas chromatography (see Chapter 10) can also be used for DLCO gas analysis. Neon (Ne) is used as the tracer gas (Figure 5-4). Helium is used as a "carrier" gas for the chromatograph. Although gas analysis using chromatography is slow (60–90 seconds), it is extremely accurate.

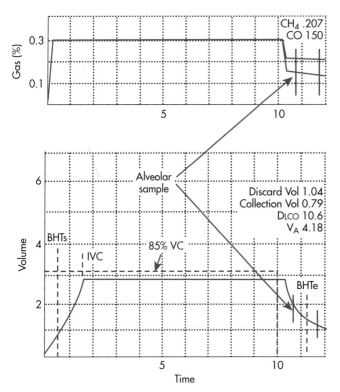

FIGURE 5-3   DLcOsb Maneuver Using Continuous Gas Analysis. Changes in gas concentrations are shown (top). Test gases (CO and CH_4) rise rapidly to their initial values of 0.3% during the breath hold. During exhalation, both gas concentrations fall as dead space is washed out. The tracer gas, CH_4, shows a plateau as alveolar gas is exhaled. CO shows a similar pattern, but with a lower concentration because of uptake (diffusion) during the breath hold. Gas concentration measurements are made from an alveolar window (gray lines) that can be adjusted. Simultaneous changes in lung volumes are shown on the bottom tracing. IVC indicates inspiratory volume (V_I). In this test, the patient failed to inspire at least 85% of the VC (dashed gray line). BHTs indicates start of breath-hold timing; BHTe indicates end of breath hold at the midpoint of the alveolar sample "window." Calculated DLCO and related measurements are displayed (computer screen), allowing inspection of changes as the alveolar sample "window" is adjusted. (Courtesy VIASYS Healthcare Critical Care Division, Palm Springs, Calif.)

The resistance of the breathing circuit should be less than 1.5 cm $H_2O/L/sec$, at a flow of 6 L/sec. This is important in allowing the patient to inspire rapidly from RV to TLC. A demand valve may be used instead of a reservoir bag for the test gas. In a demand-flow system, the maximal inspiratory pressure to maintain a flow of 6 L/sec should be less than 10 cm H_2O. Increased resistance, in either a reservoir or a demand valve system, may cause the patient to produce large subatmospheric pressures during inspiration. This has the effect of increasing pulmonary capillary blood volume, and may falsely increase DLCO.

The timing device for the maneuver should be accurate to within 100 msec over a 10-second interval (1%). Most computerized systems time the maneuver automatically. However, a means of verifying the accuracy of the breath-hold time should be available. The Jones method of timing the breath hold should be used (see Figure 5-2). The **Jones** **method** measures breath-hold time from 0.3 of the inspiratory time to the midpoint of the alveolar sample collection.

Corrections must be made for the patient's anatomic dead space (V_D) and for dead space in the valve (and sample bag, if used). Anatomic V_D should be calculated as 2.2 ml/kg (1 ml/lb) of ideal body weight. The equipment manufacturer should specify instrument V_D. Instrument V_D should not exceed 350 ml for adult subjects, including mouthpiece and any filters that might be used. Smaller instrument V_D may be necessary for pediatric patients. Anatomic and instrument V_D are subtracted from inspired volume (V_I) before the **alveolar volume** (V_A) is calculated.

All gas volumes must be corrected from ATPS to STPD for the DLCO calculations. However, when the V_A is used to calculate the ratio of DLCO to lung volume (**DL/V_A**), it is normally expressed in BTPS units. Accurate measurement of inspired volume

Time	Select	RpLp	Protocol	Dᴸcounc absolute	Dᴸcounc % predicted	Dᴸcocor absolute	Dᴸcocor % predicted	Dᴸ/Vᴀ absolute	Dᴸ/Vᴀ % predicted	Vᴀ absolute	Vᴀ % predicted	IVC absolute	BHT absolute	Fιco absolute	Feco absolute
Predicted				26.91	100	23.71	100	3.88	100	6.94	100				
Pre															
14:56:48	✓	✓	Jones-Meade (AT)	25.52	95	25.52	108	3.54		7.21	104	5.08	9.84	0.91	0.37
15:00:45	✓		Jones-Meade (AT)	24.78	92	24.78	104	3.41		7.27	105	5.18	9.83	0.91	0.38
AVG				25.15	93	25.15	106	3.47		7.24	104	5.13			

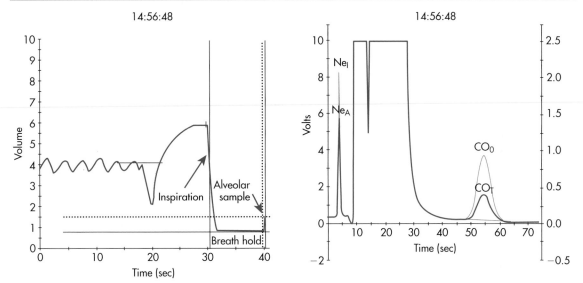

FIGURE 5-4   Dʟcosb Test Using Gas Chromatography. Volume-time tracing with inspiration, breath-hold, and alveolar sampling is shown *(left graph).* In this scheme, inspiration causes a downward deflection. Output of the gas chromatograph is shown *(right graph).* Neon (the tracer gas) and CO show distinct peaks on the gas chromatograph tracing. The alveolar sample is superimposed over a preanalysis (calibration) curve of the test gas. Neᵢ is the initial tracer concentration, and Neₐ is the concentration after the breath hold. CO concentrations of the undiluted test gas (CO_0) and end of the breath hold (CO_T) are superimposed. Calculated Dʟco and related values for multiple efforts are shown at the top. *(Courtesy Medical Graphics, Inc., St. Paul, Minn.)*

during the maneuver requires that the spirometer have an accuracy of 3.5% (3% + 0.5% for the calibration syringe itself) over a range of 8 L. Volume-based spirometer systems must also be free from leaks.

Gas analyzers that are affected by carbon dioxide (CO_2) or water vapor require appropriate absorbers. Absorption of CO_2 is usually accomplished with a chemical absorber using $Ba(OH)_2$ (baralyme) or NaOH (soda lyme). Each of these reactions produces water vapor. Therefore CO_2 absorbers should be placed upstream of an H_2O absorber. Anhydrous $CaSO_4$ is commonly used to remove water vapor. Selectively permeable tubing (PERMA PURE) can also be used to establish a known water vapor content. Gas-conditioning devices must be routinely

checked to ensure accurate gas analysis. Chemical absorbers typically add an indicator that changes color as the absorber becomes exhausted.

PF TIP

Watch the patient carefully during the Dʟcosb effort to detect either a Valsalva or Müller maneuver. Widely varying results in two or more Dʟco measurements are often caused by the patient failing to relax during the breath hold. Some pulmonary function systems provide a pressure monitor to detect large positive or negative pressures during the breath hold.

DLCOsb maneuvers should be performed after the patient has been seated for at least 5 minutes. The patient should refrain from exertion immediately before the test; exercise increases cardiac output, which increases DLCO. The patient should be instructed about the requirements of the maneuver and the technique demonstrated. Expiration to RV should be of a reasonable duration, usually 6 seconds or less. Patients who have airway obstruction may have difficulty exhaling completely in this interval. Inspiration to TLC should be rapid but not forced. Healthy subjects and patients with airway obstruction should be able to inspire at least 85% of their VC within 4 seconds (DLCO 5-1). The single-breath calculation assumes instantaneous filling of the lung. Prolonged inspiratory times will decrease the actual time of breath holding at TLC, typically resulting in a lower DLCO. The breath hold should be relaxed, against either the closed glottis or a closed valve. The patient should avoid excessive positive intrathoracic pressure (**Valsalva maneuver**) or excessive negative intrathoracic pressure (**Müller maneuver**). A Valsalva maneuver reduces pulmonary capillary blood volume and may produce a falsely low DLCO. A Müller maneuver increases pulmonary capillary blood volume and may falsely increase DLCO. Expiration after the breath hold should be smooth and uninterrupted. Exhalation should take less than 4 seconds and alveolar gas sampling should occur in less than 3 seconds (again because the calculations assume instantaneous emptying of the lung). Patients who have moderate or severe airway obstruction may have difficulty achieving these criteria. The breath-hold time, measured using the Jones method (see Figure 5-2), should be 10 seconds ± 2 seconds. Prolonged inspiratory or expiratory times may result in breath-hold times greater than 12 seconds and should be noted on the report.

PF TIP

One of the most common problems encountered when performing the DLCOsb maneuver is failure of the subjects to inspire at least 85% of their previously measured VC. Careful instruction or reinstruction of the subject usually helps to eliminate the problem. Patients who have airway obstruction may have difficulty inspiring maximally after exhalation to residual volume (RV).

DLCO 5-1

CRITERIA FOR ACCEPTABILITY
DLCOsb

1. The patient should breathe normally for several breaths, and then exhale to RV. Ideally, the exhalation should occur within 6 seconds or less.
2. Inspiration from RV to TLC should be rapid but not forced, and should occur within 4 seconds or less. Prolonged inspiratory time (e.g., because of obstruction) should be noted in the report.
3. The volume inspired (V_I or IVC) should be at least 85% of the best previously recorded VC.
4. Breath-hold time should be between 8 and 12 seconds, using the Jones method. The breath hold should be relaxed, without excessive positive or negative intrathoracic pressure.
5. Exhalation should be rapid but not forced, with total exhalation lasting 4 seconds or less. Prolonged expiratory times should be noted on the report.
6. Dead space washout should be 0.75 – 1.00 L but may be reduced to 0.5 L for patients whose VC is less than 2.0 L. If continuous analysis of expired gas is used, visual inspection of dead space washout should be made. Any adjustments to the washout volume should be noted in the report.
7. Alveolar sample volume should be 0.5 – 1.0 L and should be collected in 3 seconds or less. For patients whose VC is less than 1.0 L the sample volume may be reduced to less than 0.5 L, provided that an adequate dead space volume is cleared.
8. An interval of at least 4 minutes should elapse between repeated tests to allow clearance of the test gas from the lungs. No more than five single-breath maneuvers should be performed in one testing session to avoid back-pressure from increased COHb.
9. The average of two or more acceptable tests should be reported. Duplicate determinations should be within 3 ml/min/mm Hg of each other or within 10% of the largest observed value.
10. The unadjusted DLCOsb, DL/V_A, and V_A should be reported along with their respective predicted values and percent of predicted. Adjustments for Hb, COHb, altitude, or V_A should be included along with the values used for correction. If the DLCO is performed after inhalation of a bronchodilator, it should be reported as such.

To obtain an alveolar sample, dead space gas needs to be washed out (i.e., discarded). A washout of 0.75–1.0 L is usually sufficient to clear the patient and sampling device dead space. For patients with small vital capacities (<2.0 L), the washout volume may be reduced to 0.5 L. A sample volume of 0.5–1.0 L should be collected, but a smaller sample may be necessary in patients whose VC is less than 1 L. In DLCOsb systems that analyze expired gas continuously (see Figure 5-3), inspection of the washout of the tracer gas may be used to select an appropriate alveolar sample. Rapidly responding gas analyzers that measure the CO and tracer gas simultaneously allow adjustment of washout volume (i.e., dead space) and sample volume after completion of the maneuver. These adjustments may be particularly useful in subjects who have very small vital capacities (e.g., pediatric patients or adults with severe restrictive disease). Such adjustments assume that both the CO and tracer gas concentrations reflect changes occurring at the mouth. Alveolar sampling may be adjusted to begin at the point where the tracer gas and CO indicate an "alveolar plateau" (see Figure 5-3). In patients who have uneven mixing or emptying of the lungs, there may not be a clear demarcation between dead space and alveolar gas. Adjustments to either washout (dead space) volume or sample volume should be noted on the report.

Two or more acceptable DLCOsb maneuvers (see DLCO 5-1) should be averaged. Duplicate determinations should be within 3 ml CO/min/mm Hg of each other, or within 10% of the largest value obtained from an acceptable effort. No more than five repeated maneuvers should be performed be-

cause of the effect of increasing carboxyhemoglobin (COHb) from inhalation of the test gas. There should be a 4-minute delay between repeated maneuvers to allow for washout of the tracer gas from the lungs.

Corrections for abnormal hemoglobin (Hb) concentrations should be applied with a current Hb value. The predicted DLCO should be corrected so that it reflects the DLCO at an Hb value of 14.6 g% for adult and adolescent males, and to an Hb value of 13.4 g% for women and children of either sex younger than 15 years of age. The Hb-corrected predicted value for males may be calculated as follows:

$$DLCO\ (predicted\ for\ Hb) = DLCO\ (predicted) \times \frac{(1.7 \times Hb)}{(10.22 + Hb)}$$

Similarly, Hb correction of the predicted values for women and children younger than 15 years is calculated as follows:

$$DLCO\ (predicted\ for\ Hb) = DLCO\ (predicted) \times \frac{(1.7 \times Hb)}{(9.38 + Hb)}$$

Note that this scheme corrects the predicted value rather than the patient's measured value. For example, in an adult male patient with an Hb of 9.0 g/dl and a predicted DLCO of 25 ml/min/mm Hg, a measured DLCO of 19 ml/min/mm Hg would be reported:

	Actual	Predicted	%
DLCO ml/min/mm Hg	19.0	25.0	76
DLCO (Hb corrected) ml/min/mm Hg	19.0	19.9	95

Both uncorrected and corrected predicted DLCO values and the resulting percentages should be reported, along with the Hb value used for correction. Decreased Hb levels (anemia) will always reduce the predicted value, whereas elevated Hb (polycythemia) will increase the predicted value.

Correction for the presence of COHb in the patient's blood is also recommended. The predicted DLCO may be adjusted as follows:

$$DLCO\ (predicted\ for\ COHb) = DLCO\ (predicted) \times (102\% - COHb\%)$$

The COHb% is the fraction of carboxyhemoglobin determined by hemoximetry expressed as a percentage. This method assumes that the predicted value already includes 2% COHb in healthy subjects. For subjects who have a COHb% > 2%, the predicted value will always be reduced using this method. Patients should be asked to refrain from smoking for 24 hours before the test to reduce the CO back-pressure in the blood. For patients who continue to smoke, the time of last exposure should be recorded.

D_{LCO} varies inversely with changes in alveolar oxygen pressure (P_AO_2). P_AO_2 changes as a function of altitude, as well as with the partial pressure of oxygen in the test gas. D_{LCO} increases approximately 0.35% for each mm Hg decrease in P_AO_2, or about 0.31% for each mm Hg decrease in P_IO_2. When test gas mixtures that produce an inspired O_2 pressure of 150 mm Hg (i.e., 21% at sea level) are used, D_{LCO} values will be equivalent to those measured at sea level. Alternatively, standard test gas ($F_IO_2 = 0.21$ is typical) can be used and the predicted D_{LCO} corrected by adjusting P_IO_2. For a gas with a P_IO_2 of 150 mm Hg, the equation is as follows:

$$D_{LCO} \text{ predicted for altitude} =$$
$$D_{LCO} \text{ predicted}/(1.0 + 0.0031[P_IO_2 - 150])$$

where:
$P_IO_2 = 0.21(P_B - 47)$
and P_B is the local barometric pressure (at altitude). If the patient is breathing supplemental O_2 and the P_AO_2 is measured, the predicted D_{LCO} can be adjusted, assuming a P_AO_2 of 100 mm Hg breathing air at sea level:

$$D_{LCO} \text{ predicted for } P_AO_2 =$$
$$D_{LCO} \text{ predicted}/(1.0 + 0.0035[P_AO_2 - 100])$$

where:
P_AO_2 = Measured or estimated alveolar oxygen partial pressure

Note that corrections for altitude or elevated alveolar oxygen tensions are made to the predicted D_{LCO} values.

Corrections for Hb, COHb, and altitude or elevated P_AO_2 are recommended for all predicted D_{LCO}

values when the conditions for the corrections are known. Hb, COHb, and measured P_AO_2 may not be available for all patients; correction for altitude (P_IO_2) is easily performed for laboratories significantly above sea level. Previous guidelines recommended that corrections be applied to the patient's measured values, rather than to the predicted values. Some laboratories may prefer to use the older method.

In some instances it may be appropriate to correct the D_{LCO} for the lung volume at which it is measured. A common example would be when the subject inhales a volume that is substantially less than his or her known VC and breath holds at a V_A that is less than expected. The D_{LCO} may be corrected:

$$D_{LCO} (\text{at } V_{Am}) = D_{LCO} (\text{at } V_{Ap}) \times (0.58 + 0.42(V_{Am}/V_{Ap}))$$

where:
V_{Am} = measured alveolar volume
V_{Ap} = predicted alveolar volume (i.e., TLC-V_D)
A similar correction can be applied to the D_L/V_A:

$$D_L/V_A (\text{at } V_{Am}) = D_L/V_A (\text{at } V_{Ap}) \times (0.42 + 0.58(V_{Am}/V_{Ap}))$$

These corrections are derived from healthy subjects whose D_{LCO} was measured at alveolar volumes less than the expected value. Such corrections may not be applicable in all disease states because D_L and V_A can be altered independently of one another. In addition, some subjects may not exhale completely to RV, with the subsequent inspiration to TLC producing a V_I that is less than 85% of their VC. In such an instance the subject is actually breath holding at TLC, although the reduced V_I suggests otherwise.

Rebreathing Technique

The patient rebreathes from a reservoir containing a mixture of 0.3% CO, tracer gas, and air (or an O_2 mixture) for 30–60 seconds at a rate of approximately 30 breaths/min. The final CO, tracer, and O_2 concentrations in the reservoir are measured after this interval. An equation similar to that used for the single-breath technique is used (see DLCOsb, mentioned previously):

$$DLCOrb = \frac{V_S \times 60}{(P_B - 47)(T2 - T1)} \times Ln\left(\frac{F_ACO_{T1}}{F_ACO_{T2}}\right)$$

where:

V_S	= volume of lung reservoir system (initial volume × $F_I$tracer/$F_A$tracer)
60	= correction from seconds to minutes
P_B	= barometric pressure, mm Hg
47	= water vapor pressure, mm Hg
T2 – T1	= rebreathing interval, seconds
Ln	= natural logarithm
F_ACO_{T1}	= fraction of CO in alveolar gas at beginning of the rebreathing
F_ACO_{T2}	= fraction of CO in alveolar gas at the end of the rebreathing

The **rebreathing method** can also be implemented using a rapidly responding analyzer (for CO and tracer gas) and plotting the slope of the change in CO in relation to the slope of the tracer gas to estimate the rate of CO uptake. The rebreathing method can be used during exercise.

PF TIP

DLCO is most often measured with the single-breath (breath-hold) technique. The equipment and procedures used for the DLCOsb have been standardized by the American Thoracic Society and European Respiratory Society.

Slow Exhalation Single-Breath–Intrabreath Method

The patient inspires a vital capacity (VC) breath of test gas containing 0.3% CO, 0.3% CH_4 (methane), 21% O_2, and the balance N_2. Then the patient exhales slowly and evenly at approximately 0.5 L/sec from TLC to RV. A rapidly responding infrared analyzer monitors CO and CH_4 gas concentrations. The exponential rate of disappearance of CO can be calculated in a manner similar to the rebreathing method. Change in V_A is calculated from the change in concentration of the CH_4 tracer gas. CH_4 is used

as the tracer gas because it can be rapidly measured using an infrared analyzer. Multiple estimates of DLCO can be made during a single exhalation, recording DLCO as a function of lung volume. This is done using an equation similar to that used for the single-breath method. Instead of one estimate of V_A (equal to the lung volume at breath hold), multiple increments of V_A are made, and DLCO is plotted against lung volume. A single estimate of overall DLCO can also be obtained. The **intrabreath method** can also be used during exercise.

Membrane Diffusion Coefficient and Capillary Blood Volume

The patient performs two DLCOsb tests, each at a different level of alveolar PO_2. The first DLCOsb test is performed as described previously. The patient then breathes an elevated concentration of O_2 (balance N_2) for approximately 5 minutes, exhales to RV, and performs the second DLCOsb maneuver. DLCO values are calculated for both the air- and oxygen-breathing maneuvers. The total resistance caused by the alveolocapillary membrane (D_M) and the resistance caused by the rate of chemical combination with Hb and transfer into the red blood cell (θV_C) is calculated as follows:

$$\frac{1}{DLCO} = \frac{1}{D_M} + \frac{1}{\theta V_C}$$

where:

$1/DLCO$	= reciprocal of diffusing capacity, or resistance
$1/D_M$	= alveolocapillary membrane resistance
$1/\theta V_C$	= resistance of red blood cell membrane and rate of reaction with Hb
θ	= transfer rate of CO/milliliter of capillary blood
V_C	= capillary blood volume

Because CO and O_2 compete for binding sites on Hb, measurement of diffusion of CO at different levels of alveolar PO_2 can be used to distinguish resistance caused by the alveolocapillary membrane from resistance caused by the red blood cell membrane and Hb reaction rate. V_C is presumed to remain the same for both tests, but θ varies in response to changes in PO_2. Resistance caused by the alveolocapillary membrane ($1/D_M$) can be calculated by plotting θ at two points against $1/DLCO$ and extrapolating back to zero (as if no O_2 were present).

The membrane component of resistance to gas transfer can also be estimated by measuring the rate of uptake of nitric oxide (NO). DL_{NO} has been suggested as a direct measure of the conductance of the alveolocapillary membrane. Because NO combines with Hb approximately 280 times faster than CO, the rate of NO uptake by the blood (θ_{NO}) is very large and $1/\theta_{NO}V_C$ is negligible compared to $1/D_M$ for NO. Hence, DL_{NO} reflects the **membrane resistance** to gas diffusion in the lungs. DL_{NO} can be measured with either a single-breath or rebreathing technique. A small amount of NO is added to the diffusion mixture and the uptake measured using a chemoluminescence analyzer (see Chapter 10).

SIGNIFICANCE AND PATHOPHYSIOLOGY

See DLCO 5-2 for interpretive strategies. The average DLCO value for resting adult patients by the single-breath method is approximately 25 ml CO/min/mm Hg (STPD) with significant variability. Women have slightly lower normal values, presumably because of smaller normal lung volumes. The expected DLCO value in a healthy patient varies directly with the patient's lung volume. In some instances, it may be appropriate to adjust the predicted DLCO to account for decreased lung volume (see the section about techniques in this chapter). DLCO values can increase two to three times in healthy individuals during exercise in response to increased pulmonary capillary blood flow.

Most reference equations use age, height, sex, and race to predict DLCO. Some reference equations use body surface area (BSA) to calculate expected values. If the patient's weight is used (i.e., to calculate BSA), the ideal body weight is recommended. Using the actual body weight in obese patients can result in erroneously large predicted values unless similar subjects were included in the reference population. Significant differences exist among

---

DLCO 5-2

INTERPRETIVE STRATEGIES

DLCO

1. Were the test maneuvers performed acceptably? Were the tests repeatable within 3 ml/min/mm Hg of each other or within 10% of the largest observed value?
2. Were all appropriate corrections made to the predicted values? Hb? COHb? Altitude? V_A?
3. Are the reference values appropriate? Age? Height? Sex? Race?
4. Is DLCO less than the lower limit of normal (LLN) after appropriate corrections? If so, a gas exchange abnormality likely exists. Evaluate DL/V_A.
5. Is the DL/V_A ratio within normal limits? If so, reduced diffusing capacity is likely related to decreased lung volumes, parenchymal changes, pulmonary vascular disease, or pulmonary hypertension. Consider clinical correlation (e.g., patient's history, presentation, symptoms).
6. Is the DL/V_A ratio reduced? If so, reduced diffusing capacity is likely related to airway obstruction (uneven distribution of ventilation, $\dot{V}/\dot{Q}$ mismatch) or increased dead space. Compare V_A and TLC; a large difference suggests uneven distribution of ventilation. Look for clinical correlation.
7. Is the DLCO increased after correction for Hb or altitude? If so, consider possible causes of increased pulmonary blood volume, hemorrhage, obesity, or left-to-right shunts. Also consider undiagnosed asthma. Look for clinical correlation.
8. Is DLCO less than 50% of predicted? If so, consider additional tests (blood gases, exercise desaturation study).

---

reference equations. These discrepancies result in part from different methods used to measure DLCO in various laboratories. Laboratories should check the appropriateness of their reference equations by comparing the results obtained from healthy subjects. They should measure DLCO in a sample of healthy patients of each sex and compare the results using several reference equations. If the reference equations used are appropriate, the differences between the measured and expected values (i.e., residuals) for the healthy patients should be minimal. Predicted values for DLCO and for DL/V$_A$ should be taken from the same reference set. Regression equations for calculation of expected DLCO values are included in Appendix B.

DLCO is often decreased in restrictive lung diseases, particularly those associated with pulmonary fibrosis. Fibrotic changes in the lung parenchyma are associated with asbestosis, berylliosis, and silicosis. Many other diseases caused by inhalation of dusts also result in fibrotic changes in lung tissue. Idiopathic pulmonary fibrosis, sarcoidosis, systemic lupus erythematosus, and scleroderma are also commonly associated with reduction in DLCO. Inhalation of toxic gases or organic agents may cause inflammation of the alveoli (**alveolitis**) and decrease DLCO. These disease states are sometimes categorized as diffusion defects. The decrease in DLCO is probably more closely related to the loss of lung volume, alveolar surface area, or capillary bed than to thickening of the alveolocapillary membranes. DLCO also decreases when there is loss of lung tissue or replacement of normal parenchyma by space-occupying lesions such as tumors.

DLCO may also be reduced in the presence of pulmonary edema. Disruption of alveolar ventilation and reduction of lung volume as well as congestion of the alveoli cause the reduction in DLCO in edema. In the early stages of congestive heart failure (CHF), DLCO may be normal or slightly increased. As the left ventricle decompensates, pulmonary vessels become engorged. The increased blood volume can cause DLCO to increase, until the congestion becomes advanced. In most patients with heart failure, DLCO is decreased because of the restrictive ventilatory pattern. DLCO in patients who receive a heart transplant for chronic heart failure does not return to normal, as might be expected.

DLCO may also be decreased as a result of medical or surgical intervention for cardiopulmonary disease. Lung resection for cancer or other reasons typically results in decreased DLCO. The extent of reduction is usually directly proportional to the volume of lung removed. An exception to this pattern occurs in lung volume reduction surgery (LVRS) and in bullectomy. These surgical procedures typically resect areas of the lung that have little or no blood flow. Lack of perfusion is documented by a lung scan. Excision of tissue in such

areas reduces lung volume without necessarily reducing the surface area available for diffusion. Improved ventilation-perfusion matching in the remaining lung often results in an improvement in DLCO.

Radiation therapy that involves the lungs usually causes a decrease in DLCO. Radiation causes pneumonitis that commonly results in fibrotic changes. Drugs used in chemotherapy (e.g., bleomycin) and those used to suppress rejection in organ transplantation may cause reductions in DLCO. These drugs appear to directly affect the alveolocapillary membranes. Some drugs used in the treatment of cardiac arrhythmias (e.g., amiodarone) have been shown to decrease DLCO. For this reason, DLCO is commonly used to monitor drug toxicity.

DLCO may also be helpful in evaluating disorders such as hepatopulmonary syndrome, in which gas exchange and pulmonary vascular defects coexist. Diseases that affect the pulmonary vascular bed also typically result in decreased DLCO. These include pulmonary vasculitis and pulmonary hypertension. Pulmonary vascular disease often manifests itself as a reduced diffusing capacity with otherwise normal pulmonary function.

DLCO may be decreased in both acute and chronic obstructive lung disease. DLCO is decreased in emphysema for several reasons. Emphysematous lungs have a reduced surface area for gas exchange, with the loss of both alveolar septa and their associated capillary beds. As a result of the decreased surface area, less gas can be transferred per minute even if the remaining gas exchange units are structurally normal. In addition to loss of surface area for gas exchange, the distance from the terminal bronchiole to the alveolocapillary membrane increases in emphysema. As alveoli break down, terminal lung units become larger. Gas must diffuse farther just to reach the alveolocapillary surface. There is also mismatching of ventilation and pulmonary capillary blood flow in emphysema. Disruption of alveolar structures causes loss of support for terminal airways. Airway collapse and gas trapping result in ventilation-perfusion ($\dot{V}/\dot{Q}$) abnormalities.

Other obstructive diseases (e.g., chronic bronchitis, asthma) may not reduce DLCO unless they result in markedly abnormal $\dot{V}/\dot{Q}$ patterns. DLCO is sometimes used to differentiate among these obstructive patterns. Low D_{LCO} in the presence of obstruction is sometimes assumed to be evidence of emphysema. However, $\dot{V}/\dot{Q}$ mismatching can cause D_{LCO} to appear to be decreased in asthma, chronic bronchitis, or emphysema. Some asthmatic patients may have an increased D_{LCO}, but the cause is not completely understood.

D_{LCO} measurements at rest have been suggested to estimate the probability of **O_2 desaturation** during exercise. Not all clinicians agree that a decrease in D_{LCO} can predict desaturation. However, there does appear to be a correlation between resting D_{LCO} and gas exchange during exercise. In patients who have chronic obstructive pulmonary disease (COPD), D_{LCO} less than 50% of predicted is often accompanied by O_2 desaturation during exercise. Patients with restrictive lung disease and a low resting D_{LCO} are at risk of O_2 desaturation, even with low levels of exercise. Low resting D_{LCO} (i.e., less than 50%–60% of predicted) may indicate the need for assessment of oxygenation during exercise.

D_{LCO} is directly related to lung volume (V_A) in healthy individuals. The D_L/V_A (also termed K_{CO}) may be multiplied by the lung volume at which the measurement was obtained to express D_{LCO}. This calculation is simple because V_A must be measured to derive D_{LCO} (see Figure 5-4). In healthy subjects, and even in those with mild to moderate restriction, V_A approximates the TLC minus the assumed dead space (V_D). Analysis of this relationship can be useful to differentiate whether decreased D_{LCO} is the result of loss of lung volume (as in restriction) or from some other cause. In healthy individuals, alveolar volume and D_{LCO} are proportional to body size (height). Two patients of different height will have different D_{LCO} and V_A values, but their D_L/V_A ratios will be similar. In healthy adults, D_L/V_A is approximately 4–5 ml CO transferred/minute/liter of lung volume.

V_A is measured by the dilution of the tracer gas used (in the $D_{LCO}sb$), and reflects the same volume into which CO is distributed and diffuses across the pulmonary capillary membranes. Mismatching of ventilation and blood flow (as in obstructive disease) can cause a significant portion of the lung to not participate in gas exchange. This is usually charac-

terized by a difference between the V_A measured during the D_{LCO} maneuver and the TLC measured by plethysmography or multiple-breath gas dilution. When the D_{LCO} is reduced but the D_L/V_A is normal or near normal, the decrement in gas exchange can be assumed to be due to uneven distribution of ventilation, rather than loss of lung volume.

In the presence of pulmonary disease, both D_{LCO} and V_A may be affected. D_{LCO} goes down as the lung empties, but does so in a nonlinear fashion. In obstruction, low D_{LCO} without reduction in V_A results in a low ratio. In a purely restrictive process, a decrease in D_{LCO} reflects loss of V_A and the D_L/V_A ratio is preserved. For example, a patient who has a D_{LCO} of 12 ml CO/min/mm Hg (50% of predicted) and a V_A of 3.0 L would have a D_L/V_A ratio of 4. This reduction in D_{LCO} is roughly proportional to loss of lung volume. Some pulmonary conditions (such as pneumonectomy) may result in an increased D_L/V_A, where gas exchange is preserved and lung volume is decreased.

D_{LCO} and D_L/V_A may also be affected if the patient performs the breath-hold maneuver at a lung volume less than TLC. The predicted D_{LCO} may be corrected for the reduced V_A as described previously. There are important implications for interpretation of diffusing capacity in the complex relationship between D_{LCO} and D_L/V_A. Patients who fail to inspire fully during the maneuver will have a decreased D_{LCO}, but the D_L/V_A may appear to increase. Correcting for V_A does not correct for poor inspiratory effort (less than 85% of VC). In patients who have a low D_{LCO}, a "normal" D_L/V_A should not be confused with normal gas exchange.

The $D_{LCO}sb$ is the most widely used method because it is relatively simple to perform, is noninvasive, and is more standardized than other methods. The rapidity with which repeated maneuvers can be performed also lends to its popularity. Most automated systems use the $D_{LCO}sb$, contributing a certain degree of standardization to the methodology. Large differences in reported D_{LCO} values exist between laboratories. This variability has been attributed to different testing techniques, problems in the gas analysis involved in the test, and differences in computations. Breath holding at

TLC is not a physiologic maneuver. This and the fact that DLCO varies with lung volume cause some concerns about DLCOsb as an accurate description of diffusing capacity. DLCOsb is not practical for use during exercise. Some patients have difficulty expiring fully, inspiring fully, or holding their breath. The American Thoracic Society (ATS) and European Respiratory Society (ERS) have provided guidelines to improve standardization of the single-breath maneuver (Box 5-1).

The rebreathing method (DLCOrb) requires somewhat complicated calculations but offers the advantages of a normal breathing pattern without arterial puncture. DLCOrb is less sensitive to $\dot{V}/\dot{Q}$ abnormalities and uneven ventilation distribution than the DLCOsb. The rebreathing method is sensi-

---

BOX 5-1	DLCOsb Recommendations

A. Equipment
 1. Volume accuracy same as for spirometry: ±3.5% over 8-L range, all gases and flow conditions (includes syringe accuracy of 0.5%); checked daily.
 2. Documented analyzer linearity from 0 to full span ±0.5%, with minimal drift over test interval; checked quarterly.
 3. Circuit resistance less than 1.5 cm H_2O at 6 L/sec.
 4. Demand valve sensitivity less than 10 cm H_2O to generate 6 L/sec flow.
 5. Timing mechanism accurate to ±1% over 10 sec; checked quarterly.
 6. Instrument dead space (e.g., valves, filters) less than 0.35 L.
 7. Validate system by testing healthy nonsmokers (biologic controls) or DLCO simulator weekly.
B. Patient preparation
 1. The patient should refrain from smoking on the day of the test; time of last cigarette should be noted.
 2. No alcohol ingestion on the day of the test.
 3. No exercise immediately before test; patient should be seated for 5 minutes before DLCO maneuver.
 4. Patients on supplemental O_2 should be switched to breathing air for 10 minutes before testing, if clinically acceptable.
 5. The patient should be carefully instructed and the procedure demonstrated.
C. Technique
 1. The patient should breathe normally, and then exhale to RV within 6 seconds.
 2. Inspiration from RV to TLC should be rapid but not forced (< 4 seconds).
 3. The inspired volume (V_I) should be at least 85% of the patient's VC.

 4. The breath hold should last between 8 and 12 seconds, relaxing against closed glottis or closed valve (no Valsalva or Müller maneuver).
 5. V_D washout should be 0.75–1.0 L (0.5 L if VC less than 2.0 L); washout should last < 4 seconds.
 6. Alveolar sample volume should be 0.5–1.0 L collected in less than 3 seconds; smaller sample volume may be collected in patients whose VC is less than 1.0 L.
 7. Visual inspection of V_D washout and alveolar sampling should be used for systems that continuously analyze expired gas.
 8. Test gas should have a P_IO_2 similar to that in the reference set used for interpretation.
 9. Four minutes should elapse between repeat tests.
D. Calculations
 1. Average at least two acceptable tests; duplicate determinations should be within 3 ml/min/mm Hg of each other, or within 10% of the largest observed value.
 2. Use Jones method of timing the breath hold.
 3. Alveolar volume should be determined by single-breath dilution of tracer gas.
 4. Adjust for V_D volumes (instrument and patient).
 5. Determine inspired gas conditions (ATPS or ATPD).
 6. Correct for CO_2 and H_2O absorption.
 7. Report DLCO/V_A in ml CO (STPD)/min/mm Hg per L (BTPS).
 8. Correct predicted value for Hb, COHb, and altitude (P_IO_2) as appropriate (see text).
 9. Consider adjusting predicted value for submaximal inspiration.
 10. Use reference equations appropriate to the laboratory method and patient population.

Compiled from MacIntyre NM, Crapo RO, Viegi G et al: Standardisation of the single-breath determination of carbon monoxide uptake in the lung, *Eur Resp J* 2005; 26:720-735.

tive to the accumulation of COHb in the capillary blood and the resultant back-pressure. Capillary P_{CO} is routinely assumed to be zero. The actual alveolocapillary CO gradient at the time of testing can be estimated, although with some difficulty. The rebreathing method can be used during exercise provided the rebreathing interval is carefully controlled. An additional advantage is that acetylene can be added to the diffusion mixture to measure cardiac output simultaneously. Adding a small amount of nitric oxide (NO) to the diffusion mixture allows the $D_{L_{NO}}$ to be measured during rebreathing as well.

Measurement of DLCO by the intrabreath method (DLCOib) offers the advantage of not requiring a breath hold at TLC. However, the patient must inspire a large enough volume of test gas so that the subsequent exhalation will clear the instrument and anatomic V_D. In addition, the single-breath exhalation must be slow and even. In some systems, a flow restrictor may be necessary to limit expiratory flow. The single-breath slow-exhalation method produces values similar to those obtained by the breath-hold method in healthy patients when flow is maintained at 0.5 L/sec. Uneven distribution of ventilation may produce intrabreath DLCO values that are artificially elevated. Because the evenness of ventilation distribution can be assessed from the washout of CH_4, unacceptable DLCO values can be detected. Table 5-1 compares some advantages and disadvantages of DLCO testing methods.

Measurement of membrane (Dm) and red blood cell components (θVc) of diffusion resistance in healthy patients reveals that each factor accounts for approximately half of the total resistance to gas exchange across the alveolocapillary membranes. Difficulty in quantifying the partial pressure of O_2 in the lungs (pulmonary capillaries) restricts the use of the membrane-diffusing capacity determination. Because uptake of NO is limited almost entirely by the pulmonary capillary membranes, $D_{L_{NO}}$ can be measured to assess membrane resistance.

Numerous other physiologic factors can influence the observed DLCO:

1. *Hemoglobin and hematocrit (Hct).* Decreased Hb or Hct reduces DLCO, whereas increased Hb and Hct elevate DLCO. DLCO may be corrected if the patient's Hb is known. CO uptake varies approximately 7% for each gram of Hb. The predicted DLCO may be corrected so that the value reported is compared to a standardized Hb level of 14.6 g% for men and 13.4 g% for women and children younger than 15 years. When this correction is applied, the predicted DLCO will be reduced (and the % of predicted increased) if the patient's Hb is less than the standard value (14.6 g% or 13.4 g%, respectively). Conversely, the predicted DLCO increases (and the % of predicted decreases) if the Hb is greater than the standard value. Both corrected and uncorrected DLCO predicted values should be reported, along with the Hb value used for adjustment. Care should be taken to use Hb values that are representative of the patient's actual Hb level at the time of the DLCO test.

2. *COHb.* Increased COHb levels, often found in smokers, reduce DLCO. Smokers may have COHb levels of 10% or greater, causing significant CO back-pressure. The diffusion gradient for CO across alveolocapillary membranes is assumed to equal the alveolar pressure of CO. In healthy nonsmoking patients, very little CO (usually less than 2% COHb) is present in pulmonary capillary blood. When there is carboxyhemoglobinemia, diffusion of CO is reduced because the gradient across the membrane is reduced. COHb also shifts the oxyhemoglobin dissociation curve, further altering gas transfer. Each 1% increase in COHb causes an approximate 1% decrease in the measured DLCO. CO back-pressure corrections can also be made by estimating the partial pressure of CO in the pulmonary capillaries. This pressure can be used to correct the $F_{A}CO_0$ and the $F_{A}CO_T$. More commonly, however, the predicted DLCO is corrected for the presence of COHb in excess of 2% (see the section about techniques).

3. *Alveolar P_{CO_2}.* Increased P_{CO_2} elevates DLCO because the alveolar PO_2 is necessarily decreased. Significant increases in alveolar P_{CO_2} (i.e., moderate to severe hypoventilation) reduce the alveolar PO_2.

4. *Pulmonary capillary blood volume.* Increased blood volume in the lungs (V_C) causes increased DLCO. Increases in pulmonary capillary blood volume may result from increased cardiac output as

occurs during exercise. Patients should be seated and resting for several minutes before DLCO testing is performed. Pulmonary hemorrhage and left-to-right shunts may also cause an increase in blood volume in the lungs. In each of these cases, the increase in DLCO is related to the increased volume of Hb available for gas transfer. Excessive negative intrathoracic pressure during breath holding can increase pulmonary capillary volume and elevate the DLCO. Conversely, excessive positive intrathoracic pressure (Valsalva maneuver) can reduce pulmonary blood flow and decrease DLCO.

5. *Body position.* The supine position increases DLCO. Changes in body position affect the distribution of capillary blood flow.
6. *Altitude above sea level.* DLCO varies inversely with changes in alveolar oxygen pressure (P_AO_2). At altitudes significantly greater than sea level, DLCO increases unless corrections are made (see the section on techniques).
7. *Asthma and obesity.* Asthma and obesity have been associated with an elevated DLCO in some studies. Increased pulmonary capillary blood volume may explain these observations, but the exact physiology is unclear.

Several additional technical considerations may affect the measurement of DLCO (particularly DLCOsb). V_A is calculated from the dilution of a tracer gas during the single-breath maneuver. This technique typically underestimates lung volume in patients who have moderate or severe obstruction. Low estimated V_A results in low DLCO values. Some clinicians prefer to use a separately determined lung volume to estimate V_A. RV, measured independently by plethysmography or one of the gas dilution techniques, can be added to the inspired volume (V_I) to derive V_A. The V_A calculated by this method is usually larger in patients with airway obstruction than V_A calculated from the single-breath dilution method. The resulting estimate of DLCO is larger. The DLCO calculation, however, is based on the volume of gas into which both the inspired CO and tracer gas are distributed, but not the lung volume in which gas mixing is minimal. Some laboratories report DLCO values calculated by both methods. The ATS/ERS recommends calculation of V_A using the single-breath tracer gas method.

Comparison of the single-breath V_A measured during the DLCO maneuver with lung volumes (i.e., TLC) measured by the standard methods is often helpful in elucidating the cause for a low DLCO.

The method of timing of breath hold also influences the calculation of DLCO (see Figure 5-2). Most systems measure breath-hold time by one of three methods:
1. *Jones method:* includes 0.7 of the inspiratory time to the midpoint of the alveolar sample
2. *Epidemiology Standardization Project (ESP) method:* from the midpoint of inspiration (half of the V_I) to the beginning of alveolar sampling
3. *Ogilvie method:* from the beginning of inspiration (V_I) to the beginning of alveolar sampling

Theoretically, breath-hold time is considered the time during which diffusion occurs. That is, the DLCO equation assumes that the entire breath hold is at TLC. However, because some gas transfer takes place during inspiration and expiration, DLCO will be influenced by the proportion of time spent in these two phases. A **three-equation method** has been proposed that uses separate equations for the three phases of the maneuver (i.e., inspiration, breath hold, expiration). This method has not been widely used, however. The timing method may become significant if the reference values used for comparison were generated by one of the other methods. The Jones method is the recommended method (see Box 5-1). Rapid inspiration from RV to TLC and rapid expiration to the alveolar sampling phase reduces differences resulting from the timing methods (see Box 5-1). Conversely, patients who display prolonged inspiratory or expiratory times may have reduced DLCO values.

The volume of gas discarded before collecting the alveolar sample may affect the measured DLCO. Most automated systems allow the washout volume to be adjusted, with 0.75–1.0 L most commonly used. Washout volume may need to be reduced to 0.5 L if the patient's VC is less than 2.0 L. In patients who have obstructive disease, reducing the washout volume may result in increased dead-space gas being added to the alveolar sample. Because dead-space gas resembles the diffusion mixture, DLCO may be underestimated.

Alveolar sampling technique also affects DLCO measurement. Alveolar samples should be collected within 4 seconds, including washout and alveolar sampling. A sample volume of 0.5 – 1.0 L is recommended. Patients with a small VC (i.e., less than 2.0 L) may require a smaller volume, just as with the washout. When only a small sample is obtained, the gas may not accurately reflect alveolar concentrations of CO and tracer gas, particularly in the presence of $\dot{V}/\dot{Q}$ abnormalities. Continuous analysis of the expirate using rapidly responding analyzers allows identification of alveolar gas. Infrared analyzers that can simultaneously analyze the tracer gas and CO will allow the entire breath to be analyzed. These instruments permit adjustment of the alveolar sampling window so that a representative gas sample can be obtained (see Figure 5-3).

SUMMARY

This chapter addresses the measurement of diffusing capacity (DLCO), also referred to as transfer factor:

- DLCO can be measured by various techniques, including the single-breath, rebreathing, and intrabreath methods.

- The single-breath method, or DLCOsb, is the most commonly used. DLCOsb is noninvasive and can be repeated easily to obtain multiple measurements. Many automated DLCOsb systems are available.
- The ATS/ERS and others have published standardization guidelines for DLCOsb. Careful attention to standards and clinical practice guidelines can reduce the variability in DLCOsb measurements in different laboratories.
- DLCO measurements are used diagnostically for a variety of diseases. Because DLCO assesses gas exchange, it is useful in both obstructive and restrictive disease patterns.
- DLCO measurements may be affected by a variety of factors, such as Hb level, COHb, or altitude. Techniques for correcting DLCO for these factors include adjusting the predicted values used for interpretation.

CASE 5-1

Case Studies

 HISTORY
P.M. is a 55-year-old woman referred to the pulmonary function laboratory because of shortness of breath on exertion. She has a 38-pack-year smoking history but stopped smoking 6 months ago. She still coughs each morning, but her sputum volume has decreased since she stopped smoking. She has no significant environmental or family history of

pulmonary disease. She had been using an inhaled β-agonist but withheld it for 12 hours before the test.

PULMONARY FUNCTION TESTING

Personal Data

Age:	55
Height:	65 in (165 cm)
Weight:	137 lb (62.3 kg)
Race:	African American

Spirometry

	PREBRONCHODILATOR				POSTBRONCHODILATOR		
	Predicted	LLN*	Actual	% Predicted	Actual	% Predicted	% Change
FVC (L)	2.89	2.16	2.77	96	2.82	98	2
FEV$_1$ (L)	2.30	1.67	1.91	83	2.01	87	5
FEV$_{1\%}$ (%)	80	70	69		71		
FEF$_{25\%-75\%}$ (L/sec)	2.33	0.92	1.44	62	1.51	65	5
PEF (L/min)	6.08	4.01	4.01	66	5.13	84	28

*Lower limit of normal.

Lung Volumes

	Predicted	LLN*	Actual	% Predicted
TLC (L)	4.39	3.42	4.97	113
FRC (L)	2.45		3.10	127
RV (L)	1.58		2.20	139
VC (L)	2.89	2.16	2.77	96
IC (L)	1.94		1.87	96
ERV (L)	0.87		0.90	103
RV/TLC (%)	36		44	

*Lower limit of normal.

Diffusing Capacity

	Predicted	Actual	% Predicted
DLCOsb (ml CO/min/mm Hg)	19.7	10.0	51
DLCOsb corr (ml CO/min/mm Hg)	18.1	10.0	55
V_A (L)	4.39	3.99	91
D_L/V_A	4.49	2.51	46
Hb (g/dl)		11.0	

TECHNOLOGIST'S COMMENTS

Spirometry maneuvers met ATS/ERS criteria. Lung volumes by body plethysmography were performed acceptably and met ATS/ERS criteria. All DLCO maneuvers met ATS/ERS criteria (two tests were averaged). DLCO was corrected for an Hb of 11 g/dl.

QUESTIONS

1. What is the interpretation of:
   a. Prebronchodilator and postbronchodilator spirometry?
   b. Lung volumes?
   c. DLCO?
2. How are the pulmonary function test results related to the patient's symptoms?
3. What other tests might be indicated?
4. What treatment might be recommended based on these findings?

DISCUSSION

Interpretation

All maneuvers were performed acceptably. FVC and FEV_1 are within normal limits, but the $FEV_{1\%}$ is below the lower limit of normal, consistent with airway obstruction. After inhaled bronchodilator, there is only a minimal change in FEV_1 and FVC. Lung volumes reveal a slightly increased functional residual capacity and moderately increased RV. The RV/TLC ratio is increased, consistent with air trapping. DLCO is markedly decreased, even after correction for Hb. D_L/V_A is decreased, consistent with an obstructive process.

Impression: Mild obstruction with minimal response to bronchodilator; this should not preclude a therapeutic trial if clinically indicated. Lung volumes suggest air trapping. DLCO is severely decreased even when corrected for Hb.

Cause of Symptoms

This patient has symptoms characteristic of airway obstruction that has progressed to the point where dyspnea on exertion prompted a visit to the physician. Her obstruction appears mild. Her FEV_1 is still above the lower limit of normal (LLN) for her age and height. Her response to bronchodilator therapy seems to indicate obstruction caused by inflammation rather than reversible bronchospasm. Lung volume testing confirms that the obstruction appears to have caused some air trapping. This pattern is not unusual for patients with chronic bronchitis and emphysema.

Her gas exchange, as measured by DLCO, is markedly impaired. Emphysema reduces DLCO by reducing the alveolocapillary surface area available for diffusion. Chronic bronchitis can reduce DLCO by causing a ventilation-perfusion mismatch. The patient may have both of these disease processes disrupting gas transfer. Her V_A measured by the single-breath inhalation of tracer gas during the DLCO maneuver is about a liter less than her TLC measured in the body plethysmograph. This discrepancy suggests poor distribution of inspired gas and is typical in patients with some degree of airway obstruction.

Patients who have reduced DLCO values seldom have normal blood gases. Exertion or exercise often aggravates the gas exchange impairment. Many patients with markedly reduced DLCO (less than 50%–60% of predicted) display exercise desaturation. That is, their PaO_2 falls to levels of 55 mm Hg or less with exercise.

continued

The decrease in DLCO does not, however, accurately predict the degree of desaturation that will occur.

Other Tests

An obvious additional test for this patient would be measuring resting arterial blood gases while she breathes room air. Resting hypoxemia would explain dyspnea on exertion. The patient returned to have a blood gas sample drawn. Her PaO_2 while breathing air was 63 mm Hg, with a saturation of 91%. Because this value did not qualify her for supplemental O_2, an exercise test was performed with an arterial catheter in place (see Chapter 7). At a low workload on the treadmill, her PaO_2 decreased to 51 mm Hg. She was then retested while breathing O_2 via nasal cannula at 1 L/min. She then tolerated more exercise, and her PaO_2 never decreased below 68 mm Hg.

Treatment

On the basis of the results of the exercise evaluation, supplemental O_2 was prescribed for the patient to use during exertion. Because she showed little response to bronchodilators, her inhaled β-agonist was discontinued. However, a trial of inhaled steroids (beclomethasone) resulted in noticeable improvement in symptoms.

CASE 5-2

Case Studies

HISTORY

B.C. is a 63-year-old woman with a history of cardiomyopathy, hypertension, and pernicious anemia. She has had episodes of ventricular tachycardia that have been managed by means of an automatic implantable cardiac defibrillator (AICD). She has never smoked and denies cough or sputum production. She experiences shortness of breath with exertion. Her family history includes a sister who had asthma and chronic bronchitis. She has no history of environmental toxin exposure. To manage her arrhythmias, her physician prescribed amiodarone.

To monitor the effects of this medication, she was referred for tests before starting the drug and again after 3 months of therapy.

PULMONARY FUNCTION TESTING

Personal Data

Sex:	Female
Age:	63
Height:	62 in (157 cm)
Weight:	131 lb (59.5 kg)
Race:	White

Spirometry

	PRETREATMENT				3 MONTHS	
	Predicted	LLN	Actual	% Predicted	Actual	% Predicted
FVC (L)	2.96	2.31	2.50	84	1.97	67
FEV$_1$ (L)	2.27	1.72	2.09	92	1.81	80
FEV$_{1\%}$ (%)	77	68	84		92	
FEF$_{25\%-75\%}$ (L/sec)	2.09	0.94	2.82	135	2.77	133

Lung Volumes (He Dilution)

	PRETREATMENT				3 MONTHS	
	Predicted	LLN	Actual	% Predicted	Actual	% Predicted
TLC (L)	4.88	3.66	3.92	87	3.50	78
FRC (L)	2.54		2.26	89	2.23	88
RV (L)	1.71		1.50	87	1.52	89
VC (L)	2.96	2.31	2.42	82	1.97	67
IC (L)	1.94		1.66	85	1.26	65
ERV (L)	0.83		0.76	91	0.71	85
RV/TLC (%)	38		38		44	

Diffusing Capacity (DLCOsb)

	PRETREATMENT			3 MONTHS	
	Predicted	Actual	% Predicted	Actual	% Predicted
DLCO (ml/min/mmHg)	18.0	12.6	69	9.7	54
DLCOsb corr (ml/min/mmHg)	16.7	12.6	75	9.7	58
V_A (L)	4.48	3.26	72	3.31	95
DL/V_A	4.0	3.9		2.9	
Hb (g/dL)	13.4	11.3		11.4	

TECHNOLOGIST'S COMMENTS

Pretreatment: Spirometry and lung volumes by He dilution met ATS/ERS criteria. The inspiratory volume during the DLCO maneuver was less than 85% of the VC.

3 Months: Spirometry, lung volumes and DLCO all met ATS/ERS criteria.

QUESTIONS

1. What is the interpretation of:
   a. Pretreatment spirometry, lung volumes?
   b. DLCO before treatment?
   c. DLCO after 3 months of treatment?
2. What is the cause of change in the patient's DLCO?
3. What technical problems might have affected the interpretation of the DLCO before treatment?

DISCUSSION

Interpretation

Pretreatment, FVC is normal, as are FEV_1 and $FEV_{1\%}$. Lung volumes by He dilution are normal. The diffusing capacity was substandard in performance because the patient could not inspire fully. The best efforts show mildly reduced DLCO that is at the lower limit of normal after correction for the patient's Hb of 11.3.

After 3 months, FVC is decreased, but FEV_1 is normal. This makes the $FEV_{1\%}$ appear greater than expected. Lung volumes by He dilution show a TLC that is mildly decreased but with a normal FRC and RV. DLCO is moderately decreased, even when corrected for an Hb of 11.4 g%. Since the previous test, the patient's VC has decreased slightly, and the DLCO has decreased significantly.

CAUSE OF CHANGES IN DIFFUSING CAPACITY

This case presents a good example of one application of DLCO: monitoring drug therapy. The patient had essentially normal lung function. Initially, her DLCO was slightly reduced. However, because she had a history of anemia, her Hb level was checked. The Hb-adjusted DLCO was at the lower limit of normal (~75% for the reference equation used). Because amiodarone

has been shown to cause changes to the lung parenchyma, her cardiologist requested pulmonary function studies, including DLCO.

On her return visit after 3 months of antiarrhythmic therapy, some significant changes had occurred. As described in the interpretation of the 3-month follow-up, her FVC had decreased slightly. TLC also decreased by a similar volume (400–500 ml). Her other lung volumes (FRC, RV) remained largely unchanged. These changes suggest that something happened that primarily affected her VC.

The patient's DLCO showed the greatest decrease during the 3-month period. Her DLCO decreased by approximately 30%. The Hb corrected % of predicted fell from 75% to 58%. The DL/V_A ratio also decreased slightly. The DL/V_A ratio is often preserved when DLCO decreases simply because of loss of lung volume. When the DL/V_A ratio decreases in conjunction with a low DLCO, factors other than loss of lung volume are assumed to be responsible for the change. In this patient, it appears that drug therapy did affect DLCO. However, a pattern of pneumonitis and fibrosis causing reduced lung volumes is not clearly evident. Because of the changes in DLCO, amiodarone therapy was discontinued.

TECHNICAL FACTORS INFLUENCING DLCO

Two noteworthy technical factors are illustrated by this case. Correction of DLCO for the effects of abnormal levels of Hb is important. In this mildly anemic patient, correction for Hb resulted in a small difference in DLCO in both tests. Her pretreatment DLCO appears mildly decreased but is borderline normal when corrected for Hb. After 3 months of amiodarone therapy, both the uncorrected and corrected DLCO values are below normal. Comparison of serial DLCO measurements can be compromised if one test is Hb-adjusted and the other is not.

A second factor is that the patient's pretreatment DLCO tests did not meet established criteria for ac-

continued

ceptability. She was unable to inspire at least 85% of her VC in any of the maneuvers. This information is documented in the technologist's comments for the test. When the patient fails to inspire maximally, the breath hold may not occur at TLC. Therefore DLCO may appear low compared with predicted values. This technical difficulty may have influenced the pretreatment test results. The patient's measured V_A (3.26 L) was significantly less than the TLC assessed by He dilution (3.92 L). In this instance, it may be appropriate to correct the predicted DLCO for the effect of the reduced lung volume using the equation described previously:

$$DLCO(at\ V_{Am}) = DLCO(at\ V_{Ap}) \times (0.58 + 0.42(V_{Am}/V_{Ap}))$$

Substituting the patient's measured alveolar volume (V_{Am}) and the predicted alveolar volume (V_{Ap}),

along with the Hb-corrected predicted DLCO (16.7 ml/min/mm Hg, in this case) for the right-hand terms in the equation:

$$DLCO(at\ V_{Am}) = 16.7 \times (0.58 + 0.42(3.26/4.48))$$

$$DLCO(at\ V_{Am}) =$$
14.8 ml/min/mm Hg (predicted at the measured V_A)

When the patient's measured DLCO of 12.6 ml/min/mm Hg is compared with 14.8 ml/min/mm Hg as the expected value, the percent predicted becomes 85%. Correcting for Hb and the effect of a substandard inspired volume suggests that the patient's diffusing capacity was well within normal limits before beginning the antiarrhythmic therapy.

SELF-ASSESSMENT QUESTIONS

Entry-level

1. Correct performance of the DLCOsb requires that the subject inspire at least:
   a. 90% of the TLC
   b. 85% of the VC
   c. 80% of the IC
   d. 2–3 times the V_T

2. In which DLCO method does the patient perform slow exhalation of the VC (after inspiring diffusion test gas)?
   a. DLCOrb (rebreathing)
   b. DL_{NO} (nitric oxide)
   c. DLCOsb (single breath)
   d. DLCOib (intrabreath)

3. A patient with a VC of 2.0 L performs several DLCOsb maneuvers with these results:

Trial	DLCO	DL/V$_A$	V$_I$
1	8.0	4.0	1.8
2	7.4	3.8	1.4
3	7.3	3.6	1.4
4	6.9	4.0	1.0

The pulmonary function technologist should:
   a. Average the first two trials and report the result
   b. Report the DLCO as 8.0
   c. Average all trials and report the result
   d. Perform one more trial

4. In which of the following conditions would an increased DLCO be expected?
   I.   Pulmonary hemorrhage
   II. Sarcoidosis
   III. Pneumonectomy
   IV. Polycythemia
   a. I and III
   b. I and IV
   c. II and III
   d. II and IV

5. DLCO is often reduced in emphysema because of
   I.   Fibrotic granulomas
   II. Destruction of alveolar septa
   III. Anemia
   IV. Increased distance from the terminal bronchiole to alveolocapillary membrane
   a. I and II
   b. I and III
   c. II and IV
   d. III and IV

Advanced

6. A 52-year-old female patient has a DLCO of 15.0 ml/min/mm Hg with a predicted value of 20.0. If her Hb is 9.5 g/dl, what is her corrected % of predicted diffusing capacity?
   a. 64%
   b. 75%
   c. 88%
   d. 91%

7. A 25-year-old male has an uncorrected D_{LCO} of 24.9 ml/min/mm Hg (69% of predicted) but no history of pulmonary disease. Which of the following might explain these findings?
  I.   Left-to-right shunt
  II. Carboxyhemoglobinemia
  III. Congestive heart failure
  IV. Anemia
    a. I and II only
    b. III and IV only
    c. I, II, and III
    d. II, III, and IV

8. An adult patient whose TLC is 6.5 L (by plethysmography) performs two acceptable D_{LCOsb} maneuvers and records the following results:

D_{LCOsb}	9.1 ml/min/mm Hg
V_A	4.5 L

Which of the following interpretive statements is most consistent with these values?
    a. Normal diffusing capacity corrected for lung volume
    b. Reduced D_{LCO} consistent with airway obstruction
    c. Reduced D_{LCO} consistent with a restrictive defect
    d. Reduced D_{LCO} consistent with obesity

9. A healthy adult male has his D_{LCO} measured at two different levels of inspired oxygen to estimate his membrane diffusing capacity. Which of the following results would be expected in this subject?
    a. 1/Dm and 1/θVc approximately equal
    b. 1/Dm approximately two times larger than 1/θVc
    c. 1/θVc approximately two times larger than 1/Dm
    d. 1/Dm 5–10 times larger than 1/θVc

10. A patient has a D_{LCOsb} of 10.6 ml/min/mm Hg (STPD), which is 50% of his predicted value. His D_L/V_A ratio is 1.6. Which of the following is most consistent with these values?
    a. Pulmonary hemorrhage
    b. Pneumonectomy
    c. Pulmonary emphysema
    d. Obesity

Selected Bibliography

GENERAL REFERENCES

Crapo RO, Jensen RL, Wanger JS: Single-breath carbon monoxide diffusing capacity, *Clin Chest Med* 2001; 22:637-649.

Hadeli KO, Siegel EM, Sherrill DL et al: Predictors of oxygen desaturation during submaximal exercise in 8,000 patients, *Chest* 2001; 120:88-92.

Hsia CW: Recruitment of lung diffusing capacity, *Chest* 2006; 1222:1774-1783.

Jensen RL, Crapo RO: Diffusing capacity: how to get it right, *Respir Care* 2003; 48:777-782.

Johnson DC: Importance of adjusting carbon monoxide diffusing capacity (DLCO) and carbon monoxide transfer coefficient (KCO) for alveolar lung volume, *Respir Med* 2000; 94:28-37.

Saydain G, Beck KC, Decker PA et al: Clinical significance of elevated diffusing capacity, *Chest* 2004; 125:446-452.

Stam H, Splinter TAW, Versprille A: Evaluation of diffusing capacity in patients with a restrictive lung disease, *Chest* 2000; 117:752-757.

D_{LCOsb}

Crapo RO, Morris AH: Standardized single breath normal values for carbon monoxide diffusing capacity, *Am Rev Respir Dis* 1981; 123:185-192.

Dinakara P, Blumenthal WS, Johnston RF et al: The effect of anemia on pulmonary diffusing capacity with derivation of a correction equation, *Am Rev Respir Dis* 1970; 102:965-972.

Graham BL, Mink JT, Cotton DJ: Effect of breath hold time on D_{LCOsb} in patients with airway obstruction, *J Appl Physiol* 1985; 58:1319-1325.

Graham BL, Mink JT, Cotton DJ: Overestimation of the single breath carbon monoxide diffusing capacity in patients with air-flow obstruction, *Am Rev Respir Dis* 1984; 129:403-409.

Kanner RE, Crapo RO: The relationship between alveolar oxygen tension and the single breath carbon monoxide diffusing capacity, *Am Rev Respir Dis* 1986; 133:676-681.

Leech JA, Martz L, Liben A et al: Diffusing capacity for carbon monoxide: the effects of different durations of breath hold time and alveolar volume and of carbon monoxide back pressure on calculated results, *Am Rev Respir Dis* 1985; 132:1127-1135.

Mohsenifar Z, Tashkin DP: Effect of carboxyhemoglobin on the single breath diffusing capacity: derivation of an empirical correction factor, *Respiration* 1979; 37:185-188.

Punjabi NM, Shade D, Patel AM et al: Measurement variability in single breath diffusing capacity of the lung, *Chest* 2003; 123:1082-1089.

DLCORB

Barazanji KW, Ramanathan M, Johnson RL Jr et al: A modified rebreathing technique using an infrared gas analyzer, *J Appl Physiol* 1996; 80:1258-1262.

Hsia CCW, McBrayer DG, Ramanathan M: Reference values of pulmonary diffusing capacity during exercise by a rebreathing technique, *Am J Respir Crit Care Med* 1995; 152:658-665.

Sackner MA, Greenletch D, Heiman M et al: Diffusing capacity, membrane diffusing capacity, capillary blood volume, pulmonary tissue volume and cardiac output by a rebreathing technique, *Am Rev Respir Dis* 1975; 111:157-165.

DLCOIB

Huang Y-C, MacIntyre NR: Real-time gas analysis improves the measurement of single-breath diffusing capacity, *Am Rev Respir Dis* 1992; 146:946-950.

Newth CJL, Cotton DJ, Nadel JA: Pulmonary diffusing capacity measured at multiple intervals during a single exhalation in man, *J Appl Physiol Respir Environ Physiol* 1977; 43:617-623.

Wilson AF, Hearne J, Brennan M et al: Measurement of transfer factor during constant exhalation, *Thorax* 1994; 49:1121-1126.

STANDARDS AND GUIDELINES

American Association for Respiratory Care: Single-breath carbon monoxide diffusing capacity: 1999 Update, *Respir Care* 1999; 44:539-546.

MacIntyre N, Crapo R, Viegi G et al: Standardisation of the single-breath determination of carbon monoxide uptake in the lung, *Eur Respir J* 2005; 26:720-735.

Blood Gases and Related Tests

CHAPTER OUTLINE

OBJECTIVES

After studying this chapter you will be able to:

Entry-level

1. Describe how pH and PCO_2 are used to assess acid-base status
2. Interpret PO_2 and oxygen saturation to assess oxygenation
3. Identify the appropriate procedure for obtaining an arterial blood gas specimen
4. List situations in which pulse oximetry can be used to evaluate a patient's oxygenation

Advanced

1. Describe at least two limitations of pulse oximetry
2. Describe the use of capnography to assess changes in ventilation-perfusion patterns of the lung
3. Assess oxygenation using arterial oxygen content
4. Calculate the shunt fraction using appropriate laboratory data

KEY TERMS

A-a gradient	base excess (BE)	Hb affinity
a-v̄ content difference	capnography	hemoximetry
Allen's test	cyanosis	Henderson-Hasselbalch equation

methemoglobin	polarographic	spectrophotometer
oxygen content	pulse oximetry (SpO_2)	Swan-Ganz catheter
pH	shunt fraction	transcutaneous
phosphorescence	solubility	

Blood gas analysis is the most basic test of lung function. Evaluation of the acid-base and oxygenation status of the body provides important information about the function of the lungs themselves. Anaerobic sampling of arterial blood is required, which is an invasive procedure that carries risks involved with blood-borne pathogens. Pulse oximetry and capnography measure gas exchange parameters and have the advantage of monitoring patients noninvasively. Understanding the limitations of noninvasive techniques allows them to be used to provide appropriate patient care. Calculating **oxygen content** and the **shunt fraction** uses blood gas measurements to assess gas exchange as it applies to oxygenation.

This chapter addresses how blood gas measurements are used in the pulmonary function laboratory. A complete description of blood gas electrodes and other measuring devices is included in Chapter 10. The use of pulse oximetry and capnography as adjuncts to traditional invasive measures is discussed. Two methods of calculating shunt fraction are detailed so that the most appropriate method may be used.

pH

pH is the negative logarithm of the hydrogen ion [H^+] concentration in the blood, used as a positive number. The pH scale has no units. It is derived by converting the [H^+] to a negative exponent of 10 and calculating its logarithm. The [H^+] of water is 1×10^{-7} mol/L. The negative logarithm of 1×10^{-7} is 7. The pH of water (7) represents the midpoint of the pH scale. The physiologic range of pH in blood in clinical practice is from approximately 6.90 – 7.80.

CARBON DIOXIDE TENSION

PCO_2 is a measurement of the partial pressure exerted by CO_2 in solution in the blood. The measurement is expressed in millimeters of mercury (mm Hg) or in kilopascals (kPa) used in the International System of Units (1 mm Hg × 0.133 kPa). The normal range for PCO_2 in arterial blood is 35 – 45 mm Hg (4.66 – 5.99 kPa). In mixed venous blood, PCO_2 varies from 40 – 46 mm Hg (5.32 – 6.12 kPa).

OXYGEN TENSION

PO_2 measures the partial pressure exerted by oxygen (O_2) dissolved in the blood. Like PCO_2, it is recorded in millimeters of mercury or in kilopascals. The normal range for arterial PO_2 is 80 – 100 mm Hg (10.64 – 13.30 kPa) for healthy young adults breathing air at sea level. The normal range declines slightly in older adults. Mixed venous PO_2 averages 40 mm Hg (5.32 kPa) in healthy patients. Barometric pressure (at altitudes significantly above sea level) also influences the expected arterial PO_2 (see Appendix C).

Techniques

pH

Blood pH is measured by exposing the specimen to a glass electrode (see Figure 10-28) or by measuring light absorbance with an optical pH indicator under anaerobic conditions. pH measurements are made at 37°C. The pH of arterial blood is related to the $PaCO_2$ by the **Henderson-Hasselbalch equation**:

$$pH = pK + \log \frac{[HCO_3^-]}{[CO_2]}$$

where:

pK = negative log of dissociation constant for carbonic acid (6.1)

$[HCO_3^-]$ = molar concentration of serum bicarbonate

$[CO_2]$ = molar concentration of CO_2

$PaCO_2$ (measured directly by a CO_2 electrode or similar device) may be multiplied by 0.03 (the solubility coefficient for CO_2) to express $PaCO_2$ in milliequivalents per liter (mEq/L). The equation then may be expressed as follows:

$$pH = pK + \log \frac{[HCO_3^-]}{[0.03(PaCO_2)]}$$

Carbon Dioxide Tension

PCO_2 has been measured traditionally by exposing whole blood to a modified pH electrode contained in a jacket with a Teflon membrane at its tip (see Chapter 10). The jacket contains a bicarbonate buffer. As CO_2 diffuses through the membrane, it combines with water to form carbonic acid (H_2CO_3). The H_2CO_3 dissociates into H^+ and HCO_3^-, thereby changing the pH of the bicarbonate buffer. The change in pH is measured by the electrode and is proportional to the PCO_2. Newer blood gas analyzers use a **spectrophotometer** to measure the absorbance of CO_2 in the infrared portion of the spectrum. The blood must be anticoagulated and kept in an anaerobic state until analysis. PCO_2 may also be estimated using a **transcutaneous** electrode. Measurement of end-tidal CO_2 ($PETCO_2$) is sometimes used to track PCO_2 (see the section on capnography, later in this chapter).

pH and PCO_2 are usually measured from the same sample, so bicarbonate can be easily calculated. Automated blood gas analyzers perform this calculation along with others to derive values such as total CO_2 (dissolved CO_2 plus HCO_3^-) and stan-

dard bicarbonate (i.e., HCO_3^- corrected to a $PaCO_2$ of 40 mm Hg). If the hemoglobin (Hb) is measured or estimated, the **base excess (BE)** can be calculated. The normal buffer base at a pH of 7.40 is approximately 48 mEq/L. BE is the difference between the actual buffering capacity of the blood and the expected value (~48 mEq/L). When the buffering capacity is less than the expected value, the difference is a negative value. This is sometimes referred to as a base deficit rather than a negative base excess. The main buffers that affect the BE are HCO_3^- and Hb.

Oxygen Tension

The PO_2 (arterial or mixed venous) has been traditionally measured by exposing whole blood, obtained anaerobically, to a platinum electrode covered with a thin polypropylene membrane. This type of electrode is called a **polarographic** electrode or Clark electrode. Oxygen molecules are reduced at the platinum cathode after diffusing through the membrane (see Chapter 10). Newer blood gas analyzers use an optical system that senses the ability of O_2 to change the intensity and duration of **phosphorescence** in a phosphorescent dye. PO_2 may also be measured using a transcutaneous electrode (see Chapter 10).

PF TIP

Blood gas analyzers usually report blood gas values at 37°C. If the patient has an extreme body temperature (hypothermia or hyperthermia), correction may be useful. At low body temperatures, more gas dissolves in the blood, so PO_2 and PCO_2 show lower values when exposed to electrodes that measure their activity. At elevated temperatures, the opposite occurs; less gas dissolves and partial pressures appear higher. pH changes in relation to PCO_2.

Blood gas values (pH, PCO_2, PO_2) are influenced by the patient's temperature. Alteration of body temperature affects the partial pressure of dissolved CO_2, which influences pH as described in the previous equations. Table 6-1 describes the expected

TABLE 6-1			
Effects of Body Temperature on Blood Gas Values*			
Temperature (°C)	34°	37°	40°
pH	7.44	7.40	7.36
Pco_2	35	40	46
Po_2	79	95	114

*Temperature corrections based on algorithms from CLSI (formerly NCCLS): *C12-A Definitions of quantities and conventions related to blood pH and gas analysis; approved standard,* vol. 14, no. 11), 1994.

blood gas changes when the patient's temperature is not 37°C. Although blood gas measurements are made at 37°C, the value reported is sometimes corrected to the patient's temperature.

Technical problems with blood gas electrodes and related measuring devices include contamination by protein or blood products. In electrode-based analyzers, depletion of buffers in the electrodes may reduce accuracy and cause unacceptable drift. Tears or ruptures of the membranes used to cover the electrodes are also common malfunctions. Some newer analyzers use spectrophotometric methods that can be compromised by mechanical or electronic failure of the sampling cuvette, or by inadequate mixing of the specimen.

Specimen Collection for Blood Gases

Arterial samples are usually obtained from either the radial or the brachial artery in adults. Arterial specimens may also be drawn from the femoral or dorsalis pedis arteries. The radial artery of the nondominant hand is usually the preferred site.

Before a radial artery puncture, adequacy of collateral circulation to the hand from the ulnar artery should be established using the modified **Allen's test.** The technologist occludes both the radial and ulnar arteries by pressing down over the wrist. The patient is instructed to make a fist, then open the hand and relax the fingers. The palm of the hand is pale and bloodless because both arteries are occluded. The ulnar artery is released while the radial remains occluded. The hand should be reperfused rapidly (5–15 seconds) if the ulnar supply is

adequate. If perfusion is inadequate, an alternative site should be used.

Arterial puncture should not be performed through any type of lesion. Similarly, puncture distal to a surgical shunt (e.g., shunts used for dialysis) should be avoided. Infection or evidence of peripheral vascular disease should prompt selection of an alternative site. Some patients may be using anticoagulant drugs such as heparin, warfarin (Coumadin), or streptokinase. High doses of these drugs or a history of prolonged clotting times may be relative contraindications to arterial puncture. Box 6-1 lists some of the potential hazards associated with arterial puncture.

PF TIP

Success in obtaining an arterial specimen by radial puncture requires careful positioning of the patient's wrist. The hand should be hyperextended with good support under the wrist. A topical anesthetic may be useful for some patients, but is usually unnecessary. Always perform the modified Allen's test to ensure adequate collateral circulation before puncturing the artery. The person drawing the sample should be in a comfortable position (i.e., sitting) to maximize control of the needle during insertion. A vented syringe or similar device allows the blood to "pulse" into the syringe, ensuring that the needle is in the lumen of the artery.

Mixed venous samples are drawn from a pulmonary artery (Swan-Ganz) catheter. Contamination of the mixed venous specimen with flush solution is a common problem. Withdrawing a small volume of blood into a "waste" syringe ensures that the sample is not diluted by flush solution in the catheter. Care should be taken to limit the volume of blood removed in this process. Significant blood loss can occur with repetitive measurements. Another common problem with mixed venous specimen collection is displacement of the catheter tip. If the catheter is advanced too far, it may "wedge" into a pulmonary arteriole. Specimens drawn from this position often reflect arterialized pulmonary capillary blood. Similarly, if the catheter tip is withdrawn or "loops back," it may be in the

BOX 6-1	Complications of Arterial Puncture for Blood Gas Testing

- Pain and discomfort
- Hematoma
- Air or blood emboli
- Infection or contamination
- Inadvertent needle stick
- Vascular trauma or occlusion
- Vasovagal response
- Arterial spasm

BLOOD GASES 6-1

CRITERIA FOR ACCEPTABILITY

Blood Gases

1. Blood should be collected anaerobically. Syringe body and plunger should be tight-fitting. Commercially available blood gas kits should be used according to manufacturers' specifications. Air bubbles should be expelled immediately.
2. The specimen must be adequately anticoagulated; sodium or lithium heparin is preferred. If liquid heparin is used, all excess should be expelled. Choice of anticoagulant should be determined by analyses to be performed (e.g., electrolytes).
3. A sample volume of 2–4 ml is recommended.
4. The specimen should be analyzed as soon as possible. If immediate analysis is not available, the specimen should be drawn in a glass syringe and stored in an ice-water slurry at 0°C and analyzed within 1 hour. Specimens drawn in plastic syringes should not be placed in ice water.
5. The specimen should be adequately identified, including patient name and/or number, date/time, ordering physician, and accession number. Information provided with the specimen should be the site from which it was obtained, FIO_2 (if applicable), and ventilator settings (if applicable).
6. Analysis should be performed on an instrument that has been recently calibrated and whose function is documented by appropriate controls.

right ventricle or atrium rather than the pulmonary artery. Specimens obtained from this location may not represent true mixed venous blood.

Venous samples from peripheral veins are not useful for assessing oxygenation. Venous blood reflects only the metabolism of the area drained by that particular vein. Venous samples may be used for measurement of pH or blood lactate during exercise.

Blood is usually collected in a syringe to which an anticoagulant (e.g., heparin) has been added, and sealed from the atmosphere immediately (Blood Gases 6-1). Blood gases are typically drawn using specially designed syringes containing a dry anticoagulant (i.e., a blood gas "kit"). Dry heparin is applied to the lumen of the needle and the interior of the syringe. A small heparin pellet is often placed in the syringe to provide additional anticoagulation. Care must be taken that heparin solution (sometimes used for flushing arterial catheters) does not contaminate the sample. Contamination by flush solution may affect PO_2 and PCO_2 values by dilution, but the buffering capacity of whole blood prevents large changes in pH.

After the syringe has been capped (see Chapter 11 for safe handling of blood specimens), the sample should be thoroughly mixed by rolling or gently shaking. Mixing helps prevent the sample from clotting, whether dry or liquid heparin is used. Mixing is also important for analyzers that use spectrophotometric methods for measuring blood gases. Lithium heparin or a similar preparation should be used for specimens that will also be used for electrolyte analysis.

Air contamination of arterial or mixed venous blood specimens can seriously alter blood gas values. Room air at sea level has a PO_2 of approximately 150 mm Hg, and a PCO_2 near 0. If air bubbles are present in a blood gas specimen, equilibration of gases between the sample and air occurs (Table 6-2). Contamination commonly occurs during sampling when air is left in the syringe after the sample is collected. Small bubbles may also be introduced if the needle does not connect tightly to the syringe. Other sources of air contamination include poorly fitting plungers and failure to properly cap the syringe. Use of a vented syringe

TABLE 6-2

Air Contamination of Blood Gas Samples

	In Vivo Values	Air Contamination*
pH	7.40	7.45
P_{CO_2}	40	30
P_{O_2}	95	110

*Typical values that might occur when a blood gas specimen is exposed to air, either directly or by mixing with a solution that has been exposed to air (e.g., heparinized flush solution). The change in pH occurs because of the change in P_{CO_2}.

or one in which the pulse pressure of the blood displaces the plunger can help prevent air bubble contamination.

Sample storage depends on the type of syringe used. If a glass syringe is used, the sample may be stored in ice-water slush if analysis is not done within a few minutes. Ice water reduces the metabolism of red and white blood cells in the sample. Specimens with O_2 tensions in the normal physiologic range (50–150 mm Hg) show minimal changes over 1–2 hours for glass syringes if kept in ice water. Changes in specimens held at room temperature are related to cellular metabolism in the blood, particularly in white blood cells and platelets. Specimens with P_{O_2} values above 150 mm Hg are most susceptible to alterations resulting from gas leakage or cell metabolism. When the P_{O_2} is 150 mm Hg or more, Hb is almost completely bound with O_2. In such cases, a small change in O_2 content results in a large change in P_{O_2}.

If a plastic syringe is used, blood gas specimens should be analyzed within 30 minutes. Plastic syringes are not completely gas tight, so room air can contaminate the sample. The influx of O_2 may be counterbalanced by the consumption of O_2 if the sample is not iced. When a blood gas specimen is placed in an ice-water bath, the **solubility** of O_2 increases, as does the affinity of hemoglobin for oxygen. This lowers the partial pressure of O_2 in the sample and increases the gradient between the sample and the environment. This gradient exaggerates the leakage of O_2 into the specimen (as occurs with plastic syringes). When the sample is introduced into the analyzer at 37°C, solubility

and **Hb affinity** return to their normal values, the oxygen that leaked in is released, and the P_{O_2} is falsely increased. Because of these phenomena blood gas specimens in plastic syringes should not be placed in ice water. If specimens cannot be routinely analyzed within 30 minutes, glass syringes with ice-water storage may be preferable.

PF TIP

Blood gas specimens should be analyzed as soon as possible. Specimens drawn in plastic syringes should NOT be placed in ice water, and should be analyzed within 30 minutes. Specimens that cannot be analyzed within 30 minutes should be drawn in a glass syringe and placed in an ice-water slush to retard cellular metabolism. Blood gas specimens drawn for shunt studies and specimens with elevated white blood cell counts should be analyzed immediately to minimize changes in Pa_{O_2}.

Capillary samples are useful in infants when arterial puncture is impractical. The area for collection (the heel is commonly chosen) should be heated by a warm compress and lanced. Blood is then allowed to fill the required volume of heparinized glass capillary tubes. Squeezing the tissue should be avoided because predominately venous blood will be obtained. The capillary tubes should be carefully sealed to avoid air bubbles. Guidelines for quality control of blood gas analyzers and for the safe handling of blood specimens are included in Chapter 11.

Significance and Pathophysiology

See Blood Gases 6-2 for interpretive strategies.

pH

The pH of arterial blood in healthy adults averages 7.40 with a range of 7.35–7.45. Arterial pH below 7.35 constitutes acidemia. A pH above 7.45 constitutes alkalemia. Because of the logarithmic scale, a

BLOOD GASES 6-2

INTERPRETIVE STRATEGIES

Blood Gases

1. Was the blood gas specimen obtained acceptably? Free of air bubbles and clots? Analyzed promptly and/or iced appropriately?
2. Did the blood gas analyzer function properly? Was there a recent acceptable calibration of all electrodes or sensors? Was analyzer function validated by appropriate quality controls?
3. Is pH within normal limits (7.35–7.45)? If so, go to Step 4. If below 7.35, acidosis is present; if above 7.45, alkalosis is present. Otherwise, look for compensatory changes or combined disorders.
4. Is PCO_2 within normal limits (35–45 mm Hg)? If so, go to Step 5.
   If PCO_2 >45 and pH <7.35, then respiratory acidosis is present.
   If PCO_2 >45 and pH >7.35, then compensated respiratory acidosis is present.
   If PCO_2 <35 and pH >7.45, then respiratory alkalosis is present.
   If PCO_2 <35 and pH <7.45, then compensated respiratory alkalosis is present.
5. Is calculated HCO_3^- within normal limits (22–27 mEq/L)? If so, acid-base status is probably normal; go to Step 6.
   If HCO_3^- <22 and pH <7.35, then metabolic* acidosis is present.
   If HCO_3^- <22 and pH >7.35, then compensated metabolic* acidosis is present.
   If HCO_3^- >27 and pH >7.45, then metabolic* alkalosis is present.
   If HCO_3^- >27 and pH <7.45, then compensated metabolic* alkalosis is present.
6. Is PO_2 within normal limits (80–100 mm Hg)? If so, oxygenation status is probably normal; check O_2Hb saturation via hemoximetry. Is PO_2 appropriate for FIO_2? Is A-a gradient increased? If PO_2 <55, significant hypoxemia is present.
7. Are blood gas results consistent with patient's clinical history and status? Are additional tests indicated (hemoximetry, shunt study)?

*Metabolic = nonrespiratory.

change of 0.3 pH units represents a twofold change in $[H^+]$ concentration. If the pH decreases from 7.40 to 7.10 with no change in PCO_2, the concentration of hydrogen ions has doubled. Conversely, if the concentration of $[H^+]$ is halved, the pH increases from 7.40 to 7.70, assuming the PCO_2 remains at 40 mm Hg. Changes of this magnitude represent marked abnormalities in the acid-base status of the blood and are almost always accompanied by clinical symptoms (e.g., cardiac arrhythmias).

Acid-base disorders arising from lung disease are often related to PCO_2 and its transport as carbonic acid. If the pH is outside of its normal range (i.e., acidemia or alkalemia) but PCO_2 is within normal limits, the condition is termed nonrespiratory or metabolic (Table 6-3). The calculated HCO_3^- is a useful indicator of the relationship between pH and PCO_2. In the presence of acidemia (pH less than 7.35) and normal CO_2 (PCO_2 35–45 mm Hg), HCO_3^- will be low and a nonrespiratory acidosis is present. A PCO_2 of less than 35 mm Hg in the presence of acidosis suggests that ventilatory compensation for acidemia is occurring. The acid-base status would be considered partially compensated nonrespiratory (i.e., metabolic) acidosis. Complete compensation occurs if pH returns to the normal range. This happens when ventilation reduces PCO_2 in proportion to the HCO_3^-.

In the presence of alkalemia (pH above 7.45) and normal PCO_2 (35–45 mm Hg), calculated bicarbonate will be increased and nonrespiratory (i.e., metabolic) alkalosis is present. If ventilatory compensation occurs, PCO_2 will be slightly increased. However, decreased ventilation is required so that the CO_2 can increase. Reduced minute ventilation may interfere with oxygenation. For this reason, $PaCO_2$ seldom increases above 50–55 mm Hg to compensate for nonrespiratory (i.e., metabolic) alkalosis. Compensation may be incomplete if the alkalosis is severe.

Abnormal PCO_2 and HCO_3^- characterize combined respiratory and nonrespiratory acid-base disorders. In combined acidosis, PCO_2 is elevated (more than 45 mm Hg) and HCO_3^- is low (less than 22 mEq/L). In combined alkalosis, HCO_3^- is elevated (more than 26 mEq/L) and PCO_2 is low (less than 35 mm Hg). pH is more severely deranged (i.e.,

TABLE 6-3			
Acid-Base Disorders			
Status	pH	PCO$_2$	HCO$_3^-$
Simple Disorders			
Metabolic acidosis	Low	Normal	Low
Metabolic alkalosis	High	Normal	High
Respiratory acidosis	Low	High	Normal
Respiratory alkalosis	High	Low	Normal
Compensated Disorders			
Compensated respiratory acidosis, or metabolic alkalosis	Normal*	High	High
Compensated metabolic acidosis, or respiratory alkalosis	Normal*	Low	Low
Combined Disorders			
Metabolic/respiratory acidosis	Low	High	Low
Metabolic/respiratory alkalosis	High	Low	High

*Compensation cannot return values to within normal limits in severe acid-base disturbances. In addition, a normal pH may result in instances of respiratory and metabolic disturbances that occur together but are not compensatory.

much higher or lower) than if just one disorder were present.

Carbon Dioxide Tension

The arterial carbon dioxide tension (PaCO$_2$) in a healthy adult is approximately 40 mm Hg; it may range from 35–45 mm Hg. The PCO$_2$ of venous or mixed venous blood is seldom used clinically. Body temperature affects PaCO$_2$ as described in Table 6-1.

PaCO$_2$ is inversely proportional to alveolar ventilation ($\dot{V}_A$) (see Chapter 4). When $\dot{V}_A$ decreases, CO$_2$ may not be removed by the lungs as fast as it is produced. This causes PaCO$_2$ to increase. The pH falls (i.e., [H$^+$] increases) as CO$_2$ is hydrated to form carbonic acid:

$$CO_2 + H_2O \leftrightarrow H_2CO_3 \leftrightarrow H^+ + HCO_3^-$$

Increasing levels of CO$_2$ in the blood drive this reaction to the right. The patient has respiratory acidosis resulting from hypoventilation. Conversely, when alveolar ventilation removes CO$_2$ more rapidly than it is produced, PaCO$_2$ decreases. The pH increases (i.e., [H$^+$] falls) as the patient becomes alkalotic. This condition is called hyperventilation, or respiratory alkalosis.

If dead space increases, high minute ventilation ($\dot{V}_E$) may be required to adequately ventilate alveoli and keep PaCO$_2$ within normal limits. Respiratory dead space occurs because some lung units are ventilated but not perfused by pulmonary capillary blood. Pulmonary embolization is an example of dead space–producing disease. Emboli may block pulmonary arterioles, causing ventilation of the affected lung units to be "wasted." To maintain normal PaCO$_2$, total ventilation must be increased to compensate for wasted ventilation. PaCO$_2$ may be normal, or decreased, even though significant pulmonary disease is present.

Patients who have disorders such as lobar pneumonia may increase their $\dot{V}_E$ to provide more alveolar ventilation of functional lung units. This mechanism compensates for lung units that do not participate in gas exchange. Hypoxemia is a common cause of hyperventilation (i.e., respiratory alkalosis). Hyperventilation may be seen in patients with asthma, emphysema, bronchitis, or foreign body obstruction. Anxiety or central nervous system disorders may also cause hyperventilation.

Increased PaCO$_2$ (i.e., hypercapnia) commonly occurs in patients who have advanced obstructive or restrictive disease. These individuals are characterized by markedly abnormal ventilation-perfusion ($\dot{V}/\dot{Q}$) patterns. They are unable to maintain adequate alveolar ventilation. Not all patients with advanced pulmonary disease retain CO_2. Those who do become hypercapnic often have a low ventilatory response to CO_2 (see Chapter 4). Their response to the increased work of breathing caused by obstruction or restriction is to allow CO_2 to increase rather than increase ventilation. When respiratory acidosis results from increased P_{CO_2}, renal compensation usually occurs (see Table 6-3).

Increased Pa_{CO_2} may also be seen in patients who hypoventilate as a result of central nervous system or neuromuscular disorders. Whether CO_2 retention is the result of lung disease, central nervous system dysfunction, or neuromuscular disease, pH is usually maintained close to normal. The kidneys retain and produce bicarbonate (HCO_3^-) to match the increased Pa_{CO_2}. This response may completely compensate for a mildly elevated Pa_{CO_2}. However, it can seldom produce normal pH when the Pa_{CO_2} is greater than 65 mm Hg. If the disorder causing the increased Pa_{CO_2} is acute (e.g., foreign body aspiration), little or no renal compensation may be observed.

Some degree of hypoxemia is always present in patients who retain CO_2 while breathing air. As alveolar CO_2 increases, alveolar O_2 decreases. If the cause of hypercapnia is either obstructive or restrictive lung disease, hypoxemia may be severe because of $\dot{V}/\dot{Q}$ abnormalities. Because O_2 therapy is common in these patients, changes in P_{CO_2} while breathing supplementary O_2 must be carefully monitored. Some patients with chronic hypoxemia have a decreased ventilatory response to CO_2. O_2 administered to these patients may reduce their hypoxic stimulus to ventilation. As a result, Pa_{CO_2} may increase further. O_2 therapy is usually titrated to maintain Pa_{CO_2} values less than 60 mm Hg without hypercapnia and acidosis.

Oxygen Tension

The Pa_{O_2} of healthy young adults at sea level ranges from 85-100 mm Hg and decreases slightly with age. Breathing room air at sea level results in an inspired P_{O_2} of approximately 150 mm Hg:

$$P_IO_2 = FIO_2(P_B - 47)$$
$$= 0.21(760 - 47)$$
$$= 0.21(713)$$
$$= 149.7$$

where:
FIO_2 = fractional concentration of inspired O_2
P_B = barometric pressure
47 = partial pressure of water vapor at 37°C

The partial pressure of O_2 in alveolar gas is usually close to 100 mm Hg and can be calculated using the alveolar air equation:

$$P_AO_2 = (F_IO_2 \times [P_B - 47]) - Pa_{CO_2}\left(F_IO_2 + \frac{1 - F_IO_2}{R}\right)$$

where:
Pa_{CO_2} = arterial CO_2 tension (presumed equal to alveolar CO_2 tension)
R = respiratory exchange ratio ($\dot{V}_{CO_2}/\dot{V}_{O_2}$)
Substituting 40 mm Hg for Pa_{CO_2}, and 0.8 for R:

$$P_AO_2 = (0.21 \times [760 - 47]) - 40\left(0.21 + \frac{1 - 0.21}{0.8}\right)$$
$$= (0.21 \times 713) - 40(1.1975)$$
$$= 149.7 - 47.9$$
$$= 101.8$$

In healthy lungs with good gas exchange, arterial oxygen tension can approach the value of the alveolar P_{O_2}. The difference between the alveolar and arterial oxygen tensions is described as the alveolar-arterial gradient, or **A-a gradient.** This gradient is usually less than 20 mm Hg in healthy individuals breathing air at sea level.

Hyperventilation may increase Pa_{O_2} as high as 120 mm Hg in a patient with normal lung function (see the previous alveolar air equation). Healthy subjects breathing 100% O_2 may exhibit Pa_{O_2} values higher than 600 mm Hg. The alveolar P_{O_2} (P_AO_2) for a particular inspired O_2 fraction can be calculated as previously described. Decreased Pa_{O_2} can result from hypoventilation, diffusion abnormalities, $\dot{V}/\dot{Q}$ imbalances, and inadequate atmospheric O_2 (high altitude).

Table 6-1 lists changes that occur in PaO_2 because of body temperatures above and below normal (37°C). Changes in PO_2 and PCO_2 reflect solubility of the gas. The partial pressure of each gas is a measure of its activity. Hypothermia (low body temperature) is accompanied by decreased partial pressure as more gas dissolves. Hyperthermia (elevated body temperature) causes elevated gas tensions as gas comes out of solution. All blood gas analyzers perform analyses at 37°C and most allow temperature corrections to be made. Although blood gas tensions vary with temperature, the clinical significance of correcting measurements is unclear. Blood gas values should be reported at 37°C. Care must be taken to ensure that blood gas analyzers are maintained at 37°C. Measurements made at other temperatures can significantly alter results.

PO_2 is the pressure of O_2 dissolved in blood. The amount of Hb and whether it is capable of binding O_2 has only a minimal effect on PO_2. Hypoxemia (decreased O_2 content of the blood) may occur even if PaO_2 is normal or elevated by breathing O_2. Hypoxemia commonly results from inadequate or abnormal Hb. Many automated blood gas analyzers calculate oxygen saturation (SaO_2). Saturation may be calculated from the PaO_2 and pH, assuming a normal oxygen-hemoglobin reaction occurs (Figure 6-1). Calculated SaO_2 may differ significantly from true saturation measured by a spectrophotometer (see the section on oxygen saturation).

An example of the discrepancy between calculated and measured saturation is the patient with elevated carboxyhemoglobin (COHb) resulting from smoking or smoke inhalation. The patient's PaO_2 may be normal while O_2 saturation is markedly decreased. Calculating saturation from PO_2 in this case overestimates the O_2 content of the blood. Measured SaO_2 is preferred to a calculated value.

The severity of impaired oxygenation is indicated by the PaO_2 at rest. PaO_2 is a good index of the lungs' ability to match pulmonary capillary blood flow with adequate ventilation. If ventilation matches perfusion, pulmonary capillary blood leaves the lungs with a PO_2 close to that of the alveoli. If ventilation is adequate, pulmonary capillary blood is almost completely saturated. If either of these conditions is not met (i.e., poor ventilation or $\dot{V}/\dot{Q}$ mismatching), pulmonary capillary blood has reduced O_2 content. PaO_2 is reduced in proportion to the number of lung units contributing blood with low O_2 content. Lung units with good $\dot{V}/\dot{Q}$ cannot compensate for their poorly functioning counterparts because pulmonary capillary blood leaving them is already almost fully oxygenated. O_2 binding to Hb is almost complete when the PaO_2 is greater than 60 mm Hg (~90% saturation). As PaO_2 decreases from 60 to 40 mm Hg, saturation decreases from 90% to 75%, with increasing symptoms of hypoxia (e.g., mental confusion, shortness of breath).

Delivery of O_2 to the tissues, however, depends on Hb concentration and cardiac output as well as adequate gas transfer in the lungs. Arterial oxygen content (CaO_2 in ml/dl) is defined as follows:

$$CaO_2 = (1.34 \times Hb \times SaO_2) + (PaO_2 \times 0.0031)$$

where:
1.34   = O_2 binding capacity of Hb, ml/g
Hb   = hemoglobin concentration, g/dl
SaO_2 = arterial oxygen saturation as a fraction
PaO_2 = arterial oxygen tension, mm Hg
0.0031 = solubility coefficient for O_2 at 37°C

Because most O_2 transported is bound to Hb, there must be an adequate supply (12–15 g/dl) of functional Hb. Adequate cardiac output (4–5 L/min) is necessary to deliver the oxygenated arterial blood to the tissues. Signs and symptoms of hypoxia may be present despite adequate PaO_2 because of severe anemia and/or reduced cardiac function.

The mixed venous oxygen tension ($P\bar{v}O_2$) in healthy patients at rest ranges from approximately

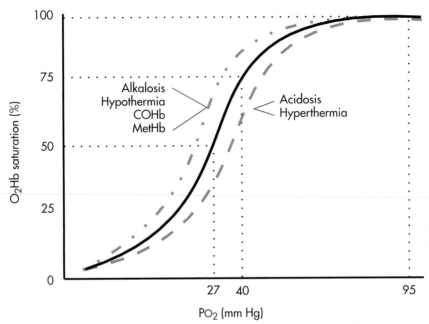

FIGURE 6-1   Oxygen-Hemoglobin Dissociation Curve. The S-shaped curve represents the relationship between partial pressure of O_2 in blood (x-axis) and Hb saturation (y-axis). The solid curve represents the reaction that occurs when hemoglobin (Hb) is normal, pH is 7.40, and temperature is 37°C. When PO_2 is 95 mm Hg, Hb is approximately 97% saturated; when PO_2 is 60 mm Hg, Hb is approximately 90% saturated; when PO_2 is 40 mm Hg (normal level for mixed venous blood), Hb is approximately 75% saturated. The P_{50} identifies the O_2 tension at which Hb is 50% saturated. For normal Hb, this is approximately 27 mm Hg. Conditions such as alkalosis, hypothermia, or elevated carboxyhemoglobin (COHb) or methemoglobin (MetHb) shift the dissociation curve to the left. This causes Hb to bind O_2 more tightly with less oxygen being unloaded as partial pressure decreases. Similarly, acidosis and hyperthermia shift the curve to the right, enhancing the delivery of O_2 as pressure decreases.

37–43, with an average of 40 mm Hg (see Figure 6-1). Mixed venous O_2 content ($C\bar{v}O_2$) averages 15 ml/dl. In healthy individuals, arterial oxygen content (CaO_2) averages 20 ml/dl. The resulting content difference, or $C(a\text{-}\bar{v})O_2$, is thus 5 ml/dl (or 5 vol%). Although PaO_2 varies with the inspired O_2 fraction and matching of $\dot{V}/\dot{Q}$, $P\bar{v}O_2$ changes in response to alterations in cardiac output and O_2 consumption. If cardiac output increases while oxygen consumption ($\dot{V}O_2$) remains constant, the $C(a\text{-}\bar{v})O_2$ decreases. Conversely, if cardiac output decreases with no change in O_2 consumption, $C(a\text{-}\bar{v})O_2$ increases. Increased cardiac output sometimes occurs in response to pulmonary shunting. This allows mixed venous oxygen content to increase, reducing the deleterious effect of the shunt. Critically ill patients often have low $P\bar{v}O_2$ values and increased $C(a\text{-}\bar{v})O_2$ as a result of poor cardiovascular performance. Alterations in $P\bar{v}O_2$ often occur even if PaO_2 is normal. $P\bar{v}O_2$ values less than 28 mm Hg in critically ill patients, accompanied by $C(a\text{-}\bar{v})O_2$ greater than 6 vol%, suggest marked cardiovascular decompensation.

Patients who have severe obstructive or restrictive diseases may have decreased PaO_2 at rest, occasionally as low as 40 mm Hg. Mild pulmonary disease may show little decrease in PaO_2 if hyperventilation is present. PaO_2 may also be relatively normal if the disease process affects ventilation and perfusion similarly. In patients with emphysema, destruction of alveolar septa may eliminate pulmonary capillaries as well, resulting in poor ventilation and equally poor blood flow. These patients may have severe airway obstruction, markedly reduced DLCO, but only a small decrease in resting PaO_2. Patients with chronic bronchitis or asthma, particularly during acute exacerbations, may have moderate or severe resting hypoxemia because of $\dot{V}/\dot{Q}$ abnormalities.

During exercise in patients with obstructive disease, PaO_2 often decreases commensurate with the extent of the disease. PaO_2 during exercise is correlated with the patient's DLCO and FEV_1, but wide variability exists. Patients with markedly decreased DLCO (less than 50%–60% of predicted) may show low PaO_2 values at rest that decrease during exercise. The degree of arterial desaturation cannot be predicted from static pulmonary function measurements.

PaO_2 may be decreased for nonpulmonary reasons such as anatomic shunts (intracardiac) or hypoventilation because of neuromuscular disease. Tissue hypoxia can occur because of inadequate or nonfunctional Hb, or because of poor cardiac output. PaO_2 should be correlated with spirometry (FEV_1), DLCO, ventilation ($\dot{V}_E$, tidal volume, dead space), and lung volumes (VC, RV, TLC) to distinguish pulmonary from nonpulmonary causes of inadequate oxygenation.

HEMOXIMETRY

Description

Hemoximetry (i.e., blood oximetry) refers to the measurement of hemoglobin (Hb) and its derivatives by spectroscopy. Oxygen saturation is the ratio of oxygenated Hb (O_2Hb) to either total available Hb or functional Hb. Functional Hb is that portion of the total Hb that is capable of binding oxygen. This ratio of content to capacity is normally expressed as a percentage but is sometimes recorded as a simple fraction. The values may differ significantly depending on the method of calculation:

1. Oxyhemoglobin fraction of total Hb:

$$\frac{O_2Hb}{(O_2Hb + rHb + COHb + MetHb)}$$

2. Oxygen saturation of available Hb:

$$\frac{O_2Hb}{O_2Hb + rHb}$$

where:

O_2Hb = oxyhemoglobin
rHb = reduced hemoglobin concentration
COHb = carboxyhemoglobin concentration
MetHb = methemoglobin concentration

The first equation is used to measure O_2 saturation with a multiple-wavelength spectrophotometer (hemoximeter); the second equation is used to measure O_2 saturation with a pulse oximeter.

Technique

O_2 saturation of Hb (O_2Hb, or SaO_2 when referring to arterial saturation) may be measured in several ways. In the first method, O_2 saturation is measured using a spectrophotometer (see Chapter 10). Whole blood is hemolyzed and the absorbances of the various components measured. The total Hb, O_2Hb, COHb, and MetHb are usually reported. Hemoximetry is usually performed in conjunction with blood gas analysis using a single specimen of blood.

An indirect method may be used to measure mixed venous oxygen saturation ($S\bar{v}O_2$). Saturation may be measured by a reflective spectrophotometer in a pulmonary artery catheter (**Swan-Ganz catheter**). In this case absorbances are measured without hemolyzing the blood. A special catheter that includes fiberoptic bundles is used to perform in vivo measurements.

Blood specimens for hemoximetry should be prepared as described for arterial blood gas specimens. Guidelines for quality control of blood gas analysis are included in Chapter 11. Measurement of percent saturation allows calculation of the O_2 content of either arterial or mixed venous blood (CaO_2 and $C\bar{v}O_2$, respectively) (see the section on oxygen tension).

Significance and Pathophysiology

See Blood Gases 6-3 for interpretive strategies. SaO_2 for a healthy young adult with a PaO_2 of 95 mm Hg is approximately 97%. The O_2Hb dissociation curve is relatively flat when the PaO_2 is above 60 mm Hg

---

BLOOD GASES 6-3

INTERPRETIVE STRATEGIES

Oxygen Saturation

1. How was the estimate of saturation obtained? Hemoximeter? Calculated saturation? Pulse oximeter?
2. For hemoximetry or calculated saturation: was the specimen obtained anaerobically and handled properly?
3. Is Hb within normal limits? If low, oxygenation may be compromised; if elevated, look for clinical correlation.
4. Is O_2Hb >90%? If so, oxygenation is probably adequate; if not, hypoxemia is likely.
5. Is O_2Hb <85%? If so, supplementary oxygen may be indicated. Correlate with PaO_2 and clinical history.
6. Is COHb >3%? If so, check for smoking history and/or environmental exposure.
7. Is MetHb >1.5%? If so, check for environmental exposure to oxidizers.

(i.e., SaO_2 is 90% or more). Saturation changes only slightly when there is a marked change in PaO_2 at partial pressures above 60 mm Hg (see Figure 6-1). Therefore PaO_2 is a more sensitive indicator of oxygenation in lungs that do not have gross abnormalities. At PaO_2 values of approximately 150 mm Hg, Hb becomes completely saturated (SaO_2 is 100%). At PaO_2 values above 150 mm Hg, further increases in O_2 content are caused by increased dissolved oxygen. Alterations in $\dot{V}/\dot{Q}$ patterns in the lungs can be monitored by allowing the patient to breathe 100% O_2, and measuring the changes in dissolved oxygen. In practice, this is accomplished by using the clinical shunt equation (see the section on shunt calculation in this chapter).

PF TIP

There are several key values to remember when assessing oxygen saturation. When SaO_2 is above 90%, PaO_2 is usually greater than 60 mm Hg. At a PaO_2 of 60, the saturation is 90% and O_2 therapy may be needed. At a PaO_2 of 55, the saturation is 85% and O_2 therapy is indicated. At a PaO_2 of 40, the saturation is approximately 75% (the same as mixed venous blood).

When PaO_2 falls below 60 mm Hg, SaO_2 decreases rapidly. Small changes in PaO_2 result in large changes in saturation. As SaO_2 falls below 90%, O_2 content decreases rapidly. At saturations less than 85% (i.e., PaO_2 <55 mm Hg), symptoms of hypoxemia increase and supplementary O_2 may be indicated.

The ability of Hb to bind O_2 may be measured by the P_{50}. P_{50} specifies the partial pressure at which Hb is 50% saturated (see Figure 6-1). The P_{50} of normal adult Hb is approximately 27 mm Hg. P_{50} may be determined by equilibrating blood with several gases at low oxygen tensions. An O_2Hb dissociation curve is then constructed to estimate the partial pressure at which Hb is 50% saturated. A second method of estimating P_{50} compares measured SaO_2 (using a spectrophotometer) with the expected saturation. Calculated saturations presume a P_{50} of 26–27 mm Hg, but it may differ significantly depending on the types of Hb and interfering substances present.

Healthy individuals have small amounts of Hb that cannot carry O_2. COHb is present in blood from metabolism and from environmental exposure to carbon monoxide (CO) gas. Normal COHb, expressed as a percentage, ranges from 0.5%–2% of the total Hb. CO comes from smoking (cigarettes, cigars, and pipes), smoke inhalation, improperly vented furnaces, automobile emissions, and other sources of combustion. In smokers, levels may increase from 3%–15%, depending on recent smoking history. Smoke inhalation or CO poisoning from other sources also results in elevated COHb levels, sometimes as high as 50%. CO combines rapidly with Hb. Exposures of short duration can cause a high level of COHb if high concentrations of CO are present. Because O_2Hb saturation decreases as COHb increases, COHb levels greater than 15% almost always result in hypoxemia. High levels of COHb are rapidly fatal because of the profound hypoxemia that occurs.

COHb absorbs light at wavelengths similar to O_2Hb. When COHb is elevated, arterial blood appears bright red. **Cyanosis,** which appears when there is an increased concentration of reduced Hb, is absent. In spite of elevated levels of COHb, PaO_2 may be close to normal limits. Blood gas analysis that includes calculated saturation will give erroneously high O_2 saturations. For this reason, O_2Hb and COHb should be measured by hemoximetry whenever possible.

COHb interferes with O_2 transport in two ways: it binds competitively to Hb, and it shifts the O_2Hb curve to the left (see Figure 6-1). Increased COHb causes reduced O_2Hb with a decrease in O_2 content. The left shift of the dissociation curve causes O_2 to be bound more tightly to Hb. The combination of these two effects can seriously reduce O_2 delivery to the tissues. COHb concentrations in blood begin to decrease once the source of CO has been removed. Removal of CO from the blood depends on the minute ventilation. Breathing air may require several hours to reduce even moderate levels to normal. Breathing 100% O_2 speeds the washout of CO. High concentrations of O_2 (often including hyperbaric therapy) are indicated whenever dangerously high levels of COHb are encountered.

Methemoglobin (MetHb) forms when iron atoms of the Hb molecule are oxidized from Fe^{++} to Fe^{+++}. The normal MetHb level is less than 1.5% of the total Hb in adults. High levels of MetHb can result from ingestion of or exposure to strong oxidizing agents. Methemoglobinemia has also been linked to high doses of medications such as lidocaine and nitroprusside. Like COHb, MetHb reduces O_2 carrying capacity of the blood by reducing the available Hb and shifting the O_2Hb dissociation curve to the left (see Figure 6-1).

The saturation of mixed venous blood ($S\bar{v}O_2$) in healthy patients averages 75% at a $P\bar{v}O_2$ of 40 mm Hg. Healthy patients have a content difference, $C(a-\bar{v})O_2$, of 5 vol%. Arterial blood, in adults with normal levels of Hb, typically carries approximately 20 vol% O_2, and mixed venous blood carries 15 vol% O_2. Pulmonary diseases that cause arterial hypoxemia may reduce $S\bar{v}O_2$ if oxygen uptake and cardiac output remain constant. Cardiac output often increases to combat arterial hypoxemia caused by intrapulmonary shunting. Increased cardiac output increases O_2 delivery to the tissues. This results in a reduced extraction of O_2 from the blood. Mixed venous blood then returns to the lungs with normal or even increased O_2 saturation. When this blood is shunted, it has a higher O_2 content, thereby reducing the shunt effect. With or without arterial

hypoxemia, $S\bar{v}O_2$ decreases if cardiac output is compromised.

$S\bar{v}O_2$ is useful in assessing cardiac function in the critical care setting and during exercise. Patients who have good cardiovascular reserves maintain a mixed venous saturation of 70%–75%. Patients whose $S\bar{v}O_2$ values are in the 60%–70% range have a limited ability to deliver more O_2 to the tissues. $S\bar{v}O_2$ values less than 60% usually indicate cardiovascular decompensation and may be associated with tissue hypoxemia. The indwelling reflective spectrophotometer (see Chapter 10) allows continuous monitoring of this important parameter. $S\bar{v}O_2$ also decreases during exercise. Despite increased cardiac output, O_2 extraction by the exercising muscles reduces the content of blood returning to the lungs.

Estimation of SaO_2 by most pulse oximeters (SpO_2) is based on absorption of light at two wavelengths. When only two wavelengths are analyzed, only two species of Hb can be detected. Absorption in the red and near-infrared portions of the visible spectrum allows measurement of the oxyhemoglobin and reduced Hb, providing an estimate of the oxygen saturation of available Hb (see the section on pulse oximetry).

PULSE OXIMETRY

Description

SpO_2 estimates SaO_2 by analyzing absorption of light passing through a capillary bed, either by transmission or reflectance. **Pulse oximetry** is noninvasive. SpO_2 is reported as percent saturation. Some pulse oximeters are also capable of measuring COHb and MetHb.

Technique

Pulse oximeters (see Chapter 10) measure the light absorption of a mixture of two forms of Hb: O_2Hb and reduced Hb (rHb). The relative absorptions at 660 nm (red) and 940 nm of light (near infrared) can be used to calculate the combination of the two

Hb forms. Absorption at two wavelengths provides an estimate of the saturation of available Hb (see the section on oxygen saturation). Most pulse oximeters use a stored calibration curve to estimate oxygen saturation.

Pulse oximetry may be used in any setting in which a noninvasive measure of oxygenation status is sufficient. This includes monitoring of O_2 therapy and ventilator management. Pulse oximetry is commonly used during diagnostic procedures such as bronchoscopy, sleep studies, or stress testing. It is also used for monitoring during patient transport or rehabilitation. Pulse oximetry may be used for continuous monitoring with inclusion of appropriate alarms to detect desaturation. Many pulse oximeter systems use memory (RAM) to record SpO_2 and heart rate for extended periods. This type of recorded monitoring allows pulse oximetry to be used for overnight studies of nocturnal desaturation. Alternatively, pulse oximetry can be used for discrete measurements or "spot checks."

Most pulse oximeters use a sensor that attaches to the finger (nail bed) or earlobe. The choice of attachment site should be dictated by the type of measurement being made. The ear site may be preferred in patients undergoing exercise testing or in whom arm movement precludes use of the finger site. Both finger and earlobe sites presume pulsatile blood flow. Most pulse oximeters adjust light output to compensate for tissue density or pigmentation. In some patients, impaired perfusion to one site determines which site is preferred. Low perfusion or poor vascularity can cause the oximeter to be unable to detect pulsatile blood flow. Rubbing or warming of the site often improves local blood flow and may be indicated to obtain reliable data. Some pulse oximeters use reflective sensors that detect light reflected from bone underlying the tissue bed. These sensors are usually placed on the patient's forehead and may function when finger or ear sensors do not.

Some pulse oximeters display a representation of the pulse waveform derived from the absorption measurements (see Chapter 10). Such waveforms may be helpful in selecting an appropriate site or troubleshooting questionable SpO_2 values. Most pulse oximeters report heart rate (HR), which is also detected from pulsatile blood flow at the sensor site. Comparison of oximeter HR with palpated pulse or with an electrocardiograph (ECG) signal can assist with selection of an appropriate site. Inability to obtain a valid HR reading or acceptable pulse waveform suggests that SpO_2 values should be interpreted cautiously (Blood Gases 6-4).

A number of factors limit the validity of SpO_2 measurements (Box 6-2). To validate pulse oximetry readings, direct measurement of arterial saturation is required. Simultaneous measurement of SpO_2 and SaO_2 can be used to confirm pulse oximeter readings. Pulse oximetry used during exercise testing has been shown to produce variable results. Hemoximetry may be necessary to validate pulse oximetry readings at peak exercise.

COHb absorbs light at wavelengths similar to oxyhemoglobin. Most pulse oximeters sense COHb as O_2Hb and overestimate the O_2 saturation; however, pulse oximeters that measure O_2Hb and COHb are available. MetHb increases absorption at each of the two wavelengths used by pulse oximeters. This causes the ratio of the two Hb forms to approach 1, which is usually represented as a saturation of 85% (see Chapter 10). Other interfering substances may cause the pulse oximeter to underestimate saturation.

BLOOD GASES 6-4

CRITERIA FOR ACCEPTABILITY

Pulse Oximetry

1. Documentation of adequate correlation with measured SaO_2 should be available. SpO_2 and SaO_2 should be within 2% from 85%–100% saturation. Elevated COHb (>3%) or MetHb (>5%) may invalidate SpO_2.
2. Adequate perfusion of the sensor site should be documented by agreement between oximeter and patient's heart rate (ECG or palpation) and reproducible pulse waveforms (if available).
3. Known interfering substances or agents should be eliminated or accounted for.
4. Pulse oximeter readings should be stable long enough to answer the clinical question being investigated. Readings should be consistent with the patient's clinical history and presentation.

INTERFERING SUBSTANCES
Carboxyhemoglobin (COHb)*
Methemoglobin (MetHb)*
Intravascular dyes (indocyanine green)
Nail polish or coverings (finger sensor)

INTERFERING FACTORS
Motion artifact, shivering
Bright ambient lighting
Hypotension, low perfusion (sensor site)
Hypothermia
Vasoconstrictor drugs
Dark skin pigmentation

*Some pulse oximeters are capable of measuring COHb and MetHb.

BLOOD GASES 6-5

INTERPRETIVE STRATEGIES

Pulse Oximetry

1. Is the SpO_2 reading supported by blood oximetry? If not, interpret cautiously.
2. Is there evidence of adequate perfusion at the sensor site? Consistent pulse waveform (if available)? Good correlation with palpated pulse or ECG heart rate? If not, consider alternate site or blood oximetry.
3. Is the patient a current smoker or smoke-inhalation victim? If so, hemoximetry is indicated.
4. Is the indicated SpO_2 >90%? If so, Hb saturation is probably adequate; correlate with clinical presentation.
5. Is indicated SpO_2 between 85% and 90%? If so, oxygen supplementation may be indicated; correlate with clinical presentation.
6. If indicated SpO_2 <85%, supplementary O_2 is indicated unless there is reason to suspect invalid SpO_2 data.
7. Does supplementary O_2 improve SpO_2 reading? If not, suspect shunt or invalid SpO_2 data.

Significance and Pathophysiology

See Blood Gases 6-5 for interpretive strategies. Arterial oxygen saturation estimated by pulse oximetry (SpO_2) should approximate that measured by hemoximetry (SaO_2) in healthy nonsmoking adults. Most pulse oximeters are capable of accuracy of ±2% of the actual saturation when SaO_2 is above 90%. For SaO_2 values of 85%–90%, accuracy may be slightly less. For very low saturations (i.e., less than 80%), pulse oximeter accuracy is less of an issue because the clinical implications are the same.

Pulse oximetry is most useful when it has been shown to correlate with blood oximetry in a patient in a known circumstance. When this is the case, pulse oximetry can be used for noninvasive monitoring, either continuously or by taking discrete measurements. Uses include monitoring of O_2 therapy, ventilatory support, pulmonary or cardiac rehabilitation, bronchoscopy, surgical procedures, sleep studies, and cardiopulmonary exercise testing. In each of these applications, careful attention must be paid to minimizing known interfering agents or substances (see Box 6-2).

Because of its limitations, pulse oximetry should be used cautiously when assessing oxygen need. This is particularly true when using pulse oximetry to detect exercise desaturation. Pulse oximetry may not accurately reflect SaO_2 during exertion. For this reason, SpO_2, even if demonstrated to correlate with SaO_2 at rest, may yield false-positive or false-negative results during exercise. Blood gas analysis with hemoximetry should be used to resolve discrepancies between the SpO_2 reading and the patient's clinical presentation.

Pulse oximetry may not be appropriate in all situations. To evaluate hyperoxemia (PaO_2 greater than 100–150 mm Hg) or acid-base status in a patient, blood gas analysis is required. Measurement of O_2 delivery, which depends on Hb concentration, cannot be adequately assessed by pulse oximetry alone.

CAPNOGRAPHY

Description

Capnography includes continuous, noninvasive monitoring of expired CO_2 and analysis of the single-breath CO_2 waveform. Continuous monitoring of expired CO_2 allows trending of changes in alveolar and dead space ventilation. Analysis of a single breath of expired CO_2 measures the uniformity of both ventilation and pulmonary blood flow. End-tidal PCO_2 ($PETCO_2$) is reported in millimeters of mercury.

Technique

Continuous monitoring of expired CO_2 is performed by sampling gas from the proximal airway. This gas may be pumped to an infrared analyzer (see Chapter 10) or to a mass spectrometer. An alternative method inserts a "mainstream" sample window directly into the expired gas stream. The analyzer signal is then passed to either a recorder or a computer. CO_2 waveforms may be displayed either individually (Figure 6-2) or as a series of deflections to form a trend plot. $PETCO_2$ may be read from the peaks of the waveforms. It can also be obtained by a simple peak detector and displayed digitally. Continuous CO_2 monitoring is commonly used in patients with artificial airways in the critical care setting. $PaCO_2$ can be measured at intervals to establish a gradient with $PETCO_2$. Respiratory rate may be determined from the

frequency of the CO_2 waveforms. The change in CO_2 concentration during a single expiration may be analyzed to detect ventilation-perfusion abnormalities (see Figure 6-2).

Technical problems involved in capnography include the necessity of accurate calibration and management of the gas sampling system (Blood Gases 6-6). Calibration using known gases (preferably two gas concentrations) is required if the system will be used to monitor $PaCO_2$. Many systems use ambient air, containing minimal CO_2, and a 5% CO_2 mixture for calibration (see Chapter 11). Condensation of water in sample tubing, connectors, or the sample chamber can affect accuracy. Some infrared analyzers may be affected if sample flow changes after calibration. Saturation of a desiccator column, if used, can also lead to inaccurate readings. Long sample lines or low sample flows can cause damping of the CO_2 waveform, invalidating analysis of the shape of the expired gas curve.

Significance and Pathophysiology

See Blood Gases 6-7 for interpretive strategies. In healthy patients, CO_2 rises to a plateau as alveolar gas is expired (see Figure 6-2). If all lung units empty

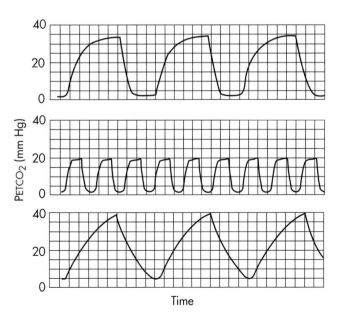

FIGURE 6-2 **Capnography Tracings.** Plots of expired CO_2 versus time for three patients are displayed. In each example, expiration is marked by a rapid increase in carbon dioxide to a peak ($PETCO_2$) followed by a return to baseline during inspiration. **Top,** Normal respiratory pattern with $PETCO_2$ near 40 mm Hg and a relatively flat alveolar phase. **Middle,** Rapid respiratory rate and low $PETCO_2$ (20 mm Hg), which may be found in a patient who is hyperventilating; the expiratory waveform has a normal configuration. **Bottom,** Abnormal expired CO_2 waveform consistent with V/Q abnormalities; no alveolar plateau is present, and the baseline does not return to zero.

BLOOD GASES 6-6

CRITERIA FOR ACCEPTABILITY

Capnography

1. CO_2 analyzer should be calibrated on a frequency consistent with the types of measurements being made. Calibration with air and 5% CO_2 is suitable for most purposes.
2. Sample flow (except in mainstream analyzers) should be high enough to prevent damping of CO_2 waveforms. Sample flow should not be changed after calibration. The sample chamber and tubing should be free of secretions or condensation that may affect the accuracy of the results.
3. $PaCO_2$ should be obtained to establish the gradient with $PETCO_2$.
4. CO_2 waveforms (if displayed) should be consistent with the patient's clinical condition.
5. CO_2 waveforms (if displayed) should return to baseline during inspiration, indicating appropriate washout of dead space.

BLOOD GASES 6-7

INTERPRETIVE STRATEGIES

Capnography

1. Was there an appropriate calibration of the CO_2 analyzer? If not, arterial–to–end-tidal CO_2 gradients may be inaccurate.
2. Are CO_2 waveforms (if available) consistent with the patient's clinical condition? Do waveforms show an obvious alveolar plateau?
3. Was $PaCO_2$ measured? If so, what is the $PaCO_2$-$PETCO_2$ gradient? If greater than 5 mm Hg, consider marked ventilation-perfusion abnormalities.
4. Has $PETCO_2$ changed (serial measurements)? Consider acute changes in dead space or cardiac output.

CO_2 evenly, the plateau appears flat. However, even healthy lungs have ventilation and blood flow imbalances. Healthy lung units empty CO_2 at varying rates. Alveolar CO_2 concentration increases slightly as the exhalation continues. $PETCO_2$ theo-

retically should not exceed $PaCO_2$. In healthy patients at rest, the $PETCO_2$ is usually close to the arterial value. During maximal exercise $PETCO_2$ may exceed $PaCO_2$. When ventilation and perfusion become grossly mismatched (e.g., in severe obstruction), end-tidal CO_2 may exceed the $PaCO_2$ as well. $PaCO_2$ reflects gas-exchange characteristics of the entire lung. Thus $PETCO_2$ may differ significantly if some lung units are poorly ventilated.

Continuous CO_2 analysis provides useful data for monitoring critically ill patients, particularly those requiring ventilatory support. $PETCO_2$ measurements allow trending of changes in $PaCO_2$ provided there is little or no change in the shape of the CO_2 waveform (indicating V/Q abnormalities). When a reference blood gas sample is obtained, $PETCO_2$ can be used as a continuous, noninvasive monitor. Respiratory rate can be measured from the frequency of expired CO_2 waveforms. Marked changes in breathing rate (e.g., hyperpnea or apnea) can be detected quickly. Analysis of the individual CO_2 waveforms, along with $PaCO_2$, may help identify abrupt changes in dead space. This can be useful in detecting pulmonary embolization or reduced cardiac output.

Problems related to ventilatory support devices can also be detected. Disconnection or leaks in breathing circuits can be quickly recognized by the loss of the CO_2 signal. Increased mechanical dead space (i.e., gas rebreathed in the ventilator circuit) can be identified by a baseline CO_2 concentration greater than zero. Irregularities in the CO_2 waveform often signal that the patient is "out of phase" with the ventilator.

The shape of the expired CO_2 curve is determined by ventilation-perfusion matching. Only lung units that are ventilated and perfused contribute CO_2 to expired gas. In patients without lung disease, the CO_2 waveform shows a flat initial segment of anatomic dead space gas containing little or no CO_2. This phase is followed by a rapid increase in CO_2 concentration, reflecting a mixture of dead space and alveolar gas. Finally, an "alveolar" plateau occurs in which gas composition changes only slightly. This slight change is caused by different emptying rates of various lung units. The absolute concentration of CO_2 at the alveolar plateau depends on factors such as minute ventilation and CO_2 production. Dead space–producing disease (e.g., pulmonary embolization or marked decrease in cardiac output) may show a profound decrease in expired CO_2 concentration. Patients who have pulmonary disease, especially obstruction, show poorly delineated phases of the CO_2 washout curve. The alveolar plateau may actually be a continuous slope throughout expiration, causing the measurement of $P_{ET}CO_2$ to be misleading.

SHUNT CALCULATION

Description

A shunt is that portion of the cardiac output that passes from one side of the heart to the other side without participating in gas exchange. This most commonly occurs from the right side to the left side. When the defect is in the lungs, it is a pulmonary shunt. If it occurs in the heart (e.g., atrial or ventricular septal defects), it is referred to as an intracardiac shunt. The shunt calculation determines the ratio of shunted blood ($\dot{Q}s$) to total perfusion ($\dot{Q}t$). Shunt is reported as a percent of total cardiac output, or sometimes as a simple fraction. Left-to-right shunting can occur when cardiac physiology is abnormal, such as patent ductus arteriosus (PDA). These types of shunts are usually detected by Doppler echocardiography rather than the shunt measurement as described.

Technique

Two methods for measuring the shunt fraction are available. The first uses O_2 content differences between arterial and mixed venous blood. This method is called the physiologic shunt equation:

1. $$\dfrac{\dot{Q}s}{\dot{Q}t} = \dfrac{CcO_2 - CaO_2}{CcO_2 - C\bar{v}O_2}$$

where:
CcO_2 = O_2 content of end-capillary blood, estimated from saturation associated with calculated P_AO_2

CaO_2 = arterial O_2 content, measured from an arterial sample
$C\bar{v}O_2$ = mixed venous O_2 content, measured from a sample obtained from a pulmonary artery catheter

The term in the denominator of this equation reflects potential arterialization of mixed venous blood. The term in the numerator reflects the actual arterialization.

The second method is more commonly used in clinical practice. The patient breathes 100% O_2 until the Hb is completely saturated (Figure 6-3). Twenty minutes of O_2 breathing is usually sufficient. Percent shunt is then calculated from differences in dissolved O_2. This method is called the clinical shunt equation:

2. $$\dfrac{\dot{Q}s}{\dot{Q}t} = \dfrac{(P_AO_2 - PaO_2) \times 0.0031}{C(a-\bar{v})O_2 + [(P_AO_2 - PaO_2) \times 0.0031]}$$

where:
P_AO_2 = alveolar O_2 tension
PaO_2 = arterial O_2 tension
$C(a\text{-}\bar{v})O_2$ = arteriovenous O_2 content difference
0.0031 = solubility factor for O_2 at 37°C

When the patient is breathing 100% O_2, P_AO_2 can be estimated from an abbreviated form of the alveolar gas equation as follows:

$$P_AO_2 = P_B - PH_2O - \left(\dfrac{PaCO_2}{0.8}\right)$$

where:
P_B = barometric pressure
PH_2O = partial pressure of water vapor at body temperature (47 mm Hg)
$PaCO_2$ = arterial CO_2 tension (as an estimate of alveolar PCO_2)
0.8 = normal (assumed) respiratory exchange ratio

This calculation of alveolar PO_2 assumes that the inspired gas is 100% O_2. If the FIO_2 is measured and found to be less than 1, the standard alveolar air equation can be used (see Appendix E).

The clinical shunt calculation is accurate only when Hb is completely saturated. This normally requires a PaO_2 greater than 150 mm Hg. A

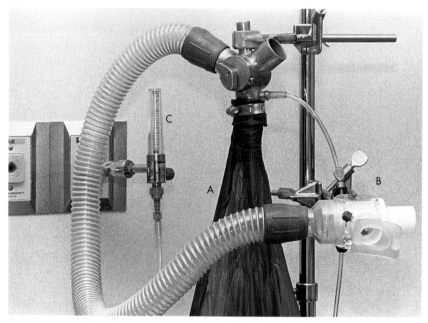

FIGURE 6-3   Equipment Used for Clinical Shunt Measurement. A, A large bag or balloon is used as a reservoir for 100% oxygen (a demand valve connected to an oxygen source may be used as well). **B,** A two-way nonrebreathing valve allows the patient to breathe gas from the balloon. **C,** An oxygen source allows the balloon to be refilled as necessary so the patient can breathe O_2 for at least 20 minutes. A blood gas syringe (not shown) is set up to obtain an arterial specimen at the end of the oxygen breathing. A pulse oximeter may be used to monitor the patient's saturation during the test. An oxygen analyzer (or blood gas analyzer capable of analyzing gas) can be used to measure the actual FIO_2.

saturation of 100% is usually easily accomplished if O_2 is breathed long enough. If breathing 100% O_2 does not increase the PaO_2 high enough to completely saturate Hb, the content difference method (physiologic method) should be used. With either method, shunt fraction may be multiplied by 100 and reported as a percentage (e.g., 0.20 ratio × 100 equals a 20% shunt).

Several technical considerations should be noted regarding shunt measurement (Blood Gases 6-8). Using O_2 content differences (equation 1) requires a pulmonary artery catheter to obtain mixed venous O_2 content. Using dissolved O_2 differences (equation 2) also relies on measured $C(a-\bar{v})O_2$. If placement of a pulmonary artery catheter is not practical, the clinical shunt equation may be used with an assumed a-$\bar{v}$ content difference (see the discussion on significance and pathophysiology in this section).

The physiologic shunt equation may be used for patients on any known FIO_2. The clinical shunt measurement requires O_2 breathing for 20 minutes or longer. Prolonged O_2 breathing may be contraindicated in patients whose respiration is driven by hypoxemia. Breathing 100% O_2 washes nitrogen (N_2) out of the lungs. Washout of N_2 combined with O_2 uptake by perfusing blood flow can reduce the size of alveoli to their critical limit. In poorly ventilated lung units, this may cause alveolar collapse. The effect of this "nitrogen shunting" may be shunt values that are falsely high because some shunting was induced by the test itself.

Significance and Pathophysiology

See Blood Gases 6-9 for interpretive strategies. In healthy individuals, approximately 5% of the cardiac output is shunted past the pulmonary system. An

BLOOD GASES 6-8

CRITERIA FOR ACCEPTABILITY

Shunt Calculation

1. For physiologic shunt, patient must have simultaneous arterial and mixed venous blood specimens drawn over a 30-second interval.
2. For clinical shunt, patient should breathe 100% O_2 for at least 20 minutes, or until Hb is completely saturated (PaO_2 >150 mm Hg). If PaO_2 >150 mm Hg cannot be achieved, clinical shunt calculation may underestimate true shunt.
3. CaO_2 and $C\bar{v}O_2$ must be measured for physiologic shunt. Measured contents should be used for clinical shunt if available; otherwise estimated a-$\bar{v}$ content difference should be based on clinical status.
4. FIO_2 should be accurately determined; this is required to calculate capillary content for physiologic shunt. FIO_2 of 1.00 can be assumed for clinical shunt calculation, but measured value improves accuracy.

BLOOD GASES 6-9

INTERPRETIVE STRATEGIES

Shunt Calculations

1. For physiologic shunt: Were arterial and mixed venous samples obtained correctly? Analyzed promptly? FIO_2 accurately determined?
2. For clinical shunt: Did patient breathe O_2 long enough to maximally saturate Hb? Was estimated or measured content difference used? Was blood gas analysis performed promptly?
3. Was calculated shunt ≤5%? If so, no significant shunting is present.
4. Was calculated shunt >5% but <10%? If so, some shunting is likely. Consider technical causes (assumed content difference, assumed FIO_2).
5. Was calculated shunt >10% but <30%? If so, significant shunting is present. Consider clinical correlation.
6. Was calculated shunt >30%? If so, severe shunting is present. Further testing is indicated to determine the site and physiologic basis for the shunt.

increased pulmonary shunt fraction indicates that some lung units have little ventilation in relation to their blood flow. These patterns may be found in both obstructive and restrictive diseases. However, even in severe obstruction or restriction, blood flow to areas of poor ventilation may be reduced by the lesions themselves. In emphysema, destruction of the alveolar septa obliterates pulmonary capillaries. As the terminal airways lose their support, they also have reduced blood flow. In poorly ventilated lung units, vasoconstriction of pulmonary arterioles redirects blood flow away from the affected area. In these cases, there may be minimal shunting, even though severe ventilatory impairment exists.

Intrapulmonary shunting is common in acute disease patterns such as atelectasis or foreign body aspiration. Diseases such as pneumonia or adult respiratory distress syndrome (ARDS) often result in a shuntlike effect. This is caused by reduced ventilation in relation to blood flow in many lung units. Foreign body aspiration may cause shunting by blocking an airway and depriving all distal lung units of ventilation. Blood flow to the affected units cannot participate in gas exchange. The degree of shunting is directly related to the number of lung units with $\dot{V}/\dot{Q}$ ratios close to zero.

Intrapulmonary shunting may also occur when the pulmonary vascular system is involved, as is the case in hepatopulmonary syndrome. Patients who have liver disease with portal hypertension commonly have arteriovenous malformations that allow significant volumes of blood to pass through the lungs without participating in gas exchange. These malformations are prominent at the lung bases and result in increased shunting when the patient is upright.

Intracardiac shunting occurs when defects in the atrial or ventricular septa allow mixed venous blood to pass from the right side of the heart to the left side of the heart without traversing the pulmonary capillaries. In the ventricles, shunting usually requires an elevated right-heart pressure to overcome the normal pressure difference between the systemic and pulmonary systems. Atrial septal defects, such as patent foramen ovale (PFO), allow blood to pass from the right atrium to the left atrium during systole.

Very large shunt values (greater than 30%) suggest that a significant volume of blood is moving from the right side of the heart to the left side of the heart without participating in gas exchange. Further testing may be required to determine whether the shunt is occurring in the lungs or in the heart. Echocardiography with contrast media or cardiac catheterization may be necessary to identify intracardiac shunts.

The accuracy of clinical shunt measurement (i.e., dissolved O_2 differences) depends on the accuracy of PO_2 determinations. In small shunts, Hb becomes 100% saturated. The difference between alveolar and arterial PO_2 values results simply from the amount of O_2 dissolved. The difference between the actual content of dissolved oxygen and the content that can potentially dissolve is the basis for the calculation. Measurements of PO_2 used for shunt calculations (200–600 mm Hg) are much higher than the normal physiologic range. Additional calibration and quality control of the PO_2 electrode may be necessary to provide accurate values for oxygen tension. Blood gases drawn for shunt studies should be analyzed immediately to avoid large changes in PaO_2 values caused by cell metabolism in the specimen.

The calculated shunt fraction also depends on the O_2 content difference between arterial and mixed venous blood. $C(a-\bar{v})O_2$ is a component of the denominator in the clinical shunt equation. The **a-$\bar{v}$ content difference** is determined not only by the lungs but also by cardiac output and perfusion status of the tissues. Ideally, the value used in the equation should be measured rather than estimated. Arterial content can be determined easily from a sample taken from a peripheral artery. However, mixed venous content can only be measured accurately from a pulmonary artery sample. In patients who do not have a pulmonary artery catheter in place, an estimated value must be used. $C(a-\bar{v})O_2$ values from 4.5–5.0 vol% are reasonable content differences in patients who have good cardiac output and perfusion status. Values of 3.5 vol% may be more realistic in patients who are critically ill.

In some instances, a-$\bar{v}$ content difference cannot be reliably estimated, or Hb cannot be maximally saturated by breathing 100% oxygen. In such cases, the alveolar-arterial oxygen gradient $P(A-a)O_2$ may be useful as an index of ventilation to blood flow. In healthy patients breathing 100% O_2 at sea level, arterial PaO_2 should increase to approximately 600 mm Hg. $\dot{Q}s/\dot{Q}t$ does not directly provide absolute values for $\dot{Q}s$, but if the cardiac output ($\dot{Q}t$) is known, $\dot{Q}s$ can be determined simply. Measurement of the shunt fraction is sometimes performed in conjunction with the determination of the V_D/V_T ratio (see Chapter 4) to assess both types of gas exchange abnormalities together.

SUMMARY

- This chapter describes the measurement of pH, PCO_2, PO_2, and blood oximetry used as part of pulmonary function testing. Technical aspects of obtaining samples are discussed in detail because accurate interpretation makes numerous assumptions regarding proper specimen handling.
- Two noninvasive methods of assessing gas exchange are commonly used: pulse oximetry and capnography. Pulse oximetry offers a simple means of assessing oxyhemoglobin saturation. Capnography is useful for monitoring changes in $PETCO_2$, particularly for patients in critical care settings.
- Shunt measurements allow estimates of severe ventilation-perfusion imbalances in the lungs. Two methods are described: the clinical and physiologic equations. The advantages and disadvantages of each are also discussed.

CASE 6-1

Case Studies

HISTORY

C.O. is a 57-year-old man referred to the pulmonary function laboratory for increasing shortness of breath. He admits having a chronic cough with production of thick white sputum, mainly upon awakening. C.O. reports that he quit smoking 3 months ago. He averaged approximately two packs of cigarettes per day for 30 years (60 pack years) before quitting. His referring physician performed pulse oximetry in the outpatient clinic and obtained read-ings of 90%–91%. Complete pulmonary function studies with arterial blood gases were requested.

PULMONARY FUNCTION TESTS

Personal Data

Sex:	Male
Age:	57 yr
Height:	66 in (168 cm)
Weight:	197 lb (89.5 kg)

Spirometry

	Before Drug	LLN*	Predicted	%	After Drug	%	%Chg
FVC (L)	3.97	3.51	4.10	97	4.04	99	2
FEV$_1$ (L)	2.31	2.35	2.99	77	2.50	84	8
FEV$_{1\%}$ (%)	58	64	73	—	62	—	7
MVV (L)	83		116	72	92	79	11

*Lower limit of normal.

Lung Volumes

	Before Drug	LLN*	Predicted	%
VC (L)	3.97	3.20	4.10	97
IC (L)	2.66		2.76	96
ERV (L)	1.31		1.35	97
FRC (L)	3.65		3.42	107
RV (L)	2.34		2.07	113
TLC (L)	6.31	4.64	6.18	102
RV/TLC (%)	37		34	—

*Lower limit of normal.

D$_{LCO}$

	Before Drug	LLN*	Predicted	%
D$_{LCO}$ (ml/min/mm Hg)	16.7	19.5	26.3	63
D$_{LCO}$ (corrected)	16.7		26.3	63
D$_L$/V$_A$	5.09		4.38	86

*Lower limit of normal.

Blood Gases

pH	7.37
P$_{CO_2}$ (mm Hg)	44
P$_{O_2}$ (mm Hg)	57
HCO$_3^-$ (mEq/L)	26.4
BE (mEq/L)	~1.7
Hb (g/dl)	16.2
O$_2$Hb (%)	80.1
COHb (%)	5.9
MetHb (%)	0.2

TECHNOLOGIST'S COMMENTS

All spirometry maneuvers were performed acceptably. Lung volumes by helium (He) dilution were also performed acceptably. D$_{LCO}$ was performed acceptably; predicted D$_{LCO}$ was corrected for an Hb of 16.2 and a COHb of 5.9.

QUESTIONS

1. What is the interpretation of:
   a. Prebronchodilator and postbronchodilator spirometry?
   b. Lung volumes?
   c. D$_{LCO}$?
   d. Blood gases?
2. What is the most likely cause of the patient's symptoms?
3. What other treatment or tests might be indicated?

DISCUSSION

Interpretation

All spirometry, lung volumes, and diffusing capacity maneuvers were performed acceptably. Spirometry reveals moderate airway obstruction with minimal response to inhaled bronchodilators. Lung volumes by He dilution show a normal TLC, but with slightly increased FRC, RV, and RV/TLC ratio. These changes are suggestive of air trapping. D$_{LCO}$ is moderately decreased even after correction for increased Hb and elevated COHb. Arterial blood gas results reveal normal acid-base status with a P$_{CO_2}$ of 44. There is moderate

continued

to severe hypoxemia as indicated by a P_{O_2} of 57 and an oxyhemoglobin saturation of 80%. The hypoxemia is further aggravated by an increased COHb consistent with cigarette smoking or environmental exposure.

Impression: Moderate obstructive airways disease with no significant improvement after inhaled bronchodilator. There is a moderate loss of diffusing capacity. There is significant hypoxemia on room air, which is further increased by an elevation of COHb. Recommend further investigation of source of CO and clinical evaluation of O_2 supplementation.

Cause of Symptoms

This case demonstrates the importance of arterial blood gas analysis in the diagnosis of pulmonary disorders. The patient's complaint of increased shortness of breath was not explained by the borderline value of pulse oximetry (Sp_{O_2}) performed in the referring physician's office. The referring physician correctly suspected a pulmonary problem resulting from the patient's previous smoking history.

The spirometric measurement shows obstruction as evidenced by the $FEV_{1\%}$ of 58%, well below the lower limit of normal (64% for this patient). The patient's FEV_1 is also below its LLN. The response of FEV_1 to inhaled bronchodilator is slightly less than 200 ml and represents only an 8% improvement over prebronchodilator values. Lung volumes are also consistent with an obstructive pattern suggesting the beginnings of air trapping.

Diffusing capacity is also reduced in a pattern consistent with mild to moderate airway obstruction. The predicted D_{LCO} has been corrected for an elevated Hb and COHb. The combination of these two corrections results in a predicted D_{LCO} that is identical to the uncorrected predicted value (see Chapter 5).

Of the pulmonary function variables measured, the arterial blood gas values are most abnormal. Although pH and P_{CO_2} are within normal limits, P_{O_2} is markedly decreased. As a result, oxygen saturation is low. Elevated COHb further complicates oxygenation. This level is characteristic of individuals who currently smoke or who are chronically exposed to low levels of CO in their environment. The patient's spouse reported that he was still smoking 5–10 cigarettes per day.

Treatment and Other Tests

The patient was referred to a smoking cessation program and prescribed a nicotine replacement medication. He was able to stop smoking. Blood gas analysis 2 weeks later confirmed his smoking cessation (i.e., COHb was 1.7%). However, his P_{O_2} improved only slightly to 61 mm Hg (Sa_{O_2} was 87%). He was referred for evaluation of possible exercise desaturation. His arterial oxygenation was shown to actually increase with exercise, so O_2 supplementation was unnecessary. His lung function continued to improve over several months, presumably because of his smoking cessation.

CASE 6-2

Case Studies

HISTORY

Y.M. is a 31-year-old woman referred to the pulmonary function laboratory for a shunt study. Her chief complaint is shortness of breath with exertion as well as at other times. Her referring physician suspected a shunt and requested a shunt study. Y.M. was in no apparent distress on arrival at the laboratory. She never smoked and had no significant environmental exposure to respiratory irritants. Her mother died of a stroke at age 50 years, but there is no heart or lung disease in her immediate family.

SHUNT STUDY
Personal Data
Age:	31 yr
Height:	69 in (175 cm)
Weight:	200 lb (91 kg)
Race:	White

Blood Gases (Drawn After 20 Minutes of O₂ Breathing)

FIO_2	1.00
P_B	752
pH	7.43
PCO_2	38
PO_2	557
HCO_3^-	24.1
BE	0.1
Hb	7.4
O_2Hb	99.6
COHb	0.3
MetHb	0.1

QUESTIONS

1. What is the patient's calculated shunt?
2. What is the interpretation of:
   a. Blood gases?
   b. Shunt?
3. What is the cause of the patient's symptoms?
4. What other treatment or tests might be indicated?

DISCUSSION

Calculations

The P_AO_2 is calculated as follows:

$$P_AO_2 = P_B - PH_2O - \left(\frac{P_ACO_2}{0.8}\right)$$

$$= 752 - 47 - \left(\frac{38}{0.8}\right)$$

$$= 705 - 48$$

$$P_AO_2 = 657$$

Substituting this value in the clinical shunt equation and assuming an a-v̄ content difference of 4.5:

$$\frac{\dot{Q}_S}{\dot{Q}_T} = \frac{(P_AO_2 - PaO_2) \times 0.0031}{C(a-\bar{v})O_2 + [(P_AO_2 - PaO_2) \times 0.0031]}$$

$$= \frac{(657 - 557) \times 0.0031}{4.5 + [(657 - 557) \times 0.0031]}$$

$$= \frac{0.31}{4.5 + (0.31)}$$

$$\frac{\dot{Q}_S}{\dot{Q}_T} = 0.06$$

Interpretation

The patient's blood gas results show a normal acid-base status. The PaO₂ reflects an appropriate increase after breathing 100% O₂ for 20 minutes. The Hb as measured by hemoximetry (7.4 mg/dl) is markedly decreased. The patient's shunt is 6% (0.06 as a fraction). This is within normal limits.

Impression: Normal arterial blood gas results and normal shunt with markedly reduced Hb. Recommend clinical correlation.

Cause of Symptoms

The patient's primary symptom of dyspnea does not appear to be caused by any significant shunting. In a shunt, blood passes from the right side of the heart to the left side without coming into contact with alveolar gas. The shunt may be in the heart or in the lungs themselves. Breathing high concentrations of oxygen will not relieve this problem. This patient increased her PaO₂ appropriately, which rules out a large shunt.

A more likely cause of the symptoms described is the patient's low Hb level. Severe anemia reduces the arterial oxygen content dramatically. Oxygen delivery to the tissues is reduced. Dyspnea can result during exertion or times of increased metabolic demand. The patient's arterial content (ml/dl) can be calculated as follows:

$$CaO_2 = (1.34 \times Hb \times O_2Hb) + (PaO_2 \times 0.0031)$$

$$= (13.4 \times 7.4 \times 0.996) + (557 \times 0.0031)$$

$$= (9.9) + (1.7)$$

$$CaO_2 = 11.6$$

This value is much lower than the normal arterial content of about 20 ml/dl. It should be noted that the term in the second parentheses represents dissolved O₂ and would be much lower if the patient were breathing room air.

Treatment and Other Tests

The patient's anemia could have been diagnosed by any test that measures total Hb. Hemoximetry, in addition to providing accurate saturation data, also provides a measurement of total Hb. The shunt study could have been performed using calculated Hb saturation, but the low arterial content would have been missed.

No treatment is indicated until the cause of anemia can be identified. Y.M. was referred to a hematologist for further evaluation. Additional testing revealed a hemolytic form of anemia, which was successfully treated.

SELF-ASSESSMENT QUESTIONS

Entry-level

1. A patient referred for a pulmonary function test has blood gases drawn, and the following data are reported:

pH	7.43
$PaCO_2$ (mm Hg)	38
HCO_3^- (mEq/L)	25.1

   These values are consistent with:
   a. Normal acid-base status
   b. Respiratory alkalosis
   c. Metabolic acidosis
   d. Compensated respiratory acidosis

2. A patient with COPD has blood gases drawn and the following values reported:

pH	7.37
PCO_2	47 mm Hg
PO_2	52 mm Hg
HCO_3^-	27.1 mEq/L
Hb	15.8 g/dl
O_2Hb	82%

   Which of the following best describes these results?
   a. Normal blood gases
   b. Compensated metabolic alkalosis
   c. Moderate to severe hypoxemia
   d. Erroneous blood gas results

3. A patient being monitored by ECG has a heart rate (HR) of 120/min. A pulse oximeter on this patient displays a saturation of 84% with a HR of 118. Which of the following should the pulmonary function technologist conclude based on these findings?
   a. The patient's COHb level is likely elevated.
   b. The pulse oximeter's sensor should be moved to an alternate site.
   c. The patient needs supplementary O_2.
   d. The pulse oximeter is malfunctioning.

4. An outpatient is referred for arterial blood gas analysis. While performing the modified Allen's test, the pulmonary function technologist notes that the patient's hand reperfuses after 30 seconds. The technologist should
   a. Use a 23-gauge or smaller needle for the puncture

b. Proceed to obtain the specimen
   c. Draw blood from an alternate site
   d. Check the patient's blood pressure before proceeding

5. A patient with interstitial lung disease has an arterial oxygen tension (PaO_2) of 60 mm Hg, but hemoximetry is not performed. What calculated SaO_2 should the pulmonary function technologist report?
   a. 95%
   b. 90%
   c. 85%
   d. 75%

Advanced

6. A patient with chronic bronchitis has a resting SpO_2 of 80%, but an arterial blood gas reveals an SaO_2 of 90%. Which of the following should the pulmonary function technologist conclude?
   a. The patient has an elevated COHb.
   b. The patient has compensated respiratory acidosis.
   c. The pulse oximeter reading is erroneous.
   d. These results are expected in patients with polycythemia.

7. A patient who has COPD performs a maximal exercise test. At peak exercise his SpO_2 is 94% and a blood gas shows an SaO_2 of 87%. Which of the following might explain these results?
   I. Carboxyhemoglobinemia
   II. Methemoglobinemia
   III. Motion artifact
   IV. Metabolic acidosis
      a. I and II only
      b. I and III only
      c. II and IV only
      d. III and IV only

8. A patient being monitored by capnography shows the following data

Time	8:35	8:40	8:45	8:50	8:55	9:00
$PETCO_2$	38	39	39	29	25	26

   Which of the following best explains the change occurring at 8:50?
   a. Hypoventilation
   b. Respiratory acidosis
   c. Acute bronchospasm
   d. Decreased cardiac output

9. A patient with dyspnea on exertion has arterial blood gases drawn at rest before beginning an exercise test and the following data are obtained:

pH	7.44
$PaCO_2$	36 mm Hg
HCO_3^-	24.4 mEq/L
PaO_2	64 mm Hg
SaO_2	91%
Hb	6.9 mg/dl
COHb	1.2%

What is the subject's arterial oxygen content (CaO_2)?
a. 10.0 ml/dl
b. 9.3 ml/dl
c. 8.6 ml/dl
d. 8.4 ml/dl

10. A patient with dyspnea at rest has a clinical shunt study performed. The following data are obtained:

P_B	761 mm Hg
FIO_2	1.00
PaO_2	597 mm Hg
$PaCO_2$	38 mm Hg
SaO_2	100%
Hb	15.1 mg/dl

On the basis of these results, the patient's Qs/Qt is approximately:
a. 5%
b. 9%
c. 12%
d. 15%

Selected Bibliography

GENERAL REFERENCES
Shapiro BA, Kozlowski-Templin R, Peruzzi WT: *Clinical application of blood gases,* ed 5, St Louis, 1994, Mosby.
West JB: *Pulmonary pathophysiology: the essentials,* ed 6, Baltimore, 2003, Lippincott, Williams & Wilkins.
West JB: *Pulmonary physiology and pathophysiology: an integrated, case-based approach,* Baltimore, 2001, Lippincott, Williams & Wilkins.

BLOOD GASES
Breen PH: Arterial blood gas and pH analysis: clinical approach and interpretation, *Anesthesiol Clin North Am* 2001; 19:885-906.
Hess D: Detection and monitoring of hypoxemia and oxygen therapy, *Respir Care* 2000; 45:65-80.
Knowles TP, Mullin RA, Hunter JA, et al: Effects of syringe material, sample storage time, and temperature on blood gases and oxygen saturation in arterialized human blood samples, *Respir Care* 2006; 51:732-736.
Mahoney JJ, Harvey JA, Wong RJ et al: Changes in oxygen measurements when whole blood is stored in iced plastic or glass syringes, *Clin Chem* 1991; 37:1244-1248.
Siggard-Anderson O: Acid-base and blood gas parameters: arterial or capillary blood? *Scand J Clin Lab Invest* 1968; 21:289-292.
Swenson ER: Metabolic acidosis, *Respir Care* 2001; 46: 342-353.

PULSE OXIMETRY
Barker SJ, Tremper KK, editors: Pulse oximetry: applications and limitations, *Int Anesthesiol Clin* 1987; 25:155-175.
Fussell KM, Ayo DS, Branca P et al: Assessing need for long-term oxygen therapy: a comparison of conventional evaluation and measures of ambulatory oximetry monitoring, *Respir Care* 2003; 48:115-119.
Gehring H, Hornberger C, Matz H et al: The effects of motion artifact and low perfusion on the performance of a new generation of pulse oximeters in volunteers undergoing hypoxemia, *Respir Care* 2002; 47:48-60.
Giuliano KK, Higgins TL: New-generation pulse oximetry in the care of critically ill patients, *Am J Crit Care* 2005; 14:26-37.
McMorrow RC, Mythen MG: Pulse oximetry, *Curr Opin Crit Care* 2006; 12:269-271.
Netzer N, Eliasson AH, Netzer C et al: Overnight pulse oximetry for sleep-disordered breathing in adults: a review, *Chest* 2001; 120:625-633.
Sinex JE: Pulse oximetry: principles and limitations, *Am J Emerg Med* 1999; 17:59-67.

CAPNOGRAPHY
Anderson CT, Breen PH: Carbon dioxide kinetics and capnography during critical care, *Crit Care* 2000; 4:207-215.
Blanch L, Romero PV, Lucangelo U: Volumetric capnography in the mechanically ventilated patient, *Minerva Anestesiol* 2006; 72:577-585.
Carlon GC, Ray C, Miodownik S et al: Capnography in mechanically ventilated patients, *Crit Care Med* 1988; 16:550-556.

Graybeal JM, Russel GB: Capnometry in the surgical ICU: an analysis of the arterial-to-end-tidal carbon dioxide difference, *Respir Care* 1993; 38:923-928.

Koulouris NG, Latsi P, Dimitroulis J et al: Noninvasive measurement of mean alveolar carbon dioxide tension and Bohr's dead space during tidal breathing, *Eur Respir J* 2001; 17:1167-1174.

St John RE, Thomson PD: Noninvasive respiratory monitoring, *Crit Care Nurs Clin North Am* 1999; 11:423-435.

Thompson JE, Jaffe MB: Capnographic waveforms in the mechanically ventilated patient, *Respir Care* 2005; 50:100-108.

SHUNT CALCULATION

Cane RD, Shapiro BA, Templin R et al: Unreliability of oxygen tension-based indices in reflecting intrapulmonary shunting in critically ill patients, *Crit Care Med* 1988; 16:1243-1245.

Cane RD, Shapiro BA, Harrison RA et al: Minimizing errors in intrapulmonary shunt calculations, *Crit Care Med* 1980; 8:294.

Harrison RA, Davison R, Shapiro BA et al: Reassessment of the assumed a-v oxygen content difference in the shunt calculation, *Anesth Analg* 1975; 54:198.

Henig NR, Pierson DJ: Mechanisms of hypoxemia, *Respir Care Clin N Am* 2000; 6:501-521.

McCarthy K, Stoller JK: Possible underestimation of shunt fraction in the hepatopulmonary syndrome, *Resp Care* 1999; 44:1486-1488.

STANDARDS AND GUIDELINES

AARC clinical practice guideline: capnography/capnometry during mechanical ventilation—2003 revision & update, *Respir Care*; 2003, 48:534-539.

AARC clinical practice guideline: blood gas analysis and hemoximetry: 2001 revision and update, *Respir Care* 2001; 46:498-505.

AARC clinical practice guideline: capillary blood gas sampling for neonatal and pediatric patients, *Respir Care* 1994; 39:1180-1183.

AARC clinical practice guideline: pulse oximetry, *Respir Care* 1991; 36:1406-1409.

AARC clinical practice guideline: sampling for arterial blood gas analysis, *Respir Care* 1992; 37:913-917.

CLSI (formerly NCCLS): *Blood gas and pH analysis and related measurements: approved guideline,* Publication C46-A, 1999.

CLSI (formerly NCCLS): *Fractional oxyhemoglobin, oxygen content and saturation, and related quantities in blood: terminology, measurement, and reporting; approved guideline,* Publication C-25A, 1997.

CLSI (formerly NCCLS): *Procedures for the collection of arterial blood specimens: approved standard,* ed 3, Publication H11-A3, 1999.

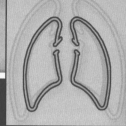

Chapter 7

Cardiopulmonary Exercise Testing

CARL MOTTRAM

CHAPTER OUTLINE

OBJECTIVES

After studying this chapter you will be able to:

Entry-level

1. Understand and select an appropriate exercise protocol based on the reason for performing the test
2. Identify the ventilatory/anaerobic threshold
3. Describe two methods for measuring ventilation, oxygen consumption, and carbon dioxide production during exercise
4. Identify indications for terminating a cardiopulmonary stress test

Advanced

1. Describe the normal physiologic changes that occur during exercise when workload is increased
2. Classify exercise limitation as caused by cardiovascular, ventilatory, gas exchange, or blood gas abnormalities or deconditioning
3. Understand the importance of evaluating breathing kinetics during exercise
4. Evaluate exercise flow-volume loop data

KEY TERMS

anaerobic threshold (AT)
Borg scale
breathing strategy
carbon dioxide production ($\dot{V}CO_2$)
lactic acid
metabolic equivalents (METs)
minute ventilation ($\dot{V}_E$)
oxygen consumption ($\dot{V}O_2$)

O_2 prescription
O_2 pulse
progressive multistage exercise tests
ramp test
ratings of perceived exertion (RPE)
6-minute walk test
steady-state tests

ventilatory equivalent for CO_2 ($\dot{V}_E/\dot{V}CO_2$)
ventilatory equivalent for oxygen ($\dot{V}_E/\dot{V}O_2$)
ventilatory threshold
V-slope method
watts
work
workload

The efficiency of the cardiopulmonary system may be different during increased metabolic demand than at rest. Tests designed to assess ventilation, gas exchange, and cardiovascular function during exercise can provide information not obtainable with the patient at rest. Cardiopulmonary exercise testing allows evaluation of the heart and lungs under conditions of increased metabolic demand. Limitations to work are not entirely predictable from any single resting measurement of pulmonary function. To define work limitations, a cardiopulmonary exercise test is necessary. In most exercise tests, cardiopulmonary variables are assessed in relation to the **workload** (i.e., the level of exercise). The patterns of change in any particular variable (e.g., heart rate) are then compared with the expected normal response.

The primary indications for performing exercise tests are dyspnea on exertion, pain (especially angina), and fatigue. Other indications include exercise-induced bronchospasm and arterial desaturation. Exercise testing can detect the following:

1. Presence and nature of ventilatory limitations to work

2. Presence and nature of cardiovascular limitations to work
3. Extent of conditioning or deconditioning
4. Maximum tolerable workload and safe levels of daily exercise
5. Extent of disability for rehabilitation purposes
6. Oxygen (O_2) desaturation and appropriate levels of supplemental O_2 therapy
7. Outcome measurement after a treatment plan (e.g., surgery or medical)

Exercise testing may be indicated in apparently healthy individuals, particularly in adults older than 40 years. Cardiopulmonary exercise testing is indicated to assess fitness before engaging in vigorous physical activities (e.g., running). Cardiopulmonary exercise testing may be useful in assessing risk of postoperative complications, particularly in patients undergoing thoracotomy.

Exercise testing and the protocols used can be diverse in purpose and complexity. This chapter deals primarily with cardiopulmonary measurements during exercise. This does not include simple cardiac stress testing during which only the electrocardiogram (ECG) and blood pressure (BP) are monitored, or more sophisticated tests involving injection of radioisotopes. However, a brief discussion of the 6-minute walk is included.

EXERCISE PROTOCOLS

Cardiopulmonary exercise tests can be divided into two general categories depending on the protocols used to perform the test: progressive multistage tests and steady-state tests. The 6-minute walk test contains elements of each of these general categories.

Progressive multistage exercise tests examine the effects of increasing workloads on various car-

diopulmonary variables, without necessarily allowing a steady state to be achieved. These protocols are often used to determine the workload at which the patient reaches a maximum oxygen uptake ($\dot{V}O_2max$). Multistage protocols can determine maximal ventilation, maximal heart rate, or a symptom limitation (e.g., chest pain) to exercise. Progressive multistage protocols (also called incremental tests) allow cardiopulmonary variables to be compared with expected patterns as workload increases.

In a typical incremental test, the patient's workload increases at predetermined intervals (Table 7-1). The workload may be increased at intervals of 1 – 6 minutes. Measurements (e.g., BP or

TABLE 7-1

Exercise Protocols

Treadmill	Speed (mph)/Grade (%)	Interval (min)	Comment
Bruce	1.7/10 2.5/12 3.4/14 4.2/16 5.0/18 5.5/20 6.0/22	3	Large workload increments; 1.7/0 and 1.7/5 may be used as preliminary stages for deconditioned patients
Balke	3.3 – 3.4/0 increasing grade by 2.5% to exhaustion	1	Small workload increments; may use 3 mph and 2-minute intervals for deconditioned subjects, or reduce slope changes to 1%
Jones	1.0/0 2.0/0 2 – 3.5/2.5 increasing grade by 2.5% to exhaustion	1	Small workload increments and low starting workload
Cycle Ergometer	**Workload**	**Interval (min)**	**Comment**
Astrand	50 W/min (300 kpm) to exhaustion	4	Large workload increments and long intervals; 33 W (200 kpm) may be used for women
"RAMP"	10 W/min to exhaustion	Continuous	Requires electronically braked ergometer; different work rates may be used to alter ramp slope
Jones	16 W/ min (100 kpm) to exhaustion	1	Smaller increments (50 kpm) may be used for deconditioned subjects
Other	**Description**	**Interval (min)**	**Comment**
Master step test	Either constant or variable step height combined with increasing step rates	Variable	Simple to perform; workload may be difficult to qualify
6-minute walk	Distance covered in 6 minutes of free walking	6	Simple; useful in patients with limited reserves or for evaluation of rehabilitation; can also be done for 12 minutes

blood gases) are usually made during the last 20–30 seconds of each interval. Complex measurements (e.g., cardiac output) may require longer intervals. Computerized systems that continuously measure ventilation, gas exchange, and cardiopulmonary variables permit shorter intervals to be used. The combination of intervals and work increments should allow the patient to reach exhaustion or symptom limitation within a reasonable period. An incremental test lasting 8–10 minutes after a warm-up is usually appropriate. If a computerized cycle ergometer is used, a "ramp" test may be performed. In a ramp protocol, the ergometer's resistance is increased continuously at a predetermined rate (usually measured in watts per minute).

During incremental tests with short intervals (1–3 minutes or a ramp protocol), a steady state of gas exchange, ventilation, and cardiovascular response may not be attained. Healthy patients may reach a steady state in 2–3 minutes at low and moderate workloads. Attainment of a steady state, however, is unnecessary if the primary objective of the evaluation is to determine the maximum values (oxygen uptake, heart rate, or ventilation). Short exercise intervals also lessen muscle fatigue that may occur with prolonged tests. Short-interval or ramp protocols may allow better delineation of gas exchange ($\dot{V}O_2$, $\dot{V}CO_2$) kinetics. Progressive multi-stage tests using intervals of 4–6 minutes may result in a steady state.

Steady-state tests are designed to assess cardiopulmonary function under conditions of constant metabolic demand. Steady-state conditions are usually defined in terms of HR, oxygen consumption ($\dot{V}O_2$), or ventilation ($\dot{V}_E$). If the HR remains unchanged for 1 minute at a given workload, a steady state may be assumed. Steady-state tests are useful for assessing responses to a known workload. Steady-state protocols may be used to evaluate the effectiveness of various therapies or pharmacologic agents on exercise ability. For example, an incremental test may be performed initially to determine a patient's maximum tolerable workload. Then a steady-state test may be used to evaluate specific variables at a submaximal level, such as 50% and 75% of the highest $\dot{V}O_2$ achieved. The patient exercises for 5–8 minutes at a prede-

termined level to allow a steady state to develop. Measurements are performed during the last 1 or 2 minutes of the period. Successive steady-state determinations at higher power outputs may be made continuously or spaced with short periods of light exercise or rest. A similar protocol may be used for evaluation of exercise-induced bronchospasm (see Chapter 9).

PF TIP

The 6-minute walk test is a simple exercise test used to assess response to a medical or surgical intervention. It is also used to assess functional capacity as well as predict morbidity and mortality. The test is performed in an unobstructed hallway that is at least 100 feet in length. The objective of the test is to have the patient cover as much ground as possible in 6 minutes. It is important to use standardized phrases of encouragement during the test. Assessment of oxygen need should be performed prior to the test and, when indicated, adequate flow rates of oxygen utilized. Documentation should include the distance walked, the oxygen flow and delivery device if used, the mode of oxygen transport (e.g., pulling an O_2 cart versus carrying a unit), and the ratings of perceived exertion (RPE). Pulse oximetry is optional.

The **6-minute walk test** is a simple test that does not require any sophisticated equipment. It is typically performed to assess response to a medical or surgical intervention but has also been used to assess functional capacity as well as to estimate morbidity and mortality. A 100-foot (minimum) hallway that is free of obstructions is needed to perform the test. Equipment needed includes the following:

- Countdown timer
- Mechanical lap counter
- A method to mark the endpoints of the course (small traffic cones)
- Chair
- Sphygmomanometer and appropriate sized cuff
- Rating of perceived exertion scale (**Borg scale**)
- Easy access to the emergency response team (e.g., telephone, nurse call light)

An oxygen delivery device should be available, if appropriate. A pulse oximeter can be used but is not required. The objective of the test is to have the patient walk as far as possible in 6 minutes. The patient should be encouraged throughout the test, and it has been recommended that standard phrases be used to reduce test-to-test variability. Resting during the tests is permitted with encouragement to continue walking as soon as possible, while the timer continues to run. If pulse oximetry is measured, it should be done at the beginning and end of exercise but not during exercise unless a telemetry-type oximeter is available. Documentation should include the distance walked, the oxygen flow and delivery device if used, the mode of oxygen transport (e.g., pulling an O_2 cart has a different impact on work than carrying a unit), and the **ratings of perceived exertion (RPE).** See Table 7-2 for an example of a data record used to record 6-minute walk data from a patient.

EXERCISE WORKLOAD

Two methods of varying exercise workload are commonly used: the treadmill and the cycle ergometer (Figures 7-1 and 7-2). Each device has advantages and disadvantages (Table 7-3). Other methods sometimes used include arm ergometers, steps, and free running or walking (as previously described for the 6-minute walk test).

Workload on a treadmill is adjusted by changing the speed and/or slope of the walking surface. The speed of the treadmill may be calibrated either in miles per hour or in kilometers per hour. Treadmill slope is registered as "percent grade." Percent grade refers to the relationship between the length of the walking surface and the elevation of one end above level. A treadmill with a 6-foot surface and one end elevated 1 foot above level would have an elevation of $1/6 \times 100$, or approximately 17%. The primary

TABLE 7-2					
6-Minute Walk Log					
Date	Distance (ft)	Inspired Gas	Mode of O_2 Transport	SpO_2 (End Exercise)	RPE (6-20)
5/18/2002	1173	3.0 L/min NC	Patient carried unit	90	17
7/26/2002	1266	3.0 L/min NC	Patient carried unit	94	18
8/15/2002	1420	2.5 L/min	Patient carried unit	92	17

FIGURE 7-1 **Treadmill with Computerized Electrocardiogram (ECG) and Controller.** The treadmill is controlled by a programmable interface so that different protocols (e.g., speeds and percent grade) can be selected. Manual control is also provided. Cardiac monitoring and exhaled gas analysis are integrated in a single computer system. The 12-lead ECG recordings or rhythm strips can be taken automatically at each exercise level. Most automated systems provide "freeze frame" technology that allows for close review during the test and storage of data for retrieval and analysis for significant arrhythmia and ST abnormalities after the test. The same system can be interfaced to a cycle ergometer (see Figure 7-2). *(Courtesy Medical Graphics Inc., St Paul, Minn.)*

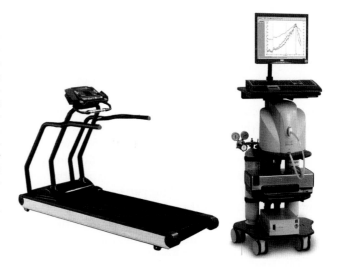

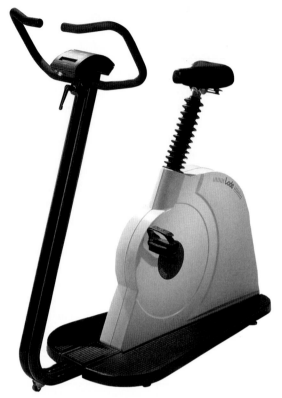

FIGURE 7-2 Electronically Braked Cycle Ergometer. Typical cycle ergometer with continuous adjustable electronic braking. Workload (i.e., resistance) is usually managed by interfacing the ergometer to a computer. The computer allows selection of various cycle ergometer protocols. Changes in pedaling rate by the patient causes a change in resistance to maintain a constant workload. *(Courtesy Medical Graphics Inc., St Paul, Minn.)*

TABLE 7-3		
Ergometers		
	Advantages	Disadvantages
Treadmill	Natural form of exercise	Risk of accidents
	Easy to calibrate	Patient anxiety
	Higher $\dot{V}O_2$max	Motion artifact
		Difficult to obtain blood
		Difficult to quantify work
Cycle ergometer	Safer than treadmill	Difficult to calibrate
	Easy to monitor	Leg fatigue more of an issue
	Easy to quantify work	Lower $\dot{V}O_2$max
	Easy to obtain blood	

advantage of a treadmill is that it elicits walking, jogging, and running, which are familiar forms of exercise. An additional advantage is that maximal levels of exercise can be easily attained, even in conditioned healthy patients. However, the actual work performed during treadmill walking is a function of the weight of the patient. Patients of different weight walking at the same speed and slope perform different work. Different walking patterns, or stride length, may also affect the actual amount of work being done. Patients who grip the handrails of the treadmill may use their arms to reduce the amount of work being performed. For these reasons, esti-

mating $\dot{V}O_2$ from a patient's weight and the speed and slope of the treadmill may produce erroneous results. $\dot{V}O_2$max has been shown to be measured slightly higher (approximately 7%–10%) on a treadmill compared with a cycle ergometer.

The cycle ergometer allows workload to be varied by adjustment of the resistance to pedaling and by the pedaling frequency, usually specified in revolutions per minute (rpm). The flywheel of a mechanical ergometer turns against a belt or strap, both ends of which are connected to a weighted physical balance. The diameter of the wheel is known, and the resistance can be easily measured. When pedaling speed (usually 50–90 rpm) is determined, the amount of work performed can be accurately calculated. One of the chief advantages of the cycle ergometer is that the workload is independent of the weight of the patient. Unlike the treadmill, $\dot{V}O_2$ can be reasonably estimated if the pedaling speed and resistance are carefully measured. In addition, workload can be changed rapidly by adjusting the tension on the flywheel. Another advantage of ergometers is better stability of the patient for gas collection, blood sampling, and blood pressure monitoring. Electronically braked cycle ergometers (see Figure 7-2) provide a smooth, rapid, and more reproducible means of changing exercise workload than mechanical ergometers. Electronically braked ergometers allow continuous adjustment of workload independent of pedaling speed. However, accuracy of the ergometer output may be dependent on a manufacturer's specified pedal cadence range (e.g., 40–100 rpm). This feature permits the exercise level to be ramped (i.e., the workload increases continuously rather than in increments). The **ramp test** allows the patient to advance from low to high workloads quickly and provides all the information normally sought during a progressive maximal exercise test. A ramp protocol typically requires electronic control (usually by a computer) for adjustment of the workload and rapid collection of physiologic data. Box 7-1 provides a systematic method of determining the desired workload increments using a cycle ergometer.

BOX 7-1	Method for Predicting Increment or Ramp Protocol

- $(\dot{V}O_2\text{max predicted} - \dot{V}O_2\text{rest})/100$ = predicted max power output (watts) to achieve in 10 minutes.
- Reduce the predicted max workload for subjects with reduced exercise tolerance.
- Increase the estimated maximal power output for very fit subjects.

Example: Predicted $\dot{V}O_2$max 2300 ml, resting $\dot{V}O_2$max 300 ml $(2300 - 300)/100$ = 20 watts/min incremental or ramp protocol

PF TIP

MET is a commonly used term to describe the level of work performed during an exercise evaluation or in relation to activities of daily living. One MET equals the O_2 uptake at rest. For clinical purposes, 1 MET is equivalent to an O_2 uptake of 3.5 ml O_2/min/kg. If O_2 consumption is measured during a cardiopulmonary exercise test, the MET level achieved can be calculated easily. For example, if a patient reaches a peak $\dot{V}O_2$ of 15 ml O_2/min/kg, the MET equivalent would be 15/3.5, or approximately 4.3 METs. Healthy sedentary patients should be able to exercise up to approximately 7 METs.

Some differences in maximal performance exist between the treadmill and the cycle ergometer. These differences primarily result from the muscle groups used. In most patients, cycling does not produce as high a maximum O_2 consumption as walking on the treadmill (approximately 7%–10% less). Ventilation and lactate production may be slightly greater on the cycle ergometer because of the different muscle groups used. Differences between the treadmill and cycle ergometer are not significant in most clinical situations. The choice of device may be dictated by the patient's clinical condition (e.g., orthopedic impairments or chief complaint only occurs with running), the types of

measurements to be made, or the space and availability of equipment in the laboratory.

Workload may be expressed quantitatively in several ways:

Work is normally expressed in kilopond-meters (kpm). One kilopond-meter equals the work of moving a 1-kg mass a vertical distance of 1 m against the force of gravity.

Power is expressed in kilopond-meters per minute (i.e., work per unit of time) or in watts. One watt equals 6.12 kpm/min (100 **watts** = $\oplus$ 600 kpm/min).

Energy is expressed by oxygen consumption ($\dot{V}O_2$), in liters or milliliters per minute (STPD) or in terms of **metabolic equivalents (METs)**. Resting or baseline $\dot{V}O_2$ can be measured as described in the following paragraphs or estimated. For purposes of standardization, 1 MET is considered equal to 3.5 ml O_2/min/kg.

For cardiopulmonary exercise evaluation, it is particularly useful to relate the ventilatory, blood gas, and hemodynamic measurements to the $\dot{V}O_2$ as the independent variable. This requires measurement of ventilation and analysis of expired gas during exercise.

A number of cardiopulmonary exercise variables may be used depending on the clinical questions to be answered. Schemes for measuring these variables are described in Table 7-4. Graded exercise with monitoring of only BP and ECG may be limited to evaluation of patients with suspected or known coronary artery disease.

Measurement of ventilation, oxygen consumption, carbon dioxide production, and related vari-

TABLE 7-4

Cardiopulmonary Exercise Variables

Variables Measured	Uses
ECG, blood pressure, SpO_2	Limited to suspected or known coronary artery disease; pulse oximetry may be misleading if used without blood gases
All of the above plus ventilation $\dot{V}O_2$, $\dot{V}CO_2$, and derived measurements	Noninvasive estimate of ventilatory threshold (AT), quantify workload; discriminate between cardiovascular and pulmonary limitation to work
All of the above plus arterial blood gases	Detailed assessment of gas exchange abnormalities; calculation of V_D/V_T; titration of O_2 in exercise desaturation; measurement of pH and lactate possible
All of the above plus mixed venous blood gases	Cardiac output by Fick method, noninvasive techniques, calculation of shunt, thermodilution cardiac output, pulmonary artery pressures, calculation of pulmonary and systemic vascular resistances

ables permits a comprehensive evaluation of the cardiovascular system. Addition of these measurements to ECG, BP, and pulse oximetry makes it possible to grade the adequacy of cardiopulmonary function. In addition, analysis of exhaled gas allows the relative contributions of cardiovascular, pulmonary, or conditioning limitations to work to be determined. All of these variables can be measured noninvasively. When using pulse oximetry to assess gas exchange, the practitioner needs to be aware of the limitations of the device that may lead to a false-positive result (e.g., motion artifact, peripheral vasoconstriction).

Adding blood gases to the exercise protocol enables detailed analysis of the pulmonary limitations to exercise. Placement of an arterial catheter is preferable to a single sample obtained at peak exercise, although this is subject to the laboratory having the skilled personnel available to place a line. Multiple specimens permit comparison of blood gases at each workload. A single sample at peak exercise may be difficult to obtain and may not adequately describe the pattern of gas exchange abnormality. However, if this technique is used, the sample should be harvested within 30 seconds of achieving the maximal workload because variables of gas exchange return to baseline rapidly in some individuals. In some patients, measurement of cardiac output (CO) using either noninvasive or invasive techniques such as a pulmonary artery (Swan-Ganz) catheter may be indicated. Noninva-

sive CO determination depends on the availability of the technology and the underlying cause of the patient's condition (e.g., may not work well in patients with chronic obstructive pulmonary disease [COPD]). Invasive techniques require the placement of a catheter that allows measurement of mixed venous blood gases, cardiac output via the Fick method, and many other derived variables. Thermal dilution cardiac output is also available with most pulmonary artery catheters.

CARDIOVASCULAR MONITORS DURING EXERCISE

Continuous monitoring of heart rate (HR) and ECG during exercise is essential to safe performance of the test. Intermittent or continuous monitoring of BP is equally important to ensure that exercise testing is safe. Recording of HR, ECG, and BP allows work limitations caused by cardiac or vascular disease to be identified and quantified. The level of fitness or conditioning can be gauged from the HR response in relation to the maximal work rate achieved during exercise.

Heart Rate and Electrocardiogram

Heart rate and rhythm should be monitored continuously using one or more modified chest leads.

Standard precordial chest lead configurations (V_1–V_6) allow comparison with resting 12-lead tracings (Exercise 7-1). Twelve-lead monitoring during exercise is practical with electrocardiographs designed for exercise testing. These instruments incorporate filters (digital or analog) that eliminate movement artifact and provide ST-segment monitoring. Limb leads normally must be moved to the torso for ergometer or treadmill testing (modified leads). A resting ECG should be performed to record both the standard and modified leads. Single-lead monitoring allows only for gross arrhythmia detection and HR determination. It may not be adequate for testing patients with known or suspected cardiac disease.

PF TIP

Exercise tests are often performed to determine a patient's maximal exercise capacity. An end point that is commonly used is the patient's predicted maximal HR. Maximal HR is easily computed as 220 – age. A subject who is 40 years old would have a predicted maximal HR of 220 – 40, or 180 beats/min. If the subject achieves at least 85% of the predicted value (153 beats/min in this case), he or she is considered to have made a maximal effort. Because maximal HR varies among individuals, some patients may reach or exceed their predicted maximum. Many patients will reach a "symptom-limited" end point before reaching 85% of the predicted maximal HR. In these cases, the patient becomes exhausted, dyspneic, or has chest pain. The technologist should always record what symptoms caused the patient's inability to continue.

EXERCISE 7-1

CRITERIA FOR ACCEPTABILITY
Cardiovascular Monitors During Exercise

1. Heart rate and rhythm (ECG) should be monitored continuously. At least one precordial lead is required; full 12-lead monitoring using modified limb leads is recommended.
2. A resting 12-lead ECG should be available for comparison with exercise tracings.
3. All exercise tracings should be free from artifact caused by motion or electrical interference.
4. ECG monitoring devices should allow manual or automated storage of arrhythmia events for later review.
5. "Raw" ECG tracings should be available for comparison with computer-averaged complexes.
6. Heart rates should be checked by visual inspection of the ECG tracing.
7. Systemic blood pressure (BP) should be monitored at appropriate intervals (i.e., at least once per exercise stage).
8. BP may be monitored using an appropriate-sized cuff or by automated noninvasive blood pressure (NIBP) monitor. A cuff/stethoscope should be available as backup for the NIBP.
9. If BP is monitored by an indwelling arterial catheter, the pressure transducer must be zeroed and calibrated appropriately. The catheter should be secured to minimize movement artifact.

The ECG monitor should allow assessment of intervals and segments up to the patient's maximal heart rate (HRmax). Computerized arrhythmia recording or manual "freeze-frame" storage allows subsequent evaluation of conduction abnormalities while the testing protocol continues (Figure 7-3). Some digital ECG systems generate computerized "median" complexes averaged from a series of beats. These may be helpful in analyzing ST-segment depression. The "raw," or nondigitized, ECG should also be available. Significant ST-segment changes should be easily identifiable from the tracing up to the predicted HRmax.

HR should be analyzed by visual inspection of the ECG, with manual measurement of the rate rather than by an automatic sensor. Most HR meters average RR intervals over multiple beats. Inaccurate HR measurements may occur with nodal or ventricular arrhythmias or because of motion artifact. Tall P or T waves may be falsely identified as R waves, causing automatic calculation of HR to be incorrect. Accurate measurement of HR is necessary to determine the patient's maximal HR in comparison with the age-related predicted value.

Motion artifact is the most common cause of unacceptable ECG recordings during exercise.

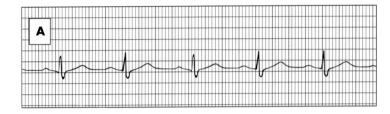

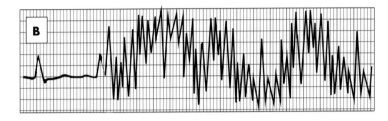

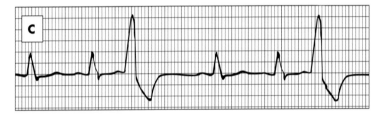

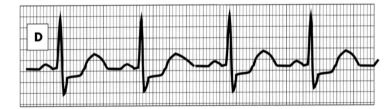

FIGURE 7-3   Electrocardiographic (ECG) Monitoring During Exercise. A, Standard rhythm lead showing normal sinus rhythm. Although testing can be done with 1–3 leads, 12-lead monitoring allows comparison with resting ECG tracings and better detection of ischemic changes. **B,** Motion artifact. The most common monitoring problem during exercise is poor ECG signals because of motion. These problems can be minimized by careful skin preparation and electrode application. Lead wires and cables should be supported so that movement and traction on electrodes is kept to a minimum. **C,** Premature ventricular contractions (PVCs). PVCs are a common occurrence during exercise in patients with underlying cardiac disease. Increased rate of PVCs, couplets (two in a row), or triplets (three in a row) may be indications for limiting the exercise test. **D,** ST-segment changes. Depression (and sometimes elevation) of the ST segment of the ECG is usually considered evidence of cardiac ischemia. Depression (or elevation) of the ST segment greater than 1–2 mm for 0.08 seconds or longer is consistent with significant ischemia. ST segments should be checked in multiple leads before, during, and after exercise.

Allowing the patient to practice pedaling on the ergometer or walking on the treadmill permits adequacy of the ECG signal to be checked. Carefully applied electrodes, proper skin preparation, and secured lead wires greatly minimize movement artifact (see Exercise 7-1). Electrodes specifically designed for exercise testing are helpful. Most of these use extra adhesive to ensure electrical contact even when the patient begins perspiring. The skin sites should be carefully prepared. Removal of surface skin cells by gentle abrasion is recommended. Patients with excessive body hair may require shaving of the electrode site to ensure good electrical contact. Lead wires must be securely attached to the electrodes. Devices that limit the movement of the lead wires can greatly reduce motion artifact. Spare electrodes and lead wires should be available to avoid test interruption in the event of an electrode failure.

HR increases linearly with increasing workload, up to an age-related maximum. Several formulas are available for predicting HRmax. For most predicted HRmax values, a variability of ±10–15 beats/min exists in healthy adult patients. Two commonly used equations for predicting HRmax are as follows:

1. $$HRmax = 220 - Age\ (years)$$

2. $$HRmax = 210 - (0.65 \times Age\ [years])$$

Equation 1 yields slightly higher predicted values in young adults. Equation 2 produces higher values in older adults. Other methods of predicting HRmax vary depending on the type of exercise protocol used in deriving the regression data. Specific criteria for terminating an exercise test should include factors based on symptom limitation as well as HR and BP changes (see the section on safety).

HR increases almost linearly with increasing $\dot{V}O_2$. The increase in cardiac output (CO) depends on both HR and stroke volume (SV) according to the following equation:

$$CO = HR \times SV$$

Increases in stroke volume account for a smaller portion of the increase in CO, primarily at low and moderate workloads (Figure 7-4). While HR increases from 70 beats/min up to 200 beats/min

in young healthy upright patients, SV increases from 80 ml to approximately 110 ml. At low workloads, increase in CO depends on the patient's ability to increase both HR and SV. At high workloads, further increases in CO result almost entirely from the increase in HR.

Deconditioned patients usually have a limited SV. High HR values occur with moderate workloads in deconditioned individuals because it is the primary mechanism for increasing CO. Training (e.g., endurance or aerobic) typically improves SV response. This allows the same cardiac output to be achieved at a lower HR. Training usually results in a lower resting HR as well as a higher tolerable maximum workload. Except in highly trained patients, maximal exercise in healthy individuals is limited by the inability to further increase the CO. Reductions in SV are usually related to the preload or afterload of the left ventricle. Increased HR response, in relation to the workload, implies that SV is compromised.

Reduced HR response may occur in patients who have ischemic heart disease or complete heart block (Exercise 7-2). Low HR is also common in patients

FIGURE 7-4 **Normal Cardiovascular Responses During Exercise.** Four cardiovascular parameters are plotted against $\dot{V}O_2$ as a measure of work rate, as they might appear in a normal healthy adult. Heart rate (HR) increases linearly with work. Maximal HR is predicted by the age of the patient. Stroke volume (SV) increases initially at low to moderate workloads but then becomes relatively constant. Cardiac output (HR × SV) increases at low and moderate workloads because of increases in both HR and SV (see text). At higher levels of work, increases in HR are responsible for increasing cardiac output. Systolic blood pressure (BP) increases by approximately 100 mm Hg in a linear fashion, whereas diastolic BP increases only slightly.

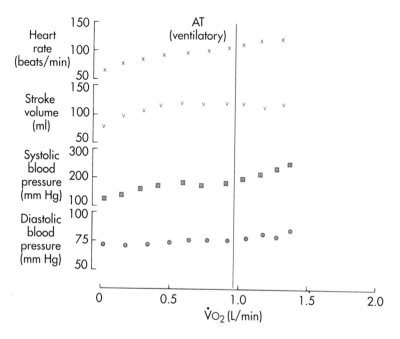

EXERCISE 7-2

INTERPRETIVE STRATEGIES

Cardiovascular Monitors During Exercise

1. Is ECG recording acceptable? Free from motion and other artifact?
2. Is resting tracing consistent with previous 12-lead ECGs? If not, are differences caused by lead placement?
3. What is the rate and rhythm at rest? Is there evidence of heart block at rest? Is there evidence of ischemia (ST-segment changes) at rest?
4. Was maximal heart rate greater than 85% of predicted? If so, patient probably exerted maximal effort. If not, what factors limited exercise? Ventilation? Pain? Fatigue? Other?
5. Did the rhythm change with exercise? Increased or decreased PVCs? Was there evidence of ischemia (ST- or T-wave changes)?
6. Was BP normal at rest? If not, consider clinical correlation.
7. Did systolic BP increase appropriately? Did it exceed 250 mm Hg at maximal exercise?
8. Did diastolic BP remain constant or increase slightly? If not, consider clinical correlation.

---

who have been treated with drugs that block the effects of the sympathetic nervous system (β-blockers, calcium channel blockers). HR response may also be reduced if the autonomic nervous system is impaired or the heart is denervated, as occurs after cardiac transplantation (e.g., chronotropic insufficiency).

In patients who have heart disease (e.g., coronary artery disease, cardiomyopathy), increased HR is typically accompanied by ECG changes such as arrhythmias or ST-segment depression. Deconditioned patients without heart disease show a high HR at lower than maximal workloads but usually without ECG abnormalities. Horizontal or down-sloping ST-segment depression greater than 1 mm (from the resting baseline) for a duration of 0.08 seconds is usually considered evidence of ischemia. ST-segment depression at low workloads that increases with HR and continues into the post-exercise period is usually indicative of multivessel coronary artery disease. ST-segment depression accompanied by exertional hypotension or marked increase in diastolic pressure is usually associated with significant coronary disease. The predictive value of ST-segment changes during exercise must be related to the patient's clinical history and risk factors for heart disease.

The most common arrhythmia that occurs during exercise testing is the premature ventricular contraction (PVC) (see Figure 7-3). Exercise-induced PVCs occurring at a rate of more than 10 per minute are often found in ischemic heart disease. Increased PVCs during exercise may also be seen in mitral valve prolapse. Coupled PVCs (couplets) often precede ventricular tachycardia or ventricular fibrillation. Occurrence of couplets or frequent PVCs may be an indication for terminating the exercise evaluation. Some patients with PVCs at rest or at low workloads may have these ectopic beats suppressed as exercise intensity increases. The most serious ventricular arrhythmias are sometimes seen in the immediate postexercise phase.

Shortness of breath (SOB) brought on by exertion is perhaps the most widespread indication for cardiopulmonary exercise evaluation. The combination of cardiovascular parameters (e.g., HR, SV) with data obtained from analysis of exhaled gas (i.e., $\dot{V}O_2$) permits assessment of dyspnea on exertion. Table 7-5 generalizes some of the basic relationships between cardiovascular and pulmonary exercise responses. These relationships help delineate whether exertional dyspnea is a result of cardiac or pulmonary disease, or whether the patient is simply deconditioned. In some instances, poor effort may mimic exertional dyspnea. Comparison of data from cardiovascular and exhaled gas variables can confirm inadequate patient effort.

Blood Pressure

Systemic BP may be monitored intermittently with the standard cuff method. Automated noninvasive cuff devices for monitoring BP are also available. Although these methods work well at rest and at low workloads, they may be difficult to implement

TABLE 7-5				
Exercise Variables and Dyspnea*				
	Cardiac	Ventilatory	Deconditioned	Poor Effort
$\dot{V}O_2max$	Less than 80% of predicted	Less than 80% of predicted	Less than 80% of predicted	Less than 80% of predicted
$\dot{V}_Emax$	Less than 70% of MVV	Greater than 90% of MVV; V_Emax less than 15 L	Less than 70% of MVV	Variable
Anaeorbic threshold	Achieved at low $\dot{V}O_2$	Usually not achieved	Achieved at low $\dot{V}O_2$	Not achieved
HR	Greater than 85% of predicted	Less than 85% of predicted	Greater than 85% of predicted	Less than 85% of predicted
ECG/signs of ischemia	ST changes, arrhythmias, chest pain	Usually normal	Normal	Normal
SaO_2	Greater than 90%	Often less than 90%, hypoxemia	Greater than 90%	Greater than 90%

*This table compares the usual findings for the exercise variables listed in subjects with dyspnea caused by cardiac disease, pulmonary disease, or deconditioning. Some subjects may have dyspnea because of combination of causes. Poor effort during exercise may result from improper instruction, lack of understanding by the subject, or lack of motivation by the subject.
MVV, Maximal voluntary ventilation; SaO_2, arterial oxygen saturation.

during high levels of exercise. BP sounds may be difficult to detect because of treadmill noise or patient movement. It is important to monitor the pattern of BP response at low and moderate workloads to establish that both systolic and diastolic pressure respond as anticipated.

Continuous monitoring of BP may be accomplished by connection of a pressure transducer to an indwelling arterial catheter (Figure 7-5). An indwelling line allows continuous display and recording of systolic, diastolic, and mean arterial pressures. In addition, the catheter provides ready access for arterial blood sampling. Arterial catheterization may be easily accomplished using either the radial or the brachial site. The catheter must be adequately secured to prevent loss of patency during vigorous exercise. Insertion of arterial catheters presents some risk of blood splashing or spills. Adequate protection for the individual inserting the catheter, as well as for those withdrawing specimens, is essential. See Chapter 6 for specific recommendations regarding arterial sampling via catheters.

Systolic BP increases in healthy patients during exercise from 120 mm Hg up to approximately 200–250 mm Hg (see Figure 7-4). Diastolic pressure normally rises only slightly (10–15 mm Hg) or not at all. The mean arterial pressure rises from approximately 90 mm Hg to approximately 110 mm Hg, depending on the changes in systolic and diastolic pressures. Increased CO, particularly the SV, causes the increase in systolic pressure almost completely. Even though CO may increase fivefold, (e.g., from 5–25 L/min), the systolic pressure only increases twofold. Systolic pressure only doubles because of the tremendous decrease in peripheral vascular resistance. Most of this decrease in resistance results from vasodilatation in exercising muscles. Increased systolic pressure (>250–300 mm Hg) should be considered an indication for terminating the exercise evaluation (Exercise 7-3). Similarly, if the systolic pressure fails to rise with increasing workload, the exercise test should be terminated and the patient's condition stabilized. Variations in BP during exercise are often caused by the patient's respiratory effort. Phasic changes with respiration are particularly common in patients who have large transpulmonary pressures because of lung disease. Differences of as much as 30 mm Hg between inspiration and expira-

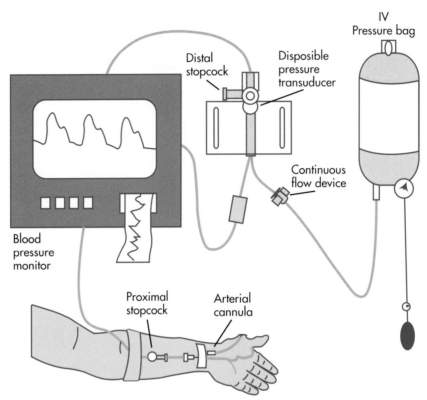

FIGURE 7-5 Pressure Transducer Setup for Continuous Arterial Monitoring. A catheter is inserted into the radial or brachial artery. Pressure tubing connects the catheter to a continuous flow device that maintains a constant pressure (and a small flow of solution) against the arterial line to prevent backflow of blood into the system. The continuous flow device also allows flushing of the system. A pressure transducer assembly is connected in line with the tubing. Pressure changes in the system are transmitted via a thin membrane to the transducer. Blood samples may be drawn by inserting a heparinized syringe at a stopcock located near the indwelling catheter (blood pressure signal is temporarily lost during sampling). A similar assembly can be used for connection to a Swan-Ganz catheter for pulmonary artery monitoring during exercise.

tion may be seen during continuous monitoring of arterial pressure.

In maximal tests (e.g., the patient reaches HRmax), it may be impossible to obtain a reliable BP at peak exercise. Even with an arterial catheter, motion artifact may prevent recording of a usable tracing. Systolic pressure may transiently drop and diastolic pressure may drop to zero at the termination of exercise. To minimize the degree of hypotension resulting from abrupt cessation of heavy exercise, the patient should "cool down." This is accomplished easily by having the patient continue exercising at a low work rate until BP and HR have stabilized at or slightly above baseline levels.

Safety

Safe and effective exercise testing for cardiopulmonary disorders requires careful pretest evaluation to identify contraindications to the test procedure (Exercise 7-4). A preliminary workup should include a complete history and physical examination by the referring physician or the physician performing the stress test. Preliminary laboratory tests should include a 12-lead ECG, chest x-ray study, baseline pulmonary function studies before and after bronchodilator therapy, and routine laboratory examinations such as complete blood count and serum electrolytes.

EXERCISE 7-3

INDICATIONS FOR TERMINATING EXERCISE TESTS

- Monitoring system failure
- 2-mm horizontal or down-sloping ST depression or elevation
- T-wave inversion or Q waves
- Sustained supraventricular tachycardia
- Ventricular tachycardia
- Increasing frequency of multifocal premature ventricular beats
- Development of second- or third-degree heart block
- Exercise-induced left or right bundle branch block
- Progressive chest pain (angina)
- Sweating and pallor
- Systolic pressure greater than 250 mm Hg
- Diastolic pressure greater than 120 mm Hg
- Failure of systolic pressure to increase or a drop of 10 mm Hg with increasing workload
- Lightheadedness, mental confusion, or headache
- Cyanosis
- Nausea or vomiting
- Muscle cramping

EXERCISE 7-4

CONTRAINDICATIONS TO EXERCISE TESTING*

- Recent (within 4 weeks) myocardial infarction
- Unstable angina pectoris
- Second- or third-degree heart block
- Rapid ventricular/atrial arrhythmias
- Orthopedic impairment
- Severe aortic stenosis
- Congestive heart failure
- Uncontrolled hypertension
- Limiting neurologic disorders
- Dissecting/ventricular aneurysms
- Severe pulmonary hypertension
- Thrombophlebitis or intracardiac thrombi
- Recent systemic or pulmonary embolus
- Acute pericarditis
- PaO_2 less than 40 mm Hg on room air (unless an oxygen environment is provided)
- $PaCO_2$ greater than 70 mm Hg

*These conditions represent relative contraindications to exercise testing; the risk to the patient must be evaluated on a case-by-case basis.

The risks and benefits of the entire exercise procedure should be explained to the patient. Appropriate informed consent should be obtained. This includes an explanation of any alternative tests that might be done and what the consequences of not performing the stress test might be. A physician experienced in exercise testing should supervise the test. Tests may be performed by qualified practitioners on patients younger than 40 years with no known risk factors provided a physician is immediately available. Criteria for terminating the exercise evaluation before the specified end point or symptom limitation occurs are listed in Exercise 7-4.

After termination of the exercise evaluation for whatever reason, the patient should be monitored until HR, BP, and ECG return to pretest levels. ECG monitoring should continue for at least 5 minutes (as recommended by the American College of Sports Medicine). Tracings should be made at frequent intervals immediately after exercise.

Personnel conducting exercise tests should be trained in handling cardiovascular emergencies and all aspects of cardiopulmonary resuscitation (e.g., advanced cardiac life support [ACLS]). The laboratory should have available resuscitation equipment, including the following:

1. Standard intravenous (IV) medications (e.g., epinephrine, atropine, lidocaine)
2. Syringes, needles, IV infusion apparatus
3. Portable O_2 and suction equipment
4. Airway equipment, endotracheal tubes, and laryngoscope
5. Direct current (DC) defibrillator and appropriate monitor

All emergency equipment should be checked daily or immediately before any cardiopulmonary exercise evaluation. Equipment such as defibrillators, laryngoscopes, and suction apparatus should be routinely evaluated for proper function according to institutional policies.

VENTILATION DURING EXERCISE

Collection and analysis of expired gas during cardiopulmonary exercise testing provides a noninvasive means of obtaining the following variables:

- Minute ventilation ($\dot{V}_E$)
- Tidal volume (V_T)
- Frequency of breathing; respiratory rate (f_b)
- Oxygen consumption; oxygen uptake ($\dot{V}O_2$)
- Carbon dioxide production ($\dot{V}CO_2$)
- Respiratory exchange ratio (RER)
- Ventilatory equivalent for oxygen ($\dot{V}_E/\dot{V}O_2$)
- Ventilatory equivalent for carbon dioxide ($\dot{V}_E/\dot{V}CO_2$)

Equipment Selection and Calibration

The two common methods of exhaled gas analysis use either a mixing chamber (Figure 7-6) or computerized breath-by-breath measurements (Figure 7-7). Pneumotachometers are used in both mixing chamber and breath-by-breath systems and should be calibrated with a known volume (3-L syringe) or flow signal (Exercise 7-5). The flow sensor's accuracy should comply with the criteria set by the American Thoracic Society and European Respiratory Society (ATS-ERS) for flow-measuring devices (e.g., ±3% or 50 ml, whichever is greater). Validation of a flow-measuring device can be performed by connecting it in series with a volume-based spiro-

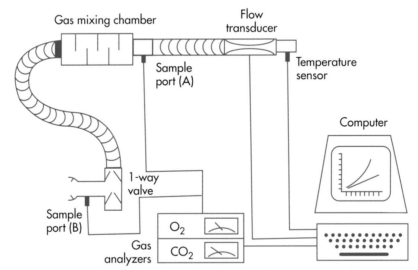

FIGURE 7-6　Mixing Chamber System for Analysis of Expired Gas. The patient inspires room air through a one-way valve and expires through large-bore tubing into a mixing chamber with a volume of approximately 5 L. Baffles in the chamber cause the gas to be thoroughly mixed so that it is representative of mixed expired gas. A small volume is extracted at *sample port A* and directed to the O_2 and CO_2 analyzers for determination of F_EO_2 and F_ECO_2. Expired gas then passes through a flow-sensing device (pneumotachometer) from which volume can be obtained by integration. A temperature probe at the flow transducer provides data for conversion of gas volume from ambient temperature to BTPS and STPD. Signals from the gas analyzers, flow transducer, and temperature sensor are recorded directly on an analog recorder or converted to digital signals for computer processing. Analysis of individual breaths of expired gas can be obtained by sampling at *port B*. This technique allows determination of respiratory rate and end-tidal CO_2 and O_2 concentrations. The mixing chamber system can be used for exercise protocols as well as for resting metabolic measurements.

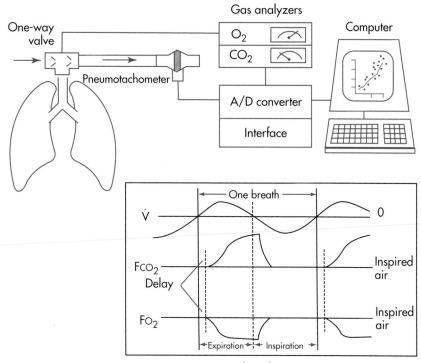

FIGURE 7-7   Breath-by-Breath System for Determination of $\dot{V}O_2$, $\dot{V}CO_2$, and Ventilation. The patient inspires and expires through a pneumotachometer or similar flow-sensing device, which may or may not require the use of a uni-directional value. Gas is continuously sampled at the patient's mouth to determine fractional concentrations of O_2 and CO_2. The flow signal and signals from the gas analyzers are integrated to measure volume, F_EO_2, and F_ECO_2, and to calculate $\dot{V}_E$, $\dot{V}O_2$, $\dot{V}CO_2$, rate, and V_T. Computerization is required to perform calculations and corrections. Simultaneous recording of flow ($\dot{V}$) and fractional concentrations of O_2 and CO_2 are shown *(insert)*. During expiration, F_{CO_2} increases and F_{O_2} decreases. Gas concentrations and flow are out of phase because of the time required to transport gas from the mouthpiece to the analyzers and the response time of the analyzers themselves. Storing appropriate phase-delay corrections (determined during calibration) in the computer can align signals. Ventilatory and gas-exchange parameters can be monitored and displayed on a breath-by-breath basis. For exercise tests or metabolic measurements, breath-by-breath data are averaged over a short interval (10–60 seconds) or specific number of breaths.

meter of known accuracy. Gas analyzers should also be calibrated and checked before each test procedure. Two-point calibration with gases that approximate the physiologic range to be tested provide the most appropriate means of ensuring accuracy. Three-point calibration is necessary to check the linearity of the analyzers. Table 7-6 lists some recommended gas concentrations for calibration of analyzers to be used for exercise tests.

If a gas collection valve (see Chapter 10) is used in the breathing circuit, it should have a low resistance (1–2 cm H_2O at 100 L/min) and a small dead space. In healthy adults, a valve dead space of 100 ml is acceptable. A valve with reduced dead space (25–50 ml) may be more appropriate for children or for patients who have dead space–producing disease or small tidal volumes. Some breath-by-breath systems can be programmed to reject small breaths (<100 ml). If this feature is used, the volume of rejected breaths should be matched to valve dead space. Breaths that do not clear valve dead space should be discarded. If valve dead space is too large for the patient, significant rebreathing may occur. In breath-by-breath exercise systems, this may show

EXERCISE 7-5

CRITERIA FOR ACCEPTABILITY

Ventilatory Measurements During Exercise

1. Volume transducer calibration before exercise measurements should be performed according to ATS-ERS standards and kept for documentation.
2. Temperature and other environment factors should be recorded.
3. Breathing valve resistance and dead space should be appropriate for the patient tested, if applicable.
4. Ventilatory variables should be measured over intervals appropriate for the type of exercise (incremental versus steady state).
5. Recent FEV_1 and MVV maneuvers should be available for interpretive purposes. The quality of the spirometry also needs to be considered.
6. Maximal flow-volume (F-V) loop should be measured before exercise if exercise F-V or tidal volume loops are to be measured.
7. Inspiratory capacity (IC) should be accurately measured in order to plot exercise flows in relation to maximal F-V loop.

TABLE 7-6

Recommended Calibration Gases for Exercise Systems

Type of Exercise Test	Suggested Calibration Gases
Maximal or submaximal with subject breathing room air	20.9% O_2, 0% CO_2 15% O_2, 5% CO_2
Maximal or submaximal with subject breathing supplementary O_2 (may also be used to check linearly)	20.9% O_2, 0% CO_2 15% O_2, 5% CO_2 26% O_2, 0% CO_2

formed after 4–6 minutes at a constant workload. For incremental protocols, sampling may be performed during the last minute of each stage. In breath-by-breath systems, sampling is done continuously, with data being displayed for each breath. Breath-by-breath data may also be averaged over several breaths.

up as an expired CO_2 level that does not decrease to zero during inspiration. Many modern exercise systems have small flow sensors that do not require a valve system, so dead space and valve resistance become less critical.

If a mixing chamber is used, the patient should be allowed to breathe through the circuit with a nose clip in place long enough to wash out room air with expired gas. The exact washout volume, or time, depends on the volume of the mixing chamber. Breath-by-breath systems (see Figure 7-7) normally require minimal washout because fractional gas concentrations are sampled directly at the mouthpiece. If supplemental O_2 is breathed, the inspiratory portion of the breathing circuit as well as the patient's lungs should be in equilibrium before gas sampling starts.

Depending on the protocol and equipment used, gas collection and analysis are performed over a specified interval during each exercise level. For steady-state protocols, gas collection is usually per-

PF TIP

Patients who have lung disease may be limited by their ventilatory capacity during exercise. The maximal voluntary ventilation (MVV) is often used as an index of ventilatory capacity during exercise. Healthy patients typically use less than 70% of their MVV during maximal exertion. Patients with lung disease often have a reduced MVV and may reach or exceed 80% of their MVV during maximal exercise. In terms of absolute volumes, if the maximal ventilation during exercise is within 10–15 L/min of the patient's MVV, a ventilatory limitation to exercise is probably present. Some individuals may have flow limitation even though their ventilation is less than their MVV.

In gas collection or mixing chamber systems, raw data collected includes the following:

1. Volume expired, in liters
2. Temperature of gas at the measuring device (°C)

3. Time of collection, seconds or minutes
4. Respiratory rate during the collection interval
5. Fraction of mixed expired O_2 (FeO_2)
6. Fraction of mixed expired CO_2 ($FeCO_2$)

These data can be recorded manually or by a multichannel recorder with appropriate analog signals. In most modern systems, the data are gathered into a computer by means of an analog-to-digital (A/D) converter (see Chapter 10). Computerized data reduction offers the advantage of immediate feedback for all measurements. Automated data collection also offers greater flexibility for using different exercise protocols (see Table 7-1). Breath-by-breath gas analysis requires that signals from the flow sensor be integrated with the gas analyzer signals for FeO_2 and $FeCO_2$. The phase delay between volume and gas concentration signals must be considered (see Figure 7-7). This is done by measuring phase delay time (for each gas analyzer) during calibration. The phase delay is then stored, and subsequent measurements use this factor to align the volume and gas signals. Sampling flow or sample lines should not be altered after calibration because phase delay values may change. Water or particulate contamination of the gas analyzer sample line or damage to the sample line can also affect phase delay. Alterations of the phase delay can have a profound effect on the accuracy of the data (up to 30% error in the calculated $\dot{V}O_2$), especially at higher respiratory rates.

Minute Ventilation

Minute ventilation ($\dot{V}_E$) is the volume of gas expired per minute by the exercising patient, expressed in liters, BTPS. For an exercise system in which gas is collected, $\dot{V}_E$ may be calculated as follows:

$$\dot{V}_E = \frac{\text{Volume expired} \times 60}{\text{Collection time (sec)}} \times \text{BTPS factor}$$

Sample calculations and BTPS factors are contained in Appendix F. Modern breath-by-breath systems measure the volume of each breath and continuously compute the minute ventilation.

Healthy adults at rest breathe 5–10 L/min. During exercise, this value may increase to more than 200 L/min in trained patients. It commonly exceeds 100 L/min in healthy adults (Figures 7-8 and 7-9). The increase in ventilation removes CO_2,

FIGURE 7-8 Normal Ventilation/Gas Exchange Responses During Exercise. Four variables as they might appear in a healthy young adult are plotted against $\dot{V}O_2$. The *dotted vertical line* represents AT. $\dot{V}_E$ increases linearly with work rate at low and moderate workloads up to the AT, as does $\dot{V}CO_2$. At higher levels, $\dot{V}_E$ and $\dot{V}CO_2$ increase at a faster rate as HCO_3^- buffers lactic acid and as CO_2 is produced. The ratio of $\dot{V}CO_2$ to $\dot{V}O_2$ (RER) follows a similar pattern as RER approaches and then exceeds 1. V_D/V_T initially decreases rapidly as V_T increases; it then continues to decrease but at a slower rate (see text).

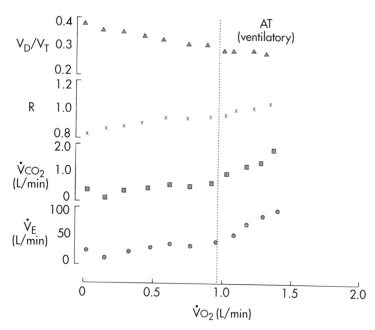

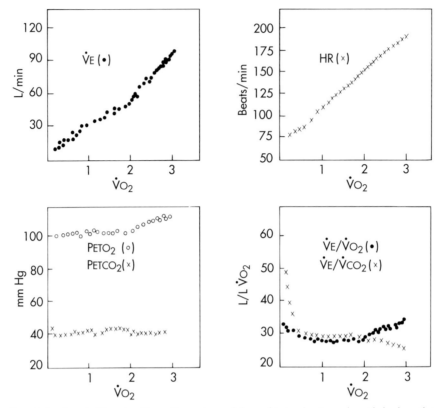

FIGURE 7-9   Breath-by-Breath Exercise Data. Four plots of data obtained using a breath-by-breath technique, as in Figure 7-7. Although data are recorded for each breath, the plots represent 30-second averages. All parameters are plotted against $\dot{V}O_2$ as the measure of work being performed. $\dot{V}_E$ increases linearly up to approximately 2 L/min $\dot{V}O_2$; HR increases linearly throughout the test. $PETO_2$ and $PETCO_2$ (end-tidal partial pressures of O_2 and CO_2, respectively) remain relatively constant up to approximately 2 L/min $\dot{V}O_2$. At this point, end-tidal O_2 begins to increase and end-tidal CO_2 begins to decrease. A similar pattern is seen on the plot of ventilatory equivalents for oxygen and carbon dioxide ($\dot{V}_E/\dot{V}O_2$ and $\dot{V}_E/\dot{V}CO_2$, respectively). A primary advantage of breath-by-breath analysis is that plots may be viewed in "real time," thus allowing modification of the testing protocol as required. Data in this example indicate the occurrence of ventilatory AT at approximately 2 L/min of $\dot{V}O_2$.

the primary product of exercising muscles, as workload increases. Ventilation increases linearly with an increasing workload (i.e., $\dot{V}O_2$) at low and moderate levels of exercise. In healthy patients, this increase in ventilation during exercise follows the rise in $\dot{V}CO_2$. Relating the $\dot{V}_E$max to resting ventilatory function provides an index of ventilatory limitations to exercise. Maximal voluntary ventilation (MVV) (see Chapter 2) can be related to the $\dot{V}_E$ achieved at the highest workload attained ($\dot{V}_E$max). Ventilatory capacity (sometimes called ventilatory ceiling) is defined by the measured MVV or the

FEV_1 (forced expiratory volume in 1 second) $\times$ 35 (some clinicians prefer $FEV_1 \times 40$). The difference between $\dot{V}_E$max and ventilatory capacity is often called the ventilatory (or breathing) reserve (Figure 7-10). Ventilatory reserve is calculated as follows:

$$\text{Ventilatory reserve} = \left[1 - \left(\frac{\dot{V}_E \text{max}}{MVV}\right)\right] \times 100$$

where:

$\dot{V}_E$max = ventilation at highest exercise level reached, liters/minute

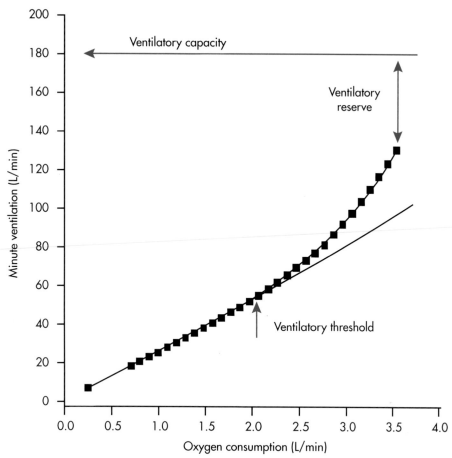

FIGURE 7-10   Ventilatory Capacity. Ventilatory capacity is defined as the measured maximal voluntary ventilation (MVV) or MVV calculated from $FEV_1 \times 35$ or 40. The difference between the $\dot{V}_Emax$ (highest level of ventilation achieved during exercise) and the ventilatory capacity is termed the ventilatory reserve or breathing reserve.

MVV = maximal voluntary ventilation, liters/minute

The ventilatory reserve is usually expressed as a percentage but can also be denoted as the actual difference. In healthy patients, the ventilatory reserve is typically 20%–40%. In patients with pulmonary disease, the reserve is less than 20% or the absolute difference between MVV and $\dot{V}_Emax$ is less than 10–15 L. This latter relationship is important in individuals with a disease process that affects their ability to perform an MVV (i.e., those who have a low or abnormal MVV). In some cases, the abnormally low MVV can yield a $\dot{V}_Emax$/MVV ratio that is in the normal range, but the actual difference is reduced (see Table 7-5). A valid MVV maneuver is essential to compare exercise ventilation with MVV. Patients who have airway obstruction may actually achieve $\dot{V}_E$ during exercise that equals or exceeds their ventilatory capacity. In both scenarios, exercise is limited by their inability to further increase ventilation and they are therefore identified as being ventilatory limited.

At high levels of ventilation in healthy patients (>120 L/min), increases in O_2 uptake gained by increased ventilation serve mainly to supply O_2 to the respiratory muscles. The same phenomenon may occur at much lower levels of ventilation in patients with severe lung disease because of the increased work of breathing. Because of the ventilatory reserve in healthy patients, exercise is seldom limited by ventilation. Maximal exercise is normally limited by inability to further increase cardiac output or inability to extract more O_2 at the tissue level in exercising muscles. Some highly trained athletes may achieve ventilatory limitation. Aerobic training can improve cardiovascular function so that ventilation, not cardiac output, limits maximal work.

Tidal Volume and Respiratory Rate

V_T during exercise may be calculated by dividing $\dot{V}_E$ by f_b. Breath-by-breath systems record individual breaths and then report an average V_T over a short interval or after a fixed number of breaths have been analyzed. Observation of the breathing kinetics or **breathing strategy** of a patient during exercise can be an important adjunct in interpretation of the exercise results. The normal response to exercise is to increase the V_T at low and moderate work-

loads. Increased V_T accounts for most of the rise in ventilation at these workloads; only a small amount results from increased f_b. This pattern continues until the V_T approaches approximately 50%–60% of vital capacity (VC). Further increases in total ventilation are accomplished by increasing f_b. These kinetic changes can be important in a patient complaining of SOB with normal lung function. A high-frequency, low–tidal volume breathing strategy will result in an increased V_D/V_T. More important, however, it may be the only physiologic reason for the patient's perceived SOB. Likewise, a patient using a large V_T and low f_b may also complain of SOB without a physiologic abnormality.

In healthy individuals, the increase in V_T is accomplished both by using the inspiratory reserve volume (IRV) and by reducing the end-expiratory lung volume (EELV) (Figure 7-11, *left panel*). This allows efficient use of the respiratory muscles and chest wall pump. In patients with chronic airflow limitation, inability to increase ventilation may be related to dynamic compression of the airways and dynamic hyperinflation (i.e., increased lung volume) that can occur during exertion. These patients have large resting lung volumes (hyperinflation). During

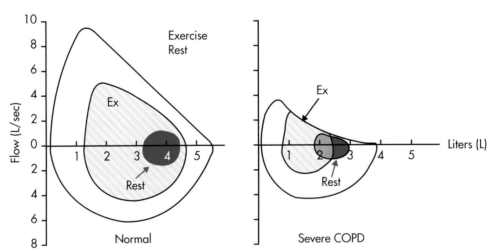

FIGURE 7-11   Flow-Volume Loop Kinetics. Normal F-V loop kinetics are shown with recruitment of exercise tidal breathing from both the IRV and the ERV, and not touching the resting maximal F-V curve (MFVC) *(left)*. Breathing kinetics of a patient with severe chronic obstructive pulmonary disease (COPD) is also shown *(right)*. The patient has to move up in absolute lung volumes to recruit tidal volume. This, along with the fact that they are flow limited throughout much of the tidal breath, increases the work of breathing.

exercise, EELV tends to increase even more as the patient attempts to optimize expiratory flow to meet ventilatory demands. The dynamic shift in lung volume places the respiratory muscles at an even greater disadvantage. The sensation of dyspnea increases tremendously, and the patient is unable to continue exercise. The consequence for these patients is an increase in the work of breathing from both flow limitation and breathing at higher lung volumes (see Figure 7-11, *right panel*). Patients who have airway obstruction may also be able to increase their $\dot{V}_E$ but cannot attain predicted values (Exercise 7-6). If VC is markedly reduced by the obstructive process, there may be little reserve to accommodate an increased V_T. Obstructed patients

who have a normal VC but increased resistance to flow may increase their V_T at a low f_b during exercise in an effort to minimize the work of breathing. This pattern continues until the V_T reaches a plateau, as described previously. Then the f_b must be augmented to further increase $\dot{V}_E$. Because of flow limitation, particularly during the expiratory phase, increases in f_b must be accomplished by shortening the inspiratory portion of each breath. Reduction of the inspiratory time in relation to the total breath time (T_i/T_{tot}) requires the inspiratory muscles to generate increasingly greater flows. The increased load placed on the muscles of inspiration typically results in dyspnea.

Unlike the pattern in obstruction, in restrictive disease V_T may remain relatively fixed. Increases in $\dot{V}_E$ during exercise are accomplished primarily by rapid respiratory rates. It is usually more efficient for patients who have "stiff" lungs to move small tidal volumes at fast rates to increase ventilation. However, these tidal volumes may still comprise a relatively large portion of their vital capacity (60%–70%). Flow-volume (F-V) loop profiles may be close to normal, whereas the work of distending the lung is increased in restrictive patterns. The mechanism of increasing ventilation primarily by increasing respiratory rate places a load on the respiratory muscles. In combination with hypoxemia, this increased load often results in extreme SOB.

Flow-Volume Loop Analysis

Another method of determining the degree of ventilatory limitation is by monitoring F-V loop dynamics during exercise. Exercise tidal-volume loops may be plotted against the resting maximal F-V loop. This technique quantifies the amount of time the patient spends on the maximal flow-volume envelope and allows the clinician to identify the percent of flow limitation (Figure 7-12). This method may better define the increased work of breathing in individuals who do not reach a classic definition of ventilatory limitation, but have a substantial component of flow limitation during exercise. Monitoring the tidal flow-volume loop

---

EXERCISE 7-6

INTERPRETIVE STRATEGIES

Ventilatory Measurements During Exercise

1. Were data collected over an interval appropriate to the type of exercise test?
2. Was resting ventilation within normal limits ≈5 to 10 L/min)? If not, why?
3. Did minute ventilation increase appropriately with workload?
4. Was $\dot{V}_E$max less than 70% of MVV or FEV$_1$ × 35–40? Was the absolute difference greater 10–15 L/min? If so, some ventilatory reserve is present. If not, ventilatory limitation to exercise is likely.
5. Was breathing kinetics appropriate? Did V_T increase to approximately 50%–60% of VC? If not, why? Was increased respiratory rate primarily responsible for increased $\dot{V}_E$? If so, suspect a restrictive ventilatory pattern or inappropriate breathing kinetics.
6. Was there flow limitation evidenced by the tidal breathing superimposed on the maximal flow-volume curve? If so, to what extent?
7. Were changes in V_T consistent with an appropriate breathing strategy?
8. What reason did the patient offer for stopping exercise (if applicable)? Was this finding consistent with the pattern of ventilation observed?

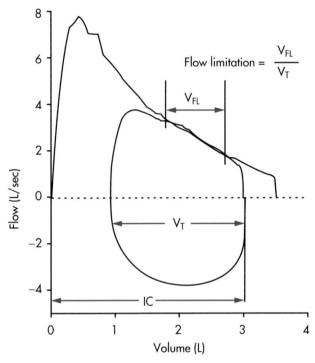

FIGURE 7-12 **Flow Limitation During Exercise.** Flow limitation can be quantified by plotting the exercise tidal breathing loop over the maximal F-V loop. The tidal loop is positioned by measuring the inspiratory capacity (IC) during exercise and positioning the end-expiratory level at an absolute lung volume equal to TLC – IC. Computer analysis can then quantify the percentage of time that the patient is breathing at or above maximal flow.

during exercise can also show dynamic changes in the flow pattern. These changes can alert the clinician to intrathoracic, extrathoracic, or fixed-airway abnormalities that are demonstrated only during exercise. This technique may also be useful in monitoring breathing kinetics during exercise. As discussed previously, the normal method of increasing tidal volume during exercise is to use both inspiratory and expiratory reserve volumes. Patients with obstructive lung disease have to "move up" in their lung volumes (see Figure 7-11) to recruit tidal volume. In some cases, individuals with normal lung function can use an inappropriate breathing strategy by moving up in their lung volumes to recruit tidal volume without evidence of flow limitation. Using these inappropriate breathing strategies may cause a concomitant sensation of dyspnea. Some patients may breathe at low lung volumes, which approach residual volume. Breathing at these low lung volumes can cause flow limitation resulting from the position of tidal breathing along the absolute lung volume scale. This breathing strategy

can elicit wheezing and SOB that can mimic asthma and has been coined a type of "pseudoasthma."

OXYGEN CONSUMPTION, CARBON DIOXIDE PRODUCTION, AND RESPIRATORY EXCHANGE RATIO DURING EXERCISE

Oxygen Consumption

Oxygen consumption ($\dot{V}O_2$) is the volume of O_2 taken up by the exercising (or resting) patient in liters, or milliliters/minute, STPD. Oxygen consumption is also commonly reported in milliliters/kilogram (ml/kg) of body weight. $\dot{V}O_2$ is the product of ventilation minute and the rate of extraction from the gas breathed (i.e., the difference between the F_IO_2 and the F_EO_2; see the following paragraph). Healthy patients at rest have a $\dot{V}O_2$ of approximately 0.25 L/min (STPD) or approximately 3.5 ml O_2/

min/kg (1 MET). During exercise, $\dot{V}O_2$ may increase to over 5.0 L/min (STPD) in trained patients. $\dot{V}O_2$ is the best single measure of external work being performed. Exercise limitation caused by ventilatory, gas exchange, or cardiovascular abnormalities may be quantified by relating exercise variables to $\dot{V}O_2$. Figures 7-4 and 7-8 provide examples of ventilatory and cardiovascular variables related to $\dot{V}O_2$ in healthy patients. The causes of work limitation may be defined by comparing these patterns in the exercising patient. Exercise limitation may be a result of pulmonary disease, cardiovascular disease, muscular abnormalities, deconditioning, poor effort, or a combination of these factors.

To calculate $\dot{V}O_2$ and $\dot{V}CO_2$, the fractional concentrations of O_2 and CO_2 in expired gas must be analyzed (Exercise 7-7). Exhaled gas is sampled from a mixing chamber (see Figure 7-6) or a breath-by-breath system (see Figure 7-7). In systems that accumulate gas (e.g., mixing chamber), a pump is used to draw the sample through the O_2 and CO_2 analyzers. Water vapor is removed from the mixed expired sample by passing the gas through a drying tube (usually containing calcium chloride). In breath-by-breath systems, fractional gas concentrations are sampled at the mouth using rapid gas analyzers. Most systems use sample tubing that is permeable to water vapor, so that the effects of humidity can be accommodated (see Chapter 10). Gas concentration signals from the analyzers are integrated with the expiratory flow signal to measure the volumes of O_2 and CO_2 exchanged for each breath (see Figure 7-7).

$\dot{V}O_2$ is calculated from an accumulated gas volume using the following equation:

$$\dot{V}O_2 = \left(\left[\frac{1-F_EO_2-F_ECO_2}{1-F_IO_2}\times F_IO_2\right]-F_EO_2\right)\times \dot{V}_E(STPD)$$

where:
F_EO_2 = fraction of O_2 in the expired sample
F_ECO_2 = fraction of CO_2 in the expired sample
F_IO_2 = fraction of O_2 in inspired gas (room air = 0.2093)

The term

$$\left(\frac{1-F_EO_2-F_ECO_2}{1-F_IO_2}\right)$$

is a factor to correct for the small differences between inspired and expired volumes when only expired volumes are measured. Ventilation is corrected to STPD as follows:

$$\dot{V}_E(STPD) = \dot{V}_E(BTPS)\times\left(\frac{P_B-47}{760}\right)\times 0.881$$

O_2 consumption at the highest level of work attainable by normal patients is termed the $\dot{V}O_2$max. $\dot{V}O_2$max is characterized by a plateau of the oxygen uptake despite increasing external workloads. $\dot{V}O_2$max is useful for comparing exercise capacity between patients. $\dot{V}O_2$max may also be used to compare a patient with his or her age-related predicted value of $\dot{V}O_2$max. Equations for deriving predicted $\dot{V}O_2$max are included in Appendix B.

EXERCISE 7-7

CRITERIA FOR ACCEPTABILITY

Oxygen Consumption and Carbon Dioxide Uptake per Minute

1. There should be documentation of appropriate gas analyzer calibrations; two-point calibration recommended for room air exercise, three-point for exercise with supplemental oxygen.
2. Phase delay calibration (breath-by-breath systems) should be documented within manufacturer's specifications.
3. Volume transducer should be calibrated before testing.
4. Breathing valve (if used) should have appropriate resistance and dead space volume for patient tested.
5. There should be evidence of appropriate washout of collection device or mixing chamber (if used).
6. RER at rest should be within the physiologic range of 0.70–1.10; RER values greater than 1.0 may be present because of hyperventilation.
7. $\dot{V}O_2$ and $\dot{V}CO_2$ should be within normal limits with the patient at rest; each should increase with increasing workloads.

One measure of impairment is the percentage of expected $\dot{V}O_2max$ attained by the exercising patient. Height, sex, age, and fitness level all affect the "normal" maximal oxygen consumption. Because of these factors, most reference equations show a large variability (±20%). Patients who have a 20%–40% reduction in their $\dot{V}O_2max$ have mild to moderate impairment. Those who have $\dot{V}O_2max$ values less than 50% of their predicted values have severe exercise impairment. Some studies have attempted to estimate $\dot{V}O_2$ based on the height and weight of the patient and the speed and slope of a treadmill. O_2 consumption estimated from treadmill walking is sufficiently variable so that its use is limited. Power output from a calibrated cycle ergometer may be used to estimate $\dot{V}O_2$ more accurately than from treadmill exercise. Workload estimated from cycle ergometry is not influenced by weight or stride. Actual $\dot{V}O_2$ may differ significantly from the estimated value, even with an ergometer. Cycle ergometry usually produces slightly lower maximal $\dot{V}O_2$ values than treadmill walking in healthy patients (see the section on exercise protocols).

Carbon Dioxide Production

Carbon dioxide production ($\dot{V}CO_2$) is a direct reflection of metabolism. It is expressed in liters or milliliters per minute, STPD. $\dot{V}CO_2$ may be calculated using the following equation:

$$\dot{V}CO_2 = (F_ECO_2 - 0.0003) \times \dot{V}_E(STPD)$$

where:
F_ECO_2 = fraction of CO_2 in expired gas
0.0003 = fraction of CO_2 in room air (may vary)
$\dot{V}_E(STPD)$ = calculated as in the equation for $\dot{V}O_2$

Pulmonary ventilation, consisting of alveolar ventilation ($\dot{V}_A$) and dead space ventilation ($\dot{V}_D$), may be related in terms of the $\dot{V}CO_2$. The fraction of alveolar carbon dioxide (F_ACO_2) is directly proportional to $\dot{V}CO_2$ and inversely proportional to $\dot{V}_A$. The

concentration of CO_2 in the lung is determined by CO_2 production and the rate of removal from the lung by ventilation. This relationship may be expressed as follows:

$$F_ACO_2 = \frac{\dot{V}CO_2}{\dot{V}_A}$$

$\dot{V}CO_2$ in a healthy patient at rest is approximately 0.20 L/min (STPD). It may increase to more than 5 L/min (STPD) during maximal exercise in trained individuals. The adequacy of $\dot{V}_A$ in response to the increase in $\dot{V}CO_2$ is indicated by how well $PaCO_2$ is maintained near normal levels. Alveolar ventilation keeps $PaCO_2$ in equilibrium with alveolar gas at low and moderate workloads. At high workloads, $\dot{V}_A$ increases dramatically to reduce $PaCO_2$ when buffering of **lactic acid** takes place. At maximal workloads, even high levels of ventilation cannot keep pace with CO_2 produced metabolically and from lactate buffering. As a result, acidosis develops.

Respiratory Exchange Ratio

The respiratory exchange ratio (RER) is defined as the ratio of $\dot{V}CO_2$ to $\dot{V}O_2$ at the mouth. RER is calculated by dividing $\dot{V}CO_2$ by $\dot{V}O_2$; it is expressed as a fraction. In some circumstances, RER at rest is assumed to be equal to 0.8. For exercise evaluation or metabolic studies, however, the actual value is calculated. RER normally varies between 0.70 and 1.00 in resting patients, depending on the nutritional substrate being metabolized (see Chapter 9). RER reflects the respiratory quotient (RQ) at the cellular level only when the patient is in a true steady state. RER may differ significantly from RQ, depending on the patient's ventilation.

RER typically increases from a resting level of between 0.75 and 0.85 as work increases. When anaerobic metabolism (see next paragraph) begins to produce CO_2 from the buffering of lactate, $\dot{V}CO_2$ approaches $\dot{V}O_2$. As exercise continues, $\dot{V}CO_2$ exceeds $\dot{V}O_2$ and the RER becomes greater than 1. RER is commonly elevated at rest because many patients hyperventilate during exhaled gas analysis before exercise begins (see Exercise 7-7). In steady-state exercise tests (i.e., 4–6 minutes at a constant workload), RER may equal RQ, and it then reflects the ratio of $\dot{V}CO_2/\dot{V}O_2$ at the cellular level. Under steady-state conditions, $\dot{V}CO_2$ reflects the CO_2 produced metabolically at the cellular level.

PF TIP

The respiratory exchange ratio (RER) is a good indicator of maximal effort during a cardiopulmonary exercise test. Patients who exert maximal effort are usually able to exceed their anaerobic threshold (AT). During exercise, the RER increases; at the highest workloads, it exceeds 1.00. An RER value greater than 1.15 is usually consistent with a maximal effort. Patients with pulmonary disease are often limited by ventilation and may not reach an RER greater than 1.

Anaerobic or Ventilatory Threshold

Measurement of and analysis of exhaled gases during exercise allows a noninvasive estimate of the **anaerobic threshold (AT).** This threshold is also termed the **ventilatory threshold** when it is denoted by a change in ventilation and CO_2 production. The AT occurs when the energy demands of the exercising muscles exceed the body's ability to produce energy by aerobic metabolism. The workload at which AT occurs is considered an index of fitness in healthy patients. The AT is also used to assess cardiac performance in patients with heart disease.

Historically, anaerobic metabolism was detected by noting an increase in the blood lactate level of an exercising patient. Analysis of $\dot{V}_E$ and $\dot{V}CO_2$ in relation to workload ($\dot{V}O_2$) can be used to detect the onset of anaerobic metabolism without drawing blood. This threshold is commonly referred to as the ventilatory threshold.

At low and moderate workloads, $\dot{V}_E$ increases linearly with increases in $\dot{V}CO_2$. When the body's energy demands exceed the capacity of aerobic pathways, further increases in energy are produced anaerobically. The primary product of anaerobic metabo-

lism is lactate. The increased lactic acid (from lactate) is buffered by HCO_3^-, resulting in an increase in CO_2 in the blood. $\dot{V}CO_2$ measured from exhaled gas increases because CO_2 is being produced by both the exercising muscles and the buffering of lactate. To maintain the pH near normal, $\dot{V}_E$ increases to match the increased $\dot{V}CO_2$. This pattern of increasing ventilation and CO_2 production can be detected when these parameters are plotted against $\dot{V}O_2$ (see Figure 7-8). Determination of the ventilatory-anaerobic threshold may be accomplished by visual inspection of an appropriate plot. Statistical analysis can also be used to determine the inflection point as displayed by the graph in Figure 7-13. Several different algorithms may be used to identify the AT. One of the most common techniques uses regression analysis to determine the "breakpoint" at which $\dot{V}O_2$ and $\dot{V}CO_2$ change abruptly (**V-slope method**).

Noninvasive AT determination may be useful in assessing cardiovascular or pulmonary diseases (Exercise 7-8). In healthy patients, AT occurs at 60%–70% of the $\dot{V}O_2$max. Patients who have cardiac disease often reach their AT at a lower workload ($\dot{V}O_2$). Early onset of anaerobic metabolism occurs when the demands of exercising muscles exceed the capacity of the heart to supply O_2. Occurrence of the anaerobic threshold at less than 40% of the $\dot{V}O_2$max is considered abnormally low. Patients who have a ventilatory limitation to exercise (i.e., pulmonary disease) may be unable to exercise at a high enough workload to reach their anaerobic threshold. In these patients, O_2 delivery is limited by the lungs, rather than by cardiac output or extraction by the exercising muscle.

Aerobic training improves cardiac performance, specifically the stroke volume (SV). Training allows more O_2 to be delivered to the tissues, resulting in a delay in the AT until higher workloads are reached. Measurement of the AT is often used to select a training level (e.g., exercise prescription). Maximum training effects seem to occur when the patient exercises at a workload slightly below the AT. In sedentary patients, deconditioning may occur. Deconditioning is characterized by reduced SV and poor O_2 extraction by the muscles from lack of use. Deconditioning may be present when the AT occurs

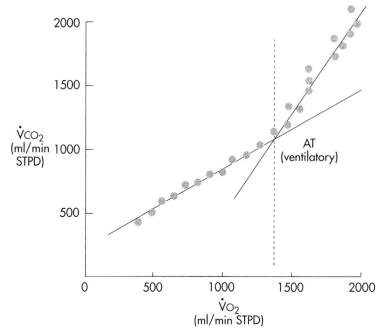

FIGURE 7-13   **V-Slope Determination of Ventilatory AT.** By plotting $\dot{V}CO_2$ against $\dot{V}O_2$, an infection point can typically be identified, indicating an abrupt increase in CO_2 production. A more precise method fits two regression lines to the data gathered. One line is a best-fit line through the low and moderate workload portion of the data; the second is fit through the high workload points. These lines are recalculated repeatedly until the best statistical "fit" is obtained. The point at which the two lines intersect represents the onset of lactate production (anaerobic threshold).

at a lower than expected workload and there is no evidence of cardiovascular disease.

The AT may also be determined by inspecting graphs of the ventilatory equivalents for O_2 and CO_2 (see the next section) plotted against workload ($\dot{V}O_2$). When $\dot{V}_E/\dot{V}CO_2$ increases without an increase in $\dot{V}_E/\dot{V}CO_2$, the AT has been reached. A similar pattern can be seen when the end-tidal O_2 and CO_2 gas tensions are plotted (see Figure 7-9). Sample calculations of $\dot{V}_E$, $\dot{V}O_2$, $\dot{V}CO_2$, and RER, as used with one of the gas collection methods, are included in Appendix F.

Ventilatory Equivalent for Oxygen

Minute ventilation during exercise may be related to the work being performed (expressed as $\dot{V}O_2$). This ratio is termed the **ventilatory equivalent for oxygen,** or $\dot{V}_E/\dot{V}O_2$. It is calculated by dividing $\dot{V}_E$ (BTPS) by $\dot{V}O_2$ (STPD) and expressing the ratio in liters of ventilation/liters of O_2 consumed per minute. The $\dot{V}_E/\dot{V}O_2$ is a measure of the efficiency of the ventilatory pump at various workloads.

During resting data collection in healthy patients, the ratio is in the range of 30 to 40 L/L depending on the degree of ventilation, including anticipatory hyperventilation. As the patient begins to exercise, this ratio decreases to about 25 ± 4 (see Figure 7-14). This initial kinetic change is assumed to be related to an improvement in $\dot{V}/\dot{Q}$ matching with increased cardiac output during exercise. At low and moderate workloads, ventilation increases linearly with increasing $\dot{V}O_2$ and $\dot{V}CO_2$. The absolute level of ventilation depends on the response to CO_2, the adequacy of $\dot{V}_A$, and the V_D/V_T ratio. At workloads above 60%–75% of the $\dot{V}O_2$max, $\dot{V}_E$ is more closely related to $\dot{V}CO_2$. As ventilation increases to match the $\dot{V}CO_2$ above the AT, the ventilatory equivalent for O_2 also increases.

Ventilation helps determine how much O_2 can be transported per minute. Therefore it is often useful to evaluate the level of total ventilation required for a particular workload to assess the role of the lungs in exercise limitations. In some pulmonary disease patterns, the $\dot{V}_E/\dot{V}O_2$ may be close to normal at rest but increases with exercise out of proportion to increases in either $\dot{V}O_2$ or $\dot{V}CO_2$. This

EXERCISE 7-8

INTERPRETIVE STRATEGIES

Oxygen Consumption and Carbon Dioxide Uptake per Minute

1. Were the data obtained acceptably? Were all calibrations appropriate? Gas analyzers? Volume transducer? Phase delay?
2. Were appropriate reference values selected? Age? Sex? Height? Weight?
3. Was $\dot{V}O_2$max (ml/kg) achieved? If so, there is no aerobic impairment.
4. Was $\dot{V}O_2$max (ml/kg) less than 80% of predicted? If so, some aerobic impairment is present. Was $\dot{V}O_2$max (ml/kg) less than 60% of predicted? If so, there is moderate to severe exercise limitation.
5. Was ventilatory AT reached? If so, at what % $\dot{V}O_2$max? If less than 50%–60%, early onset of anaerobic metabolism is likely. Consider clinical correlation.
6. What factors contributed to the reduced $\dot{V}O_2$max?
   Cardiac (arrhythmias, ischemic changes)?
   Vascular (BP response)?
   Pulmonary (ventilation, hypoxemia, V_D/V_T)?
   Other (poor effort, deconditioning, pain, orthopedic problems)?
7. What reason did the patient cite for stopping exercise (incremental tests)? Is it consistent with physiologic patterns observed?

usually occurs in individuals who have $\dot{V}/\dot{Q}$ abnormalities that worsen as cardiac output increases during exercise. Some patients who have pulmonary disease may have an elevated $\dot{V}_E/\dot{V}O_2$ at rest (i.e., greater than 40 L/L $\dot{V}O_2$) that decreases during exercise but does not return to the normal range. Many patients hyperventilate during the resting phase at the beginning of an exercise evaluation. The result is an increased $\dot{V}_E/\dot{V}O_2$ that usually returns to the normal range during exercise. This pretest hyperventilation is usually denoted by an RER of greater than 1 that returns to a normal level when the patient begins to exercise.

Ventilatory Equivalent for Carbon Dioxide

The **ventilatory equivalent for CO_2 ($\dot{V}_E/\dot{V}CO_2$)** is calculated in a manner similar to that used for the $\dot{V}_E/\dot{V}O_2$. Minute ventilation (BTPS) is divided by CO_2 production (STPD). The $\dot{V}_E/\dot{V}CO_2$ mimics the initial $\dot{V}_E/\dot{V}O_2$ kinetic change, decreasing to a normal range of 25–35 L/L $\dot{V}CO_2$. $\dot{V}_E$ tends to match $\dot{V}CO_2$ from low up to high workloads. Thus the $\dot{V}_E/\dot{V}CO_2$ remains constant in healthy patients until the highest workloads are reached. The $\dot{V}_E/\dot{V}CO_2$ may be useful for estimating the maximum tolerable workload in patients who have moderate or severe ventilatory limitations. The ventilatory equivalents for O_2 and CO_2, measured with a breath-by-breath technique, may be useful in identifying the onset of the AT. Anaerobic metabolism is usually accompanied by a steady increase in the $\dot{V}_E/\dot{V}O_2$ while the $\dot{V}_E/\dot{V}CO_2$ remains constant, or decreases slightly. The period in which $\dot{V}_E/\dot{V}O_2$ is increasing yet $\dot{V}_E/\dot{V}CO_2$ is constant is called the isocapnic buffering zone (Figure 7-14). This zone indicates the onset of metabolic acidosis, where $\dot{V}_E$ is no longer proportional to $\dot{V}O_2$ but is appropriate for $\dot{V}CO_2$. Occurrence of this pattern coincides with the buffering of the lactate ($H^+ + HCO_3^- \leftrightarrow H_2CO_3 \leftrightarrow CO_2 + H_2O$). Eventually, the buffering system cannot keep pace with the metabolic acidemia, and the $\dot{V}_E/\dot{V}CO_2$ increases as attempts to maintain pH. This same pattern may also be seen on a breath-by-breath display of $P_{ET}O_2$ and $P_{ET}CO_2$ (see Figure 7-9). A markedly elevated $\dot{V}_E/\dot{V}CO_2$ (>50) may also be observed in pulmonary hypertensive disease.

Oxygen Pulse

The efficiency of the circulatory pump may be related to the workload (i.e., $\dot{V}O_2$) during exercise by the O_2 pulse. **O_2 pulse** is defined as the volume of O_2 consumed per heartbeat and is derived from the Fick Equation:

$$\text{Cardiac output} = \frac{\dot{V}O_2}{CaO_2 - C_{\bar{v}}O_2}$$

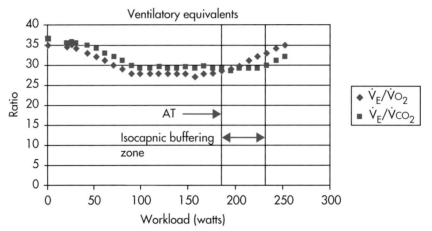

FIGURE 7-14   Determination of Ventilatory AT Using Ventilatory Equivalents Data. The ventilatory threshold is defined as the point where the $\dot{V}_E/\dot{V}_{O_2}$ begins to increase while the $\dot{V}_E/\dot{V}_{CO_2}$ remains constant or begins to decrease. The period from the onset of AT until $\dot{V}_E/\dot{V}_{CO_2}$ increases is the isocapnic buffering zone. Minute ventilation is appropriate for $\dot{V}_{CO_2}$, which now exceeds $\dot{V}_{O_2}$ because of acid buffering created by anaerobic metabolism ($H^+ + HCO_3^- \leftrightarrow H_2CO_3 \leftrightarrow H_2O + CO_2$).

$$HR \times SV = \frac{\dot{V}_{O_2}}{CaO_2 - C_{\bar{v}}O_2}$$

$$\frac{\dot{V}_{O_2}}{HR}(O_2\ pulse) = SV \times (CaO_2 - C_{\bar{v}}O_2)$$

O_2 pulse is sometimes called the "poor man's" estimate of stroke volume because of the relatively "consistent" change in the CaO_2–$C_{\bar{v}}O_2$ difference with exercise. The ratio is expressed as milliliters of O_2 per heartbeat. In healthy patients, O_2 pulse varies between 2.5 and 4.0 ml O_2/beats at rest. It increases to 10–15 ml O_2/beats during strenuous exercise.

In patients with cardiac disease, the O_2 pulse may be normal or even low at rest but does not increase to expected levels during exercise. This pattern is consistent with an inappropriately high HR for a particular level of work. Cardiac output normally increases linearly with increasing exercise (see Figure 7-4). A low O_2 pulse is consistent with an inability to increase the SV because of the relationship noted in the preceding paragraphs. O_2 pulse may even decrease in patients with poor left ventricular function. The pattern of low O_2 pulse with increasing work rate may be seen in patients with coronary artery disease or valvular insufficiency, but it is most pronounced in cardiomyopathy. Tachycardia or tachyarrhythmias tend to lower the O_2 pulse because of the abnormally elevated heart rate. Conversely, beta-blocking agents, which tend to reduce HR, may elevate the O_2 pulse.

O_2 pulse is often used as an index of fitness. At similar power outputs, a fit patient will have a higher O_2 pulse than one who is deconditioned. Fitness is generally accompanied by a lower HR, both at rest and at maximal workloads. Lower HR occurs because conditioning exercises (e.g., aerobic training) tend to increase SV. As a result, the heart beats less frequently but produces the same CO. Trained patients can thus achieve higher work rates before reaching their limiting cardiac frequency (i.e., attain a higher O_2 pulse).

EXERCISE BLOOD GASES

Arterial Catheterization

Although invasive, blood gas sampling during exercise testing is often indicated in patients with primary pulmonary disorders. An indwelling arte-

BOX 7-2	Indications for Arterial Catheterization with Exercise Testing

- Moderate or severe pulmonary disease
- Clinical suspicion of a gas exchange abnormality
- Low diffusion capacity for carbon monoxide (less than 50% predicted)
- Low or borderline PaO_2 at rest (55–60 mm Hg)
- Multiple blood specimens required (blood gases, lactate)
- Titration of supplemental O_2

EXERCISE 7-9

CRITERIA FOR ACCEPTABILITY

Exercise Blood Gases

1. Blood gases should be drawn from either a radial or a brachial catheter. Care should be taken that specimens are not contaminated with flush solution.
2. Exercise blood gas specimens should be handled like any other sample for blood gas analysis, according to the Clinical and Laboratory Standards Institute (CLSI) publication C46-A, *Blood Gas and pH Analysis and Related Measurements.*
3. Specimens from multiple exercise levels should be labeled to indicate the exercise workload and related conditions.
4. Blood obtained by a single arterial puncture at peak exercise should be obtained within 15 seconds of the observed maximal workload.
5. If pulse oximetry is used to evaluate exercise desaturation, it should be validated by correlation with co-oximetry, preferably at rest and peak exercise.
6. If pulse oximetry is used to titrate supplemental O_2 administration and SpO_2 does not increase, an arterial blood specimen may be required.

---

rial catheter permits analysis of blood gas tensions (PaO_2, $PaCO_2$), arterial saturation (SaO_2), O_2 content (CaO_2), pH, and lactate levels at various workloads. Box 7-2 lists some of the indications for arterial catheterization for exercise testing.

Arterial catheterization, at either the radial or the brachial site, has been demonstrated to be relatively safe. The modified Allen's test is performed to ascertain adequate collateral circulation (see Chapter 6). The site is cleaned with a skin preparation antiseptic, typically applied with a sterile applicator. Local anesthetic (1%–2% lidocaine [Xylocaine]) is injected subcutaneously. An appropriately sized catheter is inserted percutaneously. The catheter needs to be secured to prevent being dislodged during the exercise study. The catheter is then connected to a high-pressure flush system to maintain patency. Care must be taken when drawing blood samples from the catheter not to contaminate the specimen with flush solution (Exercise 7-9). If flush solution mixes with the specimen, dilution occurs and can affect pH, PCO_2, PO_2, and hemoglobin (Hb) values.

The catheter may also be connected to a suitable pressure transducer (see Figure 7-5) for continuous monitoring of systemic BP. The BP transducer should be balanced ("zeroed") at the level of the left ventricle during exercise. See Chapter 11 for precautions concerning insertion of arterial catheters.

Arterial Puncture

An alternate technique is to obtain a specimen by a simple arterial puncture at peak exercise. Use of a

cycle ergometer for testing allows better stabilization of the radial or brachial artery sites. The site should be identified and the modified Allen's test performed before beginning exercise. The sample should be obtained within 15 seconds of peak exercise. Blood gas tensions, particularly PaO_2, may change rapidly as blood recirculates. A serious disadvantage of the single puncture is that if the specimen cannot be obtained within 15 seconds, the procedure must be repeated. If any of the conditions listed in Box 7-2 are present, arterial catheterization should be considered.

Pulse Oximetry

Oxygen saturation during exercise may be monitored with a pulse oximeter (SpO_2) using the ear, finger, or forehead sites (see Chapter 10). Wherever the pulse oximeter is attached, the probe should be adequately secured. Motion artifact is a common problem, particularly with treadmill exercise.

An advantage of pulse oximetry is that it provides continuous measurements of saturation, compared with discrete measurements of arterial sampling. Continuous measurements can be helpful in evaluating patients who have pulmonary disease. These patients often display rapid changes in PaO_2 and SaO_2 during exercise. A decrease of 4%–5% in SaO_2 is indicative of exercise desaturation, even if some other factor (e.g., ventilation, arrhythmia) limits exercise.

Pulse oximetry may overestimate the true saturation if a significant concentration of carboxyhemoglobin (COHb) is present (see Exercise 7-9). A low total Hb level (i.e., anemia) sometimes contributes to exercise limitation. This condition may not be detected by pulse oximetry alone. Inadequate perfusion at the site of the probe (e.g., ear or finger) may also cause erroneous readings (false positive) during exercise testing. Motion artifact, light scattering within the tissue at the probe site, and dark skin pigmentation may all cause discrepancies between SpO_2 and actual SaO_2 (see Chapter 6). A single arterial sample, preferably at peak exercise, may be used to correlate the SpO_2 reading with true saturation if the specimen is analyzed with a multiwavelength blood oximeter (see Chapter 10). If adequate correlation between SaO_2 and SpO_2 during exercise is established, further blood sampling may be unnecessary.

Arterial Oxygen Tension During Exercise

In healthy patients, PaO_2 remains relatively constant even at high workloads (Exercise 7-10). Alveolar PO_2 increases at maximal exercise from the increased ventilation accompanying the increase in $\dot{V}CO_2$. The alveolar-arterial (A-a) gradient (normally approximately 10 mm Hg) widens as a result of the increase in alveolar oxygen tension. The A-a gradient also increases somewhat because of a lower mixed venous O_2 content during exercise. The A-a gradient may increase to 20–30 mm Hg in healthy patients during heavy exercise because of these mechanisms.

A decrease in PaO_2 with increasing exercise can result from increased right-to-left shunting. Similarly, inequality of $\dot{V}_A$ in relation to pulmonary capillary perfusion may result in reduced PaO_2. Diffusion limitation at the alveolocapillary interface can also affect PaO_2. Because exercise reduces the mixed venous oxygen tension ($P\bar{v}O_2$), a shunt or ventilation/perfusion inequality may result in a decrease in the PaO_2 or widening of the A-a gradient. This change in PaO_2 may occur without an absolute change in the magnitude of the shunt. Mixed venous blood with a lowered O_2 content (from extraction by the exercising muscles) passes through abnormal lung units and then mixes with normally arterialized blood.

In some patients who have decreased PaO_2 and increased $P(A-a)O_2$ at rest, oxygenation may improve with exercise. Increased cardiac output or redistribution of ventilation during exercise may actually cause an increase in PaO_2. Some improvement of PaO_2 may occur as a result of an increased PaO_2 caused by a reduction of $PaCO_2$ at moderate to high work rates.

Improved $\dot{V}/\dot{Q}$ relationships resulting directly from the changes in ventilation or cardiac output may also improve PaO_2. Because PaO_2 may either increase or decrease during exercise, measuring PaO_2 during exercise may be particularly valuable in patients with pulmonary disorders.

When PaO_2 decreases to less than 55 mm Hg or SaO_2 decreases to less than 85%, the exercise evaluation should be terminated. Patients with hypoxemia at rest or who desaturate at low work rates should be tested with supplemental O_2 (e.g., a nasal cannula) to determine an appropriate exercise **O_2 prescription**. Different flows of supplemental O_2 may be required at rest and for various levels of exertion. Correlation of PaO_2 while breathing supplemental O_2 at different exercise workloads allows precise titration of therapy to the patient's needs. Measurement of $\dot{V}O_2$ while the patient breathes supplemental O_2 presents special problems. A closed system in which the patient breathes from a reservoir containing blended gas, typically F_IO_2 0.30, is usually required.

Reported in some elite athletes at high levels of work (e.g., 400-500 watts or 9 mph/18% grade) is a widening of the A-a gradient with PaO_2 values falling into the range of 50-60 mm Hg. This phenomenon is thought to be related to the time constants of blood in the lung with very high cardiac outputs and high oxygen extraction at the cellular level.

Arterial Carbon Dioxide Tension During Exercise

In healthy patients, $PaCO_2$ remains relatively constant at low and moderate work rates (see Exercise 7-10). $\dot{V}_A$ increases to match the increase in $\dot{V}CO_2$. End-tidal CO_2 increases at submaximal workloads, indicating that less ventilation is "wasted" (V_D/V_T decreases). At workloads in excess of 50%-60% of the $\dot{V}O_2max$, metabolic acidosis from anaerobic metabolism stimulates an increase in $\dot{V}_E$. This occurs in response to the augmented $\dot{V}CO_2$ from the buffering of lactic acid as noted previously. Ventilation thus increases in excess of that required to keep $PaCO_2$ constant. A progressive decrease in $PaCO_2$ results, causing respiratory compensation for the acidosis associated with anaerobic metabolism (see Figures 7-8 and 7-9). $PETCO_2$ decreases along with $PaCO_2$ at high work rates.

Some individuals who have airway obstruction can increase $\dot{V}_A$ to maintain a normal $PaCO_2$ at low workloads. At higher workloads, however, they may be unable to reduce $PaCO_2$ to compensate for the metabolic acidosis. In many patients with airway obstruction, maximal exercise is limited by lack of ventilatory reserve. These individuals typically do not reach the AT. Ventilatory limitation prevents them from attaining a workload high enough to induce anaerobic metabolism. In patients with severe airflow obstruction, $\dot{V}_A$ may be unable to match any increment in $\dot{V}CO_2$, resulting in hypercapnia and respiratory acidosis. Increased work of breathing and reduced sensitivity to CO_2, combined with the increased $\dot{V}CO_2$ of exercise, allow $PaCO_2$ to increase.

Acid-Base Status During Exercise

The pH, like $PaCO_2$, is regulated by the $\dot{V}_A$ at low work rates. $\dot{V}_A$ increases in proportion to $\dot{V}CO_2$ up to the ventilatory AT. At work rates above AT, proportional increases in ventilation maintain the pH at near-normal levels. Most of the buffering of lactic acid is provided by HCO_3^- and a decrease in $PaCO_2$. At the highest work rates (above 80% of the $\dot{V}O_2max$), pH decreases despite hyperventilation because compensation for lactic acidosis becomes incomplete. In the presence of airway obstruction, ventilatory limitations may prevent compensation above the anaerobic threshold, with the development of significant respiratory acidosis. However, patients who have moderate or severe obstruction generally cannot exercise up to a level that elicits anaerobic metabolism. Increased $PaCO_2$ (respiratory acidosis) may be the primary cause of acidosis in these patients.

Exercise Variables Calculated from Blood Gases

Arterial blood gases drawn during exercise allow several other parameters of gas exchange to be determined (see Exercise 7-10). These include physiologic dead space, alveolar ventilation, and the V_D/V_T ratio.

Calculation of V_D, $\dot{V}_A$, and V_D/V_T requires measurement of $PaCO_2$. V_D may be calculated with the following equation:

$$V_D = \left(V_T \times \left[1 - \frac{F_ECO_2 \times (P_B - 47)}{PaCO_2} \right] \right) - V_{Dsys}$$

where:
V_T = tidal volume, liters (BTPS)
F_ECO_2 = fraction of expired CO_2
$P_B - 47$ = dry barometric pressure
$PaCO_2$ = arterial CO_2 tension
V_{Dsys} = dead space of one-way breathing valve, liters

When V_D has been determined, $\dot{V}_A$ can be calculated with the following equation:

$$\dot{V}_A = \dot{V}_E - (f_b \times V_D)$$

where:
$\dot{V}_E$ = minute ventilation (BTPS)
f_b = respiratory rate (breaths/minute)
V_D = respiratory dead space (BTPS)

V_D/V_T ratio may be calculated as the quotient of the V_D (as just determined) and the V_T, averaged from the $\dot{V}_E$ divided by f_b. Alternatively, V_D/V_T may be derived simply from the difference between arterial and mixed expired CO_2 at each exercise level:

$$V_D/V_T = \frac{(PaCO_2 - P_ECO_2)}{PaCO_2}$$

where:
P_ECO_2 = partial pressure of CO_2 in expired gas
Most breath-by-breath systems calculate V_D/V_T noninvasively by substituting end-tidal CO_2 for $PaCO_2$. This method assumes that $P_{ET}CO_2$ and $PaCO_2$ are equal. This may not be the case at higher workloads and in patients who have pulmonary disease.

V_D, which is composed of anatomic and alveolar dead space, is the part of $\dot{V}_E$ that does not participate in gas exchange. V_D/V_T expresses the relationship between "wasted" and tidal ventilation for the average breath. The healthy adult at rest has a $\dot{V}_A$ of 4–7 L/min (BTPS) and a V_D/V_T ratio of approximately 0.20–0.35. The absolute volume of dead space increases during exercise in conjunction with increased $\dot{V}_E$. Because of increases in V_T and increased perfusion of well-ventilated lung units (e.g., at the apices), the V_D/V_T ratio decreases. This pattern is expected in healthy patients (see Figure 7-8). V_D/V_T increases with age, but the kinetic change with exercise remains the same. V_D/V_T may decrease in mild or moderate pulmonary disease states as well. In severe airway obstruction or in pulmonary vascular disease, V_D/V_T remains fixed or may even increase. An increase in V_D/V_T with exertion indicates ventilation increasing in excess of perfusion. This pattern is often associated with pulmonary hypertension. The vascular "space" is fixed in pulmonary hypertension; additional lung units cannot be recruited to handle the increased CO during exercise. V_D/V_T may also be elevated in individuals who use inappropriate breathing strategies. Small tidal volumes and high respiratory rates to recruit $\dot{V}_E$ in an otherwise healthy patient can yield falsely high ratios. Coaching a patient to increase tidal volume and use a more normal breathing pattern can alleviate a falsely elevated V_D/V_T ratio.

During exercise in healthy patients $\dot{V}_A$ increases more than $\dot{V}_E$ as V_D/V_T decreases. In patients whose V_D/V_T ratio remains fixed or increases, adequacy of $\dot{V}_A$ must be assessed in terms of $PaCO_2$ and not simply by the magnitude of $\dot{V}_E$.

CARDIAC OUTPUT DURING EXERCISE

There are several methods for calculating cardiac output (CO) during exercise. Noninvasive methods include CO_2 rebreathing, soluble gas, and Doppler (ultrasound) techniques. Invasive methods measure CO by the direct Fick method or by thermal dilution. The invasive methods require placement of a pulmonary artery catheter (Swan-Ganz) (Exercise 7-11).

Noninvasive Cardiac Output Techniques

The CO_2 rebreathing technique (also termed the indirect Fick method) uses the Fick equation for CO_2:

$$\dot{Q}_T = \frac{\dot{V}CO_2}{C\bar{v}CO_2 - CaCO_2}$$

where:

$\dot{Q}_T$ = cardiac output (CO), L/min$\dot{V}CO_2$ = CO_2 production calculated from exhaled gases

$CaCO_2$ = arterial CO_2 content, calculated from $PaCO_2$

$C\bar{v}CO_2$ = mixed venous CO_2 content, calculated from alveolar PCO_2 after rebreathing to allow equilibrium of alveolar gas with mixed venous blood

The acetylene technique, also known as the soluble gas technique, can be performed with either closed-circuit or open-circuit methods. This method depends on the rate of uptake of a soluble gas (e.g., acetylene) that has a low diffusion coefficient. The rate of uptake is directly proportional to the pulmonary blood flow. As long as there is no intracardiac or pulmonary shunt, pulmonary blood flow equals cardiac output. Both of these breathing techniques correlate well with invasive techniques in healthy patients but have limited use in patients with maldistribution of ventilation.

Instrumentation with Doppler technology to estimate CO works on the principle of measuring flow with an ultrasound signal directed at the arch of the aorta. A measurement of the diameter of the aorta is also made with echocardiography. These two measurements allow for the determination of cardiac output (i.e., flow × cross-sectional area = total output). This method works well at rest and at low levels of exercise with a cycle ergometer, but

EXERCISE 7-11

CRITERIA FOR ACCEPTABILITY

Cardiac Output During Exercise

1. If a noninvasive technique (e.g., soluble gas, CO_2 rebreathing) was used, were the laboratory's quality standards for the test satisfied?
2. For the Fick cardiac output method, the pulmonary artery catheter must be properly placed. The distal port should be located in a pulmonary arteriole and must not be in the "wedge" position. For thermodilution, the catheter must also be properly placed; the proximal (injection) port must be in the right atrium with the thermistor in a pulmonary arteriole.
3. For Fick measurements, arterial and mixed venous blood should be drawn simultaneously over 15 - 30 seconds (or longer). Care should be taken to avoid dilution with flush solution; dilution can markedly alter content calculations and hence cardiac output.
4. Oxygen consumption should be measured over the same interval as blood sampling for the Fick method.
5. Thermodilution measurements should be performed according to the manufacturer's recommendations, particularly in regard to the temperature of injectate and rate of injection.
6. Two or more acceptable measurements should be averaged if possible; multiple measurements may not be practical during exercise.

motion artifact and increasing tidal volumes limit its usefulness at higher workloads.

Direct Fick Method

The direct Fick method is based on measurement of O_2 consumption and arterial-venous content difference for O_2:

$$\dot{Q}_T = \frac{\dot{V}O_2}{C(a-\bar{v})O_2} \times 100$$

where:
$\dot{Q}_T$ = cardiac output (CO), liters/minute
$\dot{V}O_2$ = oxygen consumption, liters/minute (STPD)
$C(a-\bar{v})O_2$ = arterial-mixed venous O_2 content difference, milliliters/deciliter
100 = factor to correct $C(a-\bar{v})O_2$ to liters (content differences are normally reported in vol% or milliliters/deciliter)

$\dot{V}O_2$ is measured using one of the methods described previously. $C(a-\bar{v})O_2$ is obtained by measuring or calculating oxygen content in both arterial and mixed venous blood (see Chapter 6). Arterial and mixed venous blood specimens should be drawn simultaneously during the last 15–30 seconds of each exercise level. Oxygen consumption averaged over the same interval should be used for the calculation.

Thermodilution Method

Most pulmonary artery (Swan-Ganz) catheters include circuitry for measurement of CO by thermodilution. A sensitive thermistor is placed near the tip of the catheter. A chilled saline solution (usually 10°–20°C) is injected through a catheter port that is located in the right atrium. The thermistor senses the change in temperature as the solution is pumped through the right ventricle and into the pulmonary artery. The computer then integrates the change in temperature and the time required for the change to occur, and CO is calculated.

The thermodilution method is commonly used in critical care settings. It can also be used during exercise testing. Multiple measurements (two to four) should be made at each exercise level and the results averaged. Some automated systems allow other cardiopulmonary variables (e.g., ejection fraction) to be calculated as well.

Cardiac Output During Exercise

Cardiac output in healthy adults is approximately 4–6 L/min at rest. During exercise, it may increase to 25–35 L/min (Exercise 7-12). CO is the product of HR and SV:

$$\dot{Q}_T = HR \times SV$$

where:
$\dot{Q}_T$ = cardiac output (CO), liters or milliliters
HR = heart rate, beats/minute
SV = stroke volume, liters or milliliters

EXERCISE 7-12

INTERPRETIVE STRATEGIES

Cardiac Output During Exercise

1. Were cardiac output measurements acceptable by laboratory standards? If a pulmonary artery catheter was used, were the measurements reproducible within 10% (as applicable)? If not, interpret cautiously.
2. Did cardiac output increase appropriately with increasing workloads? If not, consider cardiomyopathy, myocardial hypokinesis, valvular insufficiency, and other outflow tract abnormalities.
3. Was stroke volume normal at rest? Did it increase at low and medium workloads?
4. Was there evidence of ischemic changes or arrhythmias (on ECG) that might explain reduced cardiac output?
5. Was cardiac output compromised by increased systemic or pulmonary vascular resistance?
6. If cardiac output was not available, did the O_2 pulse (surrogate for SV) increase appropriately with exercise?

In healthy upright adults, SV is approximately 70–100 ml at rest. SV may be slightly higher if the patient is supine or semirecumbent because of increased venous return from the lower extremities. SV increases to 100–140 ml with low or moderate exercise. HR increases almost linearly with increasing work rate as described earlier, so at low workloads an increase in CO is caused by a combination of HR and SV. At moderate and high workloads, further increases in CO result mainly from increased HR. Derivation of SV (dividing $\dot{Q}_T$ by HR) is useful for quantifying poor cardiac performance in patients with coronary artery disease, cardiomyopathy, or other diseases that affect myocardial contractility.

Patients who are able to reach their predicted $\dot{V}O_2$max and their predicted HRmax typically have normal CO and SV. A patient who has a reduced $\dot{V}O_2$max but achieves maximal predicted HR often has low CO because of low SV. Limited CO with increasing workload is often accompanied by early onset of anaerobic metabolism (anaerobic or ventilatory threshold). Reduced CO may be seen in both atrial and ventricular arrhythmias, valvular insufficiency, and cardiomyopathies.

In fit patients, SV is increased both at rest and during exercise. Endurance (aerobic) training normally results in increased SV. Other benefits of aerobic training include reductions in systolic BP and ventilation. Fit patients typically have a lower resting HR than their sedentary counterparts. Because HR (i.e., cardiac output) is the factor that limits exercise in most individuals, fit patients reach a higher $\dot{V}O_2$max. Depending on the frequency, intensity, and duration of training, fit individuals are able to maintain a higher level or work for longer periods because of improved CO.

Symptoms Scales

The measurement of RPE (or Borg scale) and other symptom scales can be essential for connecting subjective symptoms and the physiologic responses to exercise. Rating scales, when they are discordant, can assist the physician in counseling the patient. There are two versions of the RPE scale, often referred as the Borg and Modified-Borg scales (Box 7-3). These scales are usually printed on a card or poster that the patient can see or point to during exercise testing. The scales should be reviewed with the patient before exercise begins. This is particularly important if exhaled gas is being collected because the patient may have a mouthpiece or facial

BOX 7-3	Ratings of Perceived Exertion (Borg) Scales		
Perceived Exertion Scale		**Modified Perceived Exertion Scale**	
6		0	Nothing at all
7	Very, very light	0.5	Very, very slight (just noticeable)
8		1	Very slight
9	Very light	2	Slight
10		3	Moderate
11	Fairly light	4	Somewhat moderate
12		5	Severe
13	Somewhat hard	6	
14		7	Very severe
15	Hard	8	
16		9	Very, very severe (almost maximal)
17	Very hard	10	Maximal
18			
19	Very, very hard		
20			

mask in place. The patient should be able to indicate his or her level of exertion even without vocalizing. General symptom scales can be adapted to any chief complaint the patient may be expressing by simply using a scale of 0–4 and grading intensity from "nothing at all" to "severe." A patient complaining of lightheadedness or chest tightness can then alert the testing staff to his or her level of discomfort during the test using hand signals.

Quality of Test

Quality assurance and quality control of instrumentation is discussed in detail in Chapter 11. However, the complexity of cardiopulmonary exercise testing warrants consideration of a quality system approach to testing. The Clinical and Laboratory Standards Institute (CLSI) has published *A Quality System Model for Health Care*. This document champions the approach that a quality model has to address the continuum of patient care, and incorporates the concept of a path of workflow process (Figure 7-15). This concept integrates pretest, test, posttest, and information management with all processes that can affect any section across the path of workflow. Pretest processes include patient assessment, test request, patient

preparation, and equipment preparation. Patient assessment, as it relates to cardiopulmonary exercise testing, might include laboratory results, current medications affecting exercise performance (e.g., β-blockers, digitalis), or orthopedic issues that may affect ergometer selection. Each quality system essential is applied to all operations in the path of workflow, which in turn allows for complete quality analysis of all processes.

Interpretation Strategies

To interpret a study appropriately, the clinician first needs to assess the degree of effort and determine whether the test is a maximal study (Box 7-4). Once the test has been qualified as maximal or submaximal, an algorithmic approach to data review and interpretation is essential (see Exercises 7-6, 7-8, 7-10, and 7-12).

The following scheme can assist in a stepwise approach to data analysis:
- Determine maximal study
- Cardiovascular response (see Exercises 7-2 and 7-11)
  - ECG, BP, CO, O_2, pulse, and symptoms
- Ventilatory response (see Exercise 7-6)
  - Ventilatory reserve, breathing kinetics

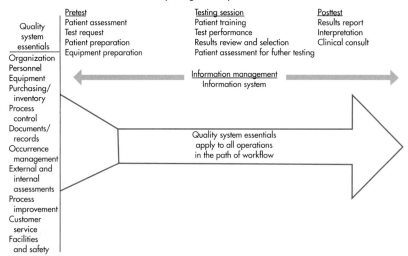

FIGURE 7-15 **Pulmonary Diagnostics Path of Workflow.** The path of workflow describes how a service is provided from the point of initiation of the request, through the delivery of those services, and any necessary follow-up.

BOX 7-4	**Determining Maximal Effort**	
***	Heart rate:	>85%–90% of predicted
***	End exercise:	50%–80% $\dot{V}_E$ of MVV or $FEV_1 \times 40$; MVV – $\dot{V}_E$max ≤15 L
**	SaO_2	<80%
*	Metabolic work:	RER >1.10 or lactate >7 mMol/L
*	Clinical investigator:	Opinion of effort or early termination criteria met

* = Weight of variable.
Once a single criterion is met, test is graded a maximal effort.

- Gas exchange (see Exercise 7-10)
  - A-a gradient, V_D/V_T, $PaCO_2$
- Metabolic and oxygen uptake (see Exercise 7-8)
  - Anaerobic/ventilatory threshold, lactate, $\dot{V}O_2$max, $\dot{V}O_2$/kg
- Impression

SUMMARY

- This chapter examines the measurement of cardiopulmonary variables during exercise.
- Various protocols for assessing exercise responses are described, including treadmill and cycle ergometry methods, as well as the 6-minute walk.
- Monitoring of the cardiovascular system with a special concern for patient safety is discussed.

- Techniques for measuring ventilation, oxygen consumption, carbon dioxide production, and the associated variables during exercise are delineated.
- The measurement of breathing kinetics and flow volume analysis during exercise are described.
- Special emphasis is given to criteria for acceptability and interpretive strategies for the various measurements described.
- Assessment of blood gases and cardiac output is also discussed.
- Case studies and self-assessment questions on the topic of cardiopulmonary exercise testing are included.

CASE 7-1	

Case Studies

HISTORY

The patient is a 54-year-old man complaining of dyspnea on exertion. Several months ago, he had an initial episode of SOB, which has worsened during the past 2 months. He has a 15–20 pack-year smoking history. He works as a foreman for a utility company and does not have any related environmental exposures. His laboratory results were all normal. His echocardiogram, chest radiograph, and CT scan of the chest were also normal. His spirometry results are as follows:

PULMONARY FUNCTION TESTS

Personal Data

Sex:	Male
Age:	54 yr
Height:	69.3 in (176 cm)
Weight:	195 lb (88.4 kg; BMI 28.6)

continued

Spirometry

| | PREDICTED | | CONTROL | |
	Normal	Range	Found	%Predicted
VC	4.73	>3.89	5.12	108
FVC	4.73	>3.89	5.03	106
FEV_1	3.74	>3.06	4.19	112
FEV_1/FVC	79.1	>69.9	83.3	
$FEF_{25\%-75\%}$	3.4	>1.9	4.0	119
FEFmax	8.7	>5.2	9.0	104
MVV	148	>115	141	95

TECHNOLOGIST'S COMMENTS

Spirometry testing was performed meeting criteria for acceptability and reproducibility.

QUESTIONS

1. What is the interpretation of the spirometry results?

Exercise Test

	Rest	AT	Max	Pred Max	%Pred Max
Exercise					
Workload (watts)		160	180		
Time (min:sec)	4:40	8:56	10:50		
$\dot{V}O_2$ (L/min)	0.167	1.938	2.108	2.424	87
$\dot{V}O_2/kg$ (ml/kg)	1.9	21.9	23.9		
R	0.80	1.07	1.13		
Cardiac function					
Heart rate (beats/min)	78	139	156	175	89
Blood pressure (direct) (mm Hg)	145/90	235/110	235/110		
Oxygen pulse (ml/beat)	2.1	13.9	13.5		
Ventilation					
Minute ventilation (L/min)	6.7	56.0	69.3	141.0	49
Respiratory rate (per min)	14	20	23		
Tidal volume (ml, BTPS)	498	2803	2975		
Tidal volume/FVC (%)	10	56	59		
Vent equiv for O_2 ($\dot{V}_E/\dot{V}O_2$)	40.5	29.2	32.8		
Blood gases					
Arterial pH	7.42		7.37		
Arterial PCO_2 (mm Hg)	38		39		
Arterial PO_2 (mm Hg)	82		98		
Arterial O_2 sat (%)	98		96		
Arterial bicarbonate (mEq/L)	24.0		22.0		
(A-a) gradient O_2 (mm Hg)	16.3		11.1		
P(ET-a) CO_2 (mm Hg)	−1.9		6.3		
V_D/V_T (%)	55		2.4		
Arterial lactate (mMol/L)	0.7		4.9		

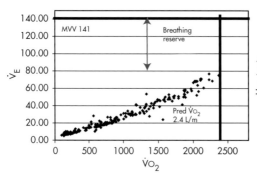

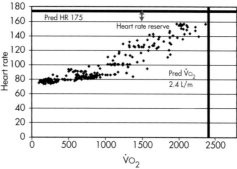

2. What is the interpretation of:
   a. Cardiovascular response?
   b. Ventilation during exercise?
   c. Gas exchange during exercise?
   d. Oxygen consumption and ventilatory threshold during exercise?
   e. Impression?
3. Discuss the patient's exercise response.
4. What treatment might be recommended based on these findings?

DISCUSSION

Interpretation (Pulmonary Function)
Normal spirometry.

Interpretation (Exercise)
The patient exercised on a cycle ergometer to a maximum workload of 180 watts using a 20-watt incremental protocol. He terminated the test complaining of SOB and leg fatigue. This appears to be a near-maximal study based on heart rate criterion.

Cardiovascular Response: Heart increased from 78–156 beats/min. Electrocardiogram showed normal sinus rhythm at rest with rare PVCs with exercise. There is no evidence of ischemic changes. Blood pressure shows exercise-induced hypertension.

Ventilatory Response: There was a normal ventilatory reserve with normal breathing kinetics. Tidal volume increased to 59% of FVC.

Gas Exchange: Arterial blood gases were normal at rest and at exercise. The V_D/V_T ratio decreased appropriately with exercise. Maximal oxygen consumption and ventilatory threshold were within normal limits.

Impression: Normal study with the exception of exercised-induced hypertension.

Discussion of Patient's Exercise Response
The testing staff selected an incremental protocol of 20 watts/min, based on what appeared to be a healthy patient with a predicted $\dot{V}O_2$max of 2.424 L (increment based on $\dot{V}O_2 = 2400 - 300/100 = 21$). The test was determined to be a near-maximal study based on a heart rate response of 89% of predicted, a large ventilatory reserve, and a lactate level of 4.9 mMol/L.

Cardiovascular Response: He had a normal heart rate response without significant ECG changes. His blood pressure showed exercise-induced hypertension, which is the only abnormality during this test. His oxygen pulse increased from 2.1 to 13.5, which is consistent with an appropriate increase in stroke volume.

Ventilatory Response: His minute ventilation increased to 69.3 liters, which was 49% of his MVV, resulting in a normal ventilatory reserve. He used appropriate breathing strategies, increasing his tidal volume to 59% of his forced vital capacity.

Gas Exchange: His resting blood gas values were within normal limits with a resting V_D/V_T at 55 being somewhat elevated. However, this is most likely secondary to a low tidal volume–high breathing frequency anticipatory response rather than a physiologic abnormality. His blood gases remained normal through exercise, and his V_D/V_T decreased appropriately with exercise. Lactate increased from 0.7–4.9 mMol/L.

Oxygen consumption and the ventilatory threshold were within normal limits.

Treatment
The primary physician was made aware of his exercise-induced hypertension. An exercise prescription was given.

CASE 7-2

Case Studies

HISTORY

A 69-year-old woman with a history of COPD seeks medical attention because of increased dyspnea on exertion. Her medical history includes a smoking history of 40 pack years. She is currently using montelukast (Singulair), salmeterol (Serevent), and budesonide (Pulmicort). Her primary care physician orders a pulmonary function test and a chest radiograph. The chest radiograph is normal.

PULMONARY FUNCTION TESTS

Personal Data

Sex:	Female
Age:	69 yr
Height:	59 in (149.9 cm)
Weight:	152 lb (68.9 kg; BMI 30.7)

Lung Volumes

	PREDICTED		CONTROL		POSTDILATOR*	
	Normal	Range	Found	%Predicted	Found	%Change
TLC (Pleth)	4.24	>3.14	4.84	114		
VC	2.41	>1.67	1.95	81	2.08	+7
RV	1.84	<2.39	2.89†	158		
RV/TLC	43.3	<56.7	59.8†	138		
FRC			3.8			

* Bronchodilator was albuterol.
† Outside normal range.

Spirometry

	PREDICTED		CONTROL		POSTDILATOR*	
	Normal	Range	Found	%Pred	Found	%Change
FVC	2.41	1.67	1.86	77	2.06	+11
FEV$_1$	1.97	>1.42	0.98†	50	1.23†	+25
FEV$_1$/FVC	81.8	>70.7	52.6†		59.5†	
FEF$_{25\%-75\%}$	2.1	>0.9	0.3†	15	0.4†	
FEFmax	4.9	>2.2	4.6	94	4.7	+3

*Bronchodilator was albuterol.
† Outside normal range.

Diffusing Capacity

	PREDICTED		CONTROL	
	Normal	Range	Found	%Pred
D$_{LCO}$sb	18.5	>12.0	11.8*	63
D$_{LCO}$ (adjusted for Hb = 14.4 g/dl)		19	11.8	62
V̇$_A$	4.09	>3.14	3.88	95

*Outside normal range.

TECHNOLOGIST'S COMMENTS

Spirometry testing was performed meeting criteria for acceptability and reproducibility.

QUESTIONS

1. What is the interpretation of:
   a. Prebronchodilator and postbronchodilator spirometry?
   b. Lung volumes and diffusing capacity?

Exercise Test

	Rest	Maximum	Pred Max	%Pred Max
Exercise				
Workload (watts)		70		
Time (min:sec)	3:20	7:01		
VO_2 (L/min)	0.266	0.863	1.368	63
VO_2/kg (ml/kg)	3.8	12.3		
R	0.80	0.95		
Cardiac function				
Heart rate (beats/min)	91	153	165	93
Blood pressure (direct) (mm Hg)	150/85	225/105		
Oxygen pulse (ml/beat)	2.9	5.6		
Ventilation				
Minute ventilation (L/min)	11.3	30.8	44.0	70
Respiratory rate (per min)	17	30		
Tidal volume (ml, BTPS)	638	1026		
Tidal volume/FVC (%)	35	56		
Vent equiv for O_2 (V_E/VO_2)	47.1	35.8		
Blood gases				
Arterial pH	7.41	7.35		
Arterial PCO_2 (mm Hg)	40	47		
Arterial PO_2 (mm Hg)	66	63		
Arterial O_2 sat (%)	91	89		
Arterial bicarbonate	25.0	25.0		
(A-a) gradient O_2 (mm Hg)	29.0	31.1		
P(ET-a) CO_2 (mm Hg)	−6.2	−3.5		
V_D/V_T (%)	60	52		
Arterial lactate (mMol/L)	0.6	3.9		

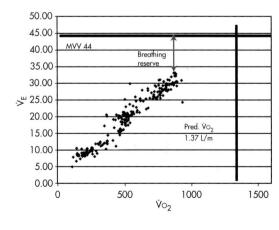

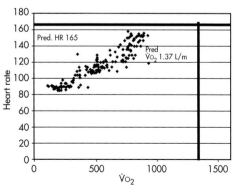

continued

2. What is the interpretation of:
   a. Cardiovascular response?
   b. Ventilation during exercise?
   c. Gas exchange during exercise?
   d. Oxygen consumption and ventilatory threshold during exercise?
   e. Impression?
3. Discuss the patient's exercise response.
4. What treatment might be recommended based on these findings?

DISCUSSION

Interpretation (Pulmonary Function)

Spirometry is consistent with moderate to severe obstruction with a significant response to bronchodilator. Her total lung capacity is within normal limits. However, there is an increase in her residual volume consistent with air trapping. Her diffusing capacity is reduced, suggesting the presence of a pulmonary parenchymal or vascular abnormality. Her primary physician ordered a cardiopulmonary exercise test to rule out an exercise gas-exchange abnormality and look for any evidence of concomitant cardiac disease.

Interpretation (Exercise)

The patient exercised on a cycle ergometer using a 10-watt incremental protocol to a maximum workload of 70 watts. She terminated the test complaining of SOB. This appears to be a maximal study based on both heart rate and ventilatory criteria.

Cardiovascular Response: The heart rate increased to a maximum of 153 beats/min, which was 93% of predicted. Blood pressure increased and showed borderline exercise-induced hypertension. The ECG displayed a normal sinus rhythm at baseline. There were no abnormalities suggestive of ischemic heart disease. Oxygen pulse increased with exercise but not to the level expected, suggesting a reduced stroke volume response to exercise.

Ventilatory Response: There is a slight reduction in the ventilatory reserve, but normal breathing kinetics with an increase in tidal volume to 56% of the vital capacity.

Gas Exchange: Arterial blood gases at rest show an increase in the A-a gradient and an elevation in V_D/V_T. Exercise blood gases show an increase in Pa_{CO_2}, consistent with ventilatory limitation and essentially no change in the A-a gradient. V_D/V_T remains high at 52%.

Oxygen consumption is moderately reduced, and it appears that the patient did not reach anaerobiosis.

Impression: (1) Moderate reduction in exercise capacity; (2) ventilatory limitation with exercise-induced hypercapnia; (3) gas exchange abnormality at rest and with exercise; and (4) exercise-induced hypertension.

Discussion of the Exercise Response

A 10-watt incremental protocol was selected based on a predicted $\dot{V}O_2$max of 1.368 L ([1300 − 300]/100 = 10). The patient terminated the test complaining of SOB. This appeared to be a maximal study based on heart rate and ventilatory criteria. Her cardiovascular response showed exercise-induced hypertension. Her oxygen pulse increased with exercise but appeared somewhat reduced. This suggests a reduced stroke volume. Another possible explanation for the reduced O_2 pulse is a defect in oxygen extraction. O_2 pulse is also directly related to arterial-venous content difference. Her ventilatory reserve was reduced with an absolute difference of 13 L (44 L expected−31 L actual). However, her $\dot{V}_E$/MVV ratio is still within normal limits. This is an excellent example of how a patient with a reduced MVV resulting from lung disease can have a normal ratio even though the overall ventilatory reserve is compromised. There should be an actual reserve of at least 10–15 L between the maximal expected and the achieved ventilation. The tidal volume increased appropriately with exercise to 56% of vital capacity, so her breathing kinetics is appropriate. She has a gas exchange abnormality at rest with an elevated V_D/V_T. Her gas exchange abnormality does not worsen with exercise. However, she does show progressive hypercapnia that is inappropriate during exercise and further supports that she is ventilation limited. Her V_D/V_T kinetics does not respond appropriately and stays essentially flat with exercise.

Treatment

The patient was enrolled in a pulmonary rehabilitation program. The following chart shows the improvement in her 6-minute walk distance after 6 weeks of enrollment.

6-Minute Walk				
	Distance (ft)	Inspired Gas	SpO₂ (End Exercise)	RPE (6–20)
Initial test	1047	Room air	91%	17
6 weeks later	1425	Room air	91%	17

CASE 7-3

Case Studies

HISTORY

The patient is a 53-year-old office worker who was referred for evaluation of SOB. She has a 44 pack-year history of smoking and continued to smoke up to the time of her test. She has a morning cough that produces thick white sputum of 50–100 ml/day. Her chest radiograph shows increased vascular markings and mild hyperinflation. She was taking no medications at the time of this test. No familial history of lung disease or cancer was found, and she had no unusual environmental exposure.

PULMONARY FUNCTION TESTS

Personal Data

Sex: Female
Age: 53 yr
Height: 65 in
Weight: 131 lb

Spirometry

	Predicted	Control	%Pred	Postdilator	%Change
FVC	3.35	3.24	97	3.34	100
FEV$_1$ (L)	2.53	1.49	59	1.56	62
FEV$_{1\%}$	75	46	—	47	—
FEF$_{25\%-75\%}$ (L/sec)	2.86	0.79	27	1.19	42
Vmax$_{50}$ (L/sec)	4.24	1.99	47	2.25	53
Vmax$_{50}$ (L/sec)	1.86	0.68	37	0.99	53
MVV (L/min)	97.9	52	53	55	56
Raw (cm H$_2$O/L/sec)	0.6 – 2.4	2.22	—	2.1	—
sGaw (L/sec/cm/H$_2$O/L)	0.14 – 0.58	0.012	—	0.13	—

Lung Volumes (by Plethysmograph)

	Predicted	Control	%Pred
VC (L)	3.35	3.27	98
IC (L)	2.31	1.80	78
ERV (L)	1.04	0.99	95
FRC (L)	2.88	3.54	123
RV (L)	1.84	2.55	136
TLC (L)	5.20	5.82	112
RV/TLC (%)	35	44	—

Diffusing Capacity (Single-Breath)

	Predicted	Control	%Pred
DLCO (ml CO/ min/mm Hg)	20	8.8	44
DLCO (adj)	18.1	8.8	49
V̇$_A$ (L)	—	5.67	—
DL/V$_A$	3.85	1.55	—

Blood Gases (FIO$_2$ 0.21)

pH	7.38
PaCO$_2$ (mm Hg)	43
PaO$_2$ (mm Hg)	59
SaO$_2$ (%)	85.1
Hb (g/dl)	11.7
COHb (%)	5.7

TECHNOLOGIST'S COMMENTS

All spirometric efforts were acceptable, both before and after bronchodilator administration. Lung volume and DLCO testing was performed acceptably. DLCO was corrected for an Hb level of 11.7 and a COHb level of 5.7.

Three days later, a treadmill test was performed with an arterial catheter in place. The test was repeated with oxygen supplementation. Gas with an FIO$_2$ of 0.28 was prepared in a meteorologic balloon for the portion of the exercise test using O$_2$ (see the Exercise Test in Case Study 7-1).

continued

QUESTIONS

1. What is the interpretation of:
   a. Prebronchodilator and postbronchodilator spirometry?
   b. Lung volumes and diffusing capacity?
   c. Room air blood gases at rest?

Exercise Test

Exercise	Air			Oxygen		
Workload						
mph	0	1.5		0	1.5	2
Grade (%)	0	0		0	0	4
Time (min)	10	3		10	3	3
Ventilation						
f (breaths/min)	16	28		13	20	31
$\dot{V}_E$ (L/BTPS)	10.20	23.40		6.23	16.59	27.81
$\dot{V}_A$ (L/BTPS)	6.02	14.74		3.74	10.45	17.80
V_T (L/BTPS)	0.638	0.836		0.479	0.830	0.897
V_D (L/BTPS)	0.262	0.309		0.190	0.307	0.323
V_D/V_T	0.41	0.37		0.40	0.37	0.36
Gas exchange						
$\dot{V}_{O_2}$ (L/STPD)	0.310	0.835		0.279	0.649	0.986
$\dot{V}_{CO_2}$ (L/STPD)	0.303	0.743		0.251	0.617	0.976
RER	0.98	0.89		0.90	0.95	0.99
$\dot{V}_E/\dot{V}_{O_2}$ (L/L)	32.90	28.00		22.33	25.50	28.20
$\dot{V}_{O_2}$/HR (ml/beat)	3.44	7.59		3.29	6.18	8.57
Pulse oximeter						
SpO_2 (%)	92	87		97	93	93
Blood gases						
pH	7.45	7.39		7.39	7.38	7.36
Pa_{CO_2} (mm/Hg)	34	39		44	45	46
Pa_{O_2} (mm/Hg)	61	47		84	71	66
Sa_{O_2} (%)	87.4	77.3		91.4	88.9	87.0
COHb (%)	5.1	4.7		4.8	4.7	4.6
$P(A-a)_{O_2}$ (mm Hg)	51	56		64	78	84
Hemodynamics						
HR (beats/min)	90	110		92	105	115
Systolic BP (mm Hg)	130	145		134	145	150
Diastolic BP (mm Hg)	85	88		90	90	90

2. What is the interpretation of:
   a. Ventilation during exercise?
   b. Gas exchange during exercise?
   c. Blood gas levels during exercise?
3. What is the cause of the patient's exercise limitation?
4. What treatment might be recommended based on these findings?

DISCUSSION

Interpretation (Pulmonary Function Tests)

All spirometry, lung volume, diffusing capacity, and blood gas measurements were acceptable.

Spirometry results show an obstructive process with a well-preserved FVC. There is only a 5% improvement in the FEV_1 after bronchodilator administration.

Lung volumes by plethysmography show increased FRC and RV consistent with air trapping. TLC is close to normal, so there is little hyperinflation. DLCOsb is decreased, even after correction for Hb and COHb. Arterial blood gases on air show hypoxemia that is complicated by an elevated COHb.

Impression: Moderately severe obstructive disease with no significant response to bronchodilators. Air trapping is present, and DLCO is severely decreased. Exercise evaluation for oxygen desaturation is recommended.

Interpretation (Cardiopulmonary Exercise Test)

The exercise test was performed in two parts; the first part of the test was stopped because the patient's Pa_{O_2}

decreased to 46 mm Hg with an SaO_2 of 77.3%. The second phase, using oxygen, was terminated because of SOB. The patient tolerated very low workloads even with supplemental O_2.

Ventilation was slightly elevated at rest but increased normally. When given O_2, the patient's ventilation was slightly lower both at rest and at similar workloads. The V_D/V_T ratio was mildly elevated but decreased with exercise, on both air and oxygen. The patient's minute ventilation was only 51% of her observed MVV after bronchodilator administration, indicating some ventilatory reserve.

The patient achieved a peak $\dot{V}O_2$ of only 0.986 L/min on oxygen, which is 53% of her age-related predicted value of 1.858 L/min. This is consistent with moderately severe exercise impairment. The ventilatory equivalent for O_2 is within normal limits, and the O_2 pulse increased normally, although not to maximal values.

Blood gas analysis during exercise shows borderline hypoxemia at rest resulting from PaO_2 of 61 mm Hg in combination with elevated COHb. PaO_2 decreased to 47 mm Hg with only slight exertion. On 28% oxygen, the PaO_2 improved to 84 mm Hg at rest but decreased as workload increased. $PaCO_2$ increased slightly during oxygen breathing, possibly because of respiratory depression. COHb was elevated, likely resulting from the patient's continued smoking. Pulse oximetry (SpO_2) during exercise shows readings higher than the actual saturation, presumably because of the elevated COHb.

The HR and BP responses were appropriate for the workloads achieved while breathing both air and oxygen. The low maximal HR suggests an exercise limitation other than cardiovascular pathology or deconditioning. The ECG was unremarkable.

Impression: Moderately severe exercise impairment primarily caused by desaturation during exercise. Some ventilatory limitation is probably present as well. Desaturation is aggravated by an elevated COHb.

Cause of the Patient's Exercise Limitation

This patient characterizes an individual with obstructive lung disease in whom derangement of blood gases limits exercise more than impaired ventilation does. Her ventilation and gas exchange are close to normal at rest and at 1.5 mph, 0% grade. PaO_2 is low, however, and decreases abruptly with just a small increase in workload. The decrease is severe enough that desaturation may occur with daily activities or during sleep. The elevated COHb further impairs O_2 delivery. Although a pulse oximeter was used during the exercise

test, its readings were falsely high because of the elevated COHb. Even if pulse oximeter readings are corrected for COHb, a discrepancy often exists between SpO_2 and SaO_2 during exercise. This error in pulse oximeter readings may result from changes in blood flow at the sensor site or motion artifact during exercise. Desaturation might be expected because of her low $DLCO$. There is some evidence that $DLCO$ values less than 50% of predicted values are accompanied by exercise desaturation.

To evaluate the effect of oxygen therapy, a controlled trial of walking while breathing supplemental O_2 was performed. The patient breathed from a balloon containing gas blended to have an FIO_2 of approximately 0.28. The most notable change was the increase in resting PaO_2 from 61 to 84 mm Hg. However, the pattern of desaturation persisted. Her O_2 tension decreased dramatically, just as when she breathed room air. Because her PaO_2 was elevated by the supplemental O_2, it remained above 55 mm Hg. This is the level at which serious symptoms of hypoxemia begin to occur. Supplemental O_2 also may be responsible for the decrease in ventilation exhibited by the patient at rest and during exercise. The mild increase in $PaCO_2$ may be evidence of increased sensitivity to hypoxemia. When she breathes O_2, her respiratory drive decreases slightly, allowing CO_2 to increase. Abnormal $\dot{V}/\dot{Q}$ is the most likely explanation of desaturation observed in the patient. The bronchitic component of her obstructive disease results in shunting and venous admixture.

While breathing oxygen, she did not desaturate to a level at which hypoxemia might be considered as a cause of the exercise limitation. She also did not increase ventilation to her maximal level. This may suggest that deconditioning was responsible for the low maximal workload achieved. However, her HR and BP did not increase as is typical in significant deconditioning. Other possible causes for the low workload achieved while breathing oxygen may be inadequate patient effort, development of bronchospasm, or greatly increased work of breathing.

Treatment

The patient began a formal effort to stop smoking and eventually quit. She was also referred for pulmonary rehabilitation, which included bronchial hygiene, breathing retraining, and exercise with supplemental O_2. She began using nasal oxygen at 1–2 L/min for exertion. A follow-up evaluation was recommended 3–6 months after smoking cessation.

CASE 7-4

Case Studies

HISTORY

The patient is a 62-year-old woman complaining of dyspnea on exertion. Her medical history includes severe subglottic stenosis, which has been managed with several rigid dilatations over the past 2 years. She had a surgically corrected endarterectomy and a significant family history of coronary artery disease. Her current medications include metoprolol (Toprol), levothyroxine (Synthroid), and amlodipine (Norvasc). On physical examination, her lungs were clear to auscultation and she was in no apparent distress. Chest radiograph showed some narrowing of the subglottic trachea with no significant change since 1 year ago.

PULMONARY FUNCTION TESTS

Personal Data

Sex:	Female
Age:	62 yr
Height:	62.5 in (158.8 cm)
Weight:	179 lb (81.3 kg; BMI 32.3)

Lung Volumes

	PREDICTED		CONTROL		POSTDILATOR*	
	Normal	Range	Found	%Pred	Found	%Change
TLC (Pleth)	4.82	>3.72	4.06	84		
VC	2.96	>2.22	2.28	77	2.42	+6
RV	1.86	<2.41	1.79	96		
RV/TLC	38.5	<50.5	44.0	114		
FRC			2.2			

*Bronchodilator was albuterol.

Spirometry

	PREDICTED		CONTROL		POSTDILATOR*	
	Normal	Range	Found	%Pred	Found	%Change
FVC	2.96	>2.22	2.07[†]	70	2.20[†]	+6
FEV_1	2.4	>1.85	1.70[†]	71	1.78[†]	+5
FEV_1/FVC	81.2	>70.0	82.3		80.9	
$FEF_{25\%-75\%}$	2.3	>1.0	1.5	67	1.5	
FEFmax	5.5	>2.9	3.1	55	3.6	+17
FIFmax					1.5	
$FEF_{50\%}/FIF_{50\%}$					1.5	

*Bronchodilator was albuterol.
[†]Outside normal range.

Airway Function

	PREDICTED		CONTROL	
	Normal	Range	Found	%Pred
SRaw	4.7	>7.9	5.5	117

Diffusing Capacity

	PREDICTED		CONTROL	
	Normal	Range	Found	%Pred
DLcosb	20.9	>14.4	14.4	69
V_A	4.64	>3.72	3.58*	77

*Outside normal range.

Oximetry

	PREDICTED			Exercise
	Normal	Range	Rest	(step 3 min)
O₂sat	96	≥93	95	97
Pulse			66	104

TECHNOLOGIST'S COMMENTS

Spirometry testing was performed meeting criteria for acceptability and reproducibility.

QUESTIONS

1. What is the interpretation of:
   a. Prebronchodilator and postbronchodilator spirometry?
   b. Lung volumes and diffusing capacity?

Exercise Test

	Rest	Maximum	Pred Max	%Pred Max
Exercise				
Workload (watts)		60		
Time (min:sec)		7:00		
Oxygen saturation (%)	99	98		
$\dot{V}O_2$ (L/min)	0.191	0.801	1.674	48
$\dot{V}O_2$/kg (ml/kg)	2.3	9.9		
R	0.68	1.05		
Cardiac function				
Heart rate (beats/min)	67	110	170	65
Blood pressure (cuff) (mm Hg)	122/60	148/72		
Oxygen pulse (ml/beat)	2.9	7.3		
Ventilation				
Minute ventilation (L/min)	6.2	29.2	68.0	43
Respiratory rate (per min)	12	20		
Tidal volume (ml, BTPS)	528	1564		
Tidal volume/FVC (%)	26	76		
Vent equiv for O_2 ($V_E/\dot{V}O_2$)	34.7	36.7		

continued

2. What is the interpretation of:
   a. Cardiovascular response?
   b. Ventilation during exercise?
   c. Gas exchange during exercise?
   d. Oxygen consumption and ventilatory threshold during exercise?
   e. Impression?
3. Discuss the patient's exercise response.
4. What treatment might be recommended based on these findings?

DISCUSSION

Interpretation (Pulmonary Function)

Spirometry results show a nonspecific reduction in vital capacity and FEV_1 with a normal FEV_1/FVC ratio. Lung volumes were within normal limits. There was no response to bronchodilator. The DLCO was at the lower limit of normal. A cardiopulmonary exercise test was ordered with F-V loop analysis to determine whether there was flow limitation that would require repeat dilation of the trachea, versus deconditioning or decreased exercise tolerance.

Interpretation (Exercise)

The patient exercised on a cycle ergometer to a maximal workload of 60 watts using a 10-watt protocol. The patient terminated the test complaining of SOB. This appears to be a submaximal study.

Cardiovascular Response: The heart rate increased to 110 beats/min, which was 65% of predicted. The ECG was a normal sinus rhythm at rest. During exercise, there were no arrhythmias and/or evidence of ischemic changes. The reduced heart rate response may also be secondary to the β-blocker the patient was taking. Blood pressure and the O_2 pulse increased appropriately with exercise.

Ventilatory Response: There was an adequate ventilatory reserve; breathing kinetics was appropriate with increasing tidal volumes to 76% of the forced vital capacity. The tidal volume to FVC ratio is somewhat elevated at 76%, but this can be seen in individuals with reduced lung volumes.

Gas Exchange: Pulse oximetry was 99% at rest and 98% at end exercise, suggesting normal oxygen saturation.

Oxygen consumption in this submaximal study was 48% of predicted, and the ventilatory threshold could not be determined.

F-V loops were performed at rest, during warm-up, and at maximal workload. There was no evidence of either inspiratory or expiratory flow limitation, when compared with either the resting maximum F-V loop or the partial loops performed during exercise.

Impression: Submaximal study with reduced exercise tolerance and no evidence of flow limitation.

Discussion of Exercise Response

A 10-watt incremental protocol was selected based on a predicted $\dot{V}O_2$max of 1.674 L ([1600 − 300]/100 = 13) and because of the patient's stated reduced exercise tolerance.

In evaluating whether a study represents maximal effort, five categories are examined. These are cardiovascular response, ventilatory response, oxygen saturation, metabolic parameters, and clinical observation (see Box 7-4). Her heart rate was 65% of predicted; $\dot{V}_E$max reached 43% of her calculated MVV. SpO_2 was 98%, and her metabolic work showed an RER of 1.05. Clinical observation revealed poor effort. These factors all suggest a submaximal study. On the basis of these findings, the study can still be interpreted accordingly.

Cardiovascular Response: Heart rate response was reduced, either related to the poor effort or secondary to a beta-blockade effect.

Ventilatory Response: There was adequate ventilatory reserve based on both a normal ratio ($\dot{V}_E$max/MVV) and an absolute difference of 39 L. Tidal volume increased appropriately with exercise; however, it did comprise a significant portion of the forced vital capacity. This is often seen in individuals with restrictive patterns and/or reduced lung volumes.

Gas exchange analysis was limited to oxygen saturation, which was normal.

Oxygen consumption was 48% of predicted in this submaximal study, and the ventilatory threshold could not be determined. This is not surprising in a submaximal test.

Flow-Volume Loops: F-V loops showed no evidence of flow limitation. The resting graph is a plot of the maximal F-V loop versus her tidal breathing. The warm-up and 60-watt graphs demonstrate her tidal breathing plotted against both her resting maximal F-V loop (dotted line, right-side graph at the bottom of page 233) and partial loops performed during exercise.

Treatment

The purpose of this test was to discover whether the patient needed another surgical dilation for subglottic stenosis. Visual inspection via bronchoscopy showed the area to be the same diameter as measured earlier. Despite this, she had an increase in dyspnea on exertion. The surgical procedure was deferred based on the results of the F-V loop analysis during exercise. The patient was enrolled in a pulmonary rehabilitation program to improve her exercise tolerance.

SELF-ASSESSMENT QUESTIONS

Entry-level

1. Which of the following is required to perform a 6-minute walk test?
   I.   Countdown timer
   II. Lap counter
   III. Pulse oximeter
   IV. Sphygmomanometer
   a. I and II
   b. I, II, and III
   c. I, II, and IV
   d. II, III, and IV

2. In an adult patient with a resting BP of 130/90, which of the following responses would be an indication to stop an exercise test?
   a. Systolic increase to 180, diastolic increase to 95
   b. Systolic increase to 255, diastolic increase to 130
   c. Systolic increase to 160, diastolic increase to 100
   d. Systolic remains at 130, diastolic decrease to 85

3. What cycle ergometer protocol should the technologist select based on the information provided?

Pred HR:	175	Pred $\dot{V}O_2$:	2.40 L/min
Height:	69 in	Weight:	190 lb
FVC:	4.65 L	FEV_1:	3.74 L

   a. 10 watts/min
   b. 15 watts/min
   c. 20 watts/min
   d. 25 watts/min

4. Which of the following is an indication for terminating a cardiopulmonary exercise test?
   a. Shortness of breath (Borg = 4)
   b. A 2-mm down-sloping ST-segment depression
   c. Five premature ventricular contractions per minute
   d. Failure of pulse oximeter sensor

5. The graph at the top of the next column plots $\dot{V}_E$ and $\dot{V}CO_2$ against $\dot{V}O_2$.
   At approximately what $\dot{V}O_2$ does the ventilatory threshold occur?
   a. 1.0 L/min
   b. 2.0 L/min
   c. 3.0 L/min
   d. 4.0 L/min

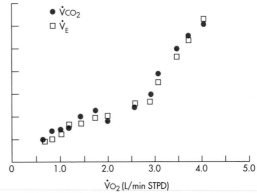

6. The "phase delay" between flow at the mouth and analysis of O_2 and CO_2 is necessary for calibration of a:
   a. Mixing chamber–type exercise system
   b. Rebreathing cardiac output system
   c. Standard Fick cardiac output determination
   d. Breath-by-breath exhaled gas analysis system

Advanced

7. Which results from a maximal exercise test would be consistent for a patient who has severe COPD?
   I. $\dot{V}_E$/MVV 90%
   II. V_T/FVC 48%
   III. V_D/V_T 12%
   IV. A-a gradient 45
   a. I and IV
   b. I and II
   c. II, III, and IV
   d. I, II, and IV

8. A 61-year-old woman with dyspnea on exertion has the following results from a cardiopulmonary exercise test.

	Rest	Maximal Exercise	Pred
HR	88	154	170
$\dot{V}O_2$ (ml/kg)	4	17	23
$\dot{V}_E$ (L)	9.0	44.0	90.0
V_T (ml)	575	685	
RR (per min)	12	64	
V_D/V_T (%)	45	50	

   These findings are most consistent with:
   a. Ventilatory limitation
   b. Pulmonary hypertension
   c. Inappropriate breathing strategy
   d. Pulmonary fibrosis

9. Tidal breathing loops at different stages of exercise are plotted against the resting maximal F-V curve. Which of the following best describes the data?

a. Inappropriate breathing strategy
b. Dynamic hyperinflation
c. No significant flow limitation
d. Fixed obstruction

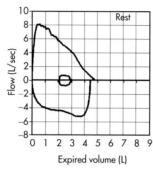
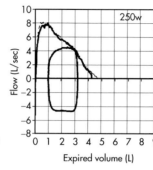
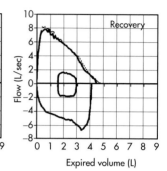

10. A patient has the following results of a cardiopulmonary exercise test (values in parentheses are percentages of predicted):

$\dot{V}O_2max$	L/min (STPD)	3.44	(97%)
HRmax	b/min	171	(95%)
V_Emax	L/min (BTPS)	60	(47%)

Which of the following best describes these results?
a. Mild aerobic impairment, consistent with deconditioning
b. Poor patient effort indicated by low maximal ventilation
c. Moderate exercise impairment with ventilatory limitation
d. Normal exercise response

11. A patient performs a symptom-limited maximal exercise test on a cycle ergometer using a ramp protocol of 20 watts/min. The ventilatory threshold is measured at 39% of the patient's peak $\dot{V}O_2$. These findings are consistent with which of the following?

a. Inappropriate ergometer protocol
b. Poor patient effort
c. Early onset of anaerobic metabolism
d. Normal cardiovascular response

12. A patient has the following results of an exercise test:

	Maximal Exercise	Predicted
HR (beats/min)	119	159
ST change (mm)	0.5	<1
$\dot{V}O_2$ (ml/min/kg)	10.2	22
$\dot{V}_E$ (L/min)	37	42
Pa_{O_2} (mm Hg)	53	>85

Which of the following clinical conditions is most consistent with these findings?
a. COPD
b. Poor patient effort
c. Exercise-induced bronchospasm
d. Coronary artery disease

Selected Bibliography

GENERAL REFERENCES

American College of Sports Medicine: *Guidelines for exercise testing and exercise prescription,* ed 6, Philadelphia, 2000, Lippincott Williams & Wilkins.

American College of Sports Medicine: *Resource manual for guidelines for exercise testing and prescription,* ed 4, Jeffrey L. Roitman (Ed), Philadelphia, 2001, Lippincott Williams & Wilkins.

Hansen JE: Exercise instruments, schemes, and protocols for evaluating the dyspneic patient, *Am Rev Respir Dis* 1984; 129(suppl):S25.

Hansen JE, Sue DY, Wasserman K: Predicted values for clinical exercise testing, *Am Rev Respir Dis* 1984; 129 (suppl):S49.

Jones NL: *Clinical exercise testing,* ed 4, Philadelphia, 1997, WB Saunders.

Wasserman K, Hansen J, Sue D et al: *Principles of exercise testing and interpretation,* ed 3, Philadelphia, 1999, Lippincott, Williams & Wilkins.

Weber KT, Janicki JS: *Cardiopulmonary exercise testing: physiologic principles and clinical applications,* Philadelphia, 1986, WB Saunders.

CARDIOVASCULAR MONITORING DURING EXERCISE

Bruce RA: Value and limitations of the electrocardiogram in progressive exercise testing, *Am Rev Respir Dis* 1984; 129(suppl):S28.

Daida H, Allison TG, Squires TW et al: Peak exercise blood pressure stratified by age and gender in apparently healthy subjects, *Mayo Clin Proc* 1996; 71:445.

Pollack ML, Bohannon RL, Cooper KH et al: A comparative analysis of four protocols for maximal stress testing, *Am Heart J* 1976; 92:39.

VENTILATION, GAS EXCHANGE, AND BLOOD GASES

Beaver WL, Wasserman K, Whipp BJ: A new method for detection of anaerobic threshold by gas exchange, *J Appl Physiol* 1986; 60:2020.

Blackie SP, Fairbarn MS, McElvaney NG et al: Normal values and ranges for ventilation and breathing pattern at maximal exercise, *Chest* 1991; 100:136-142.

Blackie SP, Fairbarn MS, McElvaney GN et al: Prediction of maximal oxygen uptake and power during cycle ergometry in subjects older than 55 years of age, *Am Rev Respir Dis* 1989; 139:1424-1429.

Eschenbacher WL, Mannina A: An algorithm for the interpretation of cardiopulmonary exercise tests, *Chest* 1990; 97:263-267.

Escourrou PJL, Delaperche MF, Visseaux A: Reliability of pulse oximetry during exercise in pulmonary patients, *Chest* 1990; 97:635-638.

Johnson BD, Beck KC, Zeballos RJ et al: Advances in pulmonary laboratory testing, *Chest* 1999; 116:1377-1387.

Johnson BD, Weisman IM, Zeballos RJ et al: Emerging concepts in the evaluation of ventilatory limitation during exercise—the exercise tidal flow-volume loop, *Chest* 1999; 116:488-503.

Jones NL: Normal values for pulmonary gas exchange during exercise, *Am Rev Respir Dis* 1984; 129 (suppl):S44.

Proctor DN, Beck KC: Delay time adjustments to minimize errors in breath-by-breath measurement of Vo_2 during exercise, *Appl Physiol* 1996; 81:2495-2499.

Whipp BJ, Ward SA, Wasserman K: Ventilatory responses to exercise and their control in man, *Am Rev Respir Dis* 1984; 129(suppl):S17.

STANDARDS AND GUIDELINES

ACC/AHA 2002 guideline update for exercise testing: a report of the American College of Cardiology/ American Heart Association Task Force on Practice Guidelines, *Circulation* 2002; 106:1883-1892.

ACC/AHA 2002 guideline update for exercise testing: a report of the American College of Cardiology/ American Heart Association Task Force on Practice Guidelines, *J Am Coll Cardiol* 2002; 40:1531-1540.

American Association for Respiratory Care: Clinical practice guideline: exercise testing for evaluation of hypoxemia and/or desaturation, *Respir Care* 2001; 46:514-522.

American Thoracic Society statement: cardiopulmonary exercise testing, *Am J Respir Crit Care Med* 2003; 167:211-277.

American Thoracic Society statement: guidelines for the six-minute walk test, *Am J Respir Crit Care Med* 2002; 166:111-117.

ATS/ACCP statement on cardiopulmonary exercise testing, *Am J Respir Crit Care Med* 2003; 167:211-277.

Clinical and Laboratory Standards Institute (CLSI): *A quality system model for health care,* approved guideline, HS01-A2, Wayne, PA, 2004, CLSI.

CLSI: *Blood gas and pH analysis and related measurements,* approved guideline, C46-A Wayne, PA, 2001, CLSI.

CLSI: *Procedures for the collection of arterial blood specimens,* approved standard, H11-A4 Wayne, PA, 2004, CLSI.

Fletcher GF, Froelicher VF, Hartley LH et al: Exercise standards: a statement for health professionals from the American Heart Association, *Circulation* 1990, 82:2286-2322.

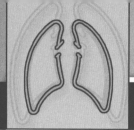

Chapter **8**

Pediatric Pulmonary Function Testing

DEBORAH K. WHITE

OBJECTIVES

After studying this chapter you will be able to:

Entry-level

1. State how recent revisions in the combined American Thoracic Society (ATS) and European Respiratory Society (ERS) task force guidelines relate to pulmonary function testing in children, and resultant interpretative strategies.
2. Suggest techniques for approaching young children and gaining their confidence.

3. Identify modifications to testing protocols for standard pulmonary function tests (PFTs) and new procedures available for testing preschool age children.
4. State limitations and considerations for equipment as related to testing in children.

Advanced
1. Relate specific pediatric disease states to anticipated changes in standard pulmonary function measurements.
2. State the physiologic and testing effects that sedation may produce in infants.
3. State differences in procedures, techniques, and terminology between pulmonary function testing in infants, toddlers, and preschool-aged children as compared with older children.

KEY TERMS

asynchrony	impedance	reactance (Xrs)
braking	impulse oscillometry	resonant frequency
dynamic FRC	interrupter technique (Rint)	respiratory inductive
exhaled nitric oxide (eNO)	passive occlusion technique	plethysmography (RIP)
forced oscillation technique	raised volume technique	respiratory system compliance
(FOT)	rapid thoracoabdominal	(Crs)
Hering-Breuer reflex	compression (RTC)	time constant

Pediatric pulmonary function testing is one of the most dynamic and challenging aspects of pulmonary physiology. Although technologic improvements have affected all areas of pulmonary function testing, the implications for pediatric testing are especially evident. Improved accuracy and precision of flow sensors, combined with user-friendly computer software, make measurements of respiratory mechanics easily obtainable. The range and sophistication of equipment is broad. Suitable systems are available for physician offices, hospital clinic settings, and clinical and research-oriented pulmonary function laboratories. Updated guidelines from the American Thoracic and European Respiratory Societies have redefined the concept of repeatability and reproducibility, and have provided recommendations for the pediatric population. Infants and toddlers, of course, are unable to follow specific instructions. Respiratory measurements in this age group are limited to techniques that are independent of effort, or that involve mechanical manipulation of the patient's chest. The specialized equipment and techniques needed for these measurements are discussed in this chapter. Preschool children present a different array of challenges for the pulmonary function technologist, and alternative techniques for measuring respiratory mechanics are now available for very young children. Standard measurements of pulmonary function are still the mainstay for children able to understand and cooperate with testing. The primary limiting factor for the pediatric patient, even into the teenage years, is the "effort and cooperation" component. This chapter focuses on practical tips, techniques, and guidelines for obtaining pulmonary function data in all age groups that are reliable and relevant in assessing pediatric respiratory ailments.

SPIROMETRY

The basics of spirometry apply to both pediatrics and adults (see Chapter 2). The same principles for testing and equipment are used. The indications for testing are similar, although disease processes in pediatrics often differ. The anatomy and physiology of the respiratory system change significantly from the infant to the young child and to the older adolescent. As for adults, the goals of spirometry are the following:

1. To identify the presence of an obstructive or restrictive defect
2. To quantify the degree of the abnormality
3. To test for a response to a bronchodilator

Spirometry in pediatrics has several pitfalls and special challenges, however. These can be addressed by posing several questions and giving specific examples.

Age Considerations for Children Performing Spirometry

Age considerations are a common concern that cannot be addressed until spirometry is attempted. Children as young as 3 years have the potential to perform the maneuver, but with limitations. It has been suggested that at least 50% of children this age can perform pulmonary function tests (PFTs). Data published by Eigen et al state that preschool children can perform technically repeatable forced vital capacity (FVC) maneuvers within 10%. Introducing spirometry to children at a young age often yields remarkable results within only a few training sessions.

Recommendations recently published from an ATS/ERS (American Thoracic Society/European Respiratory Society) focus group on preschool lung function tests more clearly define acceptable and repeatable spirometry in this young age group. The most difficult part of spirometry for a very young child is to continue to exhale once the initial blast of air occurs. Small children do not understand how to sustain applied pressure to their chest and abdomen once they feel their lungs are empty. Additional guidelines from the ATS/ERS include the following:

1. Identify premature termination of the maneuver by comparing the flow at termination to that of peak flow. If cessation of flow occurs at greater than 10% of peak flow, the vital capacity and forced expiratory flows should not be reported. $FEV_{0.5}$ or FEV_1 may still be reportable. Because vital capacity may be completely exhaled by 1 second, examining exhaled volumes closer to peak flow (e.g., $FEV_{0.5}$) may provide more accurate information regarding intrathoracic airflow obstruction.
2. As with current recommendations, the highest FVC and FEV_1 (or $FEV_{0.5}$) should be reported, and the selection of "best" curve based on the sum of FVC and $FEV_{0.5}$.
3. Additionally, a close look at extrapolated volume is recommended. Because children have smaller lung volume, extrapolated volume during spirometry may exceed the 5% (or 50 ml) criteria currently stated in ATS/ERS guidelines. In very young children, an expiratory curve with an extrapolated volume as high as 80 ml or 12.5% (whichever is greater) may be acceptable and should be re-examined.

Although it is desirable to have at least two repeatable maneuvers, even a single satisfactory trial provides important information. However, learning variability and lack of repeatability should be noted. Other testing modalities available in assessing very young children are discussed later in the chapter.

On average, by age 5 years, most children can perform spirometry with adequate technique and repeatability. Published guidelines from the ATS/ERS task force offer more realistic expectations for young children. There is not an age that all children, without exception, can perform technically acceptable spirometry. The ATS/ERS guidelines suggest that certain flow-volume curves may be "usable" if not technically acceptable. Consider Figure 8-1, A. This 5-year-old child is a first time blower. On multiple attempts, her FEV_1 was repeatable with the best curve as shown. Note, however, that exhalation is incomplete and expiratory time is very short (slightly over 1 second). Therefore the FVC values are underestimated and the FEV_1/FVC inaccurate. The curves, however, meet criteria for satisfactory start of test and are free of artifact for at least the first second. These classify as usable flow-volume loops, although not technically perfect.

Spirometry	PRED	LLN	PRE	% PRED	POST	% PRED	% CHG
			A		**B**		
FVC (L)	1.57	1.29	1.25	80	1.41	90	13
FEV$_1$ (L)	1.41	1.16	1.21	86	1.38	98	13
FEV$_1$/FVC (%)	90	81	97	**	97	**	**
FEF$_{25\%-75\%}$ (L/sec)	**	**	1.45	**	1.76	**	21
PEFR (L/sec)	3.53	2.54	2.77	79	3.46	98	25
FET 100% (sec)	**	**	1.21	**	1.54	**	**

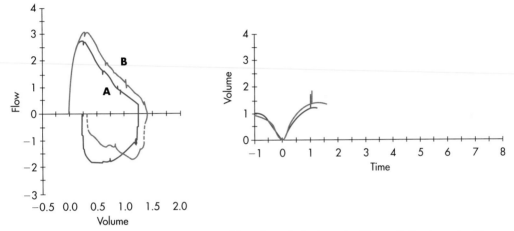

FIGURE 8-1   First-Time Spirometry in a 5-Year-Old Patient. A, Prebronchodilator. **B,** Postbronchodilator.

PF TIP

ATS/ERS guidelines now differentiate between technically "acceptable" and "usable" flow-volume loops. This is important in young children or any age patient who cannot complete the full FVC maneuver.

As long as the patient blows for at least 1 second and that first second is free of artifact, the F-V loop and values may be used for interpretation. However, caution is suggested in interpreting the FEV$_1$/FVC or any parameter based on a full expiratory maneuver.

The shape of the postbronchodilator flow-volume loop in Figure 8-1, *B*, is similar to the one in Figure 8-1, *A*, but larger. There is a proportional increase in both FVC and FEV$_1$, which suggests the

child took a deeper breath before performing the FVC maneuver. Learning effect can be seen even during the first session of working with a young child and should definitely be considered when interpreting this study. Although a bronchodilator response should not be ruled out, it is likely that learning effect was responsible for most of the improvement. It should be emphasized that spirometry is an effort-dependent test that requires cooperation and attention from the child. Equally important is the experience and patience of a well-trained pulmonary function technologist. Children who are mentally delayed or not capable of following directions may not perform adequate spirometry at any age, regardless of the coach or technologist. Patients who are not feeling well or having chest pain, for example, may follow instructions, but not perform maximally.

Ensuring Maximal Effort on the Part of the Child

First, gain the child's confidence and do not rush into testing. Children are fearful that the testing will hurt. When possible, reassure the child by carrying on a conversation that is directed toward the child. See Figure 8-2 for a list of suggestions that will "break the ice" and get things going in a positive direction. Try to demonstrate the test and reassure the child that it is easy. Prepare the child for testing. When possible, the child should be standing and the technologist at eye level with the child. The use of nose clips is recommended but depends on the age and cooperation of the child. The anatomy of the nasopharyngeal structures in younger children is such that the use of nose clips may not be necessary. If the child is willing to wear nose clips, encourage him or her to do so.

TIPS for SUCCESS with SPIROMETRY

1. Greet the child, introduce yourself, and engage in conversation
   * Compliment the child on a pretty dress or cool T-shirt
   * Ask about vacations, school, sports activities, etc.
   * Ask if the child would like to play a "blowing game" on the computer
2. Demonstrate the test
   * Blow on a tissue, pinwheel, or similar toy
   * Reassure the child how easy the test is
3. Encourage the child to stand straight and hold the flow sensor upright
   * Use nose clips if possible, but compromise if necessary
   * Get at the same eye level of the child
4. Be expressive with body language
   * Change the intonation of your voice and be enthusiastic
   * Use your hands to emphasize action
5. Use words the child can understand and keep directions simple
   * "Breathe in, breathe out"
   * "Take little baby breaths"
   * "Take a giant breath in until you feel ready to burst"
   * "Blast the air out. Keep blowing until it comes out of your toes"
6. Think like a kid!
   * "Race" with the child to see who can blow longer
   * Pretend it's the child's birthday and he or she has to blow out the same number of candles as his or her age
   * Show the child the "mountains" he or she has blown and explain how the mountains can be made taller and wider
7. Be prepared to try different techniques (open vs. closed) and offer rest periods
8. Offer praise and prizes
   * High fives
   * "Best Blower of the Day" awards
   * Small toys or stickers
   * Smiley faces or A+ on PFT reports
9. *Be patient,* and know when to quit. Repeated efforts can be frustrating and counterproductive for the next visit

FIGURE 8-2   **Tips for Success with Spirometry in Pediatric Patients.**

Many pulmonary function systems offer two mouthpiece techniques for performing spirometry: "closed" and "open" techniques. Each offers advantages and disadvantages. Attempt the technique with which laboratory personnel are most comfortable and consistent. For the closed technique, have the child stand with nose clips in place and the mouthpiece situated securely. Ask the patient to breathe tidally for several breaths. This offers the opportunity to observe the child and ensure that the seal around the mouthpiece is tight. It also gives the child a feeling of security that he or she will get plenty of air through the mouthpiece. The child should be reassured during tidal breathing that he or she is doing very well. If the spirometer permits real-time visualization of flow, the clinician may show the child that he or she is "drawing pictures" with his or her breathing. It is essential to gain the child's confidence and offer praise whenever possible. It is very important to talk the child through the maneuver. Use simple words and phrases. For example, "Breathe in, breathe out," "Take easy, little, baby breaths," or "One more little breath. Now take a giant breath in." The technologist should be vocal and use hands and arms to demonstrate. The intonation of the voice should mimic the action, for example "easy, gentle breaths" in a soft voice versus "big, fast, and long breath" in a louder tone. Sometimes having the child "race" with another technologist, both blowing tissues into the air, may be helpful. Other simple toys, such as pinwheels, may offer incentive.

If the child is having particular difficulty, changing the technique may lead to success. For example, use a different mouthpiece or try the open technique. The child may have a sensitive gag reflex, or for unclear reasons, become anxious with tidal breathing. With the open technique, the child should first be instructed to hold the mouthpiece close to his or her face, perhaps supported on the cheek. Next, open the mouth wide, take in the deepest breath possible, place the mouthpiece in the mouth, and immediately blow. The disadvantage of this technique is that air may be lost as the child tries to get the mouthpiece into his or her mouth and form a seal. It is often helpful to graduate the child from the open to the closed technique once he or she becomes more comfortable performing spirometry.

Importance of Effort

As mentioned previously, the biggest challenge with children is ensuring a maximal breath in before the forced expiration. The concept is simple: The more air in, the more air out. The technologist should strive to get the child to breathe in as deeply as possible and observe the child's chest excursion. Movement of the shoulders upward without chest excursion is common and can fool the technologist into believing it is a maximal inspiratory capacity. This may also be a pitfall when comparing prebronchodilator and postbronchodilator spirometry. Figure 8-3 is also from a 5-year-old patient performing spirometry for the first time. The prebronchodilator spirometry (see Figure 8-3, *A*) appears to be normal and was repeatable. Postbronchodilators, both FVC and FEV_1, improve significantly (see Figure 8-3, *B*). The increase in FVC and FEV_1 is very symmetrical, similar to the last example presented (see Figure 8-1, *A*). Learning effect cannot be ruled out. However, the shape of the F-V curve is very different with postbronchodilator spirometry. This is an example of a situation where the change in $FEV_{0.5}$ might be more helpful in assessing intrathoracic airflow obstruction than the change in FEV_1.

PF TIP

For spirometry, different "catch phrases" can help the child more clearly understand instructions. Examples are:
- "Take a big breath in until you feel like a balloon ready to burst!"
- "Punch that air out like a dump truck is rolling over your belly!"
- "Keep blowing until the air comes out of your toes!"

Be creative and think like a kid!

Spirometry	PRED	LLN	PRE	% PRED	POST	% PRED	% CHG
			A		**B**		
FVC (L)	1.29	1.07	1.21	94	1.36	106	13
FEV₁ (L)	1.26	0.96	1.14	98	1.31	113	15
FEV₁/FVC (%)	89	79	94	**	96	**	**
FEF$_{25\%-75\%}$ (L/sec)	**	**	1.38	**	2.29	**	65
PEFR (L/sec)	2.68	1.93	2.73	102	3.48	130	27
FET 100% (sec)	**	**	1.8	**	2.93	**	**

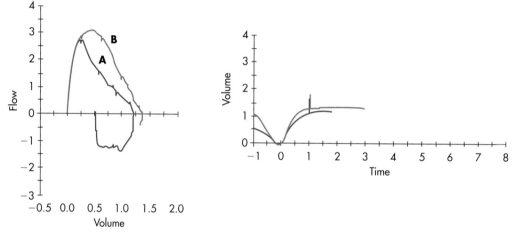

FIGURE 8-3   **First-Time Spirometry in a 5-Year-Old Patient. A,** Prebronchodilator. **B,** Postbronchodilator.

The child is at a low lung volume when 1 second is reached (close to FVC) and the FEV₁ is not reflective of airflow changes that are occurring at midlung volumes. It is critically important to realize that all the "action" has already taken place by the time 1 second has elapsed. Parameters such as FEV$_{0.5}$ or FEV$_{0.75}$ should be assessed in these young children, although guidelines for interpretation are not available. Contrast Figure 8-3 with Figure 8-4, *A* and *B*. In this example of a 7-year-old child, both FVC and FEV₁ increase with postbronchodilator spirometry; however, the increase in FEV₁ is proportionately higher, which also increases the FEV₁/FVC ratio. Although learning may have some effect in this example, it is evident that mild intrathoracic airflow obstruction is completely reversed. Once a child has learned the technique and is capable of performing spirometry, the results are remarkably repeatable. The ATS/ERS guidelines now base repeatability of

FVC and FEV₁ on lung volume. Because younger children have smaller lung volumes than adults, these revised guidelines pertain to the pediatric population as well as older patients with severe lung disease.

PF TIP

In patients with an FVC less than or equal to 1.0 L, repeatability of the largest and next largest FVC and FEV₁ should be within 100 ml. Patients with an FVC greater than 1.0 L should have repeatability for both FVC and FEV₁ within 150 ml.

Older children often are able to perform spirometry with an FVC and FEV₁ within 5%. However, for smaller children with even more reduced lung volume, the 100-ml criterion correlates with repeatability closer to 10%.

Spirometry	PRED	LLN	PRE	% PRED	POST	% PRED	% CHG
			A		**B**		
FVC (L)	1.41	1.15	1.26	89	1.36	97	9
FEV$_1$ (L)	1.26	1.02	0.96	79	1.24	98	28
FEV$_1$/FVC (%)	90	81	77	**	91	**	**
FEF$_{25\%-75\%}$ (L/sec)	**	**	0.79	**	1.65	**	109
PEFR (L/sec)	3.46	2.49	2.33	76	2.93	85	26
FET 100% (sec)	**	**	6.74	**	7.03	**	**

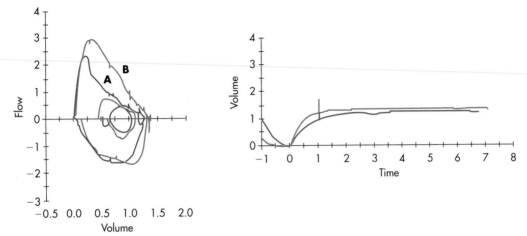

FIGURE 8-4 **Spirometry in a 7-Year-Old Patient. A,** Prebronchodilator spirometry in a child showing mild intrathoracic airflow obstruction. **B,** Postbronchodilator response.

Once a maximal inspiration is accomplished, most young children do not have difficulty blowing out forcefully. As for adult spirometry, the technologist should minimize hesitation before the forced maneuver that may create a "time zero" or back-extrapolated volume error. Do not encourage a breath hold. Delayed exhalation can result in a poor peak flow measurement and falsely raise the FEV$_1$. Figure 8-5 demonstrates this volume extrapolation or time zero error.

Figure 8-5, *A,* is an acceptable FVC maneuver. Note how the delayed exhalation in Figure 8-5, *B,* can skew the curve to the right and falsely elevate timed parameters. Young children have a desire to please and, unless they are feeling unwell, will usually respond to the direction to "blast the air out."

PF TIP

Relate the FVC maneuver to a roller coaster ride. Take a big breath in like "going up" a BIG hill and then an immediate FAST and smooth "ride" down. Don't encourage patients to hesitate or hold their breath before blowing out.

Obtaining a maximal peak flow can actually be more difficult in an adolescent. Teenage children often can be reluctant to perform maximally unless strongly encouraged to do so. This may be due to chest pain, embarrassment, or fear that something is wrong with them. Occasionally, this poor effort may be related to typical teenage angst or

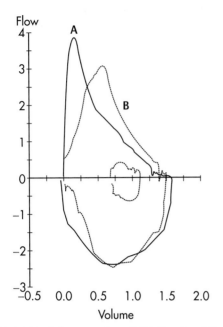

FIGURE 8-5 **Spirometry in a Child Showing Effects of Effort. A,** An acceptable FVC effort. **B,** Poor technique, resulting in delayed exhalation (see text).

PF TIP

End-of-test criteria state the subjects exhale (1) until they are unable to exhale further, or (2) the volume-time curve shows no change in volume (<25 ml for ≥1 second). Additionally, (3) in children younger than 10 years and older than 6 years, the subject should attempt to exhale for 3 or more seconds. In children older than 10 years, the subject should try to exhale for at least 6 seconds.

Because children have lung volumes that are significantly smaller than adult lung volumes, their lungs may completely empty in only 2 or 3 seconds. When a child feels empty, the natural instinct is take a breath back in. With instruction, practice, and maturing the child can learn to continue the expiration; however, this may not be possible on the first several visits to the lab. This does not invalidate the FVC maneuvers but requires that the testing be evaluated carefully. Figure 8-6, *A,* represents three prebronchodilator flow-volume (F-V) loops superimposed over each other. Although this young child does not meet the end-of-test criteria, the FEV_1 and shape of the F-V loop are remarkably repeatable. Postbronchodilator (see Figure 8-6, *B*) F-V loops are significantly improved, and repeatable. The newly adopted ATS/ERS guidelines more realistically represent what can be expected of a younger child.

Children who are severely obstructed, like their adult counterparts, may have the ability to exhale for an extended time. Figure 8-7 shows the F-V loop and volume-time tracing of a 10-year-old girl with cystic fibrosis. This child is able to sustain expiration for 15 seconds. However, the additional volume measured in this prolonged expiration is small and may exhaust the child performing the test. She approaches a flow plateau at approximately 7–8 seconds, and the maneuver can be terminated at this point. The spirometry is certainly still valid for interpretation if terminated before zero flow occurs. Many decisions regarding acceptability of PFT results require good judgment from the technologist and careful interpretation from the physician.

attention-seeking motivation. A sensitive and perceptive technologist can often combine the right amount of compassion with the necessary verbal encouragement to obtain optimal results. Variability due to effort alone may be especially important if the patient is performing serial measurements, as in a methacholine challenge. A change in treatment regimen or admission to the hospital is often based on spirometric changes; therefore repeatability is critical.

Length of Exhalation for a Child During an FVC Maneuver

Long-established criteria from the ATS suggested that an FVC maneuver should last for at least 6 seconds or until there was a plateau in the volume-time curve. Young children often cannot meet these criteria. The current ATS/ERS guidelines have added an age stipulation to the recommendations.

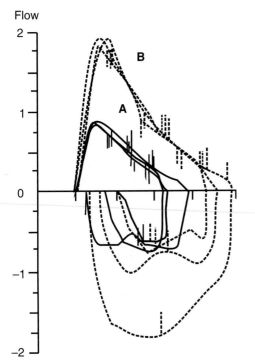

FIGURE 8-6   Repeatability of Efforts in a Young Child.
A, Prebronchodilator spirometry that is repeatable, although the end-of-test criteria are not met (see text). **B,** Postbronchodilator spirometry in the same patient, again demonstrating repeatability of improvement (see text).

Reliability of $FEF_{25\%-75\%}$ in Children

Historically, $FEF_{25\%-75\%}$ has been used to evaluate flow from the small airways. More precisely, the $FEF_{25\%-75\%}$ should be considered a measurement of flow at lower lung volumes, not merely flow from medium-sized and smaller airways. As in adults, the variability of the $FEF_{25\%-75\%}$ is greater than that of the FVC and FEV_1. Because children may be even less repeatable at baseline, the reliability of this measurement in pediatric testing may be questionable. In addition, if the child does not fully exhale to RV, $FEF_{25\%-75\%}$ may be artificially elevated because of reduced vital capacity. If it is reported, the $FEF_{25\%-75\%}$ in a pediatric subject should be interpreted with caution, especially in a very young child. A substantially greater change postbronchodilator

is needed before a change can be considered significant. Refer back to Figure 8-3, *A* and *B*. Although the exhalation times do not meet the revised 3-second guideline for a child younger than 10 years, it does appear that this patient exhaled to a volume plateau. The change in shape of the F-V loop, as well as the change in $FEF_{25\%-75\%}$ of 65%, is certainly suggestive of a reversal of intrathoracic airflow obstruction. An $FEF_{25\%-75\%}$ that improves by more than 35%–45% after bronchodilator may be indicative of reactivity, but again caution is advised when considering this parameter. Repeatability of the $FEF_{25\%-75\%}$ is more reliable in older children and teenagers. As previously noted, $FEF_{25\%-75\%}$ can be reduced for several reasons that are not always related to peripheral airway disease. Refer to Figure 8-8. This F-V loop is from a 17-year-old patient who had tracheal stenosis after a prolonged intubation as a young child. The $FEF_{25\%-75\%}$ of this curve is severely reduced, as is the FEV_1. The reduction is not due to peripheral airway obstruction but to a large central (tracheal) airway obstruction.

Other Parameters of Forced Flow Helpful in Pediatrics

Spirometry yields a variety of expiratory and inspiratory flows, including $FEF_{25\%}$, $FEF_{50\%}$, $FEF_{75\%}$, $FEF_{85\%}$, $FIF_{50\%}$, and the $FEF_{50\%}/FIF_{50\%}$ ratio. Each of these parameters relates to flow at a particular lung volume and may have some benefit for particular instances. These flows, like the $FEF_{25\%-75\%}$, are less repeatable than the FEV_1 and FVC, and do not have any reference values. The $FEF_{50\%}/FIF_{50\%}$ ratio may be helpful in identifying intrathoracic versus extrathoracic airflow obstruction (see Chapter 2). Unlike the expiratory limb of the F-V loop, the inspiratory limb has not been well characterized in pediatric subjects. There are several reasons for this; however, the most important are energy expenditure and effort dependence. Expiration from TLC is far more repeatable because of the elastic recoil of the lung. The $FEF_{50\%}$ occurs in the portion of the expiratory limb that is considered effort independent. The inspiratory limb, conversely, is effort dependent and energy dependent for the entire maneuver. Therefore optimal

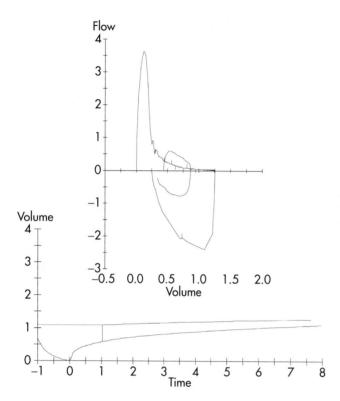

FIGURE 8-7   **F-V Loop and Volume-Time Tracing of a 10-Year-Old Girl with Cystic Fibrosis** (see text). Note prolonged exhalation and severe airflow obstruction.

patient effort is vital for analyzing the inspiratory loop. A great deal of important information can be obtained from an appropriately performed maneuver. Too often, the inspiratory limb is ignored. When teaching children how to perform spirometry, certainly the emphasis is on expiration. Once it is mastered, attention should be paid to the inspiratory maneuver as well.

PF TIP

Assuming maximal effort is given by the child for the entire maneuver, the inspiratory limb of the flow-volume loop can give valuable information regarding extrathoracic obstruction in pediatric patients.

The aperture, or opening, through the vocal cords is approximately the same at both 50% of expiratory vital capacity and 50% of inspiratory vital capacity. Hence, the $FEF_{50\%}/FIF_{50\%}$ ratio should not be greater than 1.0. A ratio greater than 1.0

suggests an extrathoracic obstruction; however, this relationship has not been closely studied or reported in pediatric patients. Conversely, an $FEF_{50\%}/FIF_{50\%}$ ratio of less than 1.0 may be normal or may represent significant intrathoracic obstruction. In addition, a ratio close to normal is possible if significant obstruction is seen on both inspiration and expiration (fixed obstruction), yielding a ratio of 1.0. This underlies the importance of correlating the F-V loop with the child's clinical picture and symptoms.

Figure 8-9 shows examples of F-V loops with differing $FEF_{50\%}/FIF_{50\%}$ ratios and the shape of the loops represented by those ratios. Although $FEF_{50\%}/FIF_{50\%}$ may not always discriminate between intrathoracic and extrathoracic airflow obstruction, the importance of extrathoracic obstruction should not be underestimated. Laryngeal webs, subglottic stenosis, tracheal malacia, and other lesions of the laryngeal-tracheal airway are important causes of upper airway obstruction in the pediatric population. In addition, the vocal cords represent a major

Spirometry	PRED	LLN	PRE	% PRED
FVC (L)	3.72	3.06	2.89	78
FEV$_1$ (L)	3.31	2.72	1.13	34
FEV$_1$/FVC (%)	89	80	39	**
FEF$_{25\%-75\%}$ (L/sec)	3.86	2.62	0.54	14
PEFR (L/sec)	6.82	4.9	1.55	23
FET 100% (sec)	**	**	8.55	**

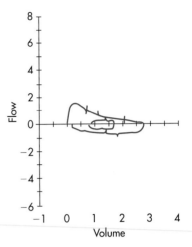

FIGURE 8-8 **Spirometry in a 17-Year-Old Girl with Severe Airflow Obstruction Resulting from Tracheal Stenosis** (see text).

"choke point" to airflow. The cords may have a structural abnormality, such as nodules or granulomas, or may become edematous, as in croup. The recurrent laryngeal nerve may be damaged, resulting in inappropriate movement or paralyzed cords. These conditions are generally easy to diagnose with direct visualization of the vocal cords. Vocal cord dysfunction (VCD) may also be responsible for poor abduction (opening) of the vocal cords during inspiration. VCD has become increasingly recognized as a reason for shortness of breath and sternal chest pain, often mimicking asthma. Adolescents who are competitive athletes or are exceptionally goal oriented and children who have stress-related disorders are at highest risk. Unfortunately, vocal cord dysfunction is highly variable and may be detectable only when the patient is stressed in a manner that provokes the condition. In very severe forms, "clipping" of the inspiratory loop with a completely normal expiratory loop is the classic presentation (see Figure 8-9, *E*). The child may or may not sound very stridorous during inspiration. The patient may try to speak while inspiring in short, gasping sentences. More common is a completely normal-appearing child with normal expiratory loops but highly variable inspiratory loops. Some inspiratory loops may be normal (FEF$_{50\%}$/FIF$_{50\%}$ < 1.0); however, often many are abnormal with an FEF$_{50\%}$/FIF$_{50\%}$ greater than 1.0. If the patient

is challenged with exercise, cold air, or methacholine, the expiratory loops remain normal while the clipping of the inspiratory loop may become more apparent. VCD is an example of a disorder in which the variability in the patient's inspiratory loop is the hallmark of the dysfunction. This variability is associated with involuntary adduction (closing) of the vocal cords. Direct visualization of the vocal cords via a laryngoscopy (during an episode) will conclusively make the diagnosis. However, laryngoscopy may not be practical or available, and a series of well-performed F-V loops are helpful in making this presumptive diagnosis. It should be emphasized that VCD, in less-than-severe cases, is primarily a diagnosis of exclusion, and absence of inspiratory clipping on F-V loops does not rule out the diagnosis.

Other Benefits of Spirometry in the Pediatric Population

The ATS/ERS recommendations emphasize the importance of repeatability of the FVC and FEV$_1$. In some instances, patients cannot reproduce these parameters, and effort is not the reason. Figure 8-10 shows an example of such an instance. If only a single (best) F-V loop (Trial 1) were reported to the physician, the interpretation would state that this

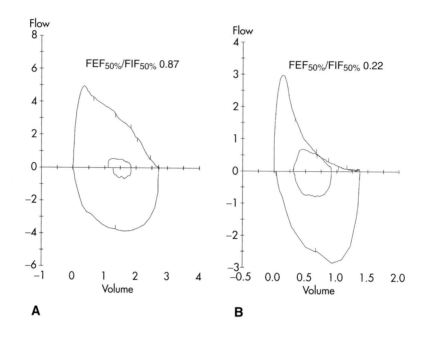

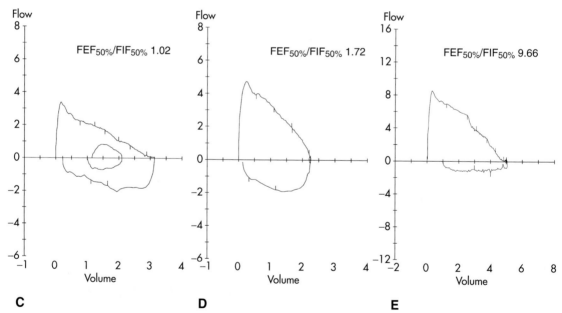

FIGURE 8-9 **F-V Loops and FEF$_{50\%}$/FIF$_{50\%}$ Ratios in Various Types of Airflow Obstruction. A,** Normal. **B,** Intrathoracic airflow obstruction. **C,** Fixed airflow obstruction. **D,** Extrathoracic airflow obstruction. **E,** Extrathoracic airflow obstruction with severe clipping of the inspiratory flow pattern (see text).

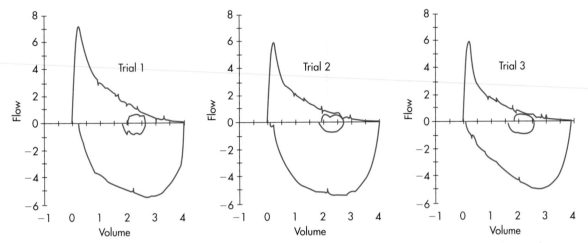

Spirometry	Trial 1	Trial 2	Trial 3
FVC (L)	4.03	3.96	3.87
FEV$_1$ (L)	2.35	1.93	1.79
FEV$_1$/FVC (%)	58	49	46
FEF$_{25\%-75\%}$ (L/sec)	1.08	0.71	0.65
PEFR (L/sec)	6.83	6.02	6.03

FIGURE 8-10   **Repeated Spirometry Maneuvers in a 15-Year-Old Patient with Asthma.** Trials 2 and 3 reveal progressively significant drops in FEV$_1$ and FEV$_1$/FVC that are not repeatable with Trial 1 (see text).

patient has mild to moderate intrathoracic airflow obstruction. However, the next two successive maneuvers performed by this 15-year-old asthmatic are also illustrated (see Figure 8-10, Trials 2 and 3). These successive trials reveal progressively significant drops in FEV$_1$ and FEV$_1$/FVC, which are not repeatable with Trial 1. This pattern is an extremely important clue to the hyperreactivity of the patient's airway. Simply performing repeated forced maneuvers may cause an asthmatic to become suddenly more obstructed and vulnerable to further bronchospasm. In such an instance, the technologist should *stop testing the patient* and administer a bronchodilator. If the patient's report included only his or her best prebronchodilator and postbronchodilator spirometry, it would completely omit this important information and might prevent necessary changes in his or her asthma medication regimen.

An interesting but opposite phenomenon may be seen in the spirometry of a mild asthmatic

patient. Deep inspirations may cause progressive bronchodilation with improving FEV$_1$ and FEV$_1$/FVC. This is a beneficial compensatory mechanism and is likely similar to the asthmatic athlete who is able to "run through" his or her asthma with bronchodilation during exercise. After exercise, tidal volumes decrease, airway temperature changes, and bronchoconstriction may be provoked.

PF TIP

Variability (or lack of repeatability) in spirometric efforts may be important for identifying diseases such as asthma and vocal cord dysfunction. Reporting or displaying all flow-volume loops can assist in the data interpretation. The technologist performing the test should look for characteristic patterns of variability and include appropriate data in the final report.

Unusual F-V curve shapes may be very helpful in providing clues to the location of fixed or variable obstruction. However, increased variability is inherent in testing children and may be effort or technique related. Conclusions based on abnormally shaped curves should be made with great care. One scenario common in pediatrics is tracheal and/or bronchial malacia. Malacia refers to an airway (or more than one airway) that is soft and pliable because of a lack of supportive connective or cartilaginous tissue. Depending on the location (intrathoracic, extrathoracic, or both), these airways may collapse during inspiration or be compressed during exhalation. Tracheal or bronchomalacia in infants may produce significant stridor and "noisy breathing," especially when the baby is excited or crying. With time and growth, the airways stiffen and are less prone to collapse. For older children, malaciac airways may produce some bizarre-shaped F-V curves. Refer to Figure 8-11. These F-V loops are from a 12-year-old girl who underwent double-lung transplantation. After transplantation, she had malacia in the left mainstem bronchus at the anastomotic site.

Trial 1 represents a forced exhalation that is normal in shape. Trial 2 is from the same patient during the same testing session. Although the PEFR in Trial 2 is slightly higher, notice the rapid drop in flow rate, followed by a "flattening" or shelflike appearance in the curve. Blowing harder caused more compression at the site of the anastomosis and resulted in a sudden decrease in flow rate. Obtaining repeatable and acceptable F-V loops in the face of malaciac airways can be challenging. Also note the reduction in $FEF_{25\%-75\%}$, as well as FEV_1, from Trial 1 to Trial 2. This represents another example of the inadequacy of looking solely at one or two parameters instead of considering the entire picture. The shape of the curve in Trial 2 is characteristic of two lungs emptying at different time constants. One lung empties normally during forced exhalation, whereas the other lung takes considerably longer to empty because of the central intrathoracic obstruction present.

Flow-volume loops that are abnormal in one phase of the breathing cycle are referred to as variable intrathoracic or variable extrathoracic obstructions (see Chapter 2). If the obstruction appears on both inspiration and expiration, it is termed a fixed obstruction and is more likely a structural abnormality. Refer again to Figure 8-8. This patient has tracheal stenosis resulting from a

Spirometry	Trial 1	Trial 2
FVC (L)	1.98	1.86
FEV_1 (L)	1.55	1.34
FEV_1/FVC (%)	78	72
$FEF_{25\%-75\%}$ (L/sec)	1.38	0.91
PEFR (L/sec)	3.45	4.06

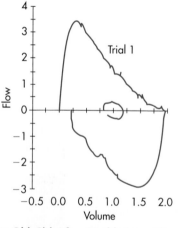
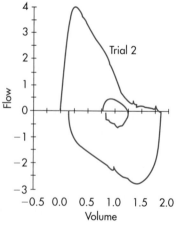

FIGURE 8-11 **Spirometry From a 12-Year-Old Girl After Double-Lung Transplantation.** After transplantation, the patient had malacia at one of the anastomotic sites (mainstem bronchus). *Trial 1,* F-V loop shows a forced exhalation that is normal in shape. *Trial 2,* F-V loop immediately following, in which the patient tried to blow harder (see text).

prolonged intubation. The square-wave nature of the loop with flow limitation evident even from the peak flow measurement is characteristic of fixed obstruction.

Challenge or Provocation Spirometry

As with adults, children can be exposed to a variety of inhaled, ingested, or topically applied substances to challenge the airways. The purpose of any challenge study is to identify and/or stage the level of airway hyperreactivity (see Chapter 9). Examples of conditions that cause bronchoconstriction in children are asthma, gastroesophageal reflux, and anaphylactic reactions. Airway hyperreactivity may range from a mild condition that produces only intermittent cough to sudden death from status asthmaticus or life-threatening anaphylaxis. Therefore it can be important to identify if a child is reactive to a substance or to stage the level of reactivity. Examples of provocative agents include methacholine, histamine, adenosine, cold air, hyperventilation, aspirin, latex, and others. The mechanism of the bronchoconstriction may differ with the agent administered; however, serial spirometry at specified time intervals and close observation of the child are required. Specific protocols for each type of challenge should be established by the pulmonary laboratory and approved by the medical director. The 1999 ATS guidelines provide specific recommendations for methacholine and exercise challenge studies. Because children can become fatigued or easily distracted with prolonged testing, abbreviated protocols have been published. It is also possible to perform challenges on young children who cannot perform spirometry. This requires very close monitoring of breath sounds, oxygen (O_2) saturation, respiratory rate, and symptoms. Challenges in pediatric patients are not recommended in any facility unfamiliar or inexperienced with children. Immediate physician availability and a fully stocked emergency cart are also essential. Patient safety and well-being are always the number-one priority.

Pulmonary Exercise Stress Testing

Pulmonary function laboratories are asked to perform exercise stress tests for two main reasons: (1) to provoke bronchoreactivity and (2) to assess level of fitness. Protocols for exercise are as varied as protocols for inhalation challenges. The protocol used is often geared toward answering a specific question such as, "Does this child have exercise-induced bronchospasm or asthma (EIB or EIA)?" An example of a protocol to evoke EIB includes pre-exercise spirometry as the first step. ECG leads are placed on the chest for heart rate (HR) assessment, and pulse oximetry is used to follow O_2 saturation. The patient performs a "free run" on a treadmill, with nose clips in place, but without a mouthpiece. Jogging on a treadmill is the most "asthmagenic" exercise because it mimics natural exercise and uses many muscle groups. This protocol also permits the technologist to watch and listen to the child without a mouthpiece in place. Evaluation of hyperventilation or stridorous respirations can be made. Vocal cord dysfunction (VCD) is very common in children during exercise. Several of the symptoms manifested (e.g., intense shortness of breath and sternal chest pain) are also symptoms of asthma. The speed and elevation of the treadmill are increased every minute to increase the patient's HR to a sustained 180 beats/min or higher for approximately 3–4 minutes. This equates to an HR of 160 or greater for at least 6 minutes, as other protocols suggest. The entire exercise study should take no more than 8–9 minutes and should end abruptly without a cool-down period. Postexercise spirometry is performed every 3–5 minutes until 20–30 minutes after exercise. Laboratories differ as to the parameter and percent decrease needed to signify EIB. A decrease in the FEV_1 of at least 15%–20% associated with a decreased FEV_1/FVC is considered diagnostic of EIB. Maximal bronchoconstriction most often occurs 6–12 minutes after exercise. Cough, desaturation, and worsening shortness of breath usually accompany changes in pulmonary function. A decrease in flow immediately after exercise with a quick return to normal is suspect and may be effort related. Children who exhibit VCD tend to recover quickly after the stress of exercise, although abnormal inspiratory flows may persist.

PF TIP

Protocols for exercise stress tests may vary according to the patient being studied and the indication for testing. Different protocols may yield differing results, and interpretation of exercise stress tests are not well standardized in pediatrics.

The indication for a maximal cardiopulmonary exercise test is to evaluate how well the respiratory and cardiovascular systems work together. The clinical question asked is often whether the child has normal exercise tolerance. If not, is the child limited by the lungs (ventilator limitation), the heart (cardiovascular limitation), or both? Maximal tests are performed with a full 12-lead ECG, pulse oximetry, and a mouthpiece in place to measure ventilation, O_2 consumption, and carbon dioxide (CO_2) production (see Chapter 7 for a detailed discussion of indications, protocols, analysis, and so on). Use of an ergometer instead of a treadmill may be a laboratory preference. Maximal O_2 consumption is usually slightly higher on a treadmill. The advantage of an ergometer, however, is that the child's upper body is relatively still while the legs cycle. This decreases movement of the head and leaks around the mouthpiece. Pulse oximetry is often problematic during exercise because of movement of the arms and fingers. With cycle ergometry, however, less whole-body motion produces less artifact. Alternatively, an oximeter probe placed above the eyebrow may yield more stable readings. The disadvantages of cycle ergometry in children are (1) modifying the equipment to fit the child, (2) keeping the child cycling consistently, and (3) obtaining true maximal O_2 consumption. Children may simply stop cycling when they feel fatigued. Unless a plateau in O_2 consumption ($\dot{V}O_2$) can be identified, the highest level reached is termed peak oxygen consumption.

LUNG VOLUMES

Lung volume measurements in the pediatric population are extremely valuable and often reveal information not obtained from spirometry only. Not all children need lung volume determination. It is preferable that the child be comfortable performing spirometry before attempting lung volumes, but many children adapt easily to a new test situation. The choice of techniques for measuring lung volume is similar to that with adults. Lung volume determination through gas dilution techniques often underestimates lung volumes in patients with obstructive airway disease. This problem becomes even more relevant in the pediatric population because the size of the airway is smaller and easier to obstruct. Helium dilution or nitrogen washout may not be as well tolerated as body plethysmography. Problems with keeping a mouth seal and breathing a dry gas for several minutes make these techniques less desirable. Conversely, a child who performs even less than optimal spirometry may "jump" into the body box and attempt the maneuvers. Many commercial body plethysmographs require minimal effort in determining thoracic gas volume (V_{TG}). Vigorous panting is no longer required to obtain V_{TG}. With most systems, limited panting or only tidal breathing is necessary. Some commercial systems permit the technologist to adjust the timing and duration of the panting to minimize patient discomfort. Technical advances in body plethysmography, the ease and versatility of making measurements, and the accuracy of the measurement make this technique the preferred choice for lung volumes in pediatric patients. A detailed description of the functioning of a body plethysmograph is included in Chapter 3.

PF TIP

Versatility and accuracy of commercially available body plethysmographs make this method of lung volume determination the preferred technique, even in the pediatric population. Children are generally *not* fearful of a plethysmograph and do not have claustrophobia as adults sometimes experience.

First Step

The first step in performing plethysmography in the pediatric population is getting the child into the body box. This is usually not a major obstacle. In many cases, the child has been to the pulmonary function laboratory on previous occasions and is familiar with the environment and personnel. The child often asks, "What's that?" This becomes an opportunity to appeal to the child's imagination. A body box, in a child's eye, can be a spaceship or Cinderella's coach. Sometimes the child only sits in the body box on the first or second visit, but ultimately this is a valuable experience. It may be possible to have the parent also sit in the body box and perform some testing until the child feels comfortable alone. The instructions should be kept simple and be demonstrated to the child. In many instances, the child will perform adequately without the need to modify instructions. Too many instructions can lead to confusion. A fitted mouthpiece and nose clips are required for testing in the body box. Some technologists suggest supporting the cheeks during the test. It may be preferable not to hold the cheeks. This may cause the child to raise his or her shoulders and not breathe at a true resting level. The child should sit up straight with hands relaxed in the lap. The instructions can be modified if the child pouches his or her cheeks, producing open loops rather than closed loops during panting. Although newer body boxes vent to the atmosphere, the door should be opened periodically to let the child rest and converse with the technologist or parent. Children requiring O_2 should also be given a break between trials to replace their cannula or mask until their oxygenation is back to baseline.

Important Plethysmographic Parameters

The tests performed and parameters examined depend on the reason for performing the study, and on the ability of the child. In very young children, obtaining a stable resting level and reproducible FRC may be all that can be accomplished. Once spirometry is mastered, the child can quickly learn to perform a full IC and VC in the body box. In a clinical setting, a skilled technologist and user-friendly software allow data to be edited as necessary to provide TLC, FRC, RV, and RV/TLC. It is important that the technologist understand when and how to average data versus deleting data and when to accept the "best test" data. This is especially true with pediatric patients who may not reproduce the entire maneuver with each trial.

Although spirometry is the first test performed in many patients, spirometry alone may not accurately predict lung volumes in children. Figure 8-12 demonstrates case presentations of obstructive and restrictive lung disease, as well as a mixed presentation. Note that predicted values, as well as the lower limit of normal (LLN), are presented. In some reference sets, the LLN is not available and is indicated with asterisks (**).

The case in Figure 8-12, *A*, is a 15-year-old white boy with advanced cystic fibrosis. Severe obstruction is evident in the spirometry data. Both FEV_1 and FEV_1/FVC are reduced, consistent with an obstructive disorder. Lung volume measurements confirm the severity of obstruction and air trapping. Although the TLC is within normal limits, FRC, RV, and RV/TLC are significantly elevated. Compare these findings with the spirometry and lung volumes in Figure 8-12, *B*. This case is a 13-year-old white girl with scoliosis. Her pulmonary function results represent a restrictive defect. FVC and FEV_1 are reduced in a symmetrical pattern; however, the ratio is normal. Restrictive disorders often present with a normal or elevated FEV_1/FVC. The lung volume measurements are also consistent with a pure restrictive defect, showing reduced volumes (TLC, FRC, RV, ERV) and a normal RV/TLC.

Many pediatric and adult diseases do not present as a purely obstructive or restrictive process, but as a combination of obstruction and restriction. Refer to Figure 8-12, *C*. This 10-year-old African American girl has systemic scleroderma. The FVC and FEV_1 are severely reduced. Her flow-volume loop has a very restrictive appearance, with a disproportionately high peak flow and increased FEV_1/FVC. A closer look at her lung volumes, however, reveals not only a moderate restrictive defect, but also an elevated RV and RV/TLC. Some elements of this pulmonary function study point to a restrictive

A

Spirometry	PRED	LLN	PRE	% PRED
FVC (L)	3.42	2.84	1.11	32
FEV$_1$ (L)	3.01	2.48	0.62	21
FEV$_1$/FVC (%)	88	78	56	**
FEF$_{25\%-75\%}$ (L/sec)	3.42	2.32	0.21	6
PEFR (L/sec)	5.99	4.31	2.07	35
FET 100% (sec)	**	**	9.2	**

Lung volumes	PRED	LLN	PRE	% PRED
VC (L)	3.42	2.84	1.11	33
TLC (L)	4.45	3.92	4.83	109
FRC$_{PL}$ (L)	2.19	1.84	3.88	177
RV (L)	1.01	0.68	3.72	368
RV/TLC (%)	24	**	77	**
IC (L)	**	**	0.95	**
ERV (L)	**	**	0.14	**

Diffusion capacity	PRED	LLN	PRE	% PRED
D$_{LCO}$ (ml/mm Hg/min)	22.9	**	14.1	61
D$_L$ Adj (ml/mm Hg/min)	22.9	**	15.2	66
D$_{LCO}$/V$_A$	6.45	**	6.06	94
V$_A$ (L)	**	**	2.31	**

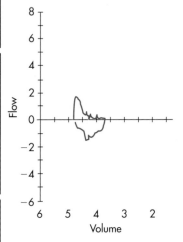

B

Spirometry	PRED	LLN	PRE	% PRED
FVC (L)	3.98	3.27	2.47	62
FEV$_1$ (L)	3.55	2.92	2.16	61
FEV$_1$/FVC (%)	89	80	87	**
FEF$_{25\%-75\%}$ (L/sec)	4.05	2.75	2.74	68
PEFR (L/sec)	7.61	5.47	5.45	81
FET 100% (sec)	**	**	6.36	**

Lung volumes	PRED	LLN	PRE	% PRED
VC (L)	3.98	3.27	2.62	66
TLC (L)	5.49	4.65	3.31	60
FRC$_{PL}$ (L)	2.72	2.12	1.66	61
RV (L)	1.33	0.91	0.69	52
RV/TLC (%)	23	**	21	**
IC (L)	**	**	1.65	**
ERV (L)	**	**	0.97	**

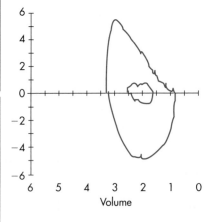

NOTE: **denotes predicted value and/or LLN not available.

FIGURE 8-12 **Pulmonary Function Studies in Obstruction, Restriction, and Mixed Disease. A,** Data from a 15-year-old boy with advanced cystic fibrosis. **B,** Data from a 13-year-old girl with scoliosis.

C

Spirometry	PRED	LLN	PRE	% PRED
FVC (L)	1.72	1.41	0.78	45
FEV$_1$ (L)	1.51	1.22	0.71	47
FEV$_1$/FVC (%)	88	79	92	**
FEF$_{25\%-75\%}$ (L/sec)	1.93	1.29	1.33	69
PEFR (L/sec)	4.14	2.97	3.15	76
FET 100% (sec)	**	**	6.98	**

Lung volumes	PRED	LLN	PRE	% PRED
VC (L)	1.72	1.41	0.78	45
TLC (L)	2.47	**	1.55	63
FRC$_{PL}$ (L)	1.21	**	0.88	73
RV (L)	0.64	**	0.77	120
RV/TLC (%)	26	**	50	**
IC (L)	**	**	0.67	**
ERV (L)	**	**	0.11	**

Diffusion capacity	PRED	LLN	PRE	% PRED
D$_{LCO}$ (ml/mm Hg/min)	16.5	**	4.4	27
D$_L$ Adj (ml/mm Hg/min)	16.5	**	4.5	27
D$_{LCO}$/V$_A$	6.41	**	4.85	76
V$_A$ (L)	**	**	0.91	**

FIGURE 8-12, cont'd   C, Data from a 10-year-old girl with systemic scleroderma. (See text for complete descriptions of each case.)

component, whereas others are consistent with obstruction. This pattern is the hallmark of a mixed obstructive and restrictive disorder. Scleroderma is a generalized disease that can cause shrinkage of any of the connective tissues in the body. When the lungs are affected, the disease initially presents as a restrictive disorder, but severe end-stage disease results in a "honeycomb lung" with obstruction in distal airways and air trapping.

Are lung volumes necessary? The cases in Figure 8-12, A and B, are straightforward presentations in which spirometry alone is very representative of the child's disease process. The lung volumes merely confirm the degree of airflow obstruction (see Figure 8-12, A) and lung restriction (see Figure 8-12, B). Mixed obstructive and restrictive disorders (see Figure 8-12, C) definitely require lung volume determination to better define the child's lung mechanics. It is not uncommon in the pediatric population to observe a seemingly restrictive spiro-

metric pattern with a proportional reduction in percent predicted FVC and FEV$_1$. However, subsequent lung volumes may identify a completely normal TLC, with an elevated RV/TLC. What appears to be a restrictive pattern on spirometry is, indeed, an obstructive disorder once lung volumes are examined. The relatively smaller size of the intrathoracic airways in the pediatric population leads to early obstruction in the peripheral airways. This may be compounded with mucus secretions in the airways or bronchoconstriction of these airways. With a forced expiration, distal airways are squeezed and occlude, resulting in significant air trapping.

Role of Measurement of Airway Resistance

Depending on the equipment and software being used, measurement of airway resistance during plethysmography may be an option. Airway resistance (Raw) is measured while having the patient pant before closing a shutter or valve to obtain the thoracic gas volume (V_{TG}). Patients, including children, have a tendency to pant at an elevated lung volume. In other words, they do not return to the resting expiratory level with every pant, and progressively increase their chest volume. If V_{TG} is measured at the very end of the maneuver, it will be artificially elevated. Although this is not the patient's true FRC, the application software makes a correction and reports separate values for V_{TG} and FRC. Raw should always be reported and interpreted at the lung volume at which it was measured (i.e., using V_{TG} to calculate specific airway resistance and specific conductance). Except in trained patients, Raw tends to be less reproducible than other pulmonary function parameters. Measurement of Raw complicates and prolongs the test and may not be necessary for routine testing. However, Raw can be significantly increased in patients with extrathoracic obstruction, central airway intrathoracic obstruction, and diffuse peripheral obstruction. Many laboratories find measurement of Raw, specific airway resistance (sRaw), and specific conductance (sGaw) helpful during methacholine challenges. Because the variability of these measurements is greater, a greater change is required to meet clinical significance. Whereas a decrease of 20% in FEV_1 is considered a positive response to methacholine, a corresponding increase of 35% – 40% in Raw is required. The measurement of Raw may be a more sensitive test and may identify changes in airflow earlier in the challenge.

DIFFUSION CAPACITY

The DLCO in the pediatric population can be an important indicator of gas transport difficulties at the alveolar level. This may be due to problems with perfusion of the pulmonary capillary bed, bleeding within the lung, or thickening of the alveolar-capillary membrane. Several serious pediatric disorders fall into these categories, and the DLCO may provide an answer to a very specific question. Examples of pediatric pulmonary diseases that may produce a reduced DLCO include pulmonary fibrosis (primary disease or secondary to radiation treatment or chemotherapy), immunologic disorders (scleroderma, systemic lupus erythematosus), bronchiolitis obliterans, pulmonary edema, and hematologic disorders. An abnormally high DLCO may be seen in acute hemorrhagenous bleeds, as in pulmonary vasculitis. The single-breath DLCO (DLCOsb) is the most common method used for assessing diffusion capacity. The problems already discussed in performing pulmonary function studies in the pediatric patient are compounded for this particular test. However, the guidelines and recommendations offered by the ATS/ERS for DLCO testing in adults are also applicable to pediatrics (see Chapter 5). Recent changes are not pediatric specific. The single-breath maneuver is difficult for very small children to perform and often requires several sessions of practice. Even older children may have difficulty accomplishing the important components of the DLCO maneuver. These components include emptying to RV before a deep inspiration, obtaining an IVC of at least 85% of FVC, a relaxed breath hold of 8 – 12 seconds, and a smooth, complete exhalation. In addition, other technical considerations may alter results, such as inappropriate mechanical or anatomic dead space corrections. Depending on the system used, if end-tidal gas is collected in a sample bag, the bag should be an appropriate size for pediatric patients. Similarly, if a demand value is used for inspiration of test gas, the triggering mechanism should be sensitive enough to be opened easily by a child. Some commercial systems also provide an option for a slow exhalation against a resistor instead of the breath hold. The advantage of this technique is that a breath hold is not necessary; however, a target flow for exhaled gas must be maintained. Unfortunately, children who cannot perform a breath hold are generally not able to perform this technique well.

Other confounders that alter the measurement of DLCO are abnormal levels or types of hemoglobin. Children who require repeated DLCO measurements may have conditions that cause anemia (e.g., chemotherapy, sickle cell disease, transplantations). Reduced circulating hemoglobin reduces the raw measurement of DLCO. Conversely, chronic hypoxemia may produce a secondary polycythemia that increases circulating hemoglobin and may increase the raw measurement of diffusion capacity. The presence of carboxyhemoglobin (COHb), methemoglobin (MetHb), or fetal hemoglobin will decrease the ability of hemoglobin to bind with carbon monoxide and reduce the diffusion capacity. It should not be assumed that pediatric patients do not smoke. Certainly teenagers should be asked if they smoke and told honestly that smoking may affect the results of the test. If the patient has been smoking before testing, a COHb level can be obtained to correct for carbon monoxide already present in the circulating blood. Correction of D_{LCO} for hemoglobin is an essential component in analyzing the diffusion capacity of the lung (see Chapter 5).

As with adults, diffusion capacity is dependent on the size of the lungs. An estimation of lung size known as the V_A (alveolar volume) is also made during the single-breath maneuver. In addition to carbon monoxide, the test gas also contains an inert gas such as helium, methane, or neon that is used to estimate V_A by a dilution method. The V_A can be compared with the TLC obtained by other methods, such as plethysmography, but should be a lesser value. Calculated V_A does not account for dead space ventilation as plethysmographic TLC measurements do. As with all gas dilution techniques, V_A will be increasingly underestimated as airflow obstruction worsens. Refer again to Figure 8-12. Recall that the patient discussed in Figure 8-12, *A*, is a young man with advanced cystic fibrosis. The raw D_{LCO} is reduced, but D_{LCO}/V_A is in the normal range. This patient's V_A is only 2.31 L as compared with the TLC of 4.83 L—more than 50% less. It is important to understand that the V_A will measure only lung volume with communicating airways (i.e., adequate ventilation). The ratio D_{LCO}/V_A also reflects diffusion capacity only in well-ventilated areas of the lung. Compare this to the patient with systemic scleroderma in Figure 8-12, *C*. The raw D_{LCO} is severely reduced, consistent with the diffusion block and fibrosis associated with scleroderma of the lung. Lung tissue less affected has a diffusion capacity within normal limits; thus the D_{LCO}/V_A is 76% predicted. The V_A of 0.91 L is closer

to the TLC value of 1.55 L, reflecting the primary restrictive component of her disease. In a purely restrictive disease, the V_A may come close to the TLC. Recall, however, that this patient also has ventilation defects.

Predictive or normative sets for the diffusion capacity in pediatrics are limited and based on small groups of children. This, unfortunately, makes interpretation of the diffusion capacity even more difficult in the pediatric population. Caution should be taken in interpreting all parameters of the diffusion capacity. Consideration should be given to the child's technique and the repeatability of the maneuvers, technical equipment limitations, and the normative sets used for comparison.

Other Measured and Clinically Followed Parameters of Pulmonary Function in Pediatrics

Maximal Respiratory Pressures

Measurement of muscle strength can be an important parameter in the pediatric population. Children have a variety of congenital and acquired neuromuscular disorders and thoracic deformities that reduce the strength of the diaphragm and intercostal muscles. Examples of neuromuscular diseases include, but are not limited to, muscular dystrophies, spinal muscle atrophy, meningomyeloceles, Guillain-Barré syndrome, myasthenia gravis, trauma-related paralysis, and steroid-induced myopathies. Thoracic deformities include scoliosis, kyphoscoliosis, pectus excavatum or carinatum, and undefined congenital syndrome abnormalities. Measuring maximal inspiratory pressure (MIP) and maximal expiratory pressure (MEP) may help (1) identify the degree of weakness and (2) follow the progression of the specific disorder. See Chapter 2 for a discussion of the technique for performing MIP and MEP. This test can be scary for children. The patient and parent should be gently warned that the measurement of the MIP might be uncomfortable and cause the child to cry. For this reason, this test should be performed after all other measurements are made. In children, it may be necessary to attach a mask and one-way valve to the pressure manometer and apply the mask snugly to the child's face. It may also be necessary to hold the mask in place until the child becomes "air hungry" and feels a need to gasp for air. It is understandable why this test is so unpopular with children. A similar measurement of spontaneous inspiratory strength may be made while a child is undergoing mechanical ventilation, and this parameter is often referred to as the negative inspiratory force (NIF). Although the measurement of inspiratory strength may ultimately be involuntary, the expiratory strength measurement (MEP) is completely effort dependent. The child cannot be forced to push as hard as possible unless he or she chooses to do so. For this reason, MEP results should be viewed cautiously. Although predicted values are available for MIP and MEP, a single measurement in time may be difficult to interpret. Rather, trending serial measurements often provides information that is more useful once the child is accustomed to the test.

Maximal Voluntary Ventilation

In a cooperative and inspired child, the maximal voluntary ventilation (MVV) can be a very useful measure of muscle strength, as well as maximal ventilation (see Chapter 2). If the child has significant muscle weakness, he or she may not be able to sustain maximal ventilation for the required 12 seconds. In this case, comparing the MVV for 6 seconds with that of 12 seconds may explain the disparity. The MVV may also be used before a maximal exercise test to identify the maximal level of ventilation of which the child is capable. Ventilatory limitation during exercise can be identified by comparing the minute ventilation at maximal O_2 consumption with the MVV obtained before exercise.

Arterial Blood Gases

An arterial blood gas is sometimes considered the most important measurement of pulmonary function. Regardless of what spirometry, lung volumes, or DLCO reveals, PaO_2 and $PaCO_2$ ultimately signify how well the lungs are performing. Arterial blood gases in children are, for obvious reasons, not popular. Pediatricians tend not to order blood gas analysis as frequently as physicians who treat adults because of the trauma of drawing arterial blood. Pulse oximetry can often be substituted for a blood gas for O_2 saturation and a capillary blood gas obtained for PCO_2. There are definite indications, however, for obtaining arterial blood gases. Examples are (1) impending ventilatory failure, (2) prior problem with anesthesia or sedation, and (3) impending thoracic surgery in a child unable to perform routine PFTs. Children tolerate arterial punctures much better with reassurance and local anesthesia at the puncture site. The use of topical lidocaine (4%)/prilocaine (EMLA) cream or subcutaneous lidocaine (1%) is extremely helpful.

INFANT, TODDLER, AND PRESCHOOL PULMONARY FUNCTION TESTING

The challenge for diagnostic testing in infants, toddlers and preschool children is their lack of comprehension of instruction. Even obtaining a value as simple as an oximetry reading may not be so simple in a crying young child or a wiggling baby. Toddlers may be capable of understanding simple instructions but can be fearful of the hospital environment, unfamiliar faces, or strange-looking equipment. Expecting full cooperation and maximal effort is unrealistic. Alternative methods of assessing pulmonary function have been developed. The ability to obtain forced flows and lung volume measurements remains the cornerstone of pulmonary function testing, even in the youngest patient. Modifications of technique and specialized equipment are necessary, however. Newer, less invasive methods of measuring tidal breathing mechanics, airway resistance, thoracoabdominal motion, **impedance,** and airway inflammation continue to be investigated and are promising techniques. Some of the techniques discussed in the following sections are available in clinical pediatric laboratories; however, other techniques are currently used primarily in the research arena. Clinical applications will be more apparent as experience and standardization of techniques are developed. Pediatric research trials grow in number yearly, and through these research trials the relevance of the following procedures will be validated.

Performance of Pulmonary Function Testing in Infants and Toddlers

Newborn babies, older infants, and young toddlers are not capable of following the directions needed to perform conscious PFTs. Placing a mask on an infant is usually not tolerated and results in a screaming baby. Even a child who permits a mask over his or her nose and mouth invariably changes his or her breathing pattern (i.e., volume and frequency of breathing). Only premature babies and young newborns will tolerate a mask while sleeping. In these specific and rare instances, it may be possible to assess passive tidal breathing mechanics. More sophisticated PFTs that measure lung volumes and forced flows require the infant to be in a quiet sleep, fully relaxed, and spontaneously breathing. To accomplish this state of sleep and cooperation, the child must be sedated.

Purpose of Pulmonary Function Tests for Infants and Toddlers

Infant and toddler PFTs provide important data regarding growth of the lungs, identification of airflow obstruction, progression of a disease state, and response to therapeutic interventions. Infant PFTs require a significant time commitment and competent and patient technologists. Sedation carries some risk, and testing should not be viewed as routine. Commercially available equipment typically uses the most technically advanced flow sensors and analyzers and may be expensive for a pulmonary laboratory to purchase. Before pursuing this type of testing, the laboratory should thoroughly evaluate its expectations, goals, and resources available to perform quality testing.

Sedation as an Important Consideration

Sedation of infants and toddlers is a common practice in pediatric hospitals because many procedures require a calm, motionless child. Procedures and protocols for sedation of children that follow The Joint Commission (TJC) guidelines are usually established by the hospital anesthesia department (see Appendix D). It is essential that established procedures be closely observed for the protection of the child, the pulmonary laboratory, and the hospital. The sedating agent chosen, the personnel needed, and the required recovery time all depend on the extent of testing needed and patient history. A straightforward test in an uncomplicated infant can be safely performed by minimal personnel with the use of an oral sedating agent, such as chloral hydrate. At the other end of the spectrum may be an infant with an unstable airway, severe pulmonary compromise, or other organ complications. This scenario may warrant an anesthesiologist and sedation nurse in addition to the technologist(s) performing the study.

Chloral hydrate is a relatively safe and easy sedating medication to administer, although several other IV agents are available with the current armamentarium of drugs. The advantages of chloral hydrate are that it is usually administered orally and may not require a "sedation team." A dose of 75–100 mg/kg of chloral hydrate is usually sufficient to provide a sedation time long enough to complete the study. If a child sleeps well during this sedation, he or she arouses easily by the end of the study. The major disadvantage is that a large dose of a very unpleasant medicine must be swallowed. A rectal suppository is available, but its absorption is quite variable. The oral dose sedation may cause vomiting, crying, and upset stomachs. Nevertheless, chloral hydrate works very well in the majority of cases.

Intravenous (IV) narcotics such as pentobarbital or secobarbital need to administered and monitored by a sedation nurse. The advantage of IV medications is that IV access is available if needed, and the medication can be titrated to the child's need. Additional options include ketamine and propofol. Both of these drugs require a physician and possibly an anesthesiologist or hospitalist to administer. The rapid onset of action and quick recovery make these attractive sedating agents but also require close monitoring for apnea. Regardless of the agent chosen, safety is the primary concern. The child must be closely monitored throughout the entire procedure, including recovery, and written documentation of the sedation procedure placed in the patient's record. A fully stocked crash cart should be nearby, and a resuscitation bag and mask should be on the patient's bed. Loss of a patent airway is always possible with any sedating agent. It is also extremely important to remember that sleep induced with sedation is not natural sleep. Changes in respiratory pattern, depth of respiration, and breathing rate should be noted. Interpretation of any test of respiratory mechanics should be made with the level of sedation in mind.

PF TIP

Sedated sleep in infants is *never* natural sleep, and respiratory measurements made during sedated sleep may be influenced by the altered sleep state.

When Children Are Too Old for Infant-Style Testing and Too Young for Standard Testing

Once toddlers reach ages 2.5–3 years, changes are occurring that make it more difficult to perform the infant-style PFTs. The most obvious is that child may "outgrow" the size of the plethysmograph. Chloral hydrate sedation may no longer be an option, therefore requiring general anesthesia. IV sedatives (narcotics, ketamine, propofol) carry more risks, and the expense of additional personnel to deliver more complicated sedations increase. The risk to benefit ratio may tip in the direction that the benefits of the test no longer outweigh the risks and cost of sedation. Physiologic changes are also occurring as the infant grows through the toddler and preschool years. The child's chest wall becomes more rigid, and the Hering-Breuer reflex disappears.

This makes several of the techniques discussed in the following sections available only to infants and small toddlers but unavailable to children in the 3-year-old to 5-year-old range. Very young children also may be able to tolerate simple passive mechanics without the need for sedation. Earlier in this chapter, spirometric measurements in young children were discussed. The following sections discuss several other available techniques to measure pulmonary mechanics. Some may be performed on any patient from infancy through adulthood, and some are developed specifically for infants, toddlers, and preschool children.

Lung Volume Measurement

As with measurement of lung volumes in adults, the lung volume compartments in the infant can be measured by several techniques, including gas dilution and whole-body plethysmography. Until recently, body plethysmography in infants was performed almost exclusively by infant pulmonary research laboratories. Only a few manufacturers produce commercially available body boxes for infants (Figure 8-13). Whole-body plethysmography in an infant presents a unique set of challenges. The theory and technical aspects of measuring V_{TG}, previously discussed in Chapter 3, are essentially the same for adults and infants but with several additional caveats. The sedated infant is placed in a supine position with nose and mouth surrounded by a tight-fitting mask with a small dead space volume. Rapidly moving valves may make airway occlusions at end-inspiration or end-expiration for determination of V_{TG} and Raw. The infant does not pant. However, tidal breaths may be shallow; therefore the pressure transducers and flow sensors must be critically precise and accurate. In addition, the infant body box is relatively small, and temperature changes can drastically alter these measurements. Therefore the temperature in the box must be controlled and the air vented. Signal-to-noise ratios are particularly critical in an infant plethysmograph. Although the child is motionless, safety features must permit rapid access to the box and the baby. The breathing apparatus should be easily remov-

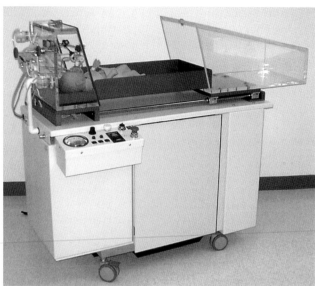

FIGURE 8-13 Infant Pulmonary Lab (IPL). Whole-body infant plethysmograph directly measures V_{TG} (FRC at resting level). The IPL also has the capability of obtaining passive mechanics and forced flows (partial and raised volume), and provides close estimation of fractional lung volumes. *(Courtesy Collins Medical [nSpire Health], Louisville, Colo.)*

able in case the child is in distress or vomits. The advantage of plethysmography in infants is that it accurately measures V_{TG}, and thus FRC may be determined. Because the infant is not capable of performing a voluntary maximal inspiration or expiration, residual volume and TLC cannot be obtained in the traditional manner. However, if the infant pulmonary function system is capable of performing raised volumes and forced thoracic compressions, then a full set of fractional lung volumes can be estimated. A forced squeeze from TLC provides a volume close to a vital capacity measurement and can be used to calculate ERV, RV, TLC, FRC/TLC, and RV/TLC.

Optional methods of determining lung volumes are available for infants, as well as toddlers and young children. These include gas equilibration techniques such as helium dilution, nitrogen washout, and SF_6 (sulfur hexafluoride) wash-in/washout techniques. Although technically easy to perform, gas equilibration techniques have several disadvantages applicable to both infants and young children. Infants will still require sedation; however, children ages 3–4 years may tolerate sitting in a chair with a mouthpiece/nose clips or facemask applied. Distractions to the awake child, such as television, reading by parent, or videos, are often necessary to obtain a quality test. Fussing and move-ment leads to leaks in the systems and may falsely elevate FRC values. When possible and practical, facemasks should be sealed with therapeutic putty. Dead space from the mask and valve switching apparatus should be taken into consideration. Adequate inspiratory flow with an appropriate inspired O_2 concentration should be available to the patient. Children with intrathoracic airflow obstruction may have poor ventilation distal to obstructed airways, causing an incomplete washout or equilibration and falsely low FRC values. The smaller the child, the smaller the radius of the airways, and superimposed obstruction from secretions or bronchospasm will further narrow the airway.

The effect of sedation in infants may compound the problem and inhibit the natural sigh mechanism, resulting in atelectasis, hypoventilation, or hypoxemia. Monitoring end-tidal CO_2 is helpful in this regard. Infants do have an incredible ability to adjust their FRC depending on their clinical status. Babies may respond to hypoxia by dynamically elevating their FRC to create a PEEP-like effect (**dynamic FRC**). Grunting is a clinical sign that an infant may be hypoxic. In this situation, further sedation and supplemental O_2 tend to relax a child. It is possible to see consecutive FRC measurements decrease as the infant falls into a deeper sedation and static lung volume decreases to a resting FRC.

Nevertheless, measurement of FRC is an important parameter in pulmonary function testing. The preceding clinical scenarios should, however, be taken into account. The normal FRC range for an infant is between 15 and 25 ml/kg of weight and 2–3 ml/cm of length. FRC serves as a reference lung volume when analyzing flows or compliance. When a parameter is referenced to a lung volume such as FRC, it is termed *specific* (e.g., specific flow at FRC, specific compliance, or specific resistance).

Passive Tidal Techniques to Measure Respiratory Mechanics

Passive Tidal Loops

Many studies have examined the passive tidal loops of infants and have attempted to differentiate normal tidal loops from loops associated with airflow obstruction. Fewer studies have concentrated on passive mechanics in preschool-aged children. Several parameters have been suggested to examine intrathoracic airflow obstruction during tidal breathing, such as t_{TPEF}/t_E (ratio of time to reach tidal peak flow to total expiratory time) and V_{PTEF}/V_E. Even recording simple measures such as tidal volume, respiratory rate, and minute ventilation may have some benefit. Passive loops are highly variable, however, and the degree of variability may differ for different age groups. They are especially subject to changes in upper airway tone, as may be seen with sedation, or with laryngeal or diaphragmatic **braking.** As mentioned previously, infants can adduct their vocal cords (grunt) during exhalation to create a physiologic PEEP. Likewise, they have the ability to modulate their diaphragms and intercostal muscles in an attempt to dynamically elevate their FRC and improve oxygenation. Therefore, the shape of tidal loops, and the parameters used to describe the shape may change from minute to minute. To assure repeatability of measures, it is advisable to express these parameters as a mean of at least 10 consecutive breaths, or at least 30 seconds of tidal breathing. The coefficient of variation should also be reported. Baseline passive measurements may then be compared to like parameters following any desired intervention (bronchodilator, for example). As with standard pulmonary function testing, passive tidal loops are not maximal maneuvers. Therefore, efforts have concentrated on techniques to identify flow limitation and quantify forced flows measurements.

Passive Compliance, Resistance, and Time Constants

The chest wall of the infant is extremely compliant, unlike that of an adult. It does not contribute significantly to the compliance of the total respiratory system. Measuring pulmonary mechanics in the infant takes advantage of this very important difference. Noninvasive measures of respiratory system compliance, therefore, directly reflect the child's lung compliance. In simplest terms, compliance is defined as change in volume divided by change in pressure ($C = \Delta V/\Delta P$) (see Chapter 2). In a quiet, relaxed baby (usually sedated), these parameters can be measured easily. The method is referred to as the **passive occlusion technique.** Rapid occlusion of the airway may occur once (single occlusion) at the end of a tidal breath, or with multiple occlusions at different lung volumes. Young infants will hold their breath when their airway is occluded. This phenomenon is known as the **Hering-Breuer reflex** and is present in children until approximately 1 year of age. During a single-breath occlusion and breath hold, alveolar pressure equalizes and can be measured by a pressure transducer at the airway opening (mouth). Once the occlusion valve opens, the child can passively exhale, and the exhaled volume can be measured by a flow sensor. The two components of **respiratory system compliance (Crs),** change in pressure and change in volume, are obtained. Respiratory system resistance (Rrs) can be easily calculated from the same maneuver. Resistance is defined as change in driving pressure divided by flow ($R = \Delta P/\dot{V}$). With the maneuver described, the driving pressure is the plateau pressure (alveolar pressure) measured at the airway opening developed during the occlusion. Flow is the peak flow (discounting pneumotach artifact) measured from the passive exhalation. Refer to Figure 8-14. The graphs on the left side of the page

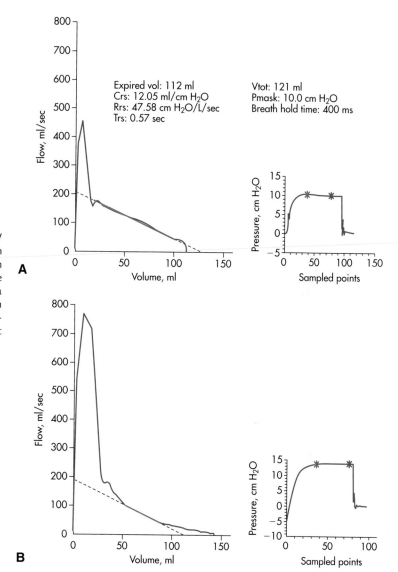

FIGURE 8-14 **Passive Occlusion/ Exhalation Mechanics in Infants. A,** An infant's passive tidal exhalation after an airway occlusion. The slope of the curve is linear, and the infant exhales to a relaxed FRC. **B,** Passive tidal exhalation showing lungs with multiple time constants, meaning that the lung does not empty homogeneously (see text).

represent passive exhalation after occlusion. The graphs on the right depict the increase in airway opening pressure to plateau (alveolar) pressure during occlusion. A normal passive exhalation after occlusion in an infant without any lung disease is shown in Figure 8-14, A.

The slope of the curve is linear as the baby exhales to a relaxed FRC. Children with airflow obstruction do not empty their lungs at a constant rate. The expiration may be forced with paradoxical movement of the diaphragm and belly. The accuracy of compliance and airway resistance measurements made under these conditions is poor. The exhaled curve may end abruptly with the child at an elevated FRC or may appear "scooped out" or curvilinear, as in Figure 8-14, B. The lungs do not empty homogeneously or uniformly and therefore have multiple time constants. One **time constant** represents the amount of time to expire approximately $2/3$ of the tidal volume. Time constant (TRS or τ) is easily calculated as compliance times resistance ($Trs = Crs \times Rrs$). Because respiratory system compliance is dependent on the lung volume at which it is measured, it may be important to "correct" the measured parameter by the infant's FRC. As mentioned earlier, dividing the raw or actual compliance by the FRC yields specific compliance.

PF TIP

Diameter of the airway is an important determinant of flow. Inflammation or secretions in the airways of a young child can cause significant intrathoracic obstruction and profound clinical symptoms.

Single-breath passive measurement of compliance is not feasible in the toddler and older age groups. The chest wall develops more rigidity as the child ages and becomes an increasingly important factor in the overall measure of respiratory system compliance. Additionally, loss of the Hering-Breuer reflex makes equilibration of pressure from the alveolus to the mouth more difficult to achieve.

Compliance in infants can also be determined by other methods, including insertion of an esophageal catheter or by weighted spirometry. Although inserting an esophageal catheter into an infant is usually not difficult, it is invasive, and the exact placement of the catheter may affect measurements. In addition, distortion of pleural pressure in children with airflow obstruction causes associated artifactual changes, yielding inaccurate compliance values. Under ideal circumstances, when accurate pleural pressures are measured, total respiratory system compliance can be subdivided into the chest wall and lung compliance components.

Children undergoing intubation and ventilation represent an additional challenge when assessing pulmonary mechanics. Several of the parameters discussed can also be obtained in babies on ventilators; however, several technical and mechanical problems must be considered. The endotracheal tube represents a resistor and can limit flow and alter pressure readings at the airway opening. Endotracheal tubes in infants are generally uncuffed, and leaks around the tubes are common. Secretions in the endotracheal tube and water condensation in the tubing easily clog pneumotachometers. Ventilators offer a variety of operational modes, such as pressure or volume control, intermittent mandatory ventilation (IMV) or synchronized IMV (SIMV), and pressure support. Depending on the mode chosen, auxiliary flow through the ventilator circuit will result in inaccurate flow measurements at the child's airway. Children on ventilators are often sedated, and passive mechanics are dependent on the sleep state. For all the reasons stated, pulmonary mechanics on children undergoing ventilation should only be done by experienced technologists who are familiar with the child and the ventilator. In addition, measurements made under artificial conditions (e.g., ventilator, PEEP) do not necessary reflect the infant's own lung mechanics when not ventilated.

Thoracoabdominal Motion Analysis

One of the main disadvantages of all the measurements discussed in the preceding sections is that they involve the use of a mask or mouthpiece. Unfortunately, the presence of any foreign body in the airway is invasive and can alter breathing, especially passive tidal breathing. An advantage to this next technique is that it does not use any device at the mouth and can be truly considered noninvasive. Although the following techniques are not commonly performed in many clinical pediatric pulmonary function laboratories, they are central to the measurements made in a sleep laboratory. Observing the motion of the respiratory system can also provide valuable qualitative and quantitative assessment of pulmonary and chest wall mechanics and are worthy of discussion. Recall the basic mechanics of breathing, and the coordination of the diaphragm and respiratory muscles during the passive breathing cycle. During inspiration, the diaphragm contracts and flattens, which causes the abdomen to rise. Simultaneously, the intercostal muscles contract, pulling the ribs upward and forward. During passive expiration, the diaphragm and intercostal muscles relax, and the abdomen and chest fall. This synchronous movement of the abdomen and rib cage can be easily monitored by placing an expandable strain gauge or band around both the abdomen and the chest wall (rib cage). These devices differ as to how they are made and the method by which they make measurements. Although the devices differ, the principle is similar. This technique is not generally limited by size or age; therefore it can apply to infants, toddlers, older children, and even adults. The length of the strain gauges or bands are appropriate for the size of the patient. A popular example of this method is known as **respiratory inductive plethysmography (RIP).** The band is elasticized and has coiled wire sewn through the band in a sinusoidal pattern. A very low-voltage alternating current is passed through the coils. As each band expands (as with inspiration), the coils are stretched, which alters the cross-sectional area of the bands and changes the inductance of the coiled wire. A positive voltage signal (upward deflection) can be visualized on the monitoring devise for both the abdominal component and rib cage component (see Figure 8-15, A). The change in the cross-sectional area is proportional to the expansion of the band, and therefore the depth of the inspiratory maneuver. As passive exhalation occurs, the bands relax, and the voltage signal drops (downward deflection), with the pattern producing a sinusoidal respiratory tracing. The movement of the rib cage (RC) and the abdomen (AB) are monitored simultaneously. Both components independently contribute to lung volume, and the sum of the two signals determines tidal volume (V_T).

The tidal volume is maximized when the rib cage and abdomen move in synchrony, or are "in phase" with one another. The phase shift, Φ or phi, describes the **asynchrony** (or lack of synchrony) of the sinusoidal relationship between these two independent components. Both qualitative and quantitative information can be obtained from these tracings. A phase shift equal to 0° denotes perfect synchrony. Figure 8-15, A, is representative of normal, quiet breathing. The movement of the rib cage and abdomen are in complete unison or synchrony. The child's resultant tidal volume is the sum of the components of rib cage and abdominal movement. Figure 8-15, B, represents a child with paradoxical breathing. Note that the rib cage tracing is moving in the opposite direction of the abdomen.

The abdominal and rib cage components are out of phase with one another. If observing this child, one would see the abdomen appear to sink while the chest was rising. This is the extreme end of asynchrony; however, there are endless variations in movement of the rib cage and abdomen between complete synchrony and asynchrony. The phase shift will increase from 0° to a maximum of 180° with complete paradoxical breathing. Refer to Figure 8-15, C. Notice the difference in the shape of the tracing of the abdominal component. There is asynchronous movement of the rib cage and abdomen in this child.

Phase shift, Φ, can also be represented on an X-Y recorder. The figures produced, known as Lissajous figures or Konno-Mead loops, graphically plot abdominal movement on the x-axis, and rib cage movement on the y-axis. The arrows on the figures represent the direction of movement of the rib cage and abdomen during the respiratory cycle. Refer back to the tracing in Figure 8-15, A. Perfect synchrony would produce a loop that appears to be a straight line oriented as depicted ($\Phi = 0°$). Figure 8-15, B, is representative of a Konno-Mead loop that demonstrates paradoxical breathing. The phase shift for this loop is 153°, approaching the maximum of 180°. The tracing in Figure 8-15, C, represents an interesting Konno-Mead loop, as one can imagine from the asynchronous movement of the rib cage and abdomen. Notice that the figure is vertical and forms a figure 8. Unfortunately, Konno-Mead loops often form figure-8 patterns, which cannot be assigned a quantitative phi value. There is also significant variation in the shape of Konno-Mead loops and phi values in patients with normal and abnormal breathing patterns. The limitations of quantifying these loops make it impractical for clinical testing in a pulmonary function laboratory. Nevertheless, there is a wealth of physiologic information in these measurements, and they are a valuable tool in illustrating the relationship of rib cage movement to abdominal movement.

An important advantage to respiratory inductance plethysmography is that it is possible to calibrate the movement of the bands in quiet breathing to a flow signal from a pneumotachometer placed over the patient's mouth. This enables quantitative

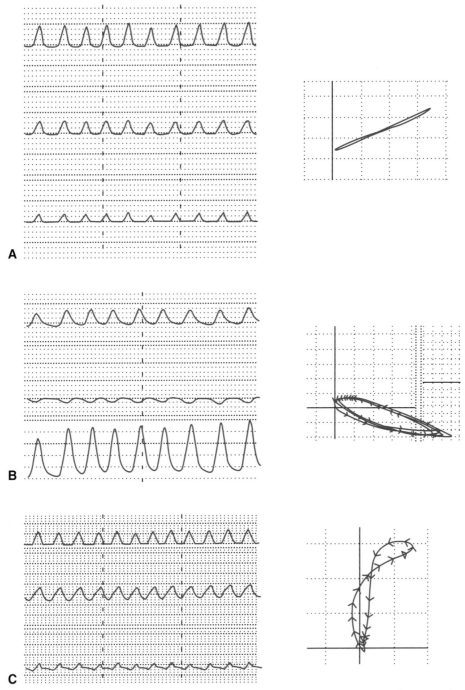

FIGURE 8-15   **Respiratory Inductive Plethysmography (RIP).** Respiratory tracings demonstrating the signals from the rib cage (RC), abdomen (AB), and sum V_T (tidal volume). Accompanying each set of tracing is the corresponding Konno-Mead loop for **A,** Normal tidal breathing, **B,** Paradoxical breathing, **C,** Asynchronous breathing and figure-8 Konno-Mead loop (see text).

measurement of tidal volumes or minute ventilation over an extended period. The calibration period is very short, and the pneumotach is removed after the calibration period.

Additional Passive Techniques Available to Measure in the Preschool Child

Impulse Oscillometry

Impulse oscillometry (IOS) is also referred to as the **forced oscillation technique (FOT).** See Chapter 9 for a detailed description. A miniature loudspeaker is placed proximal to the device's flow sensor and produces forced oscillations of flow with a range of frequencies into the airway. They are sensed as popping pulsations as the child breathes tidally. The pressure oscillations generated by the sound waves are of two types: (1) those in phase with airflow, termed *resistance* (Rrs), and (2) those out of phase with airflow, termed **reactance (Xrs).** The reactance component is complex and relates to delays of pressure change due to elastic components of the respiratory system, as well as inertia. The interaction of resistance and reactance constitutes respiratory impedance (Zrs = Rrs + Xrs).

The advantage of impulse oscillometry (IOS) is that it requires only passive tidal breathing.

The patient is asked to breathe on a mouthpiece for approximately 30–60 seconds; however, only 15–20 seconds of stable data are required. Although it is often stated that IOS is a relatively easy test to perform, even for a small child, this is not necessarily the case. The child must sit *still* with a mouthpiece in their mouth and nose clips in place. The patient's cheeks and floor of the mouth are supported by the technician's (or parent's) hands to prevent oscillations of the mouth. Gagging, swallowing, or coughing will interfere with accurate measurements. The tongue cannot move around or obstruct the mouthpiece. This can be a challenge in a 2-year-old or 3-year-old child, even for technicians experienced working with children. Often, several visits to the laboratory for practice are necessary to obtain repeatability in these very young children. Three to five trials should be collected with a mean and coefficient of variation reported. IOS should be performed before any spirometric maneuvers because the forced expirations may produce airway hyperreactivity. Several minutes should also be given between trials to allow the child to relax.

Refer to Figure 8-16 for an example of the types of graphs that IOS measurements produce. Notice there is a graph for resistance (Rrs) measurements and reactance (Xrs) measurements. In both graphs, however, the x-axis is labeled as Hz representing the multifrequency band of forced oscillations being

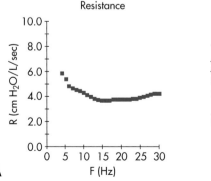
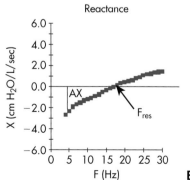

FIGURE 8-16   Impulse Oscillometry (IOS). Normal resistance and reactance tracings from a 12-year-old boy. **A,** Note the frequency dependence of the resistance curve. **B,** On the reactance curve, AX represents the area of the triangle depicted. F_{res} is the resonant frequency of the lung (see text).

emitted by the loudspeaker. Note in Figure 8-16 that the resistance in this 12-year-old child's lung is higher at lower frequencies and falls as the frequency of oscillations increase. This phenomenon is known as frequency dependence and is a characteristic pattern for a child this age. In an adult, however, this would not be normal, but more characteristic of peripheral airflow obstruction, as seen in a smoker. Caution is needed, however, in viewing resistance measurements at very low frequencies (e.g., 5 Hz) in children because of other confounding factors, such as the effect of the cardiac impulse on these measurements. Reactance measurements are even less understood. Researchers are interested in the area of the curve that is formed by the reactance curve at 5 Hz and where it crosses "zero" reactance. The triangular region highlighted in the figure is known as AX. The larger the area of this region, the more abnormal the measurement, which may be related to airflow limitation. The point (Hz) that the reactance curve crosses the zero line is known as the **resonant frequency** of the lung (F_{res}). Since reactance as this point equals zero, only resistive forces are active and contributing to impedance. The resonant frequency (F_{res}) depicted in Figure 8-16 is approximately 18 Hz.

Reference values for **impulse oscillometry** have been collected in European children, and several ongoing studies in the United States are collecting data for additional predictive purposes. The clinical significance of IOS is yet unclear. Some researchers think that it will not provide any additional information, especially regarding peripheral airflow obstruction, for children who can be trained to do spirometry. However, there may be several scenarios in which IOS is beneficial. It may be helpful for any child who cannot perform spirometry or has a significant degree of central airway malacia. Forced flows, as with spirometry, cause compression and collapse in malacic airways, whereas IOS is a passive, tidal breathing maneuver. Patients may be able to serve as their own controls and perform this procedure serially at every clinic visit. Some laboratories have performed methacholine challenges with changes in IOS parameters as the end point. The sensitivity of this test may be greater than that of the FEV_1, especially with methacholine challenges, although its variability is somewhat greater.

Interrupter Technique (Rint)

The **interrupter technique (Rint)** is another method of measuring airway resistance in the very young child. It also involves passive tidal breathing, but as the name implies, the respiratory cycle is "interrupted" during the respiratory cycle multiple times. The child is seated in a position similar to IOS, with the neck slightly extended ("sniffing" position). The cheeks are supported by a technician or parent and nose clips are in place. While the child is quietly breathing, flow is measured, and an interrupter valve closes rapidly at a preset flow or volume trigger. The value remains closed for only 100 msec, so the child is barely able to feel these occlusions but can hear the valve closing. The principle of operation assumes a rapid equilibration of mouth pressure and alveolar pressure as the occlusions occur. Each measurement is calculated by dividing the driving pressure by the flow rate immediately before the occlusion. However, as with many physiologic measurements, other factors come into play. The resistance of the chest wall and the tissues of the lung are included in Rint measurements, so the results are not purely airway resistance. Rint measurements may be obtained during either inspiration or expiration, but it is still unclear if a difference is significant. This technique has been used extensively in Europe for a considerable time but has remained primarily a research technique in the United States and abroad. Commercial devices are now available; however, predicted values are lacking in preschool children. The popularity of Rint will likely increase if the technique can show a clear clinical advantage in the pediatric population. Studies are ongoing as to the intersubject and intrasubject repeatability and reproducibility of Rint. As with IOS, this technique may serve as a clinical adjunct in assessing bronchodilator response or with inhalation challenge protocols.

Exhaled Nitric Oxide and Nasal Nitric Oxide

Measurement of **exhaled nitric oxide (eNO)** through the mouth and nasal nitric oxide are techniques now used in children. This procedure is an attractive alternative in the pediatric population because it does not involve any forced mechanics and is relatively simple to accomplish. The child is asked to take a single maximal breath in, followed by a prolonged exhalation through a restricted orifice in the mouth. Alternately, nasal nitric oxide is measured from exhaled air through the nasal passage. Abnormally low values of nasal nitric oxide are found in children with primary ciliary dyskinesia (PCD). Nitric oxide (NO) is a normally occurring substance found in reproducible levels in exhaled air. Levels of NO have been shown to significantly increase from tissues that are inflamed. The measurement of eNO has therefore been proposed as an index of airway inflammation, such as occurs in asthma. The clinical use of eNO, as well as nasal NO, in the pediatric population is still under investigation. As with IOS and Rint, eNO may be an important adjunct to serially follow asthma exacerbations in children and the effects of various drug regimens to control these exacerbations. Several limitations to this technique need to be addressed, including collection of normative data and standardization of technique. A comprehensive discussion of eNO measurements can be found in Chapter 9.

Forced Flow Techniques for Infants, Toddlers, and Preschool Children

Partial Expiratory Flow–Volume Curves

Flow is related to the volume of air in the chest during the forced exhalation. Stated simply, the larger the volume, the faster the flow. The advantage and reason for the repeatability of spirometry is that it is performed from TLC with every maneuver. As discussed earlier, with training sessions and reasonable patient effort, exhaled flows and volumes are repeatable in young children. However, if the child does not understand or cannot inhale to TLC, significant variability in flows and volumes will be observed. This is a common obstacle in the youngest of children. Traditional spirometric measurements (FVC, FEV$_1$, PEFR) may not be repeatable. These forced flows are not without merit, however. It is possible to relate these flows to a lung volume

that the child can reproduce. This can be accomplished if the child is able to breathe quietly and relaxed for several breaths. More important, if he or she returns to a stable resting level with each exhalation, then this relaxed resting level represents the child's FRC. It is not necessary to measure FRC; rather, it represents a reference point (static lung volume) to which flow can then be related. After several tidal breaths, the child is asked to take a slightly deeper breath in and blow out as hard and long as possible. It does not matter how deep the breath is, but the forced exhalation has to extend beyond the FRC point from the previous tidal breaths. Once the FRC point is identified, the flow corresponding to that point is then recorded. Because FRC is approximately 40% of TLC, flows at this relatively low lung volume correspond to flows such as FEF$_{25\%-75\%}$, FEF$_{50\%}$, and FEF$_{75\%}$ seen in standard spirometry. These flow rates are only as repeatable as the resting level FRC. The technique may be of value in a cooperative child when assessing response to bronchodilator therapy or performing a methacholine challenge, for example. If the child's tidal loops are highly variable, a stable FRC cannot be identified. The corresponding flow at FRC will not be reproducible in such instances. An additional confounding factor is the lack of predicted values for partial forced flows in the toddler age range. Because of the variability in testing, the trend has been to begin training in very young children (age 3 years) to do full FVC maneuvers from TLC or traditional spirometry.

From a historic perspective, the technique of performing partial forced F-V curves was the first attempt at obtaining forced flows in infants and dates back to the late 1970s and the work of several notable respiratory physiologists. This technique is increasing being replaced by measuring maximal forced flows from a raised lung volume close to TLC. The principle of the partial forced flows is similar to that described previously, but the infant must be sedated for complete relaxation. The child's chest is mechanically squeezed (or "hugged") by an inflatable jacket that surrounds the chest or a bladder placed over the chest and upper abdominal region. The technique is referred to as **rapid thoracoabdominal compression (RTC).** The flows that are generated are maximal flows from within tidal range (partial forced expiratory flow). They are measured by a flow sensor (usually a pneumotachometer) attached to a mask placed on the infant's face. The lung volume that can be identified and referenced is the FRC. This is the resting level that the child passively exhales to with each tidal breath. Once the FRC point is identified on the y-axis (volume), a line can be drawn upward to intersect the F-V loop. The flow as this point is referred to as the flow at FRC or V̇max FRC. Figure 8-17 identifies these points.

It is important that several tidal loops are observed before the hugging maneuver to ensure that the infant returns with each breath to a stable resting level, or FRC. The RTCs are done at progressively higher pressures until maximal flow at FRC from the child is attained. The pressures are generated from a large air reservoir connected to the hugging bag. The pressure within the hugging bag usually does not exceed 100 cm H_2O. A significantly lower pressure is transmitted across the chest wall to the lung tissue. With progressively higher hugging pressures, flow at FRC increases until flow limitation is reached. At this point, higher hugging pressures do not yield higher flows, and flow at FRC may in fact decrease. Reaching flow limitation while doing these maneuvers is an important concept and is somewhat controversial. Because infants grow (length and weight) at such different rates and because males differ from females, the question of whether flow limitation is achieved with partial forced flows often arises. This question is especially difficult in infants with normal lung function. The problem is complicated when trying to identify normal flows for any particular child. Several infant research centers have published a collaborative study combining data from healthy infants, but technique-related differences still exist. It is recommended that PFT laboratories performing infant studies test a group of infants without respiratory difficulties to confirm that the normal values obtained concur with published reference norms. Although this type of comparison is desirable, some hospital internal review boards may not permit sedation of infants for collection of normative data. Another method of standardizing flow is to compare maximal flow at FRC with the actual FRC measured. This parameter is known as the specific flow at FRC (SV̇maxFRC or V̇maxFRC/FRC). As discussed earlier, FRC serves as a static measured reference volume. Because flow increases with higher volumes, a fixed relationship or constant value, independent of age or height, can be determined for flow at that volume. This constant value is termed *specific flow,* and normal specific flow should equal or exceed 1.20.

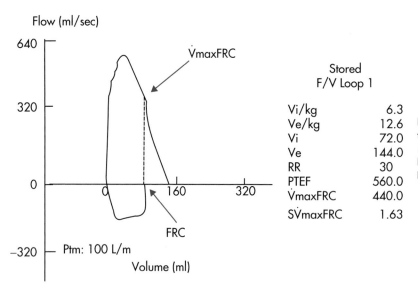

Stored F/V Loop 1	
Vi/kg	6.3
Ve/kg	12.6
Vi	72.0
Ve	144.0
RR	30
PTEF	560.0
V̇maxFRC	440.0
SV̇maxFRC	1.63

FIGURE 8-17 Partial Expiratory Forced F-V Loop in an Infant. Measurements include a V̇max FRC of 440 ml/sec and an SV̇max FRC of 1.63 (see text).

Figure 8-17 shows a partial forced expiratory flow-volume curve from an infant. A rapid thoracoabdominal compression was performed after a tidal inspiration. Parameters measured include a VmaxFRC of 440 ml/sec and an SVmaxFRC of 1.63. The specific flow at FRC was obtained by dividing the child's VmaxFRC of 440 ml/sec by a previously measured FRC of 270 ml (from nitrogen washout).

Forced Flows from Raised Lung Volume

Success in standardization of spirometry has been dependent on the patient inspiring to total lung capacity (TLC) before performing a maximal expiration. This is the key to standardization in infants as well. Techniques have been developed to *r*aise the *v*olume of the infant's lungs before a *r*apid *t*horacoabdominal *c*ompression (RVRTC). This may be accomplished by stacking inspirations or by a method known as the **raised volume technique.** For this maneuver, a bias flow of air is provided to the child during inspiration. The exhalation port is simultaneously occluded, raising the intrathoracic pressure and volume in the child's lungs. A pressure of +30 cm H_2O is required to inflate the infant's lung to near TLC. Once inflated, the child is then permitted to passively exhale. After several cycles of inflation and deflation, the child's PCO_2 decreases, relaxing the child further. The final inflation is then followed by a forced compression from the inflatable jacket. The maneuver is repeated at increasingly higher jacket pressure until expired volume and flows at mid–lung volumes maximize. The advantage of this method compared with partial forced flows is that the expired volume is nearly an FVC

measurement. The traditional FEV_1 is not measured because the infant reaches residual volume before 1 second of exhalation occurs. However, the volume expired in 0.5 seconds or 0.75 seconds can be calculated and is analogous to the FEV_1 in standard spirometry. Figure 8-18 shows several F-V curves obtained after rapid thoracic compressions (from raised lung volume) superimposed. Progressively higher squeeze pressures do not yield higher flows or volumes, indicating that flow limitation has been met. In addition, a partial F-V curve (from a lower lung volume) is superimposed on the diagram. The F-V curve in this example is from a child with normal lung function. Compare this to the F-V loop pictured in Figure 8-19. This infant PFT report is representative of a 1-year-old child with cystic fibrosis and mild intrathoracic airflow obstruction.

Note that the report resembles that of a standard PFT for an older child, except that the FEV_1 is replaced with the $FEV_{0.5}$. Although the FVC, $FEV_{0.5}$, and $FEV_{0.5}/FVC$ are within normal percent predicted range, the flows from lower lung volumes (i.e., FEF_{75} and FEF_{85}) are reduced. TLC and FRC are within percent predicted values. The RV and RV/TLC are mildly elevated, consistent with mild air trapping. Also note that the values for forced flows may be represented as a "Z" score. This is a statistical method comparing test results to normative data that is growing in popularity in the pediatric pulmonary function world and is now recommended by the ATS/ERS focus group for infants and preschool children. It is thought that Z scores more accurately reflect normative data in pediatrics because of varying growth rates for age and sex differences. Refer to Appendix G for a discussion of means, standard deviation, and confidence ranges. One standard deviation equals "1" Z score. Two (+/−) standard deviations from the mean, in a positive or negative direction, is generally considered to be within the limits of normal, or the 95% confidence range. This would be represented by a Z score of +/− 2.0. Refer again to Figure 8-19 and notice that the parameters that have normal percent predicted values also have Z scores close to zero. The FEF_{75} and FEF_{85}, however, have reduced percent predicted values, and their Z scores are greater than −2.0, both indicative of values outside of the normal range.

Overlay loops

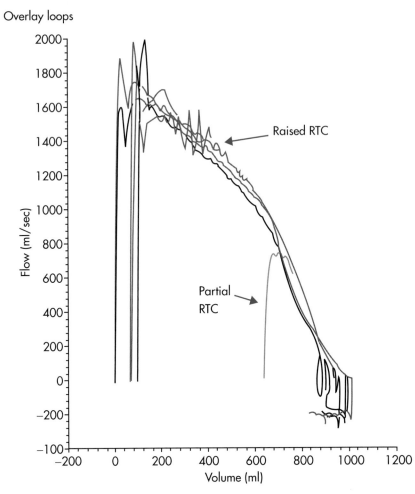

FIGURE 8-18   **Raised Lung Volume RTC.** F-V curves obtained after rapid thoracic compressions from raised lung volume (RVRTC) are superimposed. Progressively higher squeeze pressures do not yield higher flows or volumes, indicating that flow limitation has been met. In addition, a partial F-V curve (from a tidal breath) is superimposed in the diagram (see text).

PF TIP

Normative data may be viewed in a variety of statistical methods. "Z" scores are an alternative method of viewing standard deviation from the mean. A Z score of ±2.0 approximates 2 standard deviations from the mean, otherwise referred to as the 95% confidence range.

Forced Deflation Technique

As with the RTC technique, forced deflation techniques also produce maximal expiratory F-V curves (MEFV). The method, however, is exactly opposite to the positive pressure generated during the RTC

method. Instead, a negative pressure is applied to the airway opening, and the lungs are deflated quickly. This technique is usually reserved for intubated infants in a critical care setting and performed by technologists and physicians familiar with its possible complications. The size of the endotracheal tube may limit flow. The child must be maximally sedated and paralyzed, and therefore the child's lungs must be ventilated between maneuvers. Before the deflation, the lungs of the infant are manually inflated to TLC with approximately +30 to +40 cm H_2O. This inflation is performed four times with a breath hold of 2–3 seconds at TLC. The airway is then switched into a source of nega-

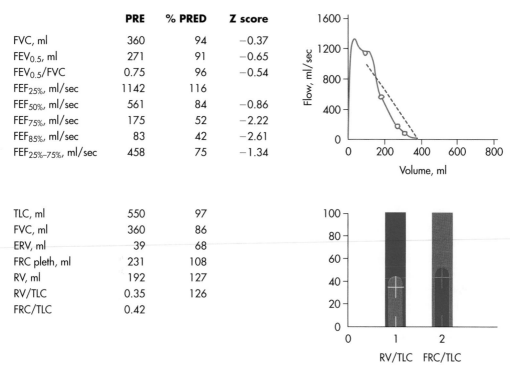

	PRE	% PRED	Z score
FVC, ml	360	94	−0.37
FEV$_{0.5}$, ml	271	91	−0.65
FEV$_{0.5}$/FVC	0.75	96	−0.54
FEF$_{25\%}$, ml/sec	1142	116	
FEF$_{50\%}$, ml/sec	561	84	−0.86
FEF$_{75\%}$, ml/sec	175	52	−2.22
FEF$_{85\%}$, ml/sec	83	42	−2.61
FEF$_{25\%-75\%}$, ml/sec	458	75	−1.34

	PRE	% PRED	
TLC, ml	550	97	
FVC, ml	360	86	
ERV, ml	39	68	
FRC pleth, ml	231	108	
RV, ml	192	127	
RV/TLC	0.35	126	
FRC/TLC	0.42		

FIGURE 8-19 **Infant Pulmonary Function Test (PFT) Report.** PFT test results from a 1-year-old child with cystic fibrosis. The report details forced flows from raised lung volumes as well as lung volume determination via plethysmography (see text).

tive pressure (approximately −30 to −40 cm H$_2$O). Air is evacuated for a maximum of 3 seconds or until expiratory flow ceases (i.e., residual volume is reached). As the lungs empty, an F-V curve is produced, and flows at lower lung volumes are analyzed. The lungs are then reinflated with 100% O$_2$, and the procedure is repeated until flow limitation is obtained.

STANDARDS FOR TESTING

For several specific PFTs, regardless of age, maximal effort and cooperation are needed to optimize results. It has often been assumed that small children are incapable of performing adequate PFTs. Laboratories that specialize in working with pediatric patients have proven this untrue. However, not every small child can or will perform up to desired expectations. Newly revised ATS/ERS criteria and recommendations have been discussed

throughout this chapter and certainly help with the standardization of many PFTs in the pediatric population. Additional guidelines for very young children have been developed by a focus group of the ATS/ERS. These recommendations are a starting point that will require worldwide acceptance and continued revisions over time. Comparing, sharing, and combining results from laboratories across the world mandate that standardization of technique be accomplished. Interpretation of PFTs should note if ATS/ERS criteria have not been reached. The physician's interpretation should state whether age, effort-related limitations, or both are evident, and these should be taken into consideration.

Variability in Reference Sets and Predicted Values for Pediatrics

Until recently, a limiting factor for interpretation of pediatric PFTs was the lack of consistent predicted values. Caution is warranted regarding the choice of an appropriate normative set. Reference sets are often named for an author or primary investigator, such as the Knudson reference set. However, normative sets may contain regression equations from one author only, or several researchers (or studies) may contribute to a single reference set. An example is the Polgar and Promadhat reference set, which is actually a compilation of regression equations from several population studies and authors. When choosing a reference set for a population of children, consideration must be given to selecting the set that most closely represents the population being tested. Several questions should be considered carefully:

- How many healthy patients were studied, and how was it determined that these patients were free of respiratory disease?
- What are the demographics of the population represented (e.g., age range, sex, race)?
- What equipment and techniques were used to collect the data?

The number of patients studied is critically important to the value of the reference set. Many common pediatric reference sets developed between the 1960s and the 1980s (e.g., Polgar, Knudson, Hsu, Zapletal) were based on relatively small numbers (several hundred children). Each child was tested only once, and therefore the sample is cross-sectional. Repeat studies were not performed on the same children as they aged and grew. By 2000, population studies on many thousands of children had been completed. In addition, these studies were longitudinal by design. *Longitudinal* means that repeated measurements were made on the same children as they grew. The power of the regression equations generated from these population studies is far greater than those of preceding decades. The ATS/ERS has recommended that, in the United States, the reference set of NHANES III (National Health and Nutrition Evaluation Survey III) be used for patients aged 8–80 years. For children younger than 8 years, the regression equations of Wang-Dockery are suggested. In a laboratory specializing in pediatrics, the Wang-Dockery reference set is appropriate for patients ages 6–18 years. Eigen has published normative data for children ages 3–6 years.

One difficulty is that these reference sets are for spirometry only. It is relatively easy to bring a portable spirometer into a school and test a group of children quickly. Repeat studies can be performed at intervals to gather longitudinal data. It is not easy to bring a large number of children into a pulmonary function laboratory and perform tests such as lung volumes and DL_{CO}. Predicted values for these PFTs are still lacking. A further problem arises when trying to combine older predicted values for lung volumes and DL_{CO} with newer, updated spirometric reference sets. Many commercial pulmonary function systems permit the user to "mix and match" regression equations and build their own reference set. Caution must be exercised when doing this. It is important that the laboratory personnel know if their reference set is a standard (unaltered) set or if it is compiled from available reference sets. It is also advisable that the reference sets be identified on the final pulmonary function reports. Consulting physicians who are not associated with the laboratory performing the studies may be interested in knowing the source of the predicted values.

Biologic variability for physiologic measurements, including pulmonary function, is critically dependent on the populations' sex, age, race, and body dimensions. Several reference sets considered only white subjects. Race correction for African Americans was applied as a constant correction factor (see Appendix B). In addition, the ages for children tested were often in the range of 8–18 years. There is tremendous growth during these years but at different rates, depending on sex and pubertal changes. Attempting to apply a simple regression for each parameter tested (e.g., FVC, FEV_1) based on one independent variable (usually height) may be misleading. Although distribution of pulmonary function values may follow the normal Gaussian (bell-shaped) curve (see Appendix B), there is increasing disparity at both ends of the age range. Further error is introduced if these regression equations are extrapolated to ages younger than the ages actually tested (e.g., down to age 6 years). This should be avoided whenever possible. Newer reference sets for spirometry now examine races separately and have even developed regression equations for each age child (Wang and Dockery).

PF TIP

In pediatric patients, lung growth is closely correlated with age, height, and sex. Trending of raw data is insufficient. Rather, the parameters being trended must account for the continually changing somatic growth pattern of the child.

Reporting of pulmonary function results is also undergoing transition. Traditionally, PFT parameters have included the patient's actual value, a predicted value, and the percent of predicted. However, the use of percent predicted to define abnormal parameters may lead to erroneous conclusions. The ATS/ERS suggests using the upper and lower limits of normal to compare test data to reference data, or the 95% confidence range. As mentioned earlier, Z scores are an alternative method of reporting data.

Measurement technique can also significantly alter physiologic data; lung volumes measured by gas dilution versus those measured by body plethysmography are one example. In pediatrics, even simple differences in performing tests may affect results. Examples include the use of nose clips versus no nose clips or standing versus sitting while performing testing. Consistency is the key, although there may be no absolutes in the correct method for a particular test. The technologist should be aware of the methods used in his or her laboratory as compared with those of the reference sets used.

FUTURE FOR PEDIATRIC PULMONARY FUNCTION LABORATORIES

It has become obvious that standardization of pulmonary function testing is a major objective of pulmonary functions laboratories worldwide, and is supported and endorsed by the American Thoracic Society and European Respiratory Society. This is vital for comparison of both pediatric and adult populations, peoples of different ethnicity, and people in good health and with pulmonary disease. Many questions are yet to be answered, and the need for further standardization is apparent for all ages, and especially for the pediatric population. Normative data continue to be collected, and there is a need to revisit tests such as lung volume determination and diffusion capacity. Although comprehensive reference sets are available for spirometry in children ages 6 years and older, this is not true for tests that require children to come to pulmonary function laboratories. One of the most difficult challenges is assessing lung function of a very young child (ages 2–4 years) because he or she may not be capable of performing standard measurements of pulmonary function. Sedation may not be an alternative, or the size or compliance of the child's chest may not be conducive to thoracoabdominal compressions. Physical examination, auscultation, and other indirect indices such as pulse oximetry are often very misleading in this age group. Presence or absence of wheezing is not necessarily correlated with O_2 status or the clinical presentation of the child. Extensive recommendations for this age group have been published by a focus group of the ATS/ERS. There is a need for continued investigation into noninvasive measurement of airflow limitation, such as IOS and exhaled nitric oxide. Other research-oriented techniques, not yet routinely performed in the United States, may have clinical applications in the future. Examples include the interrupter technique (Rint) for measurement of airway resistance and multiple-breath inert gas washout techniques helpful in identifying ventilation inequality.

Summary

- This chapter describes techniques for performing PFTs in pediatric patients.
- Spirometry, lung volumes, DLCO, blood gases, pulmonary mechanics, and challenge tests are all discussed with attention to how these measurements differ in the pediatric population.
- For each category of tests, relevant questions are posed to relate pediatric testing to adult testing.

- Special emphasis is given to how the pulmonary function technologist should approach testing in young children and adolescents.
- Measurement of lung volumes, forced flows, and passive breathing mechanics in infants and preschool children are described, along with highly specialized techniques required to obtain data from these patients.

- Special problems related to standards for testing, including newly revised guidelines from the ATS/ERS and focus groups, and the use of appropriate reference values in the pediatric population are discussed.

CASE 8-1

Case Studies

HISTORY

A.B. is an 8-year-old white girl presented to the emergency department (ED) of the Children's Hospital with severe shortness of breath and gasping respirations. Symptoms began 1 week after a fishing and camping trip and include a 1-month history of midsternal chest pain, increasing cough, and shortness of breath. Her pediatrician had been treating her with antibiotics for a presumptive left lower lobe pneumonia. In the ED, her O_2 saturation on room air was 94% and a chest radiograph revealed perihilar calcifications. After stabilization and further workup (including a negative PPD), the following tests were ordered: CT scan with contrast, ventilation-perfusion scan, and full pulmonary function studies. The PFTs revealed the following:

Spirometry	PRED	LLN	Initial	% PRED	3 mo later	% PRED
FVC (L)	1.58	1.31	1.01	64	1.71	108
FEV$_1$ (L)	1.41	1.16	0.53	37	1.46	103
FEV$_1$/FVC (%)	89	80	53	**	85	**
FEF$_{25\%-75\%}$ (L/sec)	1.83	1.24	0.39	21	1.56	85
PEFR (L/sec)	3.41	2.44	1.31	38	3.49	102
FET 100% (sec)	**	**	5.65	**	7.14	**

Lung volumes	PRED	LLN	Initial	% PRED	3 mo later	% PRED
VC (L)	1.58	1.31	1.01	64	1.71	108
TLC (L)	2.26	1.91	2.08	92	2.31	102
FRC$_{PL}$ (L)	1.11	0.88	1.47	132	0.91	82
RV (L)	0.61	0.43	1.08	177	0.61	100
RV/TLC (%)	26	**	52	**	26	**
IC (L)	**	**	0.61	**	1.42	**
ERV (L)	**	**	0.17	**	0.31	**

Diffusion capacity	PRED	LLN	Initial	% PRED	3 mo later	% PRED
D$_{LCO}$ (ml/mm Hg/min)	13.8	**	5.9	42	8.7	63
DL Adj (ml/mm Hg/min)	13.8	**	6.2	45	8.7	63
D$_{LCO}$/V$_A$	6.41	**	5.92	92	4.62	72
V$_A$ (L)	**	**	0.99	**	1.89	**
Hb (g/dl)			11.6		13.3	

Initial and 3-Month Follow-up PFTs from an 8-Year-Old Girl with Histoplasmosis.

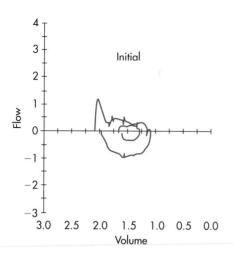

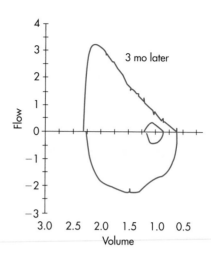

QUESTIONS

1. What do the results of the spirometry reveal?
2. What other important information does the lung volume measurement add to the interpretation?
3. How should the results of the diffusion capacity be interpreted?
4. What other studies would be helpful and why?

The chest radiograph and CT scan revealed marked hilar adenopathy with calcifications and bilateral anatomic compression of the mainstem bronchi. Once all the diagnostic information was collected, the patient was diagnosed with fibrosing mediastinitis due to a histoplasmosis infection.

5. How do her symptoms and PFT results correlate with the diagnosis of central airflow compression?

The patient began taking intraconazole (to treat histoplasmosis) and prednisone. Refer back to Figure 8-19, B, for follow-up PFTs performed 3 months after the initial PFTs.

6. Describe the changes that have occurred in the pulmonary function testing.
7. How should the PFTs be interpreted?
8. Compare the D_{LCO} and D_{LCO}/V_A before and after treatment and explain the results.

DISCUSSION

The initial spirometry has a flow-volume loop that is consistent with fixed airflow obstruction. Note that even the PEF is severely reduced, which suggests that central airway involvement is extensive. There is a rapid decline in flow rate beyond the peak flow, and the remainder of the VC is exhaled at a relatively constant, but severely decreased, flow rate until end-exhalation.

Inspiratory flow rate is also diminished but is relatively greater than expiratory flow. Both the VC and FEV_1 are reduced, as is the ratio of FEV_1/FVC. The expiratory obstruction is severe due to the FEV_1 being reduced to 37% of predicted. The lung volume data reveal that the patient's TLC is normal (92% predicted); there is not a restrictive component to this pulmonary disorder. This cannot be determined by spirometry only. When spirometry reveals such a low FVC and FEV_1, yet total lung capacity is normal, an elevated RV/TLC must also exist. It is easy to imagine that during forced maneuvers, lesions that compress the central airways can completely obstruct airflow, leading to a reduced VC. In this case, the slow vital capacity obtained in the body box is slightly greater than the forced vital capacity during spirometry. The obstruction is so significant, however, that any expiratory maneuver leads to airway closure and resulting air trapping. The D_{LCO} (corrected for hemoglobin) is also reduced to 45% of predicted, but the D_L/V_A is normal at 98%. Notice that the V_A is only 0.99 L, substantially lower than the TLC of 2.08 L. Because the V_A is determined with a gas equilibration technique, in the face of severe obstruction a reduced V_A would be expected. The D_L/V_A of 98% indicates that the areas of the lung that are well ventilated are also diffusing carbon monoxide normally. An arterial blood gas would further clarify the patient's oxygenation and acid-base status. Indeed, an ABG was drawn that revealed mild respiratory alkalosis and a mild hypoxemia (PaO_2 of 73).

After aggressive multidrug therapy, the patient's pulmonary function improved quickly and substan-

continued

tially. By 3 months after the initial PFTs, spirometry and lung volumes were all completely normal without any evidence for airflow obstruction or air trapping. The DLCO (corrected for hemoglobin) was improved to 63% of predicted. The DL/V_A decreased to 72%; however, this is directly due to the increase of the V_A to 1.89 L (much closer to the TLC of 2.31 L). Depending on the LLN for the laboratory, a DL/V_A of 72% may be within normal limits or mildly decreased.

SELF-ASSESSMENT QUESTIONS

Entry-level and Advanced

1. A 7-year-old child has an FVC of 0.95 L. ATS/ERS recommends that:
   I. The repeatability of his FVC maneuvers be within 150 ml
   II. The repeatability of his FEV_1 be within 100 ml
   III. Exhalation time should be at least 3 seconds with a flow plateau
   IV. Volume extrapolation errors are insignificant in children younger than 10 years
      a. I, II, and III
      b. II and III
      c. I only
      d. II, III, and IV

2. A 12-year-old child with advanced cystic fibrosis has lung volume determination by two methods, plethysmography and nitrogen washout. Which of the following outcomes would be expected:
   a. The FRC from the nitrogen washout and the V_{TG} from plethysmography would be comparable.
   b. The FRC from the nitrogen washout would likely underestimate V_{TG} because of poor equilibration of gas in the thorax of an obstructed patient.
   c. The V_{TG} from plethysmography would likely overestimate V_{TG} because of hyperinflation and air trapping.
   d. The FRC from nitrogen washout would likely be overestimated because of inherent leaks in the system.

3. An 11-year-old boy performs technically acceptable and repeatable spirometry. His FVC reveals a value of 3.5 L (119% of predicted) and FEV_1 is 2.30 (92% of predicted). These spirometric values indicate:

   a. Normal spirometry
   b. Mild obstructive component
   c. Mild restrictive component
   d. Severe obstructive component

4. Which of the following statements regarding ATS/ERS recommendations for spirometry most applies to older children?
   a. The best F-V curve is based on the curve with highest addition of FVC and FEV_1, but the best values for each parameter should be independently reported.
   b. The curve with the best peak flow should be reported.
   c. The F-V loop with the best FEV_1 should be reported.
   d. The best F-V curve is based on the curve with the highest addition of FVC and $FEF_{25\%-75\%}$, but the best values for each parameter should be independently reported

5. Primary pulmonary hypertension in children is characterized by decreased perfusion to the lung, but FVC and TLC are within normal limits. Assuming a normal hemoglobin of 14.0, the expected results from performing diffusing capacity would reveal:
   a. Increased raw DLCO and increased DL/V_A
   b. Normal DLCO, but reduced DL/V_A
   c. Reduced raw DLCO, but normal DL/V_A
   d. Reduced raw DLCO and reduced DL/V_A

6. A 4-year-old child is performing spirometry for the first time. The child is capable of performing similar F-V loops several times; however, his best expiratory time is 2 seconds. Which of the following statements is true regarding the spirometry?
   a. The test meets all current ATS/ERS recommendations.
   b. The F-V loops produced may be "usable" loops (i.e., FEV_1 is reportable if even the loops are not technically acceptable).

c. The loops are not usable because a true FVC cannot be obtained,

d. Only the one best PEFR is reportable.

7. Inspiratory loops in children:
   a. Should be essentially ignored because of effort limitation
   b. Are as repeatable as expiratory loops
   c. Can be a valuable component of the F-V loop when performed maximally
   d. Can be examined for evidence of intrathoracic airflow obstruction

8. Ease of obtaining repeatable forced flow measurements in infants may be affected by which of the following?
   I. Sleep state
   II. Type of sedation used
   III. Age/size of child
   IV. Technical and equipment considerations
      a. I, III, and IV
      b. II and III
      c. III and IV
      d. I, II, III, and IV

9. During tidal breathing, a sedated infant has a passive single-breath occlusion performed. The peak flow immediately after occlusion is 360 ml/sec, the occlusion plateau is 9.0 cm H_2O, and the passive exhaled volume is 144 ml. This child's respiratory system compliance can be calculated as:
   a. 4 ml/cm H_2O
   b. 13 ml/cm H_2O
   c. 16 ml/cm H_2O
   d. Not enough information available to calculate

10. Asynchrony of the respiratory system occurs:
    a. When the chest wall (rib cage) and abdomen are moving in unison
    b. During normal, passive tidal breathing
    c. During any forced maneuver
    d. With paradoxical movement of the chest wall and diaphragm

Selected Bibliography

GENERAL REFERENCES

Davis SD: Neonatal and pediatric respiratory diagnostics, *Respir Care* 2003; 48:367-385.

Hyatt RE: Forced expiration. In *Handbook of physiology: the respiratory system,* Bethesda, MD, 1986, American Physiological Society.

Mueller GA, Eigen H: Pulmonary function testing in pediatric practice, *Pediatr Rev* 1994; 15:403-411.

Pfaff JK, Morgan WJ: Pulmonary function in infants and children, *Pediatr Clin North Am* 1994; 41:401-423.

Polgar G, Promadhat V: *Pulmonary function testing in children: techniques and standards,* Philadelphia, 1971, WB Saunders.

Stocks J, Sly PD, Tepper RS et al: *Infant respiratory function testing,* New York, 1996, Wiley-Liss.

Zapletal A, Samanek M, Paul T: Lung function in children and adolescents—methods, reference values. In *Progress in respiration research,* New York, 1987, Karger.

SPIROMETRY

Brugman SM, Howell JH, Rosenburg DM et al: The spectrum of pediatric vocal cord dysfunction, *Am J Respir Crit Care Med* 1994; 149:A353.

Crenesse D, Berlioz M, Bourrier T et al: Spirometry in children aged 3 to 5 years: reliability of forced expiratory maneuvers, *Pediatr Pulmonol* 2001; 32:56-61.

Desmond KJ, Allen PD, Demizio DL et al: Redefining end of test (EOT) criteria for pulmonary testing in children, *Am J Respir Crit Care Med* 1997; 156:542-545.

Elshami AA, Tino G: Coexistent asthma and functional upper airway obstruction, *Chest* 1996; 110:1358-1361.

Krowka MJ, Enright PL, Rodarte JR et al: Effect of effort on measurement of forced expiratory volume in one second, *Am Rev Respir Dis* 1987; 136:829-833.

Landwehr LP, Wood RP, Blager FB et al: Vocal cord dysfunction mimicking exercise-induced bronchospasm in adolescents, *Pediatr* 1996; 98:971-974.

Lebowitz MD, Sherrill DL: The assessment and interpretation of spirometry during the transition from childhood to adulthood, *Pediatr Pulmonol* 1995; 19:143-149.

McFadden ER Jr, Zawadski DK: Vocal cord dysfunction masquerading as exercise-induced asthma: a physiologic cause for "choking" during athletic activities, *Am J Respir Crit Care Med* 1996; 153:942-947.

Miller RD, Hyatt RE: Evaluation of obstructing lesions of the trachea and larynx by flow-volume loops, *Am Rev Respir Dis* 1975; 108:475-482.

Wanger JS, Ikle DN, Cherniack RM: The effect of inspiratory maneuvers on expiratory flow rates in health and asthma: influences of lung elastic recoil, *Am J Respir Crit Care Med* 1996; 153:1302-1308.

PREDICTED VALUES AND REFERENCE EQUATIONS

Cook CD, Hamann JH: Relation of lung volumes to height in healthy persons between the ages of 5 and 38 years, *J Pediatr* 1961; 59:710-715.

Eigen H: Spirometric pulmonary function in healthy preschool children, *Am J Respir Crit Care Med* 2001, 163:619-623.

Hankinson JL, Odencrantz JR, Fedan KB: Spirometric reference values from a sample of the general U.S. population, *Am J Respir Crit Care Med* 1999; 159:179-187.

Hsu KHK, Jenkins DE, Hsi BP et al: Ventilatory functions of normal children and young adults—Mexican-American, white, and black—I. Spirometry, *J Pediatr* 1979; 95:14-23.

Knudson RJ, Lebowitz MD, Holberg CJ et al: Changes in the normal maximal expiratory flow-volume curve with growth and aging, *Am Rev Respir Dis* 1983; 127:725.

Pattishall EN: Pulmonary function testing references values and interpretations in pediatric training programs, *Pediatr* 1990; 85:768-773.

Pattishall EN, Helms RW, Strope GL: Noncomparability of cross-sectional and longitudinal estimates of lung growth in children, *Pediatr Pulmonol* 1989; 7:22-28.

Wang X, Dockery DW, Wypij D et al: Pulmonary function between 6 and 18 years of age, *Pediatr Pulmonol* 1993; 15:75-88.

INHALATIONAL CHALLENGES

Cockcroft DW, Killian DN, Mellon JJA et al: Bronchial reactivity to inhaled histamine: a method and clinical survey, *Clin Allergy* 1977; 7:235-243.

Eggleston PA: A comparison of the asthmatic response to methacholine and exercise, *J Allergy Clin Immunol* 1979; 63:104-110.

Hargreave FE, Ryan A, Thomson NC et al: Bronchial responsiveness to histamine or methacholine in asthma measurement and clinical significance, *J Allergy Clin Immunol* 1981; 68:345-347.

Irvin CG: Bronchial challenge testing, *Respir Clin North Am* 1995; 1:265-285.

Seiner JC, Staudenmayer H, Koepke JW et al: Vocal cord dysfunction: the importance of psychologic factors and provocation challenge testing, *J Allergy Clin Immunol* 1987; 79:726-733.

PROVOCATIONAL AND MAXIMAL EXERCISE STRESS TESTING

Cooper DM: Rethinking exercise testing in children: a challenge, *Am J Respir Crit Care Med* 1995; 152:1154-1157.

Godfrey S: Exercise-induced asthma—clinical, physiological, and therapeutic implications, *J Allergy Clin Immunol* 1975; 56:1-17.

James FW, Kaplan S, Glueck CJ et al: Responses of normal children and young adults to controlled bicycle exercise, *Circulation* 1980; 61:902-912.

McFadden ER Jr: Exercise-induced asthma—assessment of current etiologic concepts, *Chest* 1987; 91:151S-157S.

Nixon PA, Orenstein DM: Exercise testing in children, *Pediatr Pulmonol* 1988; 5:107-122.

Strauss RH, McFadden ER Jr, Ingram RH Jr et al: Enhancement of exercise-induced asthma by cold air, *N Engl J Med* 1977; 297:743-747.

Weisman IM, Zeballos RJ: Clinical exercise testing, *Clin Chest Med* 2002; 22:679-701.

PULMONARY FUNCTION TESTING IN INFANTS AND VERY YOUNG CHILDREN

Aurora P, Stocks J, Oliver C et al: Quality control for spirometry in preschool children with and without lung disease, *Am J Respir Crit Care Med* 2004; 169:1152-1159.

Castile R, Filbrun D, Flucke R et al: Adult-type pulmonary function tests in infants without respiratory disease, *Pediatr Pulmonol* 2000; 30:215-227.

Clarke JR, Aston H, Silverman M: Evaluation of a tidal expiratory flow index in healthy and diseased infants, *Pediatr Pulmonol* 1994; 17:285-290.

Hanrahan JP, Brown RW, Carey VJ et al: Passive respiratory mechanics in healthy infants, *Am J Respir Crit Care Med* 1996; 154:670-680.

Hanrahan JP, Tager IB, Castile RG et al: Pulmonary function measures in healthy infants: variability and size correction, *Am Rev Resp Dis* 1990; 141:1127.

Hoo AF, Dezateux C, Hanrahan JP et al: Sex-specific prediction equations for V_{max} FRC in infancy, *Am J Respir Crit Care Med* 2002; 165:1084-1092.

Jones M, Castile R, Davis S et al: Forced expiratory flows and volumes in infants—normative data and lung growth, *Am J Respir Crit Care Med* 2000; 161:353-359.

Jones MH, Davis SD, Grant D et al: Forced expiratory maneuvers in very young children: assessment of flow limitation, *Am J Respir Crit Care Med* 1999; 159:791-795.

LeSouef PN, England SJ, Bryan AC: Passive respiratory mechanics in newborns and children, *Am Rev Respir Dis* 1984; 129:552-556.

Lodrup KC, Mowinckel P, Carlsen KH: Lung function measurements in awake compared to sleeping newborn infants, *Pediatr Pulmonol* 1992; 12:99-104.

McCoy KS, Castile RG, Allen ED et al: Functional residual capacity (FRC) measurements by plethysmography and helium dilution in normal infants, *Pediatr Pulmonol* 1995; 19:282-290.

Morgan WJ, Geller DE, Tepper RS et al: Partial expiratory flow-volume curves in infants and young children, *Pediatr Pulmonol* 1988; 5:232-243.

Neto GS, Gerhardt T, Silberberg A et al: Nonlinear pressure/volume relationship and measurements of lung mechanics in infants, *Pediatr Pulmonol* 1992; 12:146-152.

Panitch HB, Kekklian EN, Motley RA et al: Effect of altering smooth muscle tone on maximal expiratory flows in patients with tracheomalacia, *Pediatr Pulmonol* 1990; 9:170-176.

Sivan Y, Deakers TW, Newth CJL: An automated bedside method for measuring functional residual capacity by N_2 washout in mechanically ventilated children, *Pediatr Res* 1990; 28:446-451.

Sly PD, Brown KA, Bates JHT et al: Non-invasive determination of respiratory mechanics during mechanical ventilation of neonates: a review of current and future techniques, *Pediatr Pulmonol* 1988; 4:39-47.

Stocks J: Assessment of lung function in infants, *Perfusion* 1993; 8:71-80.

Taussig LM, Landau LI, Godfrey S et al: Determinants of forced expiratory flows in newborn infants, *J Appl Physiol* 1982; 53:1220-1227.

Tepper RS, Asdell S: Comparison of helium dilution and nitrogen washout measurements of functional residual capacity in infants and very young children, *Pediatr Pulmonol* 1992; 13:250-254.

Tepper RS, Reister T: Forced expiratory flows and lung volumes in normal infants, *Pediatr Pulmonol* 1993; 15:357-361.

Turner DJ, Stick SM, LeSouef KL et al: A new technique to generate and assess forced expiration from raised lung volume in infants, *Am J Respir Crit Care Med* 1995; 51:1441-1450.

OSCILLOMETRY AND NITRIC OXIDE

Bisgaard H, Klug B: Lung function measurement in awake young children, *Eur Respir J* 1995; 8:2067-2075.

Buchvald F, Bisgaard H: FeNO measured at fixed exhalation flow rate during controlled tidal breathing in children from the age of 2 years, *Am J Respir Crit Care Med* 2001; 163:699-704.

Ducharme FM, Davis GM: Respiratory resistance in the emergency department—a reproducible and responsive measure of asthma severity, *Chest* 1998; 113:1566-1572.

Goldman M: Clinical application of forced oscillation, *Pulm Pharm & Therapeutics* 2001; 14:341-350.

Smith HJ, Reinhold P, Goldman MD: Forced oscillation technique and impulse oscillometry, *Eur Respir Mon* 2005; 31:72-105.

STANDARDS AND GUIDELINES

American Association for Respiratory Care: Clinical practice guideline: infant/toddler pulmonary function tests, *Respir Care* 1995; 40:761-768.

American Association for Respiratory Care: Clinical practice guideline: methacholine challenge testing 2001 revision and update, *Respir Care* 2001; 46:523-530.

American Thoracic Society: Guidelines for methacholine and exercise challenge testing—1999, *Am J Respir Crit Care Med* 2000; 161:309-329.

American Thoracic Society: Lung function testing: selection of reference values and interpretative strategies, *Am Rev Respir Dis* 1991; 144:1202-1218.

American Thoracic Society/European Respiratory Society: An official American Thoracic/European Respiratory Society Statement: pulmonary function testing in preschool children, *Am J Respir Crit Care Med* 2007; 175:1304-1345.

American Thoracic Society/European Respiratory Society: ATS/ERS Statement: Raised volume forced expirations in infants—Guidelines for current practise, *Am J Respir Crit Care Med* 2005; 172:1463-1471.

American Thoracic Society/European Respiratory Society: Respiratory function measurements in infants: measurement conditions, *Am J Respir Crit Care Med* 1995; 151:2058-2064.

American Thoracic Society/European Respiratory Society: Respiratory mechanics in infants: physiologic evaluation in health and disease, *Am Rev Respir Dis* 1993; 147:474-496.

ATS/ERS Taskforce: MacIntyre N, Crapo RO, Viegi G, et al: Standardisation of the single-breath determination of carbon monoxide uptake in the lung. *Eur Respir J* 2005; 26:720-735.

ATS/ERS Taskforce: Miller MR, Crapo R, Hankinson J et al: General considerations for lung function testing, *Eur Respir J* 2005; 26:153-161.

ATS/ERS Taskforce: Miller MR, Hankinson J, Brusasco V et al: Standardisation of spirometry, *Eur Respir J* 2005; 26:319-338.

ATS/ERS Taskforce: Pellegrino R, Viegi G, Brusasco V et al: Interpretative strategies for lung function tests, *Eur Respir J* 2005; 26:948-968.

ATS/ERS Taskforce: Wanger J, Clausen JL, Coates A et al: Standardisation of the measurement of lung volumes, *Eur Resp J* 2005; 26:511-522.

Official Statement of the American Thoracic Society: Recommendations for standardized procedures for the online and offline measurement of exhaled lower respiratory nitric oxide and nasal nitric oxide in adults and children—1999, *Am J Respir Crit Care Med* 1999; 160:2104-2117.

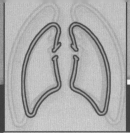

Specialized Test Regimens

CHAPTER OUTLINE

OBJECTIVES

After studying this chapter you will be able to:

Entry-level
1. Describe two methods of performing bronchial challenge tests
2. Identify a positive response to a methacholine challenge test
3. List two indications for preoperative pulmonary function testing
4. Select an appropriate protocol to test for exercise-induced asthma

Advanced
1. Judge the reliability of metabolic measurements
2. Select appropriate tests to evaluate disability in either chronic obstructive pulmonary disease (COPD) or pulmonary fibrosis
3. Identify patients in whom impulse oscillometry might be used to evaluate airway resistance
4. Evaluate the clinical implications of an elevated level of exhaled nitric oxide (eNO)

KEY TERMS

basal metabolic rate (BMR)
continuous-flow canopy
elastance

eosinophilic inflammation
eucapnic voluntary hyperventilation
exercise-induced asthma (EIA)

exhaled nitric oxide (eNO)
fast Fourier transformation (FFT)
5-breath dosimeter method

forced oscillation technique (FOT)
Harris-Benedict equations
head hood
histamine

indirect calorimetry
inertia
methacholine
nasal NO

provocative concentration (PC_{20})
pulmonary artery occlusion pressure
2-minute tidal breathing method

Diagnosis or evaluation of specific pulmonary disorders requires that appropriate tests be performed. Specialized test regimens, such as those described in this chapter, often consist of standard tests performed under special conditions. For example, forced expiratory volume (FEV_1) may be analyzed after inhalation challenge, hyperventilation, or exercise to quantify airway reactivity. The clinical question asked regarding a patient might be whether he or she qualifies for disability or whether it is safe to undergo surgery. Spirometry, lung volumes, diffusing capacity (DLCO), or blood gas analysis may be required to answer these questions.

Measurement of **exhaled nitric oxide (eNO)** provides a sensitive and highly repeatable method for evaluating airway inflammation. It can be used to detect **eosinophilic inflammation,** which is common in asthma, and to evaluate response to treatments such as inhaled corticosteroids.

Impulse oscillometry provides a unique way to evaluate airway function. It provides a measurement of airway resistance in spontaneously breathing subjects and can be used in conjunction with bronchodilator evaluation or bronchial challenge.

Metabolic measurements are widely used to assess caloric needs and nutritional support in a variety of patients. The methods used are similar to those used in gas exchange measurements during exercise. Specialized calculations allow precise description of the nutritional status of the patient.

BRONCHIAL CHALLENGE TESTING

Bronchial challenge testing is used to identify and characterize airway hyperresponsiveness. Challenge tests may be performed in patients with symptoms of bronchospasm who have normal pulmonary function studies or uncertain results of bronchodilator studies. Bronchial challenge can also be used to assess changes in hyperreactivity of the airways or to quantify its severity. Bronchial challenge tests are sometimes used to screen individuals who may be at risk from environmental or occupational exposure to toxins.

Several commonly used provocative agents can be used to assess airway hyperreactivity. These include the following:
- Methacholine challenge
- Histamine challenge
- **Eucapnic voluntary hyperventilation** (with either cold or room-temperature gas)
- Exercise

Each of these agents may trigger bronchospasm, but in slightly different ways. **Methacholine** is a chemical that increases parasympathetic tone in bronchial smooth muscle. **Histamine** triggers a similar response producing bronchoconstriction. Hyperventilation, either at rest or during exercise, results in heat and water loss from the airway. This provokes bronchospasm in susceptible patients. With each of these agents, pulmonary function variables are assessed before and after exposure to the challenge. FEV_1 is the variable most commonly used. Other flow measurements, as well as airway resistance (Raw) and specific conductance (sGaw), may also be evaluated before and after challenge. Additional parameters that have been used to assess response to bronchial challenge include breath sounds, transcutaneous PO_2 ($tcPO_2$, see Chapter 10), and forced oscillation measurements of resistance.

Methacholine Challenge

Bronchial challenge by inhalation of methacholine is performed by having the patient inhale increasing doses of the drug. All subjects will show a change in airway caliber with increasing concentrations of methacholine. Patients who have hyperresponsive airways demonstrate these changes at low doses of inhaled methacholine. This dose-response relationship permits the sensitivity of the airways to be quantified.

Spirometry, and sometimes sGaw, is measured after each dose. Most clinicians consider the test result positive when inhalation of methacholine precipitates a 20% decrease in FEV_1. The methacholine concentration at which this 20% decrease occurs is called the **provocative concentration (PC_{20}).** In the doses usually used (Box 9-1), healthy subjects do not display decreases greater than 20% in FEV_1. Therefore the methacholine challenge test is highly specific for airway hyperreactivity. Many patients who have asthma experience a 20% reduction in FEV_1 with doses of 8 mg/ml or less. However, bronchial hyperresponsiveness may also be seen in other pulmonary disorders such as COPD, cystic fibrosis, and bronchitis.

Patients to be tested should be asymptomatic, with no coughing or obvious wheezing. Recent upper or lower respiratory tract infections may alter airway responsiveness, so bronchial challenge testing may need to be deferred. Their baseline FEV_1 should be normal or at least greater than 60%–70% of their expected value. For patients with known obstruction or restriction, FEV_1 should be close to their highest previously observed value. Obvious airway obstruction (e.g., $FEV_{1\%}$ less than

the lower limit of normal) is a relative contraindication. If the patient has an FEV_1 less than 1.0–1.5 L, there is a risk that a large drop in FEV_1 after methacholine challenge might leave the individual with compromised lung function. Bronchial challenge may be indicated in obstructed patients if the clinical question is related to the degree of responsiveness. Box 9-2 lists the absolute and relative contraindications to methacholine challenge.

If the patient has been taking bronchodilators, they should be withheld according to the schedule listed in Table 9-1. Other medications or substances can affect the validity of the challenge as well. All medications being taken at the time of testing should be recorded to assist in evaluation of the test results.

Baseline spirometry is performed to establish that the patient's FEV_1 is greater than 60%–70% of predicted or the previously observed best value. Patients who demonstrate obstruction based on reduced $FEV_{1\%}$ or other flows typically do not require challenge testing. However, obstructed patients may be tested to establish the degree of hyperreactivity. Patients who have a restrictive process (i.e., reduced FEV_1, FVC [forced vital capacity], and TLC) may also be tested for co-existing airway hyperresponsiveness. If a patient is unable to perform acceptable and repeatable baseline spirometry (i.e., FEV_1), changes after inhalation chal-

BOX 9-1	Methacholine Dosing Schedules
4 × Increase*	**2 × Increase†**
0.0625 mg/ml	0.031 mg/ml
0.250 mg/ml	0.0625 mg/ml
1.0 mg/ml	0.125 mg/ml
4.0 mg/ml	0.25 mg/ml
16.0 mg/ml	1.0 mg/ml
	2.0 mg/ml
	4.0 mg/ml
	8.0 mg/ml
	16.0 mg/ml

* As used for the 5-breath dosimeter protocol.
† As used for the 2-minute tidal breathing protocol.

BOX 9-2	Contraindications to Methacholine Challenge Testing

ABSOLUTE
Heart attack or stroke within 3 months
Known or suspected aortic aneurysm
Uncontrolled hypertension
FEV_1 less than 50% predicted (or <1.0 L)

RELATIVE
Pregnancy or nursing
Use of cholinesterase inhibitors
FEV_1 less than 60% predicted (or <1.5 L)
Physical or mental handicaps that prevent acceptable performance of spirometry

American Thoracic Society: Guidelines for methacholine and exercise challenge testing—1999, *Am J Respir Crit Care Med* 2000; 161:309-329.

TABLE 9-1	
Withholding Medications Before Bronchial Challenge	
Short-acting β-adrenergic agents (inhaled)	8 hours
Long-acting β-adrenergic agents (inhaled)	48 hours (some may require longer)
Standard β-adrenergic agents (oral)	12 hours
Long-acting β-adrenergic agents (oral)	24 hours
Anticholinergic agents (ipratropium)	24 hours
Standard theophylline preparations	12–24 hours
Sustained-action theophylline preparations	48 hours
Cromolyn sodium	8 hours
Nedocromil	48 hours
Antihistamines	72–96 hours
Corticosteroids (inhaled or oral)	Patients challenged while taking a stable dosage*
Leukotriene modifiers	24 hours
Caffeine-containing drinks (cola, coffee)	6 hours
β-blocking agents	May increase the response

*Corticosteroids may decrease bronchial hyperreactivity.

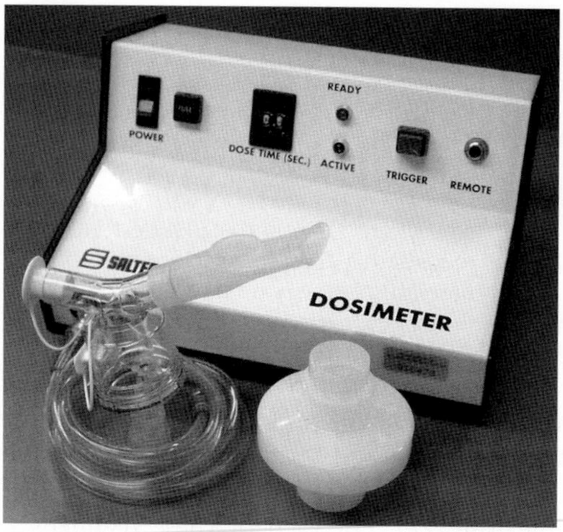

FIGURE 9-1 **Nebulizer and Dosimeter.** A DeVilbiss 646 nebulizer capable of delivering a prescribed volume of aerosol with 1-micron to 3-micron particles is shown. A dosimeter that controls the flow of gas to the nebulizer is also shown. The dosimeter provides a timer so that nebulization occurs for 0.6 seconds during inhalation. A manual trigger is shown; some dosimeters sense the patient's inspiratory effort and trigger flow automatically. Also shown is a bacteria filter that may be attached to the expiratory port of the nebulizer to reduce the volume of aerosol in the room.

lenge may be impossible to interpret. In these situations, other parameters (such as sGaw or oscillatory resistance) that are less dependent on patient effort may be preferable as an end point.

Two methods of delivering methacholine to the airway have been recommended by the American Thoracic Society (ATS): the **5-breath dosimeter method** and the **2-minute tidal breathing method.** A dosimeter can provide a true "quantitative" challenge test by delivering a consistent volume of drug. The dosimeter (or nebulizer) is activated during inspiration, either automatically (by a flow sensor) or manually (by the technologist). A standardized driving pressure (typically 20 psi) and activation time (0.5–0.6 seconds) allows a fixed volume of aerosol to be generated for each breath. By limiting the period of aerosol production, the last part of the inhalation carries the aerosol into the lung. The tidal breathing method is somewhat simpler because only a nebulizer is used.

A small-volume nebulizer is used to generate the methacholine aerosol (Figure 9-1). The nebulizer should generate an aerosol with a particle size in the range of 1.0–3.6 μm (mass median aerodynamic diameter). This particle range promotes deposition in the medium and small airways. For the tidal breathing method, the nebulizer output should be 0.13 ml/min; for use with a dosimeter (5-breath method) the output should be 0.009 ml for each 0.6-second actuation of the dosimeter. Because the output of each nebulizer varies by manufacturer and can change over time, it should be measured. This can be done by weighing the nebulizer on an accurate scale before and after a sham administration of drug. The output should be measured with the protocol to be used for testing. For the 5-breath dosimeter method, more breaths may be needed to measure the small output. The delivered dose of methacholine is standardized by using a fixed number of breaths (5) or breathing for a fixed length of time (2 minutes).

PF TIP

Despite different techniques for administering methacholine, patients who truly have asthma usually display a 20% decrease in FEV_1. The lower the dose of methacholine, the more sensitive, or hyperresponsive, the patient's airways are. Detecting a 20% decrease in FEV_1 requires that acceptable and reproducible baseline spirometry is obtained.

Two dosing routines are commonly used for methacholine challenge (see Box 9-1). One routine uses a quadrupling (4×) increase in methacholine concentration, and the other method uses a doubling dose (2×). For each of these regimens, the highest dose is 16 mg/ml, and the dilutions can be easily prepared from a stock solution starting with 100 mg of dry methacholine (Table 9-2). The stock solution is prepared by dissolving the powdered drug in a saline diluent. A preservative (0.4% phenol) may be added to the solution but is not required. Methacholine concentrations from 0.025 – 25.0 mg/ml are stable after mixing and may be kept for 5 months if refrigerated at 2–8°C. An alternate dosing scheme is provided with the

FDA-approved form of methacholine (Provocholine, Methapharm, Ontario, Canada). This dosing schedule uses methacholine concentrations of 0.025, 0.25, 2.5, 10, and 25 mg/ml and is designed for use with the 5-breath dosimeter method. Methacholine should be prepared by a pharmacist or individual trained in preparing drugs using sterile technique. Appropriate precautions should be taken when handling dry powdered methacholine. Vials of methacholine should be carefully marked with labels that clearly identify the concentration.

Five-Breath Dosimeter Method

Methacholine is prepared in five concentrations so that each dose is four times larger than the previous dose (see Table 9-2). Methacholine may be stored under refrigeration but should be brought to room temperature before administration. Baseline spirometry is performed.

The patient begins by inhaling five breaths of nebulized diluent, usually normal saline. The diluent step is optional but provides a means of checking that the patient understands the procedure and that the system is working properly. If the

TABLE 9-2

Preparation of Methacholine for Two Common Dosing Schedules*

Methacholine	Diluent (0.9% NaCl)	Dilution
Doubling Dosage, as Used in the 2-Minute Tidal Breathing Protocol		
100 mg (dry powder)	6.25 ml	16.0 mg/ml
3 ml of 16.0 mg/ml	3 ml	8.0 mg/ml
3 ml of 8.0 mg/ml	3 ml	4.0 mg/ml
3 ml of 4.0 mg/ml	3 ml	2.0 mg/ml
3 ml of 2.0 mg/ml	3 ml	1.0 mg/ml
3 ml of 1.0 mg/ml	3 ml	0.5 mg/ml
3 ml of 0.5 mg/ml	3 ml	0.25 mg/ml
3 ml of 0.25 mg/ml	3 ml	0.125 mg/ml
3 ml of 0.125 mg/ml	3 ml	0.0625 mg/ml
3 ml of 0.625 mg/ml	3 ml	0.031 mg/ml
Quadrupling Dosage, as Used in the 5-Breath Dosimeter Protocol		
100 mg (dry powder)	6.25 ml	16.0 mg/ml
3 ml of 16.0 mg/ml	9 ml	4.0 mg/ml
3 ml of 4.0 mg/ml	9 ml	1.0 mg/ml
3 ml of 1.0 mg/ml	9 ml	0.25 mg/ml
3 ml of 0.25 mg/ml	9 ml	0.0625 mg/ml

*For each schedule, 6.25 ml of saline is added to dry powdered methacholine. Subsequent dilutions then use 3 or 9 ml of saline added to 3 ml of the previous dilution.

diluent step is performed, the FEV_1 following diluent becomes the "control" and the target FEV_1 for a positive test is 80% of this value. If the diluent step is omitted, the target FEV_1 is 80% of the baseline spirometry value. The breaths should be slow and deep, and the patient should wear a nose clip. The patient should inspire from FRC to TLC. The dosimeter should be triggered as inspiration begins; this may be done manually or automatically. The nebulizer should be activated for 0.6 seconds. Inspiration should last about 5 seconds, with a 5-second breath hold at TLC to maximize aerosol deposition. Inhalations are repeated for five breaths, lasting 2 minutes or less.

Spirometry is then repeated at approximately 30 and 90 seconds after the last inhalation. A timer or stopwatch is useful for staging the maneuvers. The FVC maneuver should be acceptable and may be repeated if necessary. The number of attempts should be limited to three or four efforts so that two acceptable maneuvers are obtained within 5 minutes. Full flow-volume loop maneuvers are useful for detecting changes in inspiratory flow that may occur (e.g., vocal cord dysfunction). If Raw and sGaw are also measured, the patient should be seated in the plethysmograph and the door closed as soon as spirometry has been completed. With practice and careful timing, spirometry and resistance measurements can be completed within about 5 minutes after each dose of methacholine.

The largest FEV_1 after each dose should be reported. If airway resistance/conductance measurements are made, the average of two acceptable panting maneuvers should be reported. If FEV_1 decreases less than 20%, or specific conductance (sGaw) decreases less than 35%–40%, the next highest dose is administered. If FEV_1 decreases more than 20%, the challenge is complete. Signs and symptoms (e.g., coughing, wheezing, chest tightness) related to asthma should be recorded. A β-adrenergic bronchodilator should be administered, and spirometry repeated after a 10-minute delay.

Two-Minute Tidal Breathing Method

In this method, normal relaxed breathing is used as the patient inhales the aerosol. Methacholine is usually prepared in 10 doses of doubling concentrations (see Box 9-1 and Table 9-2). If the methacholine has been refrigerated, it should be allowed to come to room temperature for 30 minutes. A nebulizer capable of delivering 0.13 ml/min (±10%) driven by compressed air should be used. An accurate flowmeter allows adjustment to the flow necessary to deliver the desired volume.

The patient should hold the nebulizer upright and breathe quietly through the mouthpiece with nose clip in place. A facemask may be used in place of a mouthpiece, but the nose clip should not be omitted (nose clip may be placed over the mask). A filter may be placed on the expiratory limb of the nebulizer circuit to limit the amount of methacholine released in aerosol form in the testing area. A timer or stopwatch should be used to ensure that the breathing interval is exactly 2 minutes long.

As in the dosimeter method, spirometry is repeated at 30 and 90 seconds after the end of the 2-minute tidal breathing interval. If a diluent step is included, the target FEV_1 (for a positive response) is 80% of the largest value obtained after the diluent. If the diluent step is omitted, the target FEV_1 is 80% of the baseline value. Patients with highly reactive airways may have a positive response (e.g., a 20% decrease in FEV_1) to the diluent. The FVC maneuvers should be completed within about 3 minutes. If Raw or sGaw is to be measured, those measurements should be performed as quickly as possible after spirometry. If FEV_1 decreases less than 20%, the next highest dose should be administered. If FEV_1 decreases by 20% or more, the challenge is complete. A β-adrenergic bronchodilator should be administered to reverse the bronchospasm, and spirometry repeated after 10 minutes.

Spirometry or plethysmographic measurements are the most commonly used end points for bronchial challenge tests. For each parameter, the percent of decrease is calculated as follows:

$$\%Decrease = \frac{x-y}{x} \times 100$$

where:
x = control FEV_1 (baseline, or after diluent)
y = current FEV_1 after methacholine inhalation

This change is sometimes reported as a negative value (e.g., −20%) to indicate a fall in the FEV_1.

A 20% or greater decrease in the FEV_1 is considered a positive response. The decrease should be sustained. Additional spirometry efforts may be necessary to distinguish an actual decrease from variability in the maneuvers. The same equation may be used to calculate changes in airway resistance or specific conductance. A decrease of 35%–45% in sGaw is consistent with increased bronchial responsiveness. In patients suspected of having vocal cord dysfunction (VCD), complete flow-volume (F-V) loops may be helpful. VCD is sometimes mistaken for asthma in patients referred for bronchial challenge testing. Limitation of inspiratory flow (with little or no change in FEV_1) is usually observed in VCD.

Several methods of quantifying the results of the challenge are commonly used. The concentration of methacholine that results in a 20% decrease

(PC_{20}) can be calculated from the last and second-to-last doses administered:

$$PC_{20} = \text{antilog}\left[\log C_1 + \frac{(\log C_2 - \log C_1)(20 - R_1)}{R_2 - R_1}\right]$$

where:

C_1 = second-to-last methacholine concentration
C_2 = final methacholine concentration (causing 20% or greater decrease)
R_1 = percent decrease in FEV_1 after C_1
R_2 = percent decrease in FEV_1 after C_2

PC_{20} calculated this way provides a single index of bronchial responsiveness. PC_{20} may also be identified directly from a graph in which change in FEV_1 is plotted against the log concentration of methacholine (Figure 9-2). Provocative concentrations for other variables, such as sGaw, can be calculated similarly by substituting the appropriate percentage for 20 in the preceding equation and substitut-

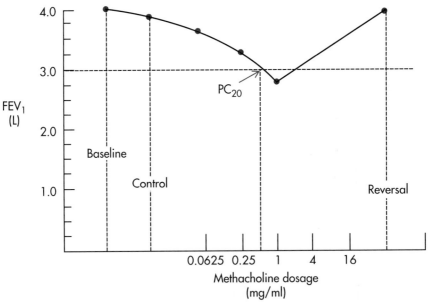

FIGURE 9-2 **Methacholine Challenge Test.** Results of data gathered during a bronchial challenge test are shown. The dosage of the challenge agent (methacholine in this case) is plotted on a logarithmic scale on the x-axis. FEV_1 (or other variable) is plotted on the y-axis. The first point represents the baseline FEV_1 (4.0 L in this example). The control value (FEV_1 after inhalation of the diluent) is plotted next. FEV_1 after each dose of methacholine is plotted until a 20% or greater decrease occurs. In this example, FEV_1 decreased by more than 20% with a dose of 1 mg/ml. A vertical line drawn from the point at which the dose response curve crosses the 20% line defines the PC_{20}. The patient is then given an inhaled bronchodilator to reverse the effect of the provocative agent, and the response is plotted.

ing the percent decrease for that variable for R_1 and R_2. Note that this calculation requires that at least two concentrations of methacholine have been given. If FEV_1 decreases 20% after the diluent or the first dose of methacholine, PC_{20} should be reported as less than the lowest concentration administered. If FEV_1 does not decrease by at least 20% after the highest dose, PC_{20} should be reported as "greater than 16 mg/ml."

See Test Regimens 9-1 for interpretive strategies. Airway responsiveness to methacholine can be described using the PC_{20}. Most patients referred for bronchial challenge testing have a history or symptoms suggestive of asthma, but not a definite diagnosis. For these patients, if FEV_1 decreases less than 20% at the highest dose ($PC_{20} > 16$ mg/ml), bronchial responsiveness is probably normal and asthma is unlikely. For patients whose FEV_1 decreases 20% or more at low doses of methacholine ($PC_{20} < 1.0$ mg/ml), the diagnosis of asthma is highly likely. For patients with PC_{20} values from $1-16$ mg/ml, the diagnosis of asthma must be considered based on the pretest probability of asthma, the history of symptoms, and other possible causes for bronchial hyperreactivity. In practice, patients who have a PC_{20} greater than $8-16$ mg/ml often do not have asthma. Patients who have a negative methacholine challenge ($PC_{20} > 16$ mg/ml) may have asthma that has been suppressed by anti-inflammatory medications or occupational asthma that is triggered by a specific agent. Conversely, some individuals who have PC_{20} values less than 8 mg/ml may not have asthma. Patients with allergic rhinitis and smokers with COPD often have bronchial hyperreactivity but not asthma.

PF TIP

Some patients whose FEV_1 drops 20% or more at low doses of methacholine may not have asthma. Hyperreactive airways are also found in some patients with COPD who smoke or in patients who have allergic rhinitis. A negative methacholine challenge (i.e., a decrease in FEV_1 <20% at the highest dose) may occur in patients who have asthma that has been suppressed by anti-inflammatory medications. Some asthmatics may have their asthma triggered by exposure to a specific agent such as cold, dry air.

TEST REGIMENS 9-1

INTERPRETIVE STRATEGIES

Bronchial Challenge Tests

1. Was the challenge agent administered appropriately?
   For methacholine or histamine, were the doses of agonist appropriate?
   Were nebulizer output, inspiratory flow, and so on, consistent for each dose?
   For exercise, did the patient maintain an appropriate workload for 6–8 minutes?
   For hyperventilation, did the patient maintain the target level of ventilation?
2. Were there any pretest factors that might influence results? Failure to withhold bronchodilators? Respiratory infection? If so, interpret cautiously or not at all.
3. Were spirometric efforts acceptable and repeatable before and during the challenge? If not, interpret very cautiously or not at all.
4. For methacholine or histamine challenge, was there a 20% decrease in FEV_1 after inhaling diluent? If so, test result is positive. Was there a 20% decrease in FEV_1 after inhalation of the agonist? If so, test result is likely positive, and PC_{20} should be used to categorize the degree of hyperresponsiveness. Was there at least a 35% decrease in sGaw (preferably 50%)? If so, test result is likely positive.
5. For exercise or hyperventilation challenge, was there a 10%–15% decrease in FEV_1 after challenge? If so, test is positive.
6. Were there signs or symptoms of airway hyperreactivity (coughing, wheezing, and shortness of breath)? If so, test suggests bronchial hyperresponsiveness.
7. Were the results borderline? If so, consider repeat testing in the future.
8. Were symptoms present despite little or no change in FEV_1? Consider additional measurements such as sGaw, or related conditions such as vocal cord dysfunction.

A number of physiologic factors affect the sensitivity and specificity of methacholine challenge testing. Methacholine causes constriction of bronchial smooth muscle. In healthy individuals, taking a deep breath before performing the FVC maneuver may cause bronchodilation for several minutes. In patients who have mild asthma, a similar response is sometimes observed. In patients who have severe asthma, the bronchodilating effect of a deep inspiration is reduced; a deep breath may actually cause bronchoconstriction. Because of this differing response, FEV_1 discriminates between those who have and those who do not have asthma.

Spirometry (i.e., FEV_1) may not detect a response in all patients. Raw or sGaw may be more sensitive in detecting hyperreactive airways in some individuals. Because Raw and sGaw are more variable than FEV_1 in healthy subjects, a larger change after methacholine challenge is required to demonstrate hyperreactive airways. A decrease in sGaw of 35%–45% may be considered a positive methacholine response. Some individuals with asthma symptoms may have primarily large airway changes in response to methacholine. These changes may manifest themselves as a decrease in sGaw or blunting of the inspiratory limb of the F-V loop. Although PEF is useful for monitoring asthma, it is less reproducible and more effort dependent than FEV_1 for detecting changes after bronchial challenge.

Technical factors can also make methacholine challenge tests difficult or impossible to interpret (Test Regimens 9-2). Changes in FEV_1 after bronchial challenge are usually not diagnostic in patients who cannot perform acceptable and reproducible baseline spirometry. Variable efforts by the patient may produce a false-positive test result (apparent reduction in FEV_1 but not asthma). FEV_1 values obtained at 30 and 90 seconds after each dose of methacholine should be similar. The maneuvers should meet criteria for an acceptable effort (see Chapter 2). However, because the primary end point is the FEV_1, it may not be necessary for the patient to exhale for 6 seconds. Using a shortened exhalation requires that the patient inspires fully to TLC, and this may be difficult to determine unless a full FVC effort is performed. The usual repeatability criteria (FEV_1 efforts within 150 ml) may not be met because of the effects of methacholine. Additional maneuvers may be needed at 30 and 90 seconds to verify that a real decrease has occurred. The FEV_1 reported for each dose of methacholine should be the largest value obtained at that level.

TEST REGIMENS 9-2

CRITERIA FOR ACCEPTABILITY
Bronchial Challenge Tests

1. The patient should withhold all bronchodilators before the test. Some long-acting bronchodilators may need to be withheld for up to a week.
2. The patient should also be free of upper or lower respiratory infection and not ingest any caffeinated beverages before the test.
3. Spirometric or plethysmographic efforts must meet standard criteria for acceptability and repeatability. For adults, the two largest FEV_1 measurements should be within 150 ml before the challenge (within 100 ml if the VC is 1.0 L or less). sGaw measurements should be within 10% before the challenge. During the challenge, acceptable efforts should be obtained; repeatability is desirable but may not be attained.
4. For methacholine and histamine challenges, a nebulizer that produces aerosol particles in the range of 1.0–3.6 μm should be used. Nebulizer output, inspiratory flow, lung volume, and breath-hold time should be consistent for all levels (doses) of challenge.
5. For exercise challenges, the patient should attain at least 80%–90% of the predicted maximal heart rate (or $\dot{V}O_2$max, if measured). This level should be maintained for 4–6 minutes. Ventilation should increase to 40%–60% of the MVV ($FEV_1 \times 35$). Measurement of $\dot{V}_E$ is recommended.
6 For hyperventilation challenges (cold or ambient air), the target ventilation level should be maintained for the specified interval (dependent on protocol used). For EVH, a target ventilation of $30 \times FEV_1$ for 6 minutes is recommended. For all challenge protocols, clinical signs and symptoms (e.g., presence or absence of coughing, wheezing) should be documented.

Adapted from ATS Guidelines for methacholine and exercise challenge testing–1999, *Am J Respir Crit Care Med* 2000; 161:309-329.

The type of nebulizer and dosimeter affects the amount of agonist reaching the airways. Factors that should be controlled as much as possible include type of nebulizer, nebulizer output, particle size, inhaled volumes, breath-hold times, and inspiratory flow. Nebulizer driving pressure or flow should be consistent throughout the test. If a single nebulizer is used, it should be thoroughly emptied between doses. If multiple nebulizers are used (one for each dose), they should be checked for similar output. Although the 5-breath dosimeter and tidal breathing techniques deliver different volumes of methacholine, the sensitivity and specificity of the test are similar for both methods in adults and in children. The spirometer used should meet the minimal standards set by the ATS/ERS (see Chapter 11). It should provide spirometric tracings or F-V loops for later evaluation.

Methacholine challenge testing is a safe procedure. The main risk to the patient is that severe bronchospasm may occur, so a physician experienced in treating acute bronchospasm should be immediately available. The technologist administering the bronchial challenge test should be thoroughly familiar with the procedure and with the signs and symptoms of bronchospasm. The technologist must know when to stop the test and how to administer bronchodilators to reverse acute bronchospasm. Medications for reversal of the bronchospasm (e.g., epinephrine, atropine) and for resuscitation should be immediately available in the event of an adverse reaction. Because of the risks involved, some laboratories require written consent from the patient. The test should be administered in a well-ventilated room to protect other patients and the technologist from exposure. The addition of a filter to the exhalation port of the nebulizer may help reduce the volume of aerosolized methacholine in the room. Technologists with known sensitivity to methacholine should not perform this procedure unless appropriate methods are used to avoid exposure to the drug.

Histamine Challenge

Aerosolized histamine extract (histamine phosphate) may be used for bronchial challenge in a manner similar to methacholine challenge. Histamine produces bronchoconstriction by an uncertain pathway. Antihistamines or H_1-receptor antagonists can block the response to histamine. Histamine-induced bronchospasm is also partially blocked by most classes of bronchodilators. Histamine differs from methacholine in its side effects, half-life, and cumulative effects. Flushing and headache are two common side effects of histamine inhalation. The peak action of histamine occurs within 30 seconds to 2 minutes, which is similar to that observed in methacholine. Recovery of baseline function is significantly shorter for histamine than for methacholine. The action of histamine, unlike that of methacholine, is thought to be less cumulative.

Patient preparation for histamine challenge is similar to that used for methacholine (see Table 9-2). Antihistamines and H_1-receptor antagonists should be withheld for 48 hours before testing.

Various dosing regimens for histamine challenge have been proposed. Box 9-3 lists one dosing protocol for histamine challenge. These increments approximately double the concentration of drug at each level. The same criteria as those used for baseline spirometry in methacholine challenge are observed. Diluent may be administered first to determine a control value for FEV_1.

If FEV_1 does not decrease by more than 10%, then five breaths of the first dilution are administered. Spirometric measurements are performed immediately, and then repeated at 3 minutes. A response is considered positive if FEV_1 decreases by 20% or more below the control at 3 minutes. If there is a negative response (FEV_1 decreases

BOX 9-3	Histamine Dosing Schedule
0.03 mg/ml	
0.06 mg/ml	
0.12 mg/ml	
0.25 mg/ml	
1.00 mg/ml	
2.50 mg/ml	
5.00 mg/ml	
10.00 mg/ml	

<20%), the next dose is given and measurements are repeated.

The results of histamine challenge are reported in a manner similar to that described for methacholine. The histamine concentration that produces a 20% decrease in FEV_1 is termed the PC_{20}. Response may also be reported by graphing the percentage of change in FEV_1 against the concentration (or its logarithm) of the drug. This type of plot is commonly called a dose-response graph. It permits interpolation of the precise concentration of drug that elicits the 20% decrease (see Figure 9-2).

Histamine, like methacholine, is relatively safe if testing follows the procedures described. Baseline and control values should always be established (see Test Regimens 9-2). Bronchial challenge should always begin with a low concentration of drug. The range of concentrations used should be appropriate for the patient tested. For adult patients in whom airway hyperreactivity is the suspected diagnosis, the dosing schedules previously described are recommended. Patients who have a positive response to histamine challenge recover more quickly than those tested with methacholine. Histamine challenge can be repeated within 2 hours after the patient has returned to baseline level of function.

Exercise Challenge

Exercise-induced asthma (EIA) is typified by bronchospasm during or immediately after vigorous exercise. EIA is related to heat and water loss from the upper airway that accompanies increased ventilation during exercise. Evaluation of exercise-induced bronchospasm (EIB) may be helpful in the following instances:

1. In patients who have shortness of breath on exertion but exhibit normal resting pulmonary function
2. In symptomatic patients in whom other bronchial provocation tests (such as methacholine challenge) produce negative or ambiguous results
3. In patients with known EIA in whom therapy is being evaluated

4. In screening patients where some risk to those with asthma might be involved (e.g., athletics, military service)

Patients referred for exercise challenge should be evaluated by means of an appropriate history and physical examination. The evaluation should include a resting electrocardiogram (ECG) to ascertain potential contraindications to exercise testing (see Chapter 7). Bronchodilators should be withheld as for methacholine challenge testing (see Table 9-1). Before exercise, the patient's FEV_1 should not be less than 65% of the predicted value. Patients with overt obstruction usually do not require an exercise challenge to demonstrate airway hyperreactivity. Patients should refrain from vigorous exercise for 4 hours before the test because there is a refractory period after exercise. Patients referred for EIB testing should be free from respiratory infections for 3–6 weeks before testing.

PF TIP

EVH testing may be a good substitute for exercise-induced asthma testing. High levels of eucapnic ventilation produce heat and water loss from the upper airway similar to the losses that occur with exercise. By setting a target ventilation that represents a significant fraction of the patient's maximal value (i.e., $FEV_1 \times 30$), airway hyperreactivity can be demonstrated. High levels of ventilation are not always achieved during exercise, especially if patients are limited by their maximal heart rate or by deconditioning.

Either a treadmill or a cycle ergometer may be used, depending on the type of physiologic measurements being made. Exercise should be vigorous enough to elicit work rates of 80%–90% of the patient's predicted heart rate (HR) for 6–8 minutes. The patient's response to an increasing workload should be monitored through continuous ECG and blood pressure (BP). A pulse oximeter should be used to determine whether oxygen (O_2) desaturation occurs with exercise. Because pulse oximetry is not always accurate during exercise, an arterial line may be indicated if there is a high probability that exercise desaturation will occur. The pulse oximeter should be left in place in the postexercise phase to detect desaturation that may occur with bronchospasm.

Measurement of variables such as minute ventilation ($\dot{V}_E$) and tidal volume (V_T) may be helpful in assessing the ventilatory load imposed by the exercise. Measurement of F-V curves during exercise may be a useful adjunct in assessing the ventilatory response to increasing workloads (see Chapter 7). A spirometer that meets ATS/ERS requirements (see Chapter 10) is necessary. Resuscitation equipment, as described in Chapter 7, should be available.

Because EIB is related to heat and water loss from the upper airway, environmental conditions should be controlled. Room temperature should be less than 25° C with relative humidity of 50% or less. The patient should wear nose clips, even if exhaled gas is not collected, to reduce gas conditioning by nasal airflow. Ambient temperature, relative humidity, and barometric pressure (P_B) should be recorded. The patient may also be allowed

to breathe dry gas from a compressed air source using a reservoir bag (Figure 9-3).

Low-intensity exercise for 1–2 minutes allows evaluation of ventilatory and cardiovascular responses to work. As soon as a normal cardiovascular response is observed, workload should be increased until the patient attains 85% of predicted maximal HR or predicted maximal O_2 consumption ($\dot{V}O_2$). Alternately, the minute ventilation ($\dot{V}_E$) may be used as a target for exercise intensity if exhaled gas is collected. Ventilation should reach 40%–60% of the patient's predicted MVV. The treadmill or cycle ergometer can be adjusted to increase or decrease the workload to maintain the correct intensity for the desired length of time.

In most instances, a short period of moderately heavy work is all that is required to trigger exercise-induced bronchospasm. The goal is to have the patient exercise at high intensity for 4–6 minutes, with total exercise duration of 6–8 minutes. Bronchospasm usually occurs immediately after the

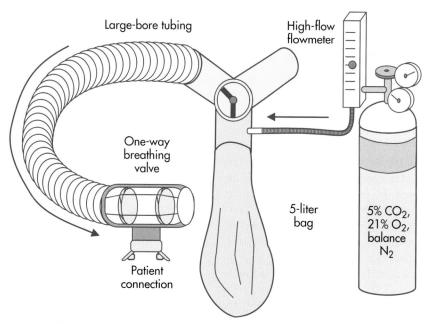

FIGURE 9-3   Breathing Circuit for Eucapnic Voluntary Hyperventilation (EVH). A gas containing 5% CO_2, 21% O_2, and balance N_2 is directed through a precision high-flow flowmeter to a reservoir bag. Flow is adjusted to a target ventilation level, such as 30 times the patient's FEV_1. The patient then breathes from the bag through a one-way valve with large-bore tubing. The patient is coached to increase ventilation to keep the bag partially deflated. The test is continued for a predetermined interval, usually 6 minutes.

exercise, not during it, unless the test is extended over a longer interval (see Test Regimens 9-2). Repeated testing should be delayed for 4 hours because of a "refractory period" during which the severity of the bronchoconstriction lessens. This response is presumably caused by the release of catecholamines during exercise. An extended warm-up period before the actual exercise may also protect the airways and lessen subsequent bronchoconstriction.

Baseline spirometry values are established before testing. The patient should be able to perform acceptable and repeatable FEV_1 measurements. Inability to perform acceptable spirometry will make interpretation of postexercise changes difficult. The baseline FEV_1 value is also the control. After exercise, spirometry is performed at 1–2 minutes, then every 5 minutes as the selected variable (usually FEV_1) decreases to a minimum. For spirometry, the highest value of acceptable measurements is recorded; FEV_1 should be repeatable. The preferred method of reporting response to exercise is the following:

$$\%Decrease = \frac{x - y}{x} \times 100$$

where:
x = baseline value (FEV_1)
y = lowest observed postexercise value

As in methacholine challenge testing, the fall in FEV_1 is sometimes presented as a negative number (e.g., −10%) to indicate a decrease. Similarly, an increase in FEV_1 (as observed in healthy subjects after exercise) may be represented as a positive value, even though the preceding calculation produces a negative number if y is greater than x. Testing should be continued until the FEV_1 returns to baseline. Maximal decreases are typically seen in the first 5–10 minutes after cessation of exercise. A decrease in FEV_1 of 10%–15% is consistent with increased airway sensitivity. Allowing the FEV_1 to fall to its lowest point provides an estimate of how severe the response to exercise has been. Spontaneous recovery usually occurs within 20–40 minutes. Some laboratories administer a β-agonist to reverse the bronchospasm as soon as a threshold (e.g.,

10–15% decrease) has been reached. The FEV_1 should return to near baseline values whether or not a bronchodilator is administered.

PF TIP

The normal response to exercise is for the FEV_1 (and specific conductance) to increase slightly. Patients who have exercise-induced bronchospasm usually have a decrease in flows (FEV_1). When an increase is expected, a decrease of 10%–15% is consistent with airway hyperreactivity. Some patients have a much greater decrease in response to even moderate exercise, so the pulmonary function technologist should be prepared to reverse severe bronchospasm.

Severe bronchospasm may occur following exercise, and the technologist performing the test should be prepared to manage it. If the bronchospasm is severe, it should be reversed using an inhaled bronchodilator. FEV_1 should return to within 10% of the pretest baseline value. Administration of a bronchodilator may also be useful in assessing borderline decreases in FEV_1 (<10%) following exercise challenge. Patients who show a minimal decrease after exercise may improve dramatically with an inhaled bronchodilator, suggesting increased airway responsiveness.

Patients who have VCD or other upper airway abnormalities are often referred for EIA tests. F-V curves (including maximal inspiratory flows) should be performed if the history or physical examination suggests these disorders. Measurement of tidal breathing loops during exercise (see Chapter 7) may also help to define the pattern of ventilatory limitation.

One potential problem with using exercise to elicit EIB is that the level of exercise chosen may not mimic real-world triggers. Sedentary patients may not attain a level of ventilation high enough to trigger EIB when exercising at 85% of their maximal HR. Patients who are very fit (e.g., elite athletes) may require high workloads to reach 85% of their predicted HR or to increase their ventilation significantly. Measurement of $\dot{V}_E$ during exercise may be needed to determine the level of ventilation attained. Patients whose asthma is triggered by cold, dry air may not show a maximal response if tested under standard laboratory conditions. Exercise-induced bronchospasm may be evaluated using hyperventilation with either cold or ambient temperature gas. These techniques eliminate the need for more complicated exercise testing. Hyperventilation (with a target ventilation level) may be more sensitive in detecting airway hyperreactivity than exercise testing.

Eucapnic Voluntary Hyperventilation

Airway hyperreactivity may also be assessed by having the patient breathe at a high level of ventilation. Heat or water loss from the upper airways has been demonstrated to provoke bronchospasm in susceptible individuals. These physiologic changes are most pronounced when the patient inhales cold, dry gas, but they can also be demonstrated with dry gas at room temperature. To prevent respiratory alkalosis (i.e., true hyperventilation), carbon dioxide (CO_2) is mixed with inspired air. This gas mixture allows high levels of ventilation with little change in pH.

Patients to be tested with **eucapnic voluntary hyperventilation** (EVH) should withhold bronchodilators as suggested in Table 9-1. Baseline spirometry is performed to ascertain that airway obstruction is not present. For ventilation challenges, the baseline FEV_1 is the control value with which subsequent measurements will be compared.

If cold air is to be used, the mixture is passed through a heat exchanger or over a cooling coil. These devices lower the temperature and remove water vapor from the gas. Gas temperatures are reduced to a subfreezing level in the range $-10°$ to $-20°$ C. The relative humidity is usually near 0%.

The patient breathes the gas at an elevated level of ventilation. In one method, the patient breathes at a fraction of his or her maximal voluntary ventilation (MVV) (e.g., 30%–70% of the MVV). CO_2 is added to the gas to maintain a stable $P_{ET}CO_2$. This is accomplished either by titrating CO_2 into the mixture or by using a gas composed of 5% CO_2, 21%

O_2, and the balance nitrogen (N_2). The patient maintains the specified level of ventilation for 4–6 minutes. Spirometry or sGaw is then measured at fixed intervals after the hyperventilation (e.g., 1, 5, and 10 minutes). A second method has the patient breathe at increasing levels of ventilation up to the MVV (e.g., 7.5, 15, 30, 60 L/min and MVV). Again CO_2 is added to the inspired gas to maintain isocapnia (i.e., $PaCO_2$ of approximately 40 mm Hg).

EVH with gas at ambient temperature also provides a stimulus for bronchospasm. In this technique, the patient breathes a mixture of 5% CO_2, 21% O_2, and the balance N_2 at room temperature. The gas is used to fill a "target" bag or balloon of approximately 5 L (see Figure 9-3). The patient breathes from the bag via a nonrebreathing valve (see Chapter 10) and large-bore tubing. The patient wears a nose clip. A high-output flowmeter is used to fill the target bag. The flowmeter is adjusted to deliver gas at approximately 30 times the patient's FEV_1. The patient breathes from the bag and tries to match his or her ventilation to keep the bag partly deflated. The high level of ventilation is continued for 6 minutes. Spirometry is performed immediately after hyperventilation and then at 5-minute intervals (i.e., at 5, 10, 15, and 20 minutes).

For both the cold-air and room-temperature protocols, if no decrease in FEV_1 occurs within 20 minutes after hyperventilation, the test may be considered negative. The percentage decrease is calculated just as for methacholine challenge testing, described previously. A decrease of 15% is consistent with some degree of airway hyperreactivity (see Test Regimens 9-2). EVH in healthy subjects usually results in bronchodilatation. Therefore a 15% decrease is abnormal and highly specific for increased bronchial responsiveness. Some asthmatic patients may experience significant decreases in FEV_1 (20%–60%). Bronchospasm should be reversed with inhaled bronchodilators, and the reversal documented with spirometry. The technologist performing the procedure should be prepared to manage severe bronchospasm if it occurs.

Raw and sGaw can be measured easily when hyperventilation tests are used. Because the airway challenge is applied once, the patient can remain in the body plethysmograph for measurements at defined intervals. Cold-air testing requires specialized equipment to refrigerate and dry inspired gas. Testing with cold air is slightly more sensitive and specific than testing with room-temperature gas. Both techniques correlate well with the results of methacholine challenge tests, although they are slightly less specific. If multiple levels of ventilation are evaluated, a dose-response curve can be constructed. However, the single challenge is less complicated and can be used to evaluate patients with suspected asthma, particularly exercise-induced asthma.

EXHALED NITRIC OXIDE

Description

Measurement of exhaled nitric oxide (eNO) provides a simple and noninvasive method for assessing airway inflammation. It is particularly useful in diagnosing and monitoring lung diseases characterized by eosinophilic inflammation, such as asthma. The fraction of eNO in an exhaled breath (FE_{NO}) can be measured with a sensitive chemoluminescent analyzer (see Chapter 10). FE_{NO} is usually reported in parts per billion (ppb). Because the measurement is dependent on flow during exhalation, the flow (in liters per second) may be subscripted to the term (e.g., $FE_{NO0.05}$ represents the FE_{NO} measured at a flow of 0.05 L/sec). NO is also sometimes measured from the nasal cavities, including the sinuses, as a marker of nasal inflammation.

PF TIP

Exhaled nitric oxide levels are typically elevated by airway inflammation in patients who have asthma. However, FE_{NO} may be reduced in patients who smoke. Smokers who also have asthma may show an elevated FE_{NO} that is not as high as it would be if they were not currently smoking. Smoking status may be an important factor in detecting airway inflammation when the FE_{NO} is near the upper limit of normal.

Techniques

FE_{NO} can be measured either online or off-line. The methods for each type of collection differ slightly in adults and children. Online measurements sample exhaled gas continuously at the mouth; off-line measurements collect exhaled air in a sampling device for later analysis.

Online FE_{NO} in Adults

Before measuring FE_{NO}, patients should refrain from smoking, eating, or drinking for at least 1 hour before testing. Measurement of eNO should be performed before other tests such as spirometry, methacholine challenge, or exercise testing. Any recent infections, as well as the current medication regimen, should be recorded at the time of testing.

Because NO is produced in the airways (and in the alveoli), it is important that the patient inhale NO-free gas. This is accomplished by having the subject inspire through an NO scrubber. The ambient NO level should be recorded as well. The patient should be instructed to exhale to RV, then insert the mouthpiece and inspire over a 2–3 second interval to TLC. A nose clip is NOT used; this lessens the possibility that the much higher **nasal NO** will accumulate and contaminate the lower airway sample.

Without breath holding, the patient then exhales slowly and evenly while exhaled gas is sampled continuously. To prevent contamination of the exhalate with nasal NO, the patient exhales against an expiratory resistance while receiving feedback to maintain a positive pressure at the mouth. This positive pressure (usually about +5 cm H_2O) causes the velum in the posterior pharynx to close, preventing nasal NO from entering the air stream. The fractional concentration of NO in the exhaled gas varies inversely with the flow. To standardize online measurements, an exhaled flow of 0.05 L/sec (i.e., 50 ml/sec) ±10% is recommended. This flow allows dead space gas to be exhaled and a plateau in NO to be observed in about 10 seconds in adults (Figure 9-4). The correct flow can be maintained by using a pressure-sensitive flow controller and providing visual feedback to the subject. The flow at which

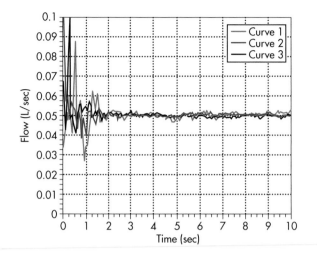

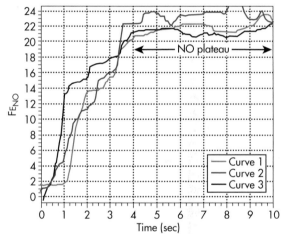

FIGURE 9-4   **Measurement of Exhaled NO (FE$_{NO}$).** The upper graph shows three efforts in which flows are measured at the mouth. The subject exhales against a slight resistance to close the velum in the oropharynx. Visual feedback in the form of a computer display helps the patient to maintain a constant pressure and thereby a constant flow at the recommended 0.05 L/sec. The lower graph displays the FE$_{NO}$ values for the three maneuvers over 10 seconds of exhalation. Exhaled NO rises to a plateau and the FE$_{NO}$ concentration is measured over a 3-second (i.e., 0.15 L) window from the plateau (see text).

FE$_{NO}$ is measured should be recorded, particularly if a nonstandard flow is used.

FE$_{NO}$ is measured from the plateau of the single-breath exhalation profile (see Figure 9-4). The plateau phase may slope up or down slightly. The exhalation should last long enough to establish this plateau (>6 seconds for adults and children older than 12 years, >4 seconds for children ages 12 years and younger). Two points should be chosen on the plateau that represent a 3-second interval (about 0.15 L) in which the FE$_{NO}$ varies less than 10%. The FE$_{NO}$ is the mean concentration over this 3-second interval. For FE$_{NO}$ values of 10 ppb or less, variability of 1 ppb NO may be used in place of the 10% criteria. A minimum of 30 seconds should elapse between repeated measurements with the subject breathing air (off the NO sampling circuit).

At least two acceptable measurements of FE$_{NO}$ that agree within 10% of each other should be averaged for the final report value. Three acceptable measurements should be averaged if FE$_{NO}$ is measured at multiple flow rates.

Off-line FE$_{NO}$ in Adults

Off-line measurements of NO allow gas to be collected away from the analyzer, making use of the analyzer more efficient. Potential problems with off-line measurements include contamination with gas from the upper airway, errors caused by storing the sample, and lack of feedback to the patient regarding technique during gas collection.

The patient inhales through an NO scrubber or from a reservoir with NO-free gas. After inhaling to TLC, the patient exhales his or her VC into an appropriate sampling device without breath holding. Expiratory resistance (+5 cm H$_2$O) is added just as is done for online measurements to minimize contamination by nasal NO. Flow is usually controlled by monitoring the back-pressure in the system; flows of 0.35 L/sec ± 10% are recommended to allow the VC to be collected in a reasonable interval. The sample is collected in a balloon made of polyester (Mylar) or a similar material that is impermeable to NO and large enough to accommodate the adult's VC. Off-line samples should be analyzed within 12 hours.

FE$_{NO}$ in Children

Online measurements in children able to perform the single-breath maneuver (typically ages 4–5 years or older) are similar to those in adults. The child inspires an NO-free gas to near TLC and then exhales at a flow of 0.05 L/sec (50 ml/sec). A dynamic flow restrictor facilitates flow control by maintaining a constant flow even though the child's mouth pressure varies. Visual or audio feedback is provided to help control the expiratory flow. Exhalation should continue for at least 4 seconds, with an observable plateau in the NO concentration that spans at least 2 seconds. Three efforts that match within 10% or two within 5% are averaged and recorded. There should be a 30-second interval between efforts.

Off-line measurements in children are similar to those for adults. The child is asked to exhale a vital capacity breath into a polyester (Mylar) balloon that is fitted with a restrictor capable of generating 5 cm H_2O back-pressure. Flow control by means of a dynamic flow restrictor greatly improves the repeatability of the measurement and allows the flow to be standardized at 50 ml/sec (i.e., same as the online method) (Test Regimens 9-3).

Nasal Nitric Oxide

Although various methods of sampling nasal NO have been described, the recommended method uses transnasal airflow in series. In this technique, air is aspirated into one naris and out the opposite side, where NO is sampled. The subject exhales against a resistance of approximately 10 cm H_2O, while air is aspirated at a constant flow rate. As for measurement of FE_{NO} from the lower airways, exhalation against resistance closes the velum in the posterior pharynx to prevent contamination of the sample. Airflow of 0.25–3.0 L/min is used for nasal NO measurements. Flows in this range allow a plateau in the NO signal within 20–30 seconds in most adults. The flow used for NO analysis, along with the transnasal flow, should be recorded.

TEST REGIMENS 9-3

CRITERIA FOR ACCEPTABILITY

Exhaled Nitric Oxide

1. Patient should be free of respiratory tract infections; no eating, drinking, or smoking for one hour prior to testing. Exhaled NO should be measured before spirometry or bronchial challenges.

ONLINE MEASUREMENT

2. Patient should inhale NO free air to TLC within 2–3 seconds.
3. Patient should exhale against +5 cm H_2O resistance at a constant flow of 0.05 L/sec (50 ml/sec) ± 10%.
4. Duration of exhalation should be more than 6 seconds for adults and children older than 12 years (>4 seconds for children ages 12 years and younger).
5. There should be a plateau in the NO signal and FE_{NO} should be measured from a 3-second window in which NO does not vary by more than 10% (1 ppb for FE_{NO} < 10 ppb).
6. Thirty seconds should elapse between repeated measurements.
7. FE_{NO} value reported should be the average of at least 2 acceptable measurements that agree within 10% of each other.

OFF-LINE MEASUREMENT

8. Patient should inspire at least two tidal breaths of NO-free air, and then a VC breath, and exhale against resistance (+5 cm H_2O) into a suitable reservoir, without breath holding.
9. Flow of 0.35 L/sec ± 10% should be maintained throughout exhalation of the VC.
10. Reservoir should be sealed immediately and NO analyzed within 12 hours.

Adapted from ATS/ERS recommendations for standardized procedures for the online and offline measurement of exhaled lower respiratory nitric oxide and nasal nitric oxide, 2005, *Am J Respir Crit Care Med* 2005; 171:912-930.

Significance and Pathophysiology

Normal values for FE_{NO} depend largely on the flow at which gas is sampled during analysis. At a standardized flow of 0.05 L/sec (50 ml/sec), healthy adults show FE_{NO} values of 10–25 ppb, whereas in children the values are slightly lower (5–15 ppb). FE_{NO} actually increases with increasing age in children. The upper limit of normal in adults is approximately 35 ppb (25 ppb in children) when FE_{NO} is measured using standardized methods and flows (50 ml/sec). FE_{NO} appears to be related to airway size; thus it tends to be slightly higher in males than in females.

Exhaled NO appears to correlate most closely with eosinophilic inflammation in the airways. Because this type of inflammation is characteristic of bronchial asthma, measurement of FE_{NO} can be viewed as a surrogate for measuring eosinophils in induced sputum samples, bronchoalveolar lavage, or bronchial biopsy in patients who have asthma. These correlations persist when inflammation is treated, making FE_{NO} an excellent tool for monitoring therapy.

Some studies have indicated a correlation between FE_{NO} and bronchial hyperresponsiveness as measured by the PC_{20} from methacholine or histamine challenge. However, many studies show little or no correlation between eNO and hyperresponsiveness. These conflicting findings may be due to the fact that eosinophilic inflammation is characteristic mainly in atopic individuals. Responsiveness to methacholine appears to correlate with FEV_1, whereas increased FE_{NO} correlates with other markers of inflammation.

Although pulmonary function tests (including bronchial challenge) are considered a standard method for diagnosing and assessing asthma, there appears to be little correlation between these measures and airway inflammation. In general, most tests of lung function do not correlate with levels of eNO. Changes in NO during periods of exacerbation tend to occur more rapidly than changes in pulmonary function indices (e.g., FEV_1). Spirometry and bronchial challenge tests can reduce the level of eNO, so that if both procedures are to be performed on a patient, FE_{NO} should be measured first.

FE_{NO} is reduced by corticosteroids' effects on airway inflammation. Numerous well-designed studies have demonstrated that steroid therapy, including inhaled corticosteroids, can be monitored and evaluated using FE_{NO} as a marker of inflammation. FE_{NO} does not appear to be reduced by either short-acting or long-acting β-agonists, either alone or in combination with inhaled corticosteroids. FE_{NO} may also be reduced in some patients treated with leukotriene modifiers.

Because of the correlation between FE_{NO} and airway inflammation, and the known anti-inflammatory effects of inhaled corticosteroids, eNO has several potential uses in asthma diagnosis and management. FE_{NO} can be used as a simple diagnostic screening tool to differentiate asthma from other conditions (such as chronic cough). Exhaled NO compares favorably with bronchial challenge tests (methacholine, exercise) in terms of sensitivity and specificity in detecting asthma. Patients who have an elevated NO level typically respond to corticosteroid therapy. FE_{NO} is therefore a good tool to evaluate response to anti-inflammatory therapy. Failure of FE_{NO} to decrease with steroid treatment suggests that the patient may be unresponsive to standard therapy or that the patient may be noncompliant with the recommended treatment. Some studies have suggested that the dosage of inhaled corticosteroids can be optimized with FE_{NO} to guide therapy.

Patients who have COPD often show normal levels of FE_{NO}. However, some studies have shown increased NO in patients with COPD. These differences may be related to the presence or absence of eosinophilic inflammation in COPD patients. Many COPD patients respond poorly to inhaled corticosteroids; measurement of FE_{NO} may provide an indicator as to whether eosinophilic inflammation is present and whether the patient may respond to steroid therapy. FE_{NO} may also be increased in pulmonary diseases that are characterized by inflammatory changes such as chronic bronchitis, chronic cough, sarcoidosis, pneumonia, alveolitis, bronchiolitis obliterans syndrome (BOS), and bronchiectasis.

FE_{NO} is typically decreased in smokers, even though smoking causes airway inflammation. The physiologic explanation for the reduction in NO levels in smokers is unclear. Cigarette smoking may decrease the production of NO by epithelial cells lining the airways. Exhaled NO levels are also usually lower than normal in patients who have cystic fibrosis (CF). As in the case of smokers, it is not clear whether the reduced levels in CF are a result of decreased production or increased metabolism of NO in the lungs.

Nasal NO levels are typically much higher than eNO. Values from 100 ppb up to more than 1000 ppb have been reported. Most of the nasal NO appears to be produced by the epithelial cells in the

INTERPRETIVE STRATEGIES

Exhaled Nitric Oxide

1. Was the measurement of FE_{NO} (online or off-line) performed acceptably? Were at least two measurements repeatable within 10%? If not, interpret cautiously or not at all.
2. Are there any pretest factors that might influence the results? Eating, drinking, or smoking within 1 hour of testing? Signs and/or symptoms of respiratory tract infection? If so, interpret cautiously or not at all.
3. If the FE_{NO} is above the upper limit of normal (>35 ppb for adults, >25 ppb for children at 0.05 L/sec) suspect eosinophilic inflammation of the airways and/or alveolitis. Consider clinical correlation, particularly if the patient is taking corticosteroids or other anti-inflammatory medications. Consider steroid unresponsiveness, inappropriate dosing, or noncompliance with prescribed therapy.
4. If FE_{NO} is much lower than normal range (15–25 ppb in adults, 5–20 ppb in children at 0.05 L/sec) consider clinical correlation (pulmonary or systemic hypertension, heart failure, ciliary dyskinesia, cystic fibrosis). Also consider other factors associated with reduced NO levels (active or passive smoking, bronchoconstriction, alcohol consumption).

paranasal sinuses. Patients with allergic rhinitis show elevated levels of NO that appear to be responsive to nasal corticosteroids. One disease in which nasal NO measurements may be particularly useful is primary ciliary dyskinesia (PCD). Patients who have PCD have much lower levels of nasal NO (Test Regimens 9-4).

FORCED OSCILLATION TECHNIQUE

One way to measure the mechanical properties of the respiratory system is to apply an oscillating flow of gas to the system and measure the resulting pressure response. This method is commonly called the **forced oscillation technique (FOT).** When the forced oscillations are applied at the mouth and the resulting pressure oscillations are measured at the mouth, the output is known as input impedance. When the oscillations are applied around the body in a closed body plethysmograph, and resulting pressures measured at the mouth, the output is known as transfer impedance. But what is impedance?

PF TIP

The forced oscillation technique (FOT) is particularly useful for measuring changes in the airways of patients who may be unable to perform spirometry or body plethysmography. This includes subjects such as young children or those with physical limitations that prevent them from performing tests that require effort and coordination (i.e., FVC).

Impedance of the respiratory system (Zrs) represents the net force that must be overcome to move gas in and out of the respiratory system (upper airway, lungs, and chest wall). Applying oscillatory flow is appropriate because that is how we breathe, in a regular in-and-out fashion. Imagine the lungs modeled as a stiff pipe (the airways) with a balloon on the end (the alveoli). The pressure required to push gas down the pipe and into the balloon must overcome three basic forces: the resistance (R) of the pipe, the **elastance** (E), or stiffness, of the balloon, and the **inertia** (I) of the gas itself. Stated mathematically, the pressure necessary to move gas down the pipe and into the balloon is as follows:

$$\text{Pressure} = R(\dot{V}) + E(V) + I(\ddot{V})$$

where:
V = volume
$\dot{V}$ = flow
$\ddot{V}$ = acceleration

This is known as the equation of motion for the system. Impedance depends not only on these three variables, R, E and I, but also on the frequency of the oscillation. At low frequencies, I is negligible, R is less important, and E is dominant. At higher fre-

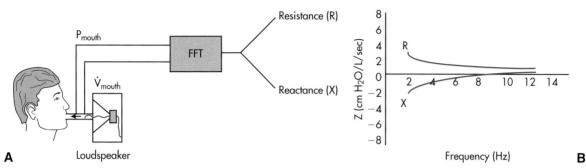

FIGURE 9-5   Measurement and Display of Respiratory System Impedance (Zrs). A, A typical apparatus for measuring input Zrs involves a loudspeaker generating a complex flow signal consisting of many, simultaneous frequencies. The flow signal is delivered to the mouth while mouth pressure (P) and flow (V̇) are measured. These measurements are then processed by computer using the fast Fourier transformation (FFT) to derive the in-phase and out-of-phase signals, which represent the real (R) and imaginary (X) part of Zrs. **B,** The real (R) and imaginary (X) parts of Zrs are shown in relation to frequency. R is frequency dependent, falling to lower values with higher frequency. This phenomenon is due to heterogeneity of lung mechanical properties as well as tissue viscoelastance. Above 5 Hz, R primarily reflects central airway resistance. X is also frequency dependent, increasing with higher frequencies. This is due to the increasing contribution of gas inertia to X as frequency gets higher. The frequency at which X crosses zero is known as the resonant frequency and is the frequency at which gas inertia and respiratory system elastance (E) are equal. This occurs at approximately 8–10 Hz in humans. With increasing bronchoconstriction, overall R increases and may become more frequency dependent, and X is reduced at any given frequency, yielding a higher resonant frequency.

quencies, R and I become more important. Frequency is also important because the lung tissues have viscoelastic mechanical properties that change with the frequency of motion.

To measure Z, one could apply flow at various single frequencies and measure the resulting pressures generated at each frequency. Alternatively, one could apply a flow signal consisting of many different frequencies at once and then use a mathematical function known as the **fast Fourier transformation (FFT)** to break down the output into unique sine waves, each of its own frequency. Despite involving complex mathematics with real and imaginary numbers, computers have made this method quick and accurate, and it has become the technique most commonly used (Figure 9-5, *A*).

Traditional devices use loudspeakers pulsating at different, predetermined frequencies to generate the broadband flow signals. One commercially available device (Figure 9-6) generates the broadband flow signal by an electronically controlled

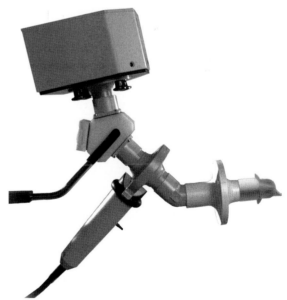

FIGURE 9-6   Commercially Available Device for FOT. A built-in loud speaker generates an impulse of flow containing a wide range of frequencies (5–35 Hz). (*Courtesy Cardinal Health, Cardiopulmonary Diagnostics, Yorba Linda, Calif.*)

deflection of an internal speaker to create an impulse of flow containing many frequencies, although the frequencies analyzed range from 5–35 Hz. For all devices, the flow signal can be applied during quiet spontaneous breathing and thus requires little subject effort or cooperation. Once performed, the output is recorded in two parts: the part of Z that is in phase with the flow signal, which represents the real part of the Z and is due to flow resistive properties of the respiratory system, R, and the part that is out of phase with the flow signal, called the reactance (X), which represents the imaginary part of Z, and encompasses E and I. These real and imaginary parts are plotted against frequency, as shown in Figure 9-5, *B*.

In most clinical applications, the FOT is used to measure R. Because the technique is noninvasive, fast, and easy, it can be applied in many situations where other methods of measuring R are difficult or cumbersome. These situations include use in pediatric patients or others who cannot perform the panting maneuvers to measure Raw by the body box technique. The R derived from the FOT has been shown to be sensitive to bronchoconstriction and bronchodilation and thus can be used to assess airway hyperresponsiveness. An important disadvantage of the technique is that, unless an esophageal balloon is placed to measure transpulmonary pressure, the R measured is not of the lungs alone but of the entire respiratory system, thus including the upper airway and chest wall. The upper airway, in particular, can markedly influence the measurement because of its high compliance and the propensity for glottic interference. Other potential problems include limited reference equations and little standardization of the technique, although recent reference sets and international guidelines are now available.

PREOPERATIVE PULMONARY FUNCTION TESTING

Preoperative pulmonary function testing is one of several means available to clinicians to evaluate surgical candidates at risk for developing respiratory complications. Preoperative testing, in conjunction with history and physical examination, ECG, and chest x-ray examination, may be indicated for any of the following reasons:

1. To estimate postoperative lung function in candidates for pneumonectomy or lobectomy
2. To plan perioperative care (preoperative preparation, type and duration of anesthetic during surgery, postoperative care) to minimize complications
3. To enhance the estimate of risk involved in the surgical procedure (i.e., morbidity and mortality) derived from history and physical examination

The need for preoperative pulmonary function testing is controversial. Some studies show increased odds of postoperative complications related to low FEV_1, hypoxemia, low D_{LCO}, hypercarbia, or low $\dot{V}_{O_2}$. Other studies show little relationship between pulmonary function and postoperative risk, especially for general surgical and cardiovascular operations. Many investigations, both prospective and retrospective, have identified that the risk of postoperative pulmonary complications is highest in thoracic procedures, followed by upper and lower abdominal procedures. Postoperative pulmonary complications may occur in as many as 25%–50% of major surgical procedures. Patients who have pulmonary disease are at higher risk in proportion to the degree of their pulmonary impairment. Specific tests, such as spirometry or D_{LCO}, seem to be most useful in candidates for lung resection or esophagectomy. Preoperative testing is also indicated for patients undergoing surgical procedures designed to alter lung function, such as lung volume reduction surgery or correction of scoliosis.

Preoperative pulmonary function testing may be indicated in patients who have the following:

1. A smoking history
2. Symptoms of pulmonary disease (e.g., cough, sputum production, shortness of breath)
3. Abnormal physical examination findings, particularly of the chest (e.g., abnormal breath sounds, ventilatory pattern, respiratory rate)
4. Abnormal chest radiographs or CT scans

Preoperative testing may also be indicated in patients who are obese (more than 30% above ideal body weight), advanced in age (usually more than 70 years of age), have a history of respiratory infections, or who are markedly debilitated or malnourished.

In surgical candidates, the primary purpose of pulmonary function testing is to reveal preexisting pulmonary impairment. VC may decrease more than 50% from the preoperative value in thoracic or upper abdominal procedures. This places individuals with compromised function at risk of having atelectasis and pneumonia. Postoperative decreases in FRC and increases in closing volume (CV) may lead to ventilation-perfusion ($\dot{V}/\dot{Q}$) abnormalities and hypoxemia. Abnormal ventilatory function related to the central control of respiration or to the ventilatory muscles may also play a role in postoperative complications.

Certain tests of pulmonary function appear to be better predictors of postoperative complications. These tests should be used both for risk evaluation and to assist in planning the perioperative care of the individual.

1. *Spirometry*. FVC, FEV_1, MVV. Obstructive disease can be easily identified with simple spirometry. A significant percentage of patients who may develop postoperative problems can be detected with minimal screening. Patients who have reduced FVC, with or without airway obstruction, typically have an impaired ability to cough effectively when VC decreases further during the immediate postoperative period. The FEV_1 is also used to predict postoperative pulmonary function in lung resection or pneumonectomy.

2. *Bronchodilator studies*. Operative candidates with airway obstruction should also be tested with bronchodilators. Postbronchodilator values for FVC, FEV_1, and MVV may be used in estimating surgical risk. There may be significantly less risk if the patient's airway obstruction is reversible. Bronchodilator studies are similarly helpful in planning perioperative care. Bronchodilator therapy or inhaled corticosteroids may improve the patient's bronchial hygiene both before and after surgery.

3. *Blood gas analysis*. Arterial blood gas analysis is helpful in assessing patients with documented lung disease to determine the response to pulmonary changes that occur postoperatively. PaO_2 is generally not a good predictor of postoperative problems. Individuals with hypoxemia at rest usually also have abnormal spirometry results, and hence are at risk. PaO_2 may improve postoperatively in patients undergoing thoracotomy for lung resection if the resected portion contributed to $\dot{V}/\dot{Q}$ abnormalities. $PaCO_2$ appears to be the most useful blood gas indicator of surgical risk. Some studies have shown that a $PaCO_2$ above 45 mm Hg, in combination with airway obstruction and pulmonary symptoms (e.g., wheezing, cough), presents an increased risk of postoperative morbidity and mortality.

4. *Exercise testing*. Exercise studies can accurately predict patients at risk. Individuals who cannot tolerate moderate workloads often have airway obstruction or similar ventilatory limitations. Patients who have an O_2 uptake ($\dot{V}O_2$) greater than 20 ml/min/kg typically have a low incidence of cardiopulmonary complications. Those unable to attain a $\dot{V}O_2$ of 15 ml/min/kg have an increased risk of postoperative complications.

5. *DLCO*. A few studies have indicated that a low percent predicted postoperative diffusing capacity is an independent indicator of increased morbidity and mortality in patients undergoing lung resection. An accurate assessment of diffusing capacity is important in selecting patients who may be candidates for lung volume reduction surgery (LVRS).

In addition to routine pulmonary function studies, several other tests are used in predicting postoperative lung function in candidates for pneumonectomy or lobectomy. These procedures are normally used in combination with spirometry and blood gas analysis.

1. *Perfusion and $\dot{V}/\dot{Q}$ scans.* Lung scans are particularly useful in estimating the remaining lung function in patients who are likely to require removal of all or part of a lung. Split-function scans are performed. These allow partitioning of lungs into right and left halves, or into multiple lung regions. Although ventilation-perfusion scans give the best estimate of overall function, simple perfusion scans yield similar information. Lung scan data, in the form of regional function percentages, are used in combination with simple spirometric indices to calculate the patient's postoperative capacity. An example follows:

Postoperative FEV_1 =

Preoperative FEV_1 × %Perfusion to unaffected regions

This calculation is termed the predicted postoperative FEV_1, or ppo-FEV_1.

Patients whose postoperative FEV_1 is less than 800 ml are typically not considered surgical candidates. Resection of any lung parenchyma resulting in an FEV_1 less than 800 ml would leave the patient more severely impaired. One exception to this general guideline occurs in patients referred for lung volume reduction surgery (LVRS). These candidates are usually end-stage COPD patients, often with FEV_1 values less than 800 ml and significant air trapping. Removal of poorly ventilated lung tissue often results in an improvement in spirometry, with significant increases in both FVC and FEV_1.

2. **Pulmonary artery occlusion pressure.** In some candidates for pneumonectomy, the development of postoperative pulmonary hypertension may be a limiting factor. To estimate the effect of redirecting the entire right ventricular output to the remaining lung, a catheter is inserted into the pulmonary artery of the affected lung and blood flow occluded by means of a balloon. The resulting pulmonary artery pressure increase in the remaining lung is then measured. A pressure increasing to less than 35 mm Hg is usually considered consistent with acceptable postoperative pressures. The effect of redirected blood flow on oxygenation may also be a consideration. This can also be examined during occlusion to estimate postoperative PaO_2.

Tests that predict the effects of resection on the remaining lung are normally done in series, with spirometry done first, followed by split-function lung scans (if spirometry results are acceptable), and then pulmonary artery occlusion pressure (if cor pulmonale is a concern). Table 9-3 summarizes general value ranges used for preoperative pulmonary function testing.

TABLE 9-3			
Preoperative Pulmonary Function			
Test	Increased Postoperative Risk	High Postoperative Risk	Candidate for Pneumonectomy*
FVC	<50% of predicted	<1.5 L	
FEV_1	<2.0 L or 50% of predicted	<1.0 L	>2.0 L
MVV		<50 L/min or 50% of predicted	>50 L/min or 50% of predicted
$PaCO_2$		>45 mm Hg	
$\dot{V}O_2$max	15–20 ml/min/kg	<15 L/min/kg	
Predicted postoperative FEV_1			>0.8 L/min
Pulmonary artery occlusion			>35 mm Hg

*Values in this column determine whether the patient is to be considered a candidate for lung resection (see text).

PULMONARY FUNCTION TESTING FOR DISABILITY

Pulmonary function tests are one of several means of determining a patient's inability to perform certain tasks. Respiratory impairment and disability, however, are not synonymous. Respiratory impairment relates to the failure of one or more of the functions of the lungs, as measured by pulmonary function studies. Disability is the inability to perform tasks required for employment and includes medically determinable physical or mental impairment. The impairment must be expected to either result in death or last for at least 12 months. Impairment in children must be comparable to that which would disable an adult.

Pulmonary function tests used to determine impairment leading to disability should characterize the type, extent, and cause of impairment. Pulmonary function testing may not completely describe all factors involved in the disabling impairment. Other factors involved may be age, educational background, and patient motivation. The energy requirements of the task in question also affect the level of disability.

Determination of the level of impairment caused by pulmonary disease usually includes history and physical examination, chest x-ray examination, other appropriate imaging techniques, and pulmonary function tests.

PF TIP

Pulmonary function tests are often used in assessing disability from lung disease. Because tests such as FVC and FEV_1 are effort dependent, it is important that all tests meet established criteria for acceptability and repeatability. Decreased values for FVC and FEV_1 may be due to lung disease or poor effort. Careful attention to test acceptability and repeatability can help distinguish pathophysiology from poor effort.

Physical examination does not allow measurement of disabling symptoms but is useful in grading shortness of breath. Shortness of breath is the most prominent feature of respiratory impairment.

Shortness of breath, like pain, is subjective. Tachypnea, cyanosis, and abnormal respiratory patterns are not indicative of the extent of impairment but may be helpful in interpreting pulmonary function studies.

Chest x-ray studies do not correlate well with shortness of breath or pulmonary function studies, except in advanced cases of pneumoconioses (i.e., "dust" diseases). Absence of usual findings in the pneumoconioses may be helpful in excluding occupational exposure to toxins as part of the impairment.

Pulmonary function studies should be objective and reproducible and, most important, specific to the disorder being investigated. Impairments caused by chronic respiratory disorders usually produce irreversible loss of function because of ventilatory impairment, gas exchange abnormalities, or a combination of both.

Forced Vital Capacity and Forced Expiratory Volume

Spirometry is the most useful index for the assessment of impairment caused by airway obstruction. The test should not be performed unless the patient is stable. The reported FVC and FEV_1 should be the largest values obtained from at least three acceptable maneuvers. The two largest FVC values and FEV_1 values should be repeatable within 5% or 0.1 L, whichever is greater. Peak flow should be achieved early in the expiration and the spirogram should show gradually decreasing flow throughout the breath. Spirometry should be repeated after inhaled bronchodilator if the patient's FEV_1 is less than 70% of the predicted value. Spirometric efforts, before and after bronchodilators, should meet these repeatability criteria. Standing height, without shoes, should be used for comparison of measured values with limits for disability (Table 9-4). In case of marked spinal deformity, arm-span measurement should be used (see Chapter 1).

Computation of the FEV_1 should be done with back-extrapolated volumes (see Chapter 2). The spirogram is acceptable if the back-extrapolated volume is less than 5% of the FVC, or 0.1 L, which-

TABLE 9-4

Forced Expiratory Volume and Forced Vital Capacity Values for Disability Determinations

Height Without Shoes (in)	FEV₁ Equal to or Less Than (L/BTPS)	FVC Equal to or Less Than (L/BTPS)
60 or less	1.05	1.25
61–63	1.15	1.35
64–65	1.25	1.45
66–67	1.35	1.55
68–69	1.45	1.65
70–71	1.55	1.75
72 to more	1.65	1.85

Adapted from Disability Evaluation Under Social Security (Blue Book, January 2005) 3.00 Respiratory System—Adult.

ever is greater. Each maneuver should be continued for 6 seconds or until there is no detectable change in volume for the last 2 seconds of the maneuver. It is unacceptable to report FEV_1 when only an F-V curve is recorded. A volume-time tracing from which FEV_1 can be measured is *required*. All lung volumes and flows must be reported at body temperature, pressure, and saturation (BTPS).

Volume calibration of the spirometer should agree to within 1% of a 3-L syringe. If spirometer accuracy is less than 99% but within 3% of the calibration syringe, a calibration correction factor should be used (see Chapter 11). If a flow-sensing spirometer is used, linearity should be documented by performing calibration at three different flows (3 L/6 sec, 3 L/3 sec, and 3 L/1 sec). The volume-time tracing should have the time sensitivity marked on the horizontal axis and the volume sensitivity marked on the vertical axis. The paper speed should be at least 20 mm/sec and the volume excursion at least 10 mm/L to allow manual calculation of the FEV_1 and FVC. The manufacturer and model of the spirometer should be stated in the report (see Test Regimens 9-3).

Diffusing Capacity

The DLCO is useful in determining impairment because of chronic impairment of gas exchange in both obstructive and restrictive disorders. The single-breath method should be used. The standard criteria for acceptability and repeatability for the DLCO maneuver may be applied (see Chapter 5). However, the IVC should be at least 90% of the

patient's best VC, and the breath-hold time between 9 and 11 seconds. The reported value should be uncorrected for hemoglobin (Hb), but abnormal Hb or carboxyhemoglobin (COHb) values should be reported. Correction for altitude should be made if the P_IO_2 is significantly different from 150 mm Hg. If the DLCO is greater than 40% of predicted but less than 60%, resting blood gas analysis is indicated.

Arterial Blood Gases

Although blood gas results are objective, they are largely nonspecific in determining impairment. Blood gases should be obtained while the subject is breathing air, either sitting or standing. The A-aO₂ gradient may not be reliable because it can be affected by hyperventilation (Table 9-5). Blood gas analysis may be required in diffuse pulmonary fibrosis and should include PaO_2 and $PaCO_2$. Blood gases (and A-a gradient) may also be assessed during exercise. The requirement for supplemental O_2 may also be quantified by exercise blood gas analysis. Pulse oximetry or capillary blood gas analysis is not an acceptable substitute for arterial blood gas analysis. Blood gas analysis should be performed by a laboratory certified by a state or federal agency.

Exercise Testing

Patients considered for exercise evaluation should first have resting blood gas evaluation, either sitting or standing. A steady-state exercise test (see Chapter 7) is then performed, preferably with a treadmill. The patient should exercise for 4–6 minutes at an O_2 consumption rate ($\dot{V}O_2$) of approximately

TABLE 9-5			
Arterial Oxygen Tension for Disability Determinations			
	Less Than 3000 ft Above Sea Level	3000 to 6000 ft Above Sea Level	More Than 6000 ft Above Sea Level
P_{CO_2} (mm Hg)	P_{O_2} (mm Hg)	P_{O_2} (mm Hg)	P_{O_2} (mm Hg)
30 or below	≤65	≤60	≤55
31	≤64	≤59	≤54
32	≤63	≤58	≤53
33	≤62	≤57	≤52
34	≤61	≤56	≤51
35	≤60	≤55	≤50
36	≤59	≤54	≤49
37	≤58	≤53	≤48
38	≤57	≤52	≤47
39	≤56	≤51	≤46
40 or above	≤55	≤50	≤45

Adapted from Disability Evaluation Under Social Security (Blue Book, January 2005) 3.00 Respiratory System—Adult.

17.5 ml/min/kg (approximately 5 METS) breathing room air. An equivalent workload should be used for cycle ergometry (e.g., 75 W for a 175-lb patient). Blood gas samples should be drawn at this workload to determine whether significant hypoxemia is present (see Table 9-5). If the patient does not desaturate at this level, a higher workload can be used to determine exercise capacity. If the patient cannot achieve a workload of 5 METS, a lower workload can be selected to determine exercise capacity.

ECG should be monitored continuously throughout the exercise evaluation, and blood gases drawn during the final 2 minutes of the test. It may be helpful to measure $\dot{V}_{O_2}$, $\dot{V}_{CO_2}$, and $\dot{V}_E$. The altitude of the test site and barometric pressure should be included in the report to assist with interpretation of blood gas values.

In reporting impairment for the purpose of determining disability, the remaining functional capacity is as important in determining the patient's ability to perform a certain task as the percentage of lost function. Some statement of the patient's ability to understand and cooperate during pulmonary function measurements should accompany the tabular and graphic data.

Limits for determining disability based on respiratory impairment have been set for the United States by the Social Security Administration. Criteria are set according to the disease category (see

Test Regimens 9-4). COPD is evaluated by comparing FEV_1 with the values in Table 9-4. Restrictive ventilatory disorders are evaluated by comparing FVC with the values in Table 9-4. Impaired gas exchange is evaluated by comparing PaO_2 with the values in Table 9-5. Disability caused by asthma is also evaluated with FEV_1. Episodes of asthma (requiring emergency treatment or hospitalization) occurring at least every 2 months or at least six times per year may also be evidence of disability (Test Regimens 9-5 and 9-6).

METABOLIC MEASUREMENTS: INDIRECT CALORIMETRY

Description

Measurements of $\dot{V}_{O_2}$, $\dot{V}_{CO_2}$, and the respiratory exchange ratio (RER, $\dot{V}_{CO_2}/\dot{V}_{O_2}$) may be used to determine resting energy expenditure (REE). REE is usually expressed in kilocalories/day (kcal/day). These measurements allow nutritional assessment and management. In combination with measurements of urinary nitrogen (UN), **indirect calorimetry** allows calories to be partitioned among various substrates (e.g., fat, carbohydrate, protein).

TEST REGIMENS 9-5

CRITERIA FOR ACCEPTABILITY

Disability Testing

1. Spirometer must show a 3-L calibration that is within 1% or corrected within 3%. Flow-based spirometers should be calibrated at three different flows to demonstrate linearity. The manufacturer and model of spirometer should be stated.
2. All FVC maneuvers should be recorded before and after bronchodilator challenge. Time scale must be at least 20 mm/sec, volume scale at least 10 mm/L. FEV_1 may not be calculated from a flow-volume tracing.
3. There must be at least three acceptable FVC maneuvers before bronchodilator; the two largest values (FVC, FEV_1) should be within 5% or 0.1 L, whichever is greater.
4. The spirogram must show peak flow early in expiration with a smooth, gradually decreasing flow. The maneuver is acceptable if the effort continues for 6 seconds or if there is a plateau with no change in volume for 2 seconds. The FEV_1 should be measured using back-extrapolation; the back-extrapolated volume should be less than 5% of FVC or 0.1 L, whichever is greater.
5. Postbronchodilator studies should be performed if FEV_1 is less than 70% of predicted. Postbronchodilator testing should be done 10 minutes after administration of the drug. The name of the drug should be included.
6. DLCO testing (if performed) should meet all current American Thoracic Society recommendations. DLCO uncorrected for Hb is reported.
7. Exercise testing (if performed) should be for 6–8 minutes at a workload of approximately 5 METS. Blood gas samples should be obtained at rest and during exercise.
8. Statements regarding the patient's ability to understand directions, as well as effort and cooperation, should be included with all tests.

Adapted from U.S. Department of Health and Human Services: *Guide to pulmonary function studies under the Social Security disability programs: disability evaluation under Social Security,* SSA Publication No 64-055, 1999.

TEST REGIMENS 9-6

INTERPRETIVE STRATEGIES

Disability Testing

1. Were spirometry, diffusing capacity, blood gases, and exercise tests performed acceptably? If not, interpret very cautiously or not at all.
2. Was FEV_1 less than the predicted limit for the patient's height? If so, disabling obstruction is very likely.
3. Was FVC less than the predicted limit for the patient's height? If so, disabling restrictive disease is likely.
4. Was the DLCO (if measured) less than 10.5 ml/min/mm Hg or less than 40% of predicted? If so, the patient has a marked gas exchange abnormality.
5. Was the patient's PaO_2, measured while clinically stable on two occasions at least 3 weeks apart but within 6 months, equal to or less than published limits (adjusted for $PaCO_2$ and altitude)? If so disabling hypoxemia is present.
6. Was PaO_2 equal to or less than published limits during steady-state exercise (less than or equivalent to 5 METS) breathing air? If so, disabling hypoxemia is present.
7. Are lung function measurements consistent with history, physical examination, chest x-ray study, and other imaging techniques?

Techniques

Indirect calorimetry may be performed with either an open-circuit or a closed-circuit system to measure O_2 consumption, CO_2 production, and RER. The open circuit method is more commonly used in clinical practice.

Open-Circuit Calorimetry

Exchange of O_2 and CO_2 may be measured by recording the fractional differences of O_2 and CO_2 between inspired and expired gas. These measurements are accomplished with a mixing chamber, a dilution system, or a breath-by-breath system similar to those used for expired gas analysis during exercise (see Chapter 7). $\dot{V}O_2$ and $\dot{V}CO_2$ are measured as described for exercise testing with mixing chamber and breath-by-breath systems. $\dot{V}_E$, V_T, and f_B (respiratory rate) may be measured simultaneously. In systems that use the dilution principle, a constant flow of gas is mixed with expired air. The dilution of CO_2 is then used to calculate ventilation. Connection to the patient may be made by a standard directional breathing valve with mouthpiece and nose clips. A ventilated hood or canopy (Figure 9-7) may also be used. Almost all metabolic measurement systems provide for connection to a mechanical ventilator circuit.

A hood or canopy allows long-term measurements without direct connection to the patient's airway. The hood is ventilated by drawing a flow of gas through it that exceeds the patient's peak inspiratory demand (40 L/min is usually adequate). Ventilation can be calculated by measuring the change in flow into and out of the hood during breathing ("bias" flow).

Connection to a ventilator requires a means of measuring exhaled volume along with fractional concentrations of both inspired and expired gas. Breath-by-breath metabolic measurement systems usually sample gas at the patient-ventilator connection.

Closed-Circuit Calorimetry

The simplest type of closed-circuit calorimeter is one that measures $\dot{V}O_2$ volumetrically. The patient rebreathes from a closed system that contains a spirometer filled with O_2. CO_2 is scrubbed from the circuit using a chemical absorber. A recorder is used to measure the decrease in spirometer volume, equal to the rate of O_2 uptake ($\dot{V}O_2$). A similar approach uses a closed spirometer system to measure the volume of O_2 added as the patient rebreathes and consumes O_2. $\dot{V}O_2$ is equal to the volume of O_2 that must be added per minute to maintain a constant volume. CO_2 production

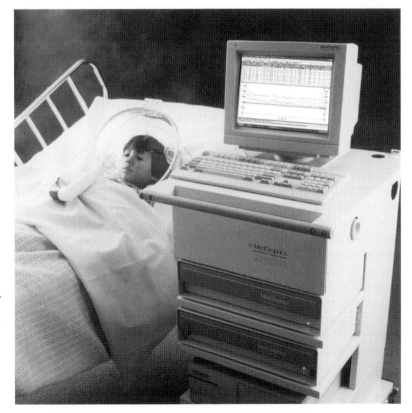

FIGURE 9-7 Canopy for Metabolic Measurements (Indirect Calorimetry). Resting energy expenditure (REE) may be measured from changes in gas flow and fractional concentrations of expired air drawn from a hood or canopy. A continuous or "bias" flow of gas is drawn through the canopy. Changes (increases or decreases) in the bias flow are measured to determine ventilation. Fractional gas concentrations are determined from the gas drawn from the hood. The canopy offers the advantage of not requiring direct connection to the patient's airway, which may affect ventilation and the measurement of REE. For patients requiring mechanical support of ventilation, the measuring apparatus samples gas from the ventilator circuit. (*Courtesy Medical Graphics Corporation, St. Paul, Minn.*)

cannot be measured with a closed-circuit system unless a CO_2 analyzer is added to the device. $\dot{V}_E$, V_T, and respiratory rate may all be determined from volume excursions of the spirometer. Closed-circuit systems may be used with spontaneously breathing patients by means of a simple breathing valve and mouthpiece. Use of a closed-circuit calorimeter with a mechanical ventilator requires that the spirometer system be connected between the patient and ventilator. The ventilator then "ventilates" the spirometer, which in turn ventilates the patient. This technique usually requires a bellows-type spirometer in a fixed container so that the positive pressure generated by the ventilator can compress the bellows. The volume delivered by the ventilator (V_I) must be increased to compensate for the volume of gas compressed in the closed-circuit spirometer during positive pressure breaths.

PF TIP

Estimation of caloric needs for a 24-hour period from a metabolic study requires that the measurements be made with the patient in a steady state. The short interval during which measurements are made (usually 5–20 minutes) should be free of interruptions that may alter the patient's metabolic rate. These include ventilator changes or suctioning. Nutritional support (if given) should be continuous, and the patient should be resting.

Performing Metabolic Measurements

The primary purpose of indirect calorimetry is to estimate REE over an extended period, usually 24 hours. To extrapolate the values obtained during the sampling period, the patient's condition during the measurement is critical (Test Regimens 9-7). The following guidelines help ensure that measurements are made under steady-state conditions:

1. The patient should be recumbent or supine for 20–30 minutes before beginning measurements and should stay quiet during the test. Ideally, the patient should be awake and alert during testing. The testing apparatus should not cause discomfort or exertion for the patient. Breathing valves, mouthpieces, and nose clips may alter the patient's breathing pattern.

TEST REGIMENS 9-7

CRITERIA FOR ACCEPTABILITY

Indirect Calorimetry

1. Appropriate calibration of gas analyzers and volume transducers should be documented before each test.
2. RQ should be within the normal physiologic range of 0.67–1.30.
3. Measured $\dot{V}O_2$ and $\dot{V}CO_2$ values should vary by no more than 5% or less for a 5-minute data collection; longer data collection intervals may be necessary if the variability is greater than 5%.
4. Data should be collected for a minimum of 5 minutes with minimal variability.
5. RQ values should be consistent with the patient's current nutritional intake.
6. Documentation should include the patient's medications, nutritional support, body temperature at time of test, and ventilatory support setting (if applicable).
7. The patient should be resting; no bolus feedings or pharmacologic stimulants or depressants. There should be no physical therapy, airway care, or major ventilator changes immediately before assessment.
8. If a stable FIO_2 cannot be achieved, REE may be estimated from the $\dot{V}CO_2$ with an assumed RQ of 0.85.
9. If a 24-hour urinary urea nitrogen (UUN) is collected for substrate use, it should be concurrent with the metabolic study.

Adapted from American Association for Respiratory Care: Clinical practice guideline: metabolic measurements using indirect calorimetry during mechanical ventilation—2004 Revision & Update, *Respir Care* 2004; 49:1073-1079.

---

2. The patient should fast for 2–4 hours before the test starts. If the patient is receiving either enteral or parenteral feedings, the feedings should be continuous rather than in bolus form. Information about the type and amount of nutritional support in the previous 24 hours may be helpful in interpreting test results.
3. The patient should be in a neutral thermal environment. Special corrections may be required for patients who are febrile or hypothermic. The patient's temperature at the time of the test should be recorded along with a temperature history of the previous 24 hours. Tempera-

ture changes of 1° C can result in a 13% change in REE.

4. Drugs or substances that alter metabolism should be avoided. Substances such as caffeine and nicotine are particularly common stimulants. Theophylline-based drugs may also increase metabolic rate.

5. Data collection should continue long enough to establish a stable baseline and verify steady-state conditions (Figure 9-8). Ten to fifteen minutes of stable readings for $\dot{V}O_2$ and $\dot{V}CO_2$ may be required, but an adequate measurement can be obtained in as short an interval as 5 minutes. Common indicators of steady-state conditions are the parameters assessed as part of the metabolic study. $\dot{V}O_2$ and $\dot{V}CO_2$ should not vary more than 5% from the mean value measured during the test (at least 5 minutes). Respiratory quotient (RQ) values should be within the normal physiologic range (0.67–1.30). If the patient does not achieve steady-state conditions, a longer test interval may be required to average representative periods of metabolic activity.

6. Patients on ventilators should be in a stable condition. Leaks in the ventilator circuit, around cuffed endotracheal tubes, or from chest tubes or bronchopleural fistulas may invalidate measurements of RQ and REE. No ventilator adjustments should be made 1–2 hours before the test period. Modifications in minute ventilation or FIO_2 settings can cause gross changes in the patterns of gas exchange, particularly in patients with pulmonary disease. The ventilator must have a stable delivered O_2 concentration; FIO_2 settings greater than 0.60 may result in erroneous $\dot{V}O_2$ measurements. Appropriate valves may need to be used for ventilator modes that involve continuous gas flow.

7. The calorimeter or metabolic cart should be calibrated at least daily, preferably before each test. Gas analyzers should be calibrated using gas concentrations appropriate for the clinical situation. Sample lines and gas-conditioning devices (absorbers) should be checked before each test. If calibration or testing produces questionable values, the device should be checked against a known standard. Burning ethanol or other material with a fixed RQ can be used. A large-volume syringe can be used to simulate a patient with $\dot{V}O_2$ and $\dot{V}CO_2$ values near zero.

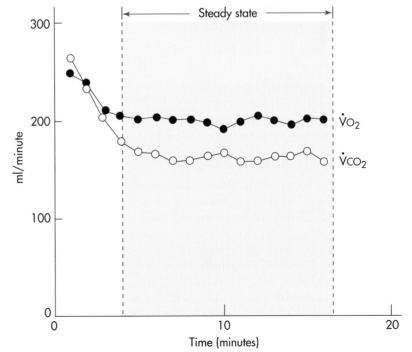

FIGURE 9-8 Indirect Calorimetry. Typical tracing of continuous measurement of $\dot{V}O_2$ and $\dot{V}CO_2$ as performed during open-circuit indirect calorimetry. The patient's expired gas is analyzed to determine O_2 consumption, CO_2 production, and RQ during a resting state. Measurements are observed until a metabolic steady state can be determined (minimum of 5 minutes). During the steady-state interval, values representing REE are measured. Daily caloric requirements are estimated from these measurements. If a 24-hour urinary urea nitrogen (UUN) sample is obtained, the percentages of energy derived from fats, carbohydrates, and proteins can be calculated (see text).

Alternately, biologic controls can be used to check the precision of the calorimeter.

Metabolic Calculations

The **Harris-Benedict equations** are commonly used to estimate REE:

Men:

$$REE(kcal/24\,hr) = 66.47 + 13.75W + 5H - 6.76A$$

Women:

$$REE(kcal/24\,hr) = 655.1 + 9.56W + 1.85H - 4.68A$$

where:
W = weight, kilograms
H = height, centimeters
A = age, years

The REE by these formulas was originally described as the **basal metabolic rate (BMR).** These equations may be used to estimate the caloric expenditure in normal individuals under conditions of minimal activity. BMR in these circumstances is related to lean body mass. To determine the optimum level of caloric intake, BMR must be adjusted upward because trauma, surgery, infections, and burns all cause the REE to increase.

The Weir equation is used to calculate REE from respiratory gas exchange and urinary nitrogen:

$$REE(kcal/24\,hr) = 5.68\,\dot{V}O_2 + 1.59\,\dot{V}CO_2 - 2.17\,UN$$

where:
$\dot{V}O_2$ is expressed in ml/min (STPD)
$\dot{V}CO_2$ is expressed in ml/min (STPD)
UN = urinary nitrogen (g/24 hr)

If UN is unknown, REE may be calculated:

$$REE(kcal/24\,hr) = 5.46\,\dot{V}O_2 + 1.75\,\dot{V}CO_2$$

Indirect calorimetry by the open-circuit method provides measures of both O_2 consumption and CO_2 production. As previously mentioned, RER is the ratio $\dot{V}CO_2/\dot{V}O_2$. Under steady-state conditions, RER approximates the mean respiratory quotient (RQ) at the cell level. RQ normally varies from 0.71–1.00, depending on the substrates being metabolized. Carbohydrate oxidation produces an RQ near 1.0, fat oxidation produces an RQ near 0.71, and protein oxidation produces an RQ of 0.82. RQ

attributable to carbohydrates and fats may be determined by subtracting $\dot{V}O_2$ and $\dot{V}CO_2$ derived from protein. This form of the RQ is termed the nonprotein RQ or RQnp and is calculated as follows:

$$RQnp = \frac{1.44\,\dot{V}CO_2 - 4.754\,UN}{1.44\,\dot{V}O_2 - 5.923\,UN}$$

where:
$\dot{V}CO_2$ is expressed in ml/min
$\dot{V}O_2$ is expressed in ml/min
UN = urinary nitrogen (g/24 hr)
1.44 = factor to convert ml/min to L/24 hr

Because CO_2 production varies with O_2 uptake, deviations of the RQ from the average value of 0.85 result in differences of less than 5% in the calculation of REE if only $\dot{V}O_2$ and RQ are used. Indirect calorimetry by the closed-circuit (volumetric) method takes advantage of this small difference by assuming a fixed RQ (usually 0.85) and measuring only $\dot{V}O_2$. Open-circuit calorimetry is usually limited to measurements on patients whose FIO_2 is 0.6 or less. However, $\dot{V}CO_2$ can be measured on these patients and $\dot{V}O_2$ estimated, again by assuming an RQ of 0.85. This method provides a means of estimating caloric needs, even though $\dot{V}O_2$ cannot be measured accurately.

UN is obtained from a 24-hour urine collection. Because protein metabolism accounts for only a small portion of total calories per day (approximately 12%), omission of the UN in the Weir equation changes the calculated REE by only 2%.

The Consolazio equations can be used to determine energy expenditure from gas exchange ($\dot{V}O_2$, $\dot{V}CO_2$), UN, and the caloric equivalents of carbohydrates, fats, and proteins:

$$CHO = 5.926\,\dot{V}CO_2 - 4.189\,\dot{V}O_2 - 1.539\,UN$$

$$FAT = 2.432\,\dot{V}O_2 - 2.432\,\dot{V}CO_2 - 1.943\,UN$$

$$PRO = 6.250\,UN$$

where:
CHO = Carbohydrates oxidized in grams/24 hours
FAT = Fat oxidized in grams/24 hours
PRO = Protein oxidized in grams/24 hours

From the grams of each substrate used, the kilocalories derived from that source can be computed:

$$carbohydrates\ (in\ kcal) = 4.18\ carbohydrates\ (in\ g)$$
$$fat\ (in\ kcal) = 9.46\ fat\ (in\ g)$$
$$protein\ (in\ kcal) = 4.32\ protein\ (in\ g)$$
$$total\ (in\ Kcal) = carbohydrate + fat + protein$$

The percentage of calories from each substrate may also be calculated by dividing the kilocalories derived from that substrate by the total kilocalories. Because the Consolazio equations are intended for analysis of normal substrate partitioning, RQ values outside of the range of 0.71 – 1.00 will result in negative values for either carbohydrates or lipids (fat). These negative values are erroneous if RER does not equal RQ (i.e., the patient is not in a metabolic steady state).

Significance and Pathophysiology

See Test Regimens 9-8 for interpretive strategies. Indirect calorimetry assesses nutritional status in patients whose daily energy needs are altered by disease, injury, or therapeutic interventions. REE accounts for approximately two thirds of the daily energy requirements in healthy patients. The Harris-Benedict equations, or similar predictive equations, are commonly used to estimate REE. Various factors can be used to adjust estimated REE to account for additional caloric needs imposed by the patient's clinical status. This approach works well in many patients. However, metabolic requirements of critically ill patients vary widely. Indirect calorimetry is indicated for patients who do not respond favorably to traditional methods of nutritional assessment and support. Indirect calorimetry can be used to detect undernourishment, overnourishment, or use of inappropriate substrates (Box 9-4).

Undernourishment or starvation can occur during acute or chronic illness. It may be detected by caloric expenditure in excess of caloric intake (negative energy balance). Both fat stores and protein from muscle breakdown may contribute to metabolism during periods of undernourishment. Indirect calorimetry is often used along with measurement of body weight, triceps skinfold measurements, and other approximations of energy reserves. These measurements allow plan-

---

TEST REGIMENS 9-8

INTERPRETIVE STRATEGIES

Indirect Calorimetry

1. Were metabolic data collected acceptably? Did $\dot{V}O_2$ and $\dot{V}CO_2$ values vary by less than 5%? If not, interpret cautiously. Was RQ between 0.67 and 1.30? If not, interpret very cautiously or not at all.
2. Was measured REE less than predicted (Harris-Benedict or similar equation)? If so, consider technical error or hypometabolic state.
3. Was RQ less than 0.70? If so, consider ketosis or starvation.
4. Was RQ greater than 1.00? If so, consider lipogenesis or non–steady state (hyperventilation).
5. Is the measured REE significantly greater than the patient's intake in the previous 24 hours? If so, the patient is probably being underfed or may be febrile.
6. Is the measured REE significantly less than the patient's intake in the previous 24 hours? If so, the patient is probably being overfed.
7. Is the nonprotein RQ near 1.00? If so, the main substrate being used is carbohydrate. Is the nonprotein RQ near 0.70? If so, the main substrate is fat.
8. Are metabolic measurements consistent with the patient's clinical status? Is nutritional support (if provided) appropriate for metabolic needs?

BOX 9-4	Indications for Indirect Calorimetry*

- Head trauma or paralysis
- COPD
- Multiple trauma
- Acute pancreatitis
- Patients in whom height or weight is indeterminate
- Poor response to enteral or parenteral support
- Patients receiving total parenteral nutrition at home
- Transplant patients
- Morbidly obese patients
- Patients with demonstrated hypermetabolism or hypometabolism
- Patients on prolonged mechanical ventilation who are unable to eat

*Risk or stress factors known to interfere with calculation of energy expenditure.

ning of nutritional therapy to replenish diminished reserves.

Overnourishment occurs when any substrate is supplied in excess of the energy requirements. Overfeeding is most deleterious when the patient's nutritional status is already adequate. Excess lipid or carbohydrate calories are stored as fat, which may place stress on one or more organ systems (e.g., liver).

Patients who have pulmonary disease present a special dilemma. Excessive carbohydrate intake results in increased CO_2 production because the RQ of carbohydrates is 1. For patients in respiratory failure, excess CO_2 production increases the ventilatory load on the respiratory system. Adjustments in substrate use can be made after the non-protein RQ is determined by indirect calorimetry. Lipids (i.e., fats) are typically substituted for glucose so that the RQ can be reduced while the caloric intake is maintained. Patients in respiratory failure may also experience atrophy of ventilatory muscles. Substrate analysis can be used to assess N_2 balance related to the breakdown of muscle protein. Substrate analysis permits measurement of nutritional requirements necessary to maintain N_2 balance.

Technical considerations involved in indirect calorimetry include the accuracy of gas analysis and measurement of expired volume during the test (open-circuit methods). The most common problem during metabolic measurements is attainment of a true steady state. Only if the measurements are made under steady-state conditions is the metabolic rate representative of caloric expenditure over 24 hours. Hyperventilation resulting from connection to a mask or mouthpiece, or from ventilator manipulation, occurs frequently. **Head hoods** or **continuous-flow canopies** can eliminate much of the stimulation associated with connection to the metabolic measurement system (see Figure 9-7) but cannot be used for patients on mechanical ventilators. Hoods or canopies may also cause hyperventilation in awake, alert patients. An RER greater than 1.0 should always be evaluated in relation to $\dot{V}_E$ and end-tidal CO_2. Abnormally high $\dot{V}_E$ and low end-tidal CO_2 values may indicate hyperventilation. RER values in excess of 1 that cannot be explained as hyperventilation may be caused by storage of excess calories as fat (lipogenesis). RER values

between 0.67 and 0.70 may occur in ketosis caused by extreme fasting or diabetic ketoacidosis. However, more commonly, low RER values (<0.67) signal improper calibration of the CO_2 or O_2 analyzers. Inaccurate calibration or improper performance of gas analyzers can result in RER values outside of the usual metabolic range of 0.70–1.

Special problems may be encountered in performing metabolic measurements on patients requiring mechanical ventilatory support. A common difficulty relates to measurements of O_2 consumption in patients receiving supplemental O_2. Measurement of $\dot{V}O_2$ by respiratory gas exchange requires analysis of the difference between inspired and expired O_2 along with $\dot{V}_E$. In patients who are breathing air, inspired FIO_2 is constant. Many O_2-blending systems, such as those used on ventilators, may not provide a constant fraction of inspired O_2. Large differences in calculated $\dot{V}O_2$ may result from small fluctuations in FIO_2, even if F_EO_2 remains relatively constant. Small differences in inspired and expired volumes (resulting from the RER) are corrected by adjusting the inspired fraction of O_2 according to the following equation:

$$\frac{(1 - F_EO_2 - F_ECO_2)}{1 - FIO_2} \times FIO_2$$

This correction of inspired FIO_2 for gas balance in the lung (i.e., the Haldane transformation) limits the accuracy of the open-circuit method of determining $\dot{V}O_2$. As FIO_2 increases, the value in the denominator of the equation becomes smaller. Even with very accurate gas analyzers, measurement of differences between FIO_2 and F_EO_2 (when FIO_2 is above 0.60) is variable. Breath-by-breath analysis of exhaled gas can reduce the problem of variable FIO_2 by measuring the fractional gas concentrations at the patient's airway and computing $\dot{V}O_2$ and $\dot{V}CO_2$ for individual breaths. Indirect calorimetry by the volumetric method (i.e., a closed system) avoids this problem by measuring the actual volume of O_2 removed during rebreathing. Allowing the patient to breathe from a reservoir bag containing an elevated FIO_2 (typically <0.60) can usually accommodate measurement of $\dot{V}O_2$ and $\dot{V}CO_2$ in spontaneously breathing patients who require supplemental O_2.

If a stable FIO_2 cannot be achieved (as is often the case when it is >0.60), REE can be estimated from the $\dot{V}CO_2$. If an RQ of 0.85 is assumed, $\dot{V}O_2$ can be estimated by dividing the $\dot{V}CO_2$ by the RQ, and then solving the Weir equation (see the section on techniques). This method will underestimate the REE when the RQ is greater than 0.85, with a maximal error of about 25% if the RQ is really 1.20. Similarly, the REE will be overestimated for RQ values less than 0.85, with a maximal error of approximately 19% if the RQ is 0.67.

Other considerations involved in metabolic measurements of ventilated patients include the effects of positive pressure on gas analysis and on volume determination. Analysis of O_2 and CO_2 in the ventilator circuit must take into account the effect of positive pressure breaths on the gas analyzers. Depending on the sampling method used, positive pressure swings during each breath may generate falsely high partial pressure readings. Closed-circuit calorimetry places a volumetric device in the breathing circuit between the ventilator and the patient. The volume delivered by the ventilator must be increased to accommodate the higher compressible gas volume in the circuit, approximately 1 ml/cm H_2O for each liter of added volume.

Summary

- Bronchial challenge tests can be done with several different agents, all of which test the airway responsiveness in slightly different ways.

- Methacholine challenge is the most commonly used and best-standardized test of airway hyperreactivity. Histamine and antigenic agents are also used.
- Exercise testing can be specifically used to evaluate exercise-induced bronchospasm. Hyperventilation tests, with cold or room-temperature air, mimic the ventilatory load that occurs with exercise.
- Exhaled nitric oxide (FE_{NO}) provides a noninvasive means of measuring eosinophilic inflammation of the airways. FE_{NO} may be useful in the diagnosis and management of diseases characterized by inflammation such as asthma.
- Impulse oscillometry uses high frequency oscillations to measure the mechanical properties of the respiratory system, in particular, resistance and impedance. It is especially useful in children or subjects who cannot perform conventional pulmonary function tests such as spirometry.
- Preoperative and disability testing use spirometry, lung volumes, diffusing capacity, blood gases, and exercise testing. Each test examines a specific aspect of either preoperative risk or respiratory impairment that prevents work.
- Metabolic measurements, specifically indirect calorimetry, provide a means of assessing nutritional status and support. They may be particularly useful in the evaluation of patients who do not respond adequately to estimated nutritional needs.

CASE 9-1

Case Studies

HISTORY
M.M. is a 39-year-old white woman who has recently experienced episodes of "choking and coughing." She was referred by her primary care physician, who suspected reactive airway involvement. M.M. relates that cigarette smoke and strong odors seem to bring on the episodes. She has never smoked and has no history of lung disease. She had some childhood allergies that disappeared at puberty. There is no history of lung disease in her immediate family. M.M. was not taking any medications at the time of she was tested.

PULMONARY FUNCTION TESTS
Personal Data

Sex:	Female
Age:	39 yr
Height:	66 in (168 cm)
Weight:	130 lb (59 kg)

continued

Exhaled NO*

	Actual	Pred
FE$_{NO}$ (ppb)	97	<35

*Measured at 50 ml/sec.

Spirometry

	Pre Drug	LLN	Pred	%
FVC (L)	3.71	3.24	3.97	93
FEV$_1$ (L)	2.96	2.62	3.24	91
FEV$_{1\%}$ (%)	80	73	83	
MVV (L/min)	106		110	96
Raw (cm H$_2$O/L/sec)	2.37		0.6–2.4	
sGaw (L/sec/cm H$_2$O/L)	0.14	0.12		

Methacholine Challenge*

Methacholine (mg/ml)	FEV$_1$	%Control	sGaw	%Control
Baseline	2.96	—	0.14	—
Control	2.92	100	0.14	—
0.0625	2.93	100	0.13	93
0.25	2.90	99	0.11	79
1.0	2.75	94	0.11	79
4.0	2.41	83	0.09	64
16.0	1.99	68	0.08	57

*5-breath dosimeter method.

TECHNOLOGIST'S COMMENTS

Exhaled NO measurements were acceptable and repeatable. All spirometry and body box efforts were acceptable and reproducible. The patient complained of "chest tightness" near the end of the test; some scattered wheezes were heard on auscultation.

QUESTIONS

1. What is the interpretation of:
   a. Exhaled nitric oxide (FE$_{NO}$)?
   b. Spirometry?
   c. Airway resistance and specific conductance?
2. What is the interpretation of the methacholine challenge?
3. Are these findings related to the patient's symptoms?
4. What treatment might be recommended based on these findings?

DISCUSSION

Interpretation (Prechallenge FE$_{NO}$ and Pulmonary Function)

Analysis of the patient's eNO is consistent with significant airway inflammation. Spirometry before and during the inhalation challenge was performed acceptably, as were maneuvers in the body plethysmograph. Spirometry results are within normal limits. Raw and sGaw are close to the limits of normal, suggestive of airflow obstruction.

Interpretation (Methacholine Challenge)

The methacholine challenge test is positive with a PC$_{20}$ of approximately 5.2 mg/ml. The test was terminated because the patient's FEV$_1$ decreased below 80% of the control value with the final dose of methacholine. sGaw decreased in a similar fashion, with a 36% decrease (64% of control) at the 4 mg/ml dose and a 43% decrease (57% of control) at the maximal inhaled dose. Wheezing was present on auscultation for the last two methacholine doses, and the patient experienced symptoms similar to her chief complaint when the test became positive.

Impression: Normal lung function with a positive methacholine challenge, consistent with hyperreactive airway disease.

Cause of Symptoms

This patient is an ideal candidate for a bronchial challenge test. Her baseline pulmonary function studies are within normal limits but her exhaled nitric oxide level strongly suggests inflammation of the airways. Her complaint of episodic coughing and choking suggests some form of hyperreactive airway abnormality. Many patients who have an asthmatic response to inhaled irritants complain of cough as the primary symptom; wheezing may or may not be present.

If obvious airway obstruction were present on the baseline spirometry, the challenge test would have been contraindicated. A simple before-bronchodilator and after-bronchodilator trial may have been sufficient to demonstrate reversible obstruction. Methacholine challenge testing may be used in patients with known obstruction to quantify the degree of airway hyperreactivity. In this case, the objective of the test was to determine whether the patient had hyperreactivity.

FEV$_1$ is commonly used as the index of obstruction for inhalation challenge tests because it is simple to perform and highly reproducible. Raw and sGaw are sometimes used to define the extent of airway reactivity. sGaw is sensitive and reproducible and may be used to quantify changes occurring during challenge testing. A decrease of at least 35%–45% in sGaw may be considered indicative of a positive response. As was observed in this patient, sGaw may actually decrease more rapidly than FEV_1. In some instances, PEF may decrease as the challenge is performed, particularly if the large airways are involved.

Results of a methacholine challenge test should be interpreted cautiously. The patient should be free of symptoms at the time of the test. β-Adrenergic, anticholinergic, or methylxanthine bronchodilators that may influence the results must be withheld before testing (see Table 9-3). Some long-acting β-agonists may need to be withheld for several days before testing. These conditions were met in this patient because she was not taking any medications. Because both FEV_1 and sGaw fell markedly with a PC_{20} less than 8 mg/ml, the test can be interpreted as positive with some certainty. The patient appears to have airway inflammation. The cause of the patient's symptoms appears to be asthma triggered by inhaled irritants as described in her history.

Treatment

The patient was started on an inhaled corticosteroid (fluticasone). She was also given a portable peak-flow meter. The patient was instructed in its use and her PEF correlated well with that measured during spirometry. She was told to use the device every morning and evening or when symptoms appeared. Any significant change in PEF was treated with a β-adrenergic bronchodilator through a metered-dose inhaler. Subsequent reports indicated that her peak flow fell in excess of the level demonstrated on the challenge, but symptoms were promptly relieved with use of the inhaler. Her FE_{NO} while taking inhaled corticosteroids was measured during a follow-up visit at 25 ppb. This finding suggests that her underlying airway inflammation was being adequately managed at her current dose.

CASE 9-2

Case Studies

HISTORY

R.I. is a 38-year-old woman whose presenting complaint is shortness of breath while jogging or playing tennis. She has been physically active for several years but recently had a "chest cold" that took 4 weeks to resolve. She smoked for approximately 2 years while in high school. She works as a teacher and has no unusual environmental exposures. Family history includes an older sister who has chronic bronchitis. She is not currently taking any medications. Her HMO referred her for evaluation of possible exercise-induced bronchospasm.

PULMONARY FUNCTION TESTS

Personal Data

Sex:	Female
Age:	38 yr
Height:	62 in (158 cm)
Weight:	119 lb (54 kg)

Eucapnic Voluntary Hyperventilation

	Baseline	5 min	10 min	Postbronchodilator
FEV₁ (Pred: 2.64 L)	1.97	1.25		1.92
% Predicted	75	47		73
% Change	0	−37		−3
FVC (Pred: 3.37 L)	2.71	2.07		2.8
% Predicted	81	61		83
% Change	0	−24		3
PEF (Pred: 6.0 L/sec)	5.5	2.8		3.65
% Predicted	91	46		61
% Change	0	−49		−33

continued

TECHNOLOGIST'S COMMENTS

All spirometry maneuvers were performed acceptably before and after hyperventilation. The patient hyperventilated at 60 L/min for 6 minutes. There were audible wheezes immediately after hyperventilation.

QUESTIONS

1. What is the interpretation of:
    a. Baseline spirometry?
    b. Response to EVH?
    c. Response to bronchodilator?
2. Are the findings related to the cause of the patient's symptoms?
3. What other tests might be indicated?
4. What treatment might be recommended based on these findings?

DISCUSSION

Interpretation

All spirometric maneuvers were performed acceptably. Baseline spirometry results are close to the lower limit of normal, with a mildly decreased FEV_1. After EVH, there were significant decreases in FEV_1, FVC,

and peak flow at 5 minutes. After an inhaled bronchodilator, FEV_1 returned to prechallenge levels and FVC increased. Peak-flow recovery was somewhat slower.

Impression: Borderline normal spirometry results with a positive EVH test consistent with hyperreactive airways.

Cause of Symptoms

This patient is typical of an adult who begins experiencing breathlessness with increased physical activity and seeks medical attention. Her complaints suggest exercise-induced bronchospasm. The development of this problem may or may not be related to her recent chest infection.

EVH is an appropriate way to challenge the airways in cases such as this. The patient breathed a mixture of 5% CO_2, 21% O_2, and balance N_2 for 6 minutes. The target level of ventilation was set at 30 times her FEV_1, or approximately 60 L/min. Spirometry was repeated 5 minutes after hyperventilation. In this case, the patient experienced a significant decrease in FEV_1, FVC, and PEF (Figure 9-9). Because of the marked decrease in FEV_1, additional postchallenge measurements (at

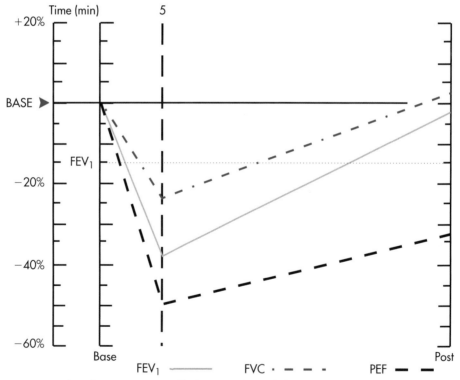

FIGURE 9-9   Eucapnic Voluntary Hyperventilation (EVH) Graph for Case 9-2. FVC, FEV_1, and PEF are plotted after a bronchial challenge maneuver. In this patient, there was a marked decrease in all three variables at 5 minutes (a positive test result). The graph also plots the reversal of the induced bronchospasm by inhaled bronchodilator.

10 and 15 minutes) were omitted. Four inhalations of albuterol through a metered-dose inhaler with a spacer reversed the obstruction, although PEF recovered only partially.

Other Tests

EVH challenges the airways by inducing heat and water loss with increased ventilation. This is the same physical stimulus that may be responsible for exercise-induced bronchospasm. The patient in this case could have been tested using exercise as the challenge agent. However, EVH is simpler and takes less time. In addition, EVH may be more sensitive in detecting exercise-induced asthma than exercise testing itself. Exercise tests are often performed with patients working at 80%–90% of their maximal HR for 6–8 minutes. In many patients, particularly if they are sedentary, the workload that produces this elevation in HR may not induce a high enough level of ventilation to provoke bronchospasm. EVH, using a target of 30 times the FEV_1, produces a level of ventilation that is approximately 75% of MVV.

Treatment

The patient was given a β-adrenergic bronchodilator to be used as pretreatment before exercise. She reported significant improvement in her symptoms. A trial regimen of cromolyn sodium also reduced the occurrence of symptoms associated with athletic activities.

CASE 9-3

Case Studies

HISTORY

J.P. is a 53-year-old woman who had multiple abdominal injuries in a motor vehicle accident. After surgical repair of a perforated bowel, acute renal failure developed, followed by respiratory failure. She was placed on mechanically supported ventilation and became increasingly dependent on the ventilator. After 13 days, a metabolic study was requested to assess the adequacy of parenteral nutrition.

METABOLIC ASSESSMENT

Personal Data

Sex:	Female
Age:	53 yr
Height:	62 in (157.5 cm)
Weight:	110 lb (50 kg)

Nutritional Information

	Total Calories	Nonprotein Calories	Protein (g)
Parenteral	1717	1393	75
Enteral	(None)		
24-hour UN	9 g		
Basal metabolic rate	1176 kcal/24 hours (estimated)		

Ventilator Settings

FIO_2	0.35
V_T	750 ml
Rate	10
Mode	SIMV (synchronized intermittent mandatory ventilation)
Status	Awake, resting

Metabolic Measurements

$\dot{V}CO_2$ (ml/min)	205
$\dot{V}O_2$ (ml/min)	200
RER (RQ)	1.03
$\dot{V}_E$ (L/min)	10.2
REE (kcal/day)	1442
RQ_{NP} (nonprotein RQ) (see text)	1.07

Energy Substrate Use

Carbohydrate	1480 kcal/day
Fat	−289 kcal/day
Protein	243 kcal/day

Blood Gases

pH	7.37
$PaCO_2$	51
PaO_2	71
HCO_3^-	29

continued

QUESTIONS

1. What is the interpretation of:
   a. REE?
   b. Substrate utilization?
2. Why does the patient have an RER (RQ) greater than 1?
3. Are the data representative of the patient's caloric requirements?
4. What changes in therapy (ventilator settings, nutritional support) are indicated?

DISCUSSION

Interpretation

Exhaled gases for this study were collected over 15 minutes and appear to represent a steady state. A UN sample was collected for 24 hours before the test. The patient was receiving 1717 kcal/day of parenteral nutrition. REE as determined by metabolic assessment indicates a requirement of 1442 kcal/24 hours. Substrate utilization showed carbohydrate oxidation (104%). The negative value for fat utilization is consistent with lipogenesis. Replacement of glucose with lipids and reduction of total calories to approximately 1450 kcal/day is recommended. The patient should be reassessed within 24 hours.

Cause of Elevated RER (RQ)

This study involves factors commonly encountered in the nutritional support of critically ill patients. These elements include the patient's clinical status, estimated and actual caloric requirements, and the role of nutritional status in ventilatory support.

The patient was critically ill and required ventilatory support. Parenteral nutrition was being supplied approximately 45% above the estimated resting caloric requirements. Estimation of caloric requirements is often performed by calculating the basal rate using the Harris-Benedict equations (see the section on metabolic measurements: indirect calorimetry). BMR is then adjusted with factors that consider the clinical status of the patient (e.g., disease state, trauma).

The metabolic study indicated that the patient required fewer calories per day than were currently being given. In addition, carbohydrates were supplying the entire caloric need. The negative value calculated for fat utilization indicates that some of the carbohydrates were probably being stored as fat (i.e., lipogenesis). When carbohydrates are oxidized, CO_2

is produced. The RER of 1.03 supports an excess CO_2 production in relation to metabolic demands.

The metabolic assessment was performed with the patient on a ventilator. The patient's $\dot{V}_E$ during the assessment was 10.2 L, slightly higher than the ventilator settings. Difficulty weaning this patient from mechanically supported ventilation may have been caused by the CO_2 load induced by parenteral nutrition in excess of metabolic demand. The arterial blood gas analysis supports increased CO_2 production. Pa_{CO_2} is increased in spite of mechanical support of ventilation. The patient was unable to ventilate enough to return her $PaCO_2$ to near 40 mm Hg. Excess CO_2 apparently contributed to the difficulty weaning the patient from mechanical ventilation.

Valid Data (Steady State)

The interpretation notes that the data were representative of a steady state. Steady-state measurements are essential to estimate caloric requirements for an entire 24-hour period. Each metabolic assessment should include adequate data so that steady-state conditions can be verified. The length of the study should be appropriate to establish that a steady state existed. Analysis of the variability of $\dot{V}_{O_2}$ and $\dot{V}_{CO_2}$ may be helpful. O_2 consumption and CO_2 production during measurements ideally should vary less than 5%. RER values outside the normal range of 0.70–1.00 should be carefully evaluated to ensure that measurement errors did not occur. Difficulty measuring $\dot{V}_{O_2}$ in patients receiving supplemental O_2 is well documented. Calorimetry using open-circuit methods is usually limited to measurements when F_{IO_2} is 0.60 or less.

Changes in Therapy

J.P. was switched to a 50/50 mixture of lipid and carbohydrate. The total caloric intake was also reduced to 1450 kcal/day. Her ventilation decreased, and ventilatory support was gradually reduced. An additional metabolic study indicated agreement between the prescribed nutritional support and her metabolic demands. RER on the subsequent study was 0.79 with an REE of 1395 kcal/day. This RER value compares favorably with 0.82, which is a target value for metabolism of appropriate amounts of carbohydrate, fat, and protein. She was successfully weaned from the ventilator 4 days after the initial assessment.

SELF-ASSESSMENT QUESTIONS

Entry-level

1. A patient with symptoms of chest tightness and cough while playing basketball is referred for bronchial challenge. In addition to spirometry before/after the challenge, which of the following protocols would be most appropriate?
   I. Treadmill exercise for 4–6 minutes at 85% of predicted maximal HR
   II. Cycle ergometer ramp test at 50 W/min
   III. Eucapnic voluntary hyperventilation at $30 \times FEV_1$ for 6 minutes
   IV. Eucapnic voluntary hyperventilation at $MVV \times 5$ minutes
      a. I and III only
      b. II and IV only
      c. II and III only
      d. I and IV only

2. A 35-year-old woman performs a methacholine challenge using the 5-breath dosimeter protocol. The following data are recorded:

	FEV_1
Baseline	2.95 L
Diluent	3.01 L
0.0625 mg/ml	2.89 L
0.250 mg/ml	2.75 L
1.0 mg/ml	2.70 L
4.0 mg/ml	2.51 L
16.0 mg/ml	2.35 L

   Based on these results the PC_{20} is
   a. Less than 0.0625 mg/ml
   b. Between 1.0 and 4.0 mg/ml
   c. Between 4.0 and 16.0 mg/ml
   d. Greater than 16.0 mg/ml

3. A patient who complains of shortness of breath is referred for a bronchial challenge test. Baseline spirometry shows the following results:

	Pred	LLN	Actual
FVC (L)	3.56	2.75	3.01
FEV_1 (L)	2.89	2.18	2.12
FEV_1/FVC (%)	81	71	70
PEF (L/sec)	7.8	5.5	5.7
Raw (cm H_2O/L/sec)	1.5		2.4
sGaw (L/sec/cm H_2O/L)		0.12	0.10

Based on these results the pulmonary function technologist should
   a. Perform a methacholine challenge using the 5-breath dosimeter method
   b. Perform a methacholine challenge using the 2-minute tidal breathing method
   c. Do an exercise test for 6–8 minutes with postexercise spirometry
   d. Administer a bronchodilator and repeat spirometry after 15 minutes

4. After inhalation of methacholine, a patient has spirometry and specific conductance measured. Which of the following changes are consistent with a positive methacholine challenge test?
   a. FEV_1 decreased 10%, sGaw increased 10%
   b. FEV_1 decreased 15%, sGaw increased 35%
   c. FEV_1 decreased 25%, sGaw decreased 50%
   d. FEV_1 increased 5%, sGaw decreased 25%

5. Which of the following would be considered indications for preoperative testing in a patient scheduled for lung resection?
   I. Age greater than 40 years
   II. Current smoker
   III. Shortness of breath on exertion
   IV. BMI of 26.6
      a. I and III only
      b. I and IV only
      c. II and III only
      d. II and IV only

Advanced

6. A patient with a history of COPD is being evaluated for disability. His FEV_1 is 1.44 L (43% of predicted), and his D_{LCO} is 14.5 ml CO/min/mm Hg (61% of predicted). Which of the following tests is most appropriate to perform next?
   a. Lung volumes by plethysmography
   b. Room air arterial blood gases
   c. Treadmill exercise test with pulse oximetry
   d. Postbronchodilator spirometry

7. A 50-kg patient in respiratory failure on a ventilator has a metabolic study performed at an FIO_2 of 0.30 (30%); the following data are reported:

continued

Time (min)	1	2	3	4	5	6
$\dot{V}O_2$ ml/min	244	255	259	256	250	255
$\dot{V}CO_2$ ml/min	150	155	160	153	151	154
RQ	0.61	0.61	0.62	0.60	0.60	0.60
REE kcal/24	1596	1665	1695	1667	1631	1663

Which of the following statements best describe these results?
  a. A steady state was not achieved.
  b. The patient is being overfed.
  c. There is a gas analyzer malfunction.
  d. The REE was calculated incorrectly.

8. Bronchoconstriction may result in which of the following changes in respiratory system impedance as measured by the forced oscillation technique (FOT)?
  I. Rise in the real part of impedance
  II. Increase in the frequency dependence of resistance
  III. Increase in resonant frequency
  a. I only
  b. II and III only
  c. I and III only
  d. I, II, and III

9. A 39 year-old patient has her exhaled nitric oxide level (FE_{NO}) measured at a flow of 0.05 L/sec; the average of three repeatable efforts is reported as 65 ppb. She then performs spirometry, and her FVC, FEV_1 and FEV_1/FVC are all within normal limits. Which of the following should the pulmonary function technologist conclude from these results?
  a. The patient has eosinophilic inflammation in her airways and/or alveoli.
  b. The patient is malingering.
  c. The FE_{NO} was measured at the incorrect flow.
  d. All results are within normal limits.

10. Which of the following results suggest that a patient may have asthma:
  I. 10% or 100-ml increase in postbronchodilator FEV_1 (whichever is greater)
  II. 20% decrease in FEV_1 after inhaling 4 mg/ml of methacholine
  III. 14% fall in FEV_1 after 8 minutes of exercise at 90% of the predicted HR
  IV. FE_{NO} of 100 ppb measured at a flow of 50 ml/sec
  a. I and IV only
  b. II and III only
  c. I, II, and III
  d. II, III, and IV

Selected Bibliography

BRONCHIAL CHALLENGE

Allen ND, Davis BE, Hurst TS, Cockcroft DW: Difference between dosimeter and tidal breathing methacholine challenge: contributions of dose and deep inspiration bronchoprotection, Chest 2005; 128:4018-4023.

Anderson SD, Branman JD: Methods for "indirect" challenge tests including exercise, eucapnic voluntary hyperpnea, and hypertonic aerosols, Clin Rev Allergy Immunol 2003; 24:27-54.

Anderson SD, Argyros GJ, Magnussen H et al: Provocation by eucapnic voluntary hyperpnoea to identify exercise induced bronchonstriction, Br J Sports Med 2001; 35:344-347.

Argyros GJ, Roach JM, Hurwitz KM et al: Eucapnic voluntary hyperventilation as a bronchoprovocation technique, Chest 1996; 109:1520-1524.

Assoufi BK, Dally MB, Newman-Taylor AJ et al: Cold-air test: a simplified standard method for airway reactivity, Clin Respir Physiol 1986; 22:349-357.

Cockcroft DW, Davis BE, Todd DC, Smycniuk AJ: Methacholine challenge: comparison of two methods, Chest 2005; 127:839-844.

Cockcroft DW: Bronchoprovocation methods: direct challenges, Clin Rev Allergy Immunol 2003; 24:19-26.

Cockcroft DW, Killian DN, Mellon JJA et al: Bronchial reactivity to inhaled histamine: a method and clinical survey, Clin Allergy 1977; 7:235-243.

Eliasson AH, Phillips YY, Rajagopal KR et al: Sensitivity and specificity of bronchial provocation testing: an evaluation of four techniques in exercise induced bronchospasm, Chest 1992; 102:347.

Haas F, Axen K, Schicchi JS: Use of maximum expiratory flow-volume curve parameters in the assessment of exercise induced bronchospasm, Chest 1993; 103:64-68.

Irvin CG: Bronchial challenge testing, Respir Clin North Am 1995; 1:265-285.

Joos GF, O'Conner B, Anderson SD, Chung F et al: Indirect airway challenges, Eur Respir J 2003; 21:1050-1068.

Storms WW: Review of exercise-induced asthma, *Med Sci Sports Exerc* 2003; 35:1464-1470.

EXHALED NITRIC OXIDE

Berkman N, Avital A, Breuer R et al: Exhaled nitric oxide in the diagnosis of asthma: comparison with bronchial provocation tests, *Thorax* 2005; 60:383-388.

Deykin A, Halpern O, Massaro AF et al: Expired nitric oxide after bronchoprovocation and repeated spirometry in patients with asthma, *Am J Resp Crit Care Med* 1998; 157:769-775.

Franklin PJ, Stick SM, LeSouef PN et al: Measuring exhaled nitric oxide levels in adults; the importance of atopy and airway responsiveness, *Chest* 2004, 126:1540-1545.

Kissoon N, Duckworth LJ, Blake KV et al: Effect of β2-agonist treatment and spirometry on exhaled nitric oxide in healthy children and children with asthma, *Pediatr Pulmonol* 2002; 34:203-208.

Lim AY, Chambers DC, Ayres JG et al: Exhaled nitric oxide in cystic fibrosis patients with allergic bronchopulmonary aspergillosis, *Respir Med* 2003; 97:331-336.

Reid DW, Johns DP, Feltis B et al: Exhaled nitric oxide continues to reflect airway hyperresponsiveness and disease activity in inhaled corticosteroid-treated adult asthmatic patients, *Respirology* 2003; 8:479-486.

Silikoff PE, McClean PA, Slutsky AS et al: Marked flow-dependence of exhaled nitric oxide using a new technique to exclude nasal nitric oxide, *Am J Resp Crit Care Med* 1997, 155:260-267.

Smith AD, Cowan JO, Brassert KP et al: Use of exhaled nitric oxide measurements to guide treatment in chronic asthma, *N Engl J Med* 2005; 352:2163-2173.

Zitt M: Clinical applications of exhaled nitric oxide for the diagnosis and management of asthma: a consensus report, *Clin Ther* 2005; 27:1238-1250.

FORCED OSCILLATION TECHNIQUE

Dencker M, Malmberg LP, Valind S et al: Reference values for respiratory system impedance by using impulse oscillometry in children aged 2-11 years, *Clin Physiol Funct Imaging* 2006; 26:247-250.

Marotta A, Klinnert MD, Price MR et al: Impulse oscillometry provides an effective measure of lung dysfunction in 4 year old children at risk for persistent asthma, *J Allergy Clin Immunol* 2003; 112:317-322.

Oostveen E, Macleod D, Lorino H et al: The forced oscillation technique in clinical practice: methodology, recommendations and future developments, *Eur Respir J* 2003; 22:10 26-1041.

PREOPERATIVE PULMONARY FUNCTION TESTING

Algar FJ, Alvarez A, Salvatierra A et al: Predicting pulmonary complications after pneumonectomy for lung cancer, *Eur J Cardiothorac Surg* 2003; 23:201-208.

Beckles MA, Spiro SG, Colice GL et al: The physiologic evaluation of patients with lung cancer being considered for resectional surgery, *Chest* 2003; 123 (suppl):105S-114S.

Behr J: Optimizing preoperative lung function, *Curr Opin Anaesthesiol* 2001; 14:65-69.

Epstein SK, Faling LJ, Daly BD et al: Predicting complications after pulmonary resection: preoperative exercise testing vs a multifactorial cardiopulmonary risk index, *Chest* 1993; 104:694-700.

Ferguson MK, Durkin AE: Preoperative prediction of the risk of pulmonary complications after esophagectomy for cancer, *J Thorac Cardiovasc Surg* 2002; 123:661-669.

Fisher BW, Majumdar SR, McAlister FA: Predicting pulmonary complications after nonthoracic surgery: a systematic review of blinded studies, *Am J Med* 2002; 112:219-225.

Fuso L, Cisternino L, Di Napoli A et al: Role of spirometric and arterial gas data in predicting pulmonary complications after abdominal surgery, *Respir Med* 2000; 94:1171-1176.

Kearney DJ, Lee TH, Reilly JJ et al: Assessment of operative risk in patients undergoing lung resection: importance of predicted pulmonary function, *Chest* 1994; 105:753-759.

Older P, Smith R, Hall A, French C: Preoperative cardiopulmonary risk assessment by cardiopulmonary exercise testing, *Crit Care Resusc* 2000; 2:198-208.

RESPIRATORY IMPAIRMENT FOR DISABILITY

Sood A, Beckett WS: Determination of disability for patients with advanced lung disease, *Clin Chest Med* 1997; 18:471-482.

Taiwo OA, Cain HC: Pulmonary impairment and disability, *Clin Chest Med* 2002; 23:841-851.

U.S. Department of Health and Human Services: *Guide to pulmonary function studies under the Social Security disability programs: disability evaluation under Social Security,* SSA Publication No 64-055, 1999. http://www.ssa.gov/disability/professionals/pfs-pub055.htm, Last modified 12/13/2006; accessed 12/16/2006.

U.S. Department of Health and Human Services: *Disability evaluation under Social Security (Blue Book-January 2005)—3.00 respiratory system—adult.* http://www.ssa.gov/disability/professionals/bluebook/3.00-Respiratory-Adult.htm, Last modified 12/13/2006, last accessed 12/16/2006.

U.S. Department of Health and Human Services: *Disability evaluation under Social Security (Blue Book-January 2005)—103.00 respiratory system—childhood.* http://www.ssa.gov/disability/professionals/bluebook/103.00-Respiratory-Childhood.htm, Last modified 12/13/2006, last accessed 12/16/2006.

METABOLIC MEASUREMENTS (INDIRECT CALORIMETRY)

Battezzati A, Vigano R: Indirect calorimetry and nutritional problems in clinical practice, *Acta Diabetol* 2001; 38:1-5.

Branson RD: The measurement of energy expenditure: instrumentation, practical considerations and clinical application, *Respir Care* 1990; 35:640-659.

Compher C, Frankenfield D, Keim N et al: Best practice methods to apply to measurement of resting metabolic rate in adults: a systematic review, *J Am Diet Assoc* 2006; 106:881-903.

Consolazio CF, Johnson RE, Pecora LJ: *Physiological measurements of metabolic functions in man,* New York, 1963, McGraw-Hill.

Da Rocha EE, Alves VG, da Fonseca RB: Indirect calorimetry: methodology, instruments and clinical application, *Curr Opin Clin Nutr Metab Care* 2006; 9:247-256.

Harris JA, Benedict FG: *Biometric studies of basal metabolism in man,* Carnegie Institute of Washington 1919; Publication No 279.

Miles JM: Energy expenditure in hospitalized patients: implications for nutritional support, *Mayo Clin Proc* 2006; 81:809-816.

Roffey DM, Byrne NM, Hills AP: Day-today variance in measurement of resting metabolic rate using ventilated-hood and mouthpiece & nose-clip indirect calorimetry systems, *J Parenter Enteral Nutr* 2006; 30:426-432.

Stewart CL, Goody CM, Branson R: Comparison of two systems of measuring energy expenditure, *J Parenter Enteral Nutr* 2005; 29:212-217.

Weir JB: New methods for calculating metabolic rate with special reference to protein metabolism, *J Physiol* 1949; 109:1-9.

Weissman C, Kemper MA, Askanazi J et al: Resting metabolic rate of the critically ill patient: measured versus predicted, *Anesthesiology* 1986; 64:673-679.

GUIDELINES AND STANDARDS

American Association for Respiratory Care: Clinical practice guideline: Metabolic measurements using indirect calorimetry during mechanical ventilation—2004 Revision & Update, *Respir Care* 2004; 49:1073-1079.

American Association for Respiratory Care: Clinical practice guideline: methacholine challenge testing—2001 revision & update, *Respir Care* 2001; 46:523-530.

American Thoracic Society/European Respiratory Society: Recommendations for standardized procedures for the online and offline measurement of exhaled lower respiratory nitric oxide and nasal nitric oxide, 2005, *Am J Resp Crit Care Med* 2005; 171:912-930.

American Thoracic Society: Guidelines for methacholine and exercise challenge testing—1999, *Am J Respir Crit Care Med* 2000; 161:309-329.

Sterk PJ, Fabbri LM, Quanjer PH et al: Airway responsiveness: standardized challenge testing with pharmacological, physical and sensitizing stimuli in adults: Statement of the European Respiratory Society, *Eur Respir J* 1993; 6 (suppl 16):53-83.

Pulmonary Function Testing Equipment

OBJECTIVES

After studying this chapter you will be able to:

Entry-level

1. Describe two types of volume displacement spirometers
2. List at least two principles used by flow-sensing spirometers to measure volume
3. Select a directional breathing valve for a specific testing situation
4. Identify the types of gas analyzers used for diffusing capacity and dilutional lung volume tests
5. Describe the function of commonly used gas conditioning devices

Advanced
1. Select and set up the basic components of a body plethysmograph
2. Contrast and compare measurement of oxygen saturation by multiwavelength and pulse oximeters
3. Identify the measurement principles of pH, PCO_2, and PO_2 blood gas devices
4. Describe the important characteristics of an "office" spirometer
5. Discuss various types of data storage applicable to pulmonary function data

KEY TERMS

ambient temperature, pressure, and saturation (ATPS)
chemoluminescence analyzers
co-oximeter
dry rolling-seal spirometer
emission spectroscopy
Fleisch-type pneumotachometer
flow-sensing spirometer
fluorescence quenching
free breathing valves
gas chromotography

heated-wire flow sensors
hemoximeter
light-emitting diode (LED)
office spirometer
peak flow meter
Pitot tube flow sensor
polarographic electrode
potentiometer
pressure differential flow sensor
pressure plethysmograph
pulse oximeter

reflective spectrophotometry
resistive element
Silverman pneumotachometer
spectrophotometric oximeter
thermal conductivity analyzers
turbine
volume-displacement spirometer
water-seal spirometer
wedge bellows spirometer

This chapter describes pulmonary function equipment used for common testing applications. Included are **volume-displacement spirometers** and **flow-sensing spirometers**, peak flow meters, body plethysmographs, breathing valves, pulmonary gas analyzers, gas conditioning devices, blood gas analyzers and oximeters, and computerized pulmonary function systems.

Hutchinson introduced the precursor of the modern spirometer around 1844. This spirometer was a water-sealed volume-displacement device. Some aspects of the original device are still evident in today's spirometers. Flow-sensing spirometers have become much more common with the advent of sophisticated electronics and software that can integrate flow signals to measure volume by a variety of methods. Microprocessor-based spirometers are now small enough to be handheld.

Analysis of respiratory gases by volumetric methods was pioneered by Haldane in the early part of the 20th century. However, modern gas analyzers use indirect means (e.g., electrodes or sensors) to measure partial pressures of gases, or physical separation of gases to measure fractional concentrations (gas chromatography). Almost every instrument in the pulmonary function laboratory today combines signal transducers, analog-to-digital converters, and computer software to process and record physiologic data. Some devices, such as the pulse oximeter, are based almost entirely on electronic components. Computers eliminate many tedious calculations, allowing the technologist to concentrate on obtaining high-quality, repeatable data.

VOLUME DISPLACEMENT SPIROMETERS

Water-Seal Spirometers

For more than 100 years, the **water-seal spirometer** was the basic tool used to measure lung volumes and flows. The spirometer consists of a large bell

(7 – 10 L) suspended in a container of water with the open end of the bell below the surface of the water (Figure 10-1). A breathing circuit into the interior of the bell allows for accurate measurement of gas volumes. The patient breathes into the spirometer, moving the bell up during expiration and down with inspiration. Each spirometer bell has a "**bell factor**" relating the vertical distance moved to a specific volume (milliliters or liters). For many years movement of the bell was recorded using a pen to make a tracing on a rotating drum called a **kymograph**. Volumes were measured from the kymograph tracing by using paper that incorporated the bell factor for the spirometer. Volumes measured in this way reflect the gas in the spirometer that is at **ambient temperature, pressure, and saturation (ATPS)**. These volumes, such as vital capacity (VC), had to be corrected to BTPS.

This type of spirometer bell is more commonly used to activate a potentiometer. The **potentiometer** is a device that produces an analog DC voltage signal proportional to its position or displacement. For example, an output of 10 volts might equal a volume of 10 L in the spirometer. This analog signal can be used to drive a mechanical recorder such as a strip-chart recorder. More commonly, however, the analog signal is digitized with an analog-to-digital (A/D) converter. The digitized signal from the spirometer can then be stored and processed by a computer. Some potentiometers also produce analog signals representing the speed of movement of a volume displacement spirometer. This signal is proportional to flow. All volume displacement spirometers use some type of potentiometer or position encoder to produce signals that can be digitized and stored by a computer.

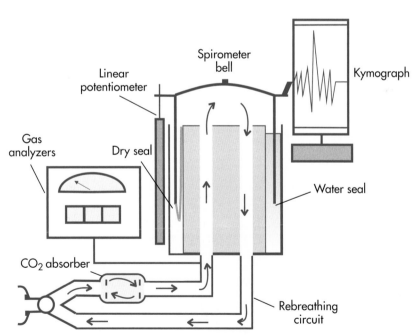

FIGURE 10-1   Cutaway View of Water-Seal and Dry-Seal Spirometers. The spirometer bell "floats" in a well. A water seal *(right side)* and a dry rolling seal *(left side)* are shown (see text). Also shown is a rebreathing circuit with CO_2 absorber and gas analyzers, as might be used for closed-circuit FRC determination. Although not widely used, a kymograph was often attached so that excursions of the bell traced a volume-time spirogram on moving graph paper. The convention of plotting expiratory volume in an upward direction can be traced to this type of spirometer/kymograph setup. A linear potentiometer provides analog outputs for volume and flow.

For simple spirometry, a single large-bore tube can be used for both inspiration and expiration. For rebreathing studies, the breathing circuit incorporates a carbon dioxide (CO_2) absorber (usually soda lime). Inspiratory and expiratory circuits are separated with one-way valves to reduce dead space. Water-seal spirometers are typically used for spirometry. They may also be used to measure ventilation, including $\dot{V}_E$, V_T, and respiratory rate. Water-seal spirometers can be used to obtain flow-volume (F-V) curves, although their frequency response may be limited by their physical characteristics. By including the rebreathing apparatus described (see Figure 10-1), lung volumes by helium

dilution can be obtained. In combination with an appropriate reservoir for the test gas, water-sealed spirometers can be used to perform diffusing capacity tests, both single-breath and rebreathing. The water-seal spirometer can be used as a reservoir for special gas mixtures such as those used for DLCO tests.

The Stead-Wells water-seal or **dry-seal spirometer** is still used, although not commonly. The Stead-Wells spirometer uses a lightweight plastic bell (Figure 10-2). The water-sealed bell "floats" in the water well, rising and falling with breathing excursions. In the dry-seal version, a rubberized seal connects the bell to the internal wall of the spirom-

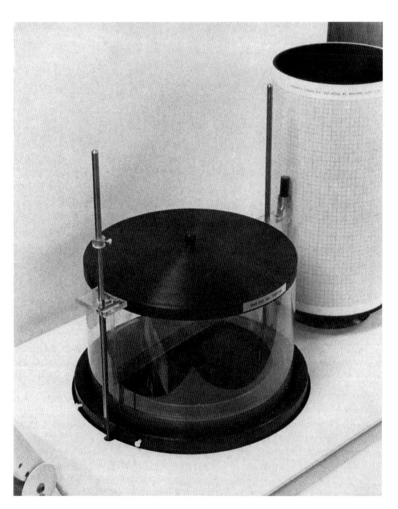

FIGURE 10-2 **Stead-Wells Dry-Seal Spirometer.** The conventional Stead-Wells spirometer used a lightweight plastic bell that floated in water. This version uses a silicon seal similar to that found in the dry rolling-seal spirometer. The spirometer bell carries a pen that traces directly on a rotating kymograph (rarely used today). With appropriate circuitry and gas analyzers, helium (He) dilution FRC determinations and DLCO measurements are easily performed. *(Courtesy Warren E. Collins, Inc., Braintree, Mass.)*

eter well. The rubber seal then "rolls" over itself, much the same as the dry rolling-seal spirometer (see next section). The Stead-Wells bell is usually attached to a linear potentiometer that provides analog signals proportional to volume and flow. These signals are passed to a computer through an A/D converter. The Stead-Wells design is capable of meeting the minimum requirements for flow and volume accuracy recommended by the American Thoracic Society and European Respiratory Society (ATS/ERS) (see Chapter 11).

Problems with water-seal (and dry-seal) spirometers are usually caused by leaks in the bell or in the breathing circuit. Gravity causes the spirometer to lose volume in the presence of leaks. Leaks in the spirometer, tubing, or valves can be detected by raising the bell and plugging the patient connection. Any change in volume can be detected easily by recording the spirometer volume over several minutes. Weights can be added to the top of the bell to enhance detection of small leaks. During patient testing, improper positioning of the spirometer can cause inaccurate measurements. If positioned too high, the bell can rise out of the water or reach the top of its travel range. This causes the volume-time tracing to appear abruptly flattened. The pattern observed may be mistaken for a normal end-of-expiration. If a Stead-Wells spirometer is positioned too low, it may empty completely. This may result in water being drawn into the breathing circuit, gas analyzer, or other system components. Inadequate water in the device may also lead to erroneous readings that are sometimes difficult to detect. The size of the water-seal spirometer and its weight when filled with water make it somewhat difficult to transport. The waterless version of the spirometer eliminates the last consideration.

Because lung volumes and flows are corrected to BTPS conditions, careful attention to the ambient conditions of volume-displacement spirometers is required. Although the temperature of gas in the spirometer can be easily measured, the temperature may change significantly during maneuvers such as a forced vital capacity (FVC). These changes can be difficult to monitor, resulting in volumes and flows that are not representative of lung physiology.

PF TIP

The use of volume-displacement spirometers accounts for some of the conventions used in spirometry today. Plotting expiratory volume in the upward direction mimics the graph made by the pen of a Stead-Wells–type spirometer on a rotating kymograph. Plotting MVV as an accumulated volume over time originated from the chain-driven pulley of a water-sealed bell.

Maintenance of water-seal spirometers includes routine draining of the water well. Both wet and dry versions of the Stead-Wells spirometer must be checked for cracks or leaks in the bell. Chemical absorbers for water vapor must be routinely checked. Water absorbers can be rapidly exhausted because the gas in the spirometer is almost completely saturated with water vapor.

Infection control of water-seal spirometers typically involves replacing breathing hoses and mouthpieces after each patient. Although the patient's expired gas comes into direct contact with the water in the spirometer, cross-contamination is uncommon. Some systems allow use of low-resistance bacteria filters to protect from contamination those parts of the breathing circuit that are not changed after patient use. Such filters should be used with caution for flow-dependent maneuvers. Water condensation in the filter element may significantly alter its resistance. The volume of these filters may need to be considered when calculating system volume or system dead space, as is required for dilutional measurements of lung volumes.

Because of problems such as leaks and maintenance required for water-seal spirometers, these devices have become relatively rare in clinical practice. Water-seal or dry-seal spirometers may be used in longitudinal studies that were begun before other types of spirometers was available.

Dry Rolling-Seal Spirometers

Another type of volume-displacement spirometer is the **dry rolling-seal spirometer**. A typical unit consists of a lightweight piston mounted horizontally in a cylinder. A rod that rests on frictionless bearings supports the piston (Figure 10-3). The piston is coupled to the cylinder wall by a flexible plastic seal. The seal rolls on itself rather than sliding as the piston moves. A similar type of rolling-seal may also be used with a vertically mounted, lightweight piston that rises and falls with breathing (as in the dry-seal Stead-Wells described in the preceding section). The maximum volume of the cylinder with the piston fully displaced is usually 10–12 L. The piston has a large diameter so that excursions of just a few inches are all that is necessary to record large volume changes. The piston is normally constructed of lightweight aluminum to reduce inertia. Mechanical resistance is kept to a minimum by the bearings supporting the piston rod and by the rolling seal itself.

Although they can be used with a mechanical recorder, most dry rolling-seal spirometers use linear or rotary potentiometers. The potentiometer responds to piston movement to produce DC voltage outputs for volume and flow. For example, a 10-V potentiometer attached to a 10-L spirometer may produce an output of 1 V/L. On a separate channel, a flow of 1 L/sec may produce an output of 1 V. Flow in this case is proportional to the speed of the moving piston. These analog outputs for volume and flow are digitized so that a computer can store and manipulate the data.

The piston of the standard dry rolling-seal spirometer (Figure 10-4) travels horizontally, eliminating the need for counterbalancing. The vertically mounted version (see Figure 10-2) depends on a lightweight piston and the rolling seal to reduce resistance to breathing. Temperature corrections (from ATPS to BTPS) are made by applying a correction factor to the digital value stored in the computer. A one-way breathing circuit and CO_2 scrubber may be added so that dry rolling-seal spirometers can be used for rebreathing tests in much the same way as water-seal spirometers.

To perform studies such as the open-circuit nitrogen washout test, a "dumping" mechanism is attached to the spirometer. The dumping device empties the spirometer after each breath or after a predetermined volume has been reached. Addition of an automated valve and alveolar sampling device allows the dry rolling-seal spirometer to be used

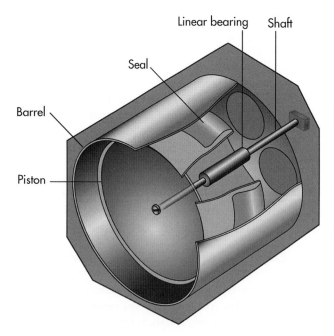

FIGURE 10-3   Cutaway View of a Dry Rolling-Seal Spirometer. A flexible seal attaches the piston to the wall of the cylinder and rolls on itself. The piston has a large surface area, so horizontal movement is minimized. This allows recording of normal breaths and maximal respiratory excursions with little resistance. The piston is supported by a shaft that rides on a linear bearing. The shaft activates a rotary potentiometer (not shown). Rotation of the potentiometer generates analog signals for flow and volume. *(Illustration by Jennifer Pryll, Courtesy Morgan Scientific, Haverhill, Mass.)*

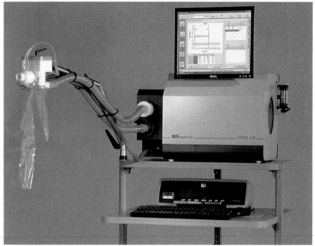

FIGURE 10-4 **Dry Rolling-Seal Spirometer.** A pulmonary function system designed around a dry rolling-seal spirometer. Two ports to accommodate simple spirometry, as well as rebreathing maneuvers with a CO_2 absorber (see also Figure 10-3). *(Courtesy Morgan Scientific, Haverhill, Mass.)*

for single-breath diffusion studies. Dry rolling-seal spirometers are typically capable of meeting the minimum standards recommended by the ATS/ERS (see Chapter 11).

Common problems encountered with dry rolling-seal spirometers are sticking of the rolling-seal and increased mechanical resistance in the piston-cylinder assembly. These difficulties can usually be avoided by adequate maintenance of the spirometer. As for other types of volume-displacement spirometers, simple correction of volumes from ATPS to BTPS may not completely reflect physiologic flow or volume changes. Infection control of the dry rolling-seal involves disassembling the piston-cylinder. The interior of the cylinder and the face of the piston are usually wiped with a mild antibacterial solution. The rolling-seal itself is also wiped with disinfectant. Alcohol or similar drying agents may cause deterioration of the seal and should not be used. The seal should be routinely checked for leaks or tears. After reassembly, the piston should be positioned at the maximum volume position. When the rolling-seal is extended completely, the material of the seal is less likely to develop creases that can result in uneven movement of the piston. With the previously described reservations, bacteria filters may be used to avoid contamination of the spirometer.

Bellows-Type Spirometers

A third type of volume-displacement spirometer is the bellows or **wedge bellows spirometer**. Both devices consist of a collapsible bellows that folds or unfolds in response to breathing excursions. The conventional bellows design is a flexible accordion-type container. One end is stationary and the other end is displaced in proportion to the volume inspired or expired. The wedge bellows operates similarly except that it expands and contracts like a fan (Figure 10-5). One side of the bellows remains stationary; the other side moves with a pivotal motion around an axis through the fixed side. Displacement of the bellows by a volume of gas is translated either to movement of a pen on chart paper or to a potentiometer. For mechanical recording, chart paper moves at a fixed speed under the pen while a spirogram is traced. For computerized testing, displacement of the bellows is transformed into a DC voltage by a linear or rotary potentiometer. The analog signal is routed to an A/D converter and then to a computer.

The conventional and wedge bellows may be mounted either horizontally or vertically. The horizontal bellows is mounted so that the primary direction of travel is on a horizontal plane. This design minimizes the effects of gravity on bellows

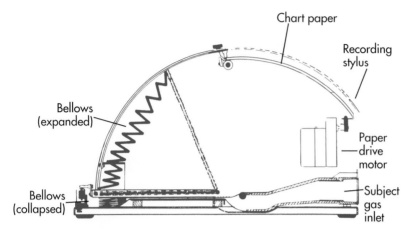

FIGURE 10-5 **Cross-sectional Diagram of a Wedge Bellows Spirometer.** Fanlike movements of the wedge bellows carries the recording stylus across moving graph paper. Some manufacturers suspend the bellows so that the primary movement is in a horizontal rather than vertical plane. Large wedge bellows offer little resistance and are comparable to dry-seal or water-seal spirometers in accuracy and linearity. *(Modified from Vitalograph Medical Instrumentation, Product Brochure, Lenexa, Kan.)*

movement. The horizontal bellows (either conventional or wedge) with a large surface area offers little mechanical resistance. This type is normally used in conjunction with a potentiometer to produce analog volume and flow signals. Small (approximately 7–8 L), vertically mounted bellows are available and may be used for portable spirometry and bedside testing. Most of these types offer simple mechanical recording, digital data reduction, or both by means of a small, dedicated microprocessor.

Both bellows-type spirometers (Figure 10-6) can be used to measure vital capacity and its subdivisions, as well as FVC, FEV_1, expiratory flows, and MVV. Some bellows-type spirometers, especially those that are mounted vertically, are designed to measure expiratory flows only. These types expand upward when gas is injected, then empty spontaneously under their own weight. Horizontally mounted bellows can usually be set in a mid-range to record both inspiratory and expiratory maneuvers. This allows F-V loops to be recorded. With appropriate gas analyzers and breathing circuitry, bellows systems may be used for gas dilution FRC determinations and DLCO measurements. Most bellows-type spirometers meet ATS recommendations for flow and volume accuracy.

One problem that may occur with bellows-type spirometers is inaccuracy resulting from sticking of the bellows. The folds of the bellows may adhere

because of dirt, moisture, or aging of the bellows material. Some bellows-type spirometers require the bellows to be partially distended when not in use. This technique allows moisture from exhaled gas to evaporate and prevents deterioration of the bellows. Leaks may also develop in the bellows material or at the point where the bellows is mounted. Leaks can usually be detected by filling the bellows with air, plugging the breathing port, and attaching a weight or spring to pressurize the contained gas.

Infection control of bellows-type spirometers depends on the method of construction. In some instruments, the bellows can be entirely removed; in others, the interior of the bellows must be wiped clean. Many bellows are made from rubberized or plastic-based material that can be cleaned with a mild detergent and dried thoroughly before reassembly. Bacteria filters may be used to avoid contamination of the bellows, with the reservations described previously.

Volume-displacement spirometers were once the main devices used for pulmonary function testing. Many such devices are still in use, and some manufacturers continue to produce sophisticated spirometers based on the volume-displacement principle. However, use of flow-sensing spirometers has become increasingly common, both in the pulmonary function laboratory and in small, portable devices for bedside or clinic use.

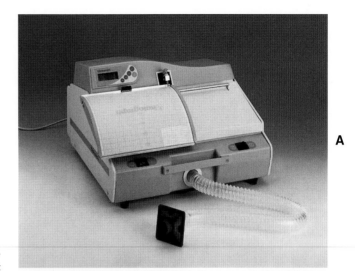

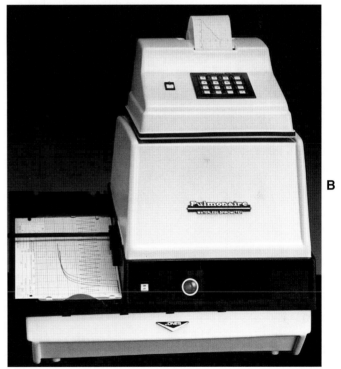

FIGURE 10-6 Two Types of Bellows Spirometers. A, Wedge-bellows spirometer with direct writing recorder, and a dedicated microprocessor for displaying flows and volumes. **B,** Conventional bellows-type spirometer, with the bellows mounted horizontally and driving a pen across moving graph papers. A potentiometer allows analog output to a dedicated microprocessor with built-in printer for automatic data reduction. (*A courtesy Vitalograph, Inc., Lenexa, Kan.; B courtesy Jones Medical Instrument Co., Oakbrook, Ill.*)

FLOW-SENSING SPIROMETERS

In contrast to the volume-displacement spirometer is the flow-sensing spirometer, or pneumotachometer. The term *pneumotachometer* describes a device that measures gas flow. Flow-sensing spirometers use various physical principles to produce a signal proportional to gas flow. This signal is then integrated to measure volume in addition to flow. **Integration** is a process in which flow (volume per unit of time) is divided into a large number of small intervals (time). The volume from each interval is summed (Figure 10-7). Integration can be performed easily by an electronic circuit or by computer software. Accurate volume measurement by flow integration requires an accurate flow signal, accurate timing, and sensitive detection of low flow.

One type of device that responds to bulk flow of gas is the turbine or impeller. Integration may be unnecessary because the turbine directly measures gas volumes. Some turbine spirometers produce volume pulses in which each "pulse" equals a fixed volume. These spirometers count pulses very accurately. Most flow-sensing spirometers use tubes through which laminar airflow is possible (see Appendix E). Five basic types of flow sensors are commonly used: turbines, pressure-differential flow sensors, heated-wire flow sensors, Pitot tube flow sensors, and ultrasonic flow sensors.

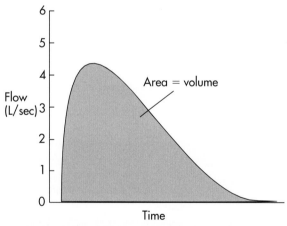

FIGURE 10-7 Volume Measurement by Flow Integration. The flow signal from many types of flow-sensing spirometers is integrated to compute volume. Flow is measured against time. The area under the flow-time curve is subdivided into a large number of small sections. Each section represents a small interval of time. Volume is equal to the sum of the areas of all sections. By dividing the curve into a large number of sections, even irregular flow curves can be accurately integrated. Integration is usually performed by a dedicated electronic circuit or by software.

PF TIP

Most spirometers use flow sensors. Flow-sensing spirometers have several advantages over volume-displacement devices. They are smaller, easier to maintain, easier to clean, and can even use disposable sensors. Their small size makes them ideal for portable systems, making simple spirometry a powerful diagnostic tool that can be used in settings such as the primary care practitioner's office.

Turbines

The simplest type of flow-sensing device is the **turbine**, or respirometer. This instrument consists of a vane connected to a series of precision gears. Gas flowing through the body of the instrument causes the vane to rotate, registering a volume (Figure 10-8). The respirometer can be used to measure slow vital capacity (VC). It can also be used for ventilation tests such as V_T and $\dot{V}_E$. One such device is the **Wright respirometer**. This respirometer can measure volumes accurately at flows between 3 and 300 L/min. At flows greater than 300 L/min (5 L/sec), the vane is subject to distortion. Because of this limitation, it should not be used to measure FVC when the patient is capable of flows greater than 300 L/min. At low flows (less than 3 L/min), inertia of the vane-gear system may underestimate volume.

A special advantage of this type of respirometer is its compact size and usefulness at the bedside. Most respirometers can register a wide range of volumes using multiple scales. The standard Wright respirometer measures 0.1 – 1 L on one scale and up to 100 L on another scale. Turbine devices are also widely used for measurements of bulk flow in various dry gas meters.

An adaptation of the turbine flow device includes a photo cell and light source that is interrupted by the movement of the vane or impeller (Figure 10-9, D). Rotation of the vane interrupts a light beam between its source and the photo cell. This produces a pulse, with each pulse equivalent to a fixed gas volume. The pulse count is summed to obtain the volume of gas flowing through the device. The

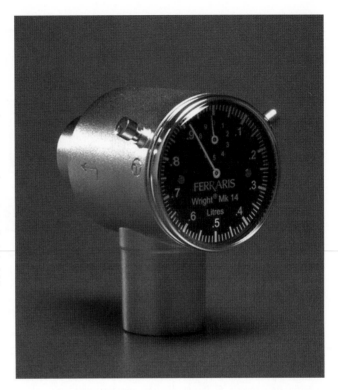

FIGURE 10-8 **Turbine-Type Flow Sensor.** The Wright Mk14 respirometer is shown. A rotating vane mounted on jeweled bearings drives reduction gears connected to the main dial. Two gas ports (bottom and rear in the photo) allow flow through the housing for measurement of volume. Although the vane turns in only one direction, inspired or expired volumes can be measured by attachment to the appropriate port. The main dial indicator measures volumes in hundredths of a liter. The small dial indicator marks volumes larger than 1 L on the face, so that accumulated volumes can be measured. The instrument also features controls for engaging or disengaging the vane and for resetting the indicators to zero. *(Courtesy Ferraris Respiratory Inc., Louisville, Colo.)*

signal produced may not be linear across a wide range of flows because of inertia or distortion of the rotating vane.

The accuracy of turbine flow devices is usually limited by the factors described. For this reason, turbine devices often do not meet the ATS minimum recommendations for spirometers. These devices may be used for monitoring or screening. Because of their simplicity and small size, several such devices are marketed for home use. This type of spirometer allows FVC, FEV_1, and peak expiratory flow (PEF) to be monitored outside the usual clinical setting.

Infection control of turbine-type respirometers depends on their construction and intended use. Devices such as the Wright respirometer usually must be gas sterilized. Water condensation from exhaled gas can damage the vane-gear mechanisms. Some turbine spirometers use disposable impellers. This avoids cross-contamination, but accuracy may be limited by the quality of the disposable sensor.

Pressure Differential Flow Sensors

Pressure differential flow sensors are among the most common implementations of flow sensing. They consist of a tube containing a **resistive element**. The resistive element allows gas to flow through it but causes a pressure drop (see Figure 10-9, *A*). The pressure difference across the resistive element is measured by means of a sensitive pressure transducer. The transducer usually has pressure taps on either side of the element (Figure 10-10, *A*). The pressure differential across the resistive element is proportional to gas flow as long as flow is laminar. This flow signal is integrated to measure volume (see Figure 10-7). Turbulent gas flow upstream or downstream of the resistive element may interfere with development of true laminar flow. Most pneumotachometers attempt to reduce turbulent flow by tapering the tubes in which the resistive elements are mounted.

Although there are many designs for resistive elements, two types are commonly used. The

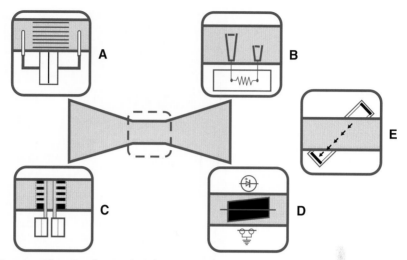

FIGURE 10-9   Common Flow-Sensing Devices (Pneumotachometers). Each flow-sensing device is mounted in a tube that promotes laminar flow *(center)*. **A,** Pressure-differential pneumotachometer in which a resistive element causes a pressure drop proportional to the flow of gas through the tube. A sensitive pressure transducer monitors the pressure drop across the resistive element and converts the differential to an analog signal. The resistive element may be a mesh screen or capillary tube; it is usually heated to 37°C or higher to prevent condensation of water from expired gas. **B,** Heated-wire pneumotachometer contains heated elements of small mass that respond to gas flow by heat loss. An electric current heats the elements (thin wires). Gas flow past the elements causes cooling. In one element, current is increased to maintain a constant temperature; the other element acts as a reference (see also Figure 10-11). The current change is proportional to gas flow, and a continuous signal is supplied to an integrating circuit as for the pressure differential flow sensor. **C,** Pitot tube flow sensor uses a series of small tubes that are placed at right angles to the direction of gas flow. Sensitive pressure transducers detect changes in gas velocity. The Pitot tubes are mounted in struts in the flow tube; separate devices face either way so that bidirectional flow can be measured (see also Figure 10-12). **D,** Electronic rotating-vane flow sensor. A vane or impeller is mounted in the flow tube. A light-emitting diode (LED) is mounted on one side of the vane, and a photodetector on the other side. Each time the vane rotates, it interrupts the light from the LED reaching the detector. These pulses are counted and summed to calculate gas volume. **E,** Ultrasonic flow sensor. High-frequency sound waves pass through membranes on either side of a flow tube at an angle to the stream of gas. The sound waves speed up or slow down depending on which direction the gas is flowing. By measuring the transit time of the sound waves, gas flow can be measured very accurately and integrated to compute volume. (See also Figure 10-13.)

Fleisch-type pneumotachometer uses a bundle of capillary tubes (or similar material) as the resistive element. Laminar flow is ensured by size and arrangement of the capillary tubes. The cross-sectional area and length of the capillary tubes determines the actual resistance to flow through the Fleisch pneumotachometer. The dynamic range of the Fleisch device must be matched to the range of flows to be measured. Different sizes (i.e., resistances) of pneumotachometers may be used to accurately measure high or low flows.

The other common type of pressure differential flow sensor is the Silverman (or Lilly) type. The

Silverman pneumotachometer uses one or more screens to act as a resistive element. A typical arrangement has three screens mounted parallel to one another. The middle screen acts as the resistive element with the pressure taps on either side, whereas the outer screens protect the middle screen and help ensure laminar flow. The Silverman pneumotachometer usually has a wider dynamic flow range than the Fleisch type. As a result, it is better suited for measuring widely varying flows.

Most Fleisch and Silverman pneumotachometers use a heating mechanism to warm the resistive element to 37°C or higher. Heating the resistive

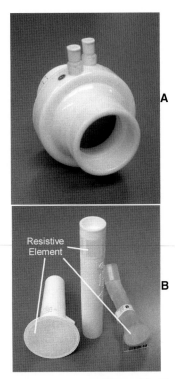

A

B

Resistive
Element

FIGURE 10-10 Pressure Differential Flow Sensors (Pneumotachometers). A, Small reusable pressure differential flow sensor is shown. This pneumotachometer consists of an unheated screen that acts as a resistive element. Two Luer-type fittings provide for connection to a pressure transducer so that the pressure drop across the resistive element can be measured. **B,** Three types of disposable pressure differential flow sensors are shown. Each device uses a porous paper or plastic screenlike material to act as a resistive element. A single pressure tap upstream of the resistive element allows pressure to be measured and compared to ambient pressure. Disposable flow sensors are calibrated at the time of manufacture. Some manufacturers print a calibration code or calibration bar code on the disposable sensor that can be used by the spirometer software to achieve accurate measurement of flow and volume.

element prevents condensation of water vapor from exhaled gas on the element. Condensation or other debris lodging in the resistive element changes the resistance across it, thus changing its calibration. A change in the resistive element such as condensation or a hole causes a change in the pressure-flow relationship. Pneumotachometers need to be recalibrated after cleaning or similar maintenance.

Some flow-sensing spirometers use resistive elements such as porous paper, rendering the flow sensor disposable (see Figure 10-10, *B*). These devices usually have a single pressure tap upstream of the resistive element. Pressure measured in front of the resistive element is referenced against ambient pressure. This design requires that the flow sensor be carefully "zeroed" before making any flow measurements. The accuracy of spirometers using this type of flow sensor often depends on how carefully the disposable resistive elements are manufactured. If the resistance varies widely from sensor to sensor, each unit may need to be calibrated before use to ensure accuracy. Some manufacturers calibrate their disposable sensors and then provide a calibration code with each sensor. This code is used to identify a particular sensor by the software in the spirometer. One method of identifying the correct calibration factor for individual flow sensors is to imprint the sensor with a bar code (see Figure 10-10, *B*). The spirometer then includes a simple bar code reader to identify the appropriate calibration factors. Some portable spirometer systems that use precalibrated flow sensors do not provide for user calibration. However, verification of accuracy (using a 3-L syringe) is usually possible, even if the manufacturer has not provided for this in the software accompanying the spirometer.

Systems that use permanent pressure-differential flow sensors usually meet or exceed the ATS/ERS minimal recommendations for spirometers. Spirometers that use disposable sensors can meet or exceed the minimal requirements, depending on the quality of the sensor and the application software responsible for signal processing. Gas composition affects the accuracy of flow measurements in pressure-differential pneumotachometers. Correction factors for gases other than air can be applied by software so that these types of flow sensors can be used for most types of pulmonary function tests.

Infection control of pressure-differential flow sensors depends on their placement in the spirometer. In open-circuit systems in which only exhaled gas is measured, only the mouthpiece needs to be changed between patients. If inspiratory and expiratory flows are measured, the flow sensor itself may need to be disinfected between patients. Disassembly and cleaning of flow sensors usually require that the spirometer be recalibrated. Disposable or single-use sensors avoid this problem. In-line bacteria filters may be used to isolate the pneumotachometer from potential contamination. The spirometer should meet all ATS/ERS requirements for range, accuracy, and flow resistance with the filter in place (see Chapter 11). If a filter is used, calibration with the filter in-line is usually required. The effect of bacteria filters on spirometric measurements has not been well defined, but proper use of filters typically causes only small errors in measured flows and volumes.

Heated-Wire Flow Sensors

Heated-wire flow sensors are a third type of flow-sensing spirometer. They are based on the cooling effect of gas flow. A heated element, usually a thin platinum wire, is situated in a laminar flow tube (see Figure 10-9, *B*). Gas flow past the wire causes a temperature decrease so that more current must be supplied to maintain a preset temperature. The current needed to maintain the temperature is proportional to gas flow. The heated element usually has a small mass so that slight changes in gas flow can be detected. The flow signal is integrated electronically or by software to obtain volume measurements. The heated wire is usually protected behind a screen to prevent impaction of debris on the element. Debris or moisture droplets on the element can change its thermal characteristics. Some systems use two wires (Figure 10-11). One measures gas flow, and the second serves as a reference. Most heated-wire flow sensors maintain a temperature higher than 37°C. Heating prevents condensation from expired air that might interfere with sensitivity of the element.

Most heated-wire flow sensors meet or exceed ATS/ERS recommendations for accuracy and precision. Gas composition may affect the accuracy of flow measurements. Correction factors for gases other than room air can be applied via software. This allows heated-wire devices to accurately measure gases for pulmonary function tests using helium, oxygen (O_2), and other gases. Heated-wire sensors can be used for routine pulmonary function tests, exercise testing, and metabolic studies. Infection control for heated-wire sensors is similar to that for pressure- differential devices. Disposable or single-use devices avoid cross-contamination even when the sensor is located proximal to the patient's airway.

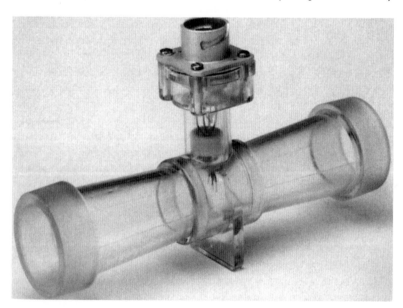

FIGURE 10-11   Heated-Wire Flow Sensor. A flow tube contains very thin, paired stainless steel wires. The wires are maintained at two temperatures exceeding body temperature and are connected by a Wheatstone bridge. The tube streamlines gas flow into laminar flow. The temperature of the wires decreases in proportion to the mass of the gas and its flow. Two wires are used; one measures expiratory flow and the other serves as a reference. *(Courtesy VIASYS Healthcare Critical Care Division, Palm Springs, Calif.)*

Pitot Tube Flow Sensors

Pitot tube flow sensors are a fourth type of flow sensor. They use the Pitot tube principle. The pressure of gas flowing against a small tube is related to the gas's density and velocity. Flow can be measured by placing a series of small tubes in a flow sensor and connecting them to a sensitive pressure transducer (see Figure 10-9, C). The pressure signal must be linearized and integrated as described for other flow-sensing devices. In practice, two sets of Pitot tubes are mounted in the same sensor so that bidirectional flow can be measured (Figure 10-12). A wide range of flows can be accommodated by using two or more pressure transducers with different sensitivities. Because this type of flow-sensing device is affected by gas density, software correction for different gas compositions is necessary. This is accomplished by sampling the gas, analyzing O_2 and CO_2, and applying the necessary correction factors. Software corrections for test gases used for various pulmonary function tests (e.g., DLCO) can be easily applied.

Pitot tube flow sensors meet or exceed ATS recommendations for accuracy and precision. Their practical applications include routine pulmonary function tests, metabolic measurements, and exercise testing. Infection control for this type of device includes single-use, or disposable flow meters. If Pitot tube flow sensors are cleaned, care must be taken that disinfectant solution or rinse water is completely removed from the small tubes used to sense flow.

Ultrasonic Flow Sensors

Gas flow can be detected and measured by passing high-frequency sound waves across the stream of gas. Ultrasonic transducers on either side of the flow tube transmit sound waves alternately across the tube. By passing the sound waves at an angle to the flow of gas in two different directions, bidirectional flow can be measured (see Figure 10-9, E). The sound waves are sped up by gas flowing in one direction and slowed down by gas flowing in the opposite direction. By measuring the "transit time" of the pulses with a very accurate digital clock, flow can be integrated to measure volume. Analyzing the change in frequency of the sound waves passing through the flowing gas has the advantage of not being affected by the gas composition, temperatures, or humidity. In addition, there are no moving parts or elements to become occluded when measuring exhaled gas.

A distinct advantage of measuring gas flow by means of ultrasonic pulses is that a disposable flow tube can be inserted between the transducers, thus eliminating problems with cross-contamination between subjects. A further advantage of this design is that the disposable flow tube does not require calibration because it simply acts as a transparent barrier separating exhaled gas from the sensing transducers (Figure 10-13).

Flow-sensing spirometers have some advantages over volume-displacement systems. When combined with appropriate gas analyzers and breathing circuits, flow-sensing spirometers can be used to perform lung volume determinations by the open-circuit method. Diffusing capacity can be measured with flow-sensing spirometers as well. Pressure-differential, heated-wire, and Pitot tube pneumotachometers are used to measure flow and volume

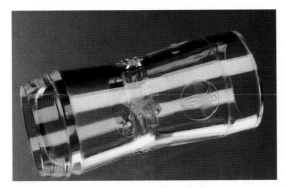

FIGURE 10-12 Pitot Tube Flow Sensor. A series of small tubes is mounted on struts in the flow tube. The tubes are connected to very sensitive pressure transducers (not shown). Using a series of transducers allows a wide range of flows to be accurately measured. Pitot tubes are mounted with struts facing both directions so that inspiratory and expiratory flow can be detected. *(Courtesy Medical Graphics, Inc., St. Paul, Minn.)*

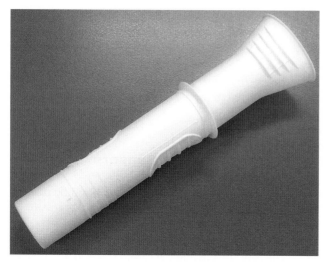

FIGURE 10-13   Ultrasonic Flow-Sensor Tube. A tube with membranous ports on either side permits high-frequency sound waves to be passed through the stream of gas. The ports are angled so that the sound waves speed up or slow down depending on the direction of gas flow. By measuring the transit time of the sound pulses compared to conditions of no flow, flow can be accurately measured. This method allows an inexpensive disposable tube to be used and prevents contamination of the ultrasonic transducers themselves. *(Courtesy ndd Medical Technologies, Inc., Andover, Mass.)*

in body plethysmographs, exercise testing systems, and metabolic carts. Because flow sensors require electronic circuitry to integrate flow or sum volume pulses, flow-based spirometers are microprocessor controlled. Some flow-sensing spirometers provide their analog signal (flow, volume, or both) to a strip chart or X-Y recorder. However, most flow sensors are integrated into a spirometer system and use computer-generated graphics to produce volume-time or flow-volume tracings.

Most flow-based spirometers can be easily cleaned and disinfected. Some flow sensors can be immersed in a disinfectant without disassembly. As noted, many systems use inexpensive, disposable sensors that can be discarded after one use. The use of in-line bacteria filters to prevent contamination of flow-based spirometers may result in changes in the operating characteristics of the spirometer. Any resistance to airflow through the filter will be added to the resistance of the spirometer. For this reason, the spirometer may need to be calibrated with the filter in place. Although the resistance offered by most filters is low, it may change with use. This may occur if water vapor from expired gas condenses on the filter media. Use of barrier filters does not eliminate the need for routine decontamination of spirometers.

Most types of the flow sensors produce a signal that is not linear across a wide range of flows. Some systems use two separate flow sensors (or variable orifices) to accommodate both low and high flows. Better accuracy can be obtained for flow and volume by matching the flow range of the sensor to the physiologic signal. Most flow-based spirometers "linearize" the flow signal electronically or by means of software corrections. In many systems, a simple "look-up table" is stored in the computer. The flow signal is continuously checked against the table and corrected. By combining a calibration factor (see Chapter 11) with the look-up table corrections, very accurate flow and integrated volume measurements are possible. Flows and volumes are corrected before variables such as FEV_1 are measured.

Turbine, pressure-differential, heated-wire, and Pitot tube flow-sensing spirometers are affected by the composition of the gas being measured. Changes in gas density or viscosity require correction of the transducer signal to obtain accurate flows and volumes. In most systems, these corrections are performed by computer software with a stored table. A flow-sensing spirometer may be calibrated with air but then used to measure mixtures containing helium, neon, oxygen, or other test gases. Some gases cause a linear shift in flow proportional to their concentrations. Corrections are usually made by applying a simple multiplier to the signal.

The accuracy of flow-based spirometers depends on the electronics, software, or both that process the flow signal. Pulmonary function variables measured on a time base (e.g., FEV_1 or FEV_6) require precise timing and accurate flow measurement. Detection of the start or end of the test is critical in flow-based spirometers. Timing is usually triggered by a minimum flow or pressure change. Signal integration begins when flow reaches a threshold limit, usually 0.1–0.2 L/sec. Spirometers that initiate timing in response to volume pulses usually have a similar threshold that must be achieved to begin recording. Contamination of resistive elements, thermistors, or Pitot tubes by moisture or other debris can alter the flow-sensing characteristics of the transducer and interfere with the spirometer's ability to detect the start or end of test. Similar problems can occur when flow drops to very low levels near the end of a forced expiration, causing measurement of flow (and volume) to be terminated prematurely. As a result, the volume (e.g., FVC or VC) may be underestimated.

Problems related to electronic "drift" require flow sensors to be "zeroed" frequently. Zeroing is simply a one-point calibration in which the output of the transducer is set to zero under a condition of no flow. Many systems "zero" the flow signal immediately before a measurement. Zeroing corrects for much of the electronic drift that occurs. A true zero requires no flow through the flow sensor. Thus the flow sensor must be held still or occluded during the zero maneuvers. Most flow-based systems use a 3-L syringe for calibration. By calibrating with a known volume signal, the accuracy of the flow sensor and the integrator can be checked with one input. Calibration and quality-control techniques for volume-displacement and flow-sensing spirometers are included in Chapter 11.

Many flow-sensing spirometers interface directly with personal computers (Figure 10-14), typically a laptop computer. Some spirometers use an interface card that plugs directly into a personal computer (PC). With the appropriate software installed on the PC, spirometry can be performed. Other spirometers place the necessary electronic components in the flow sensor head or in an external adapter. This implementation allows the flow sensor to be connected to a serial port or USB (universal serial bus) port, both of which are standard on most computers. The pressure transducer and electronics for flow-based spirometry can also be mounted on a removable card. These cards allow spirometry to be performed with handheld computers, laptop computers, or personal digital assistants (PDAs). Many flow-based spirometers use dedicated microprocessors (Figure 10-15). Some of these are very compact (Figure 10-16) so that the entire device is not much larger than a calculator. These designs allow the units to be handheld and portable.

Many portable spirometers use disposable flow sensors. Disposable sensors can provide accurate measurements if they are manufactured according to rigid specifications. Disposable flow sensors are usually precalibrated at the time of manufacture. Some manufacturers include calibration codes (or bar codes) on the sensor to be used in conjunction with the spirometer software. Ideally, each spirometer should provide a means for calibration using a 3-L syringe. As a minimum, the software in portable spirometers should allow verification of volumes, even if precalibrated flow sensors are used.

Portable (Office) Spirometers

The widespread availability of microprocessors has resulted in a large number of small, portable spirometers based on various flow-sensing principles. These spirometers can be separated into two general categories: (1) those that interface with a laptop or desktop computer and (2) stand-alone devices that incorporate a dedicated microprocessor. In both cases, these devices may be referred to as portable or **office spirometers.**

PF TIP

Most office spirometers include software features to help the user obtain high-quality data. These features include prompts to direct the patient's efforts, along with messages regarding the quality of data obtained. These quality indicators are usually based on ATS/ERS recommendations for spirometry. Many spirometers also include a grading system to assess the overall acceptability and repeatability of the patient's efforts.

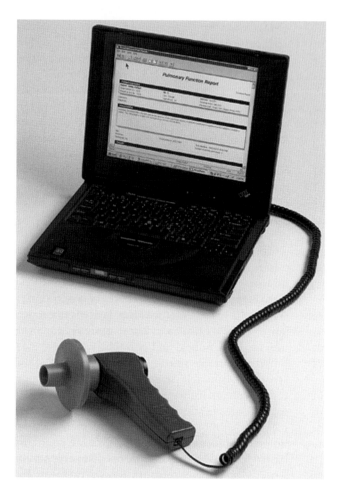

FIGURE 10-14   Flow-Sensing Spirometer Interfaced to a Laptop Computer. A pressure-differential pneumotachometer with its interface electronics connects to a laptop personal computer (PC). The laptop computer runs software that provides calculations, data storage, and printing of results. *(Courtesy Ferraris Respiratory, Inc., Louisville, Colo.)*

Interfacing a flow sensor to a PC or laptop computer makes spirometry available in a variety of clinical settings. Handheld or PC-based systems provide a relatively inexpensive way to perform spirometry, before and after bronchodilator studies, and even bronchial challenges. Increasingly sophisticated software allows spirometric data to be stored, manipulated, and displayed graphically. In spite of the availability of small, accurate spirometers, spirometry is still not widely used in primary care. Because spirometry is effort dependent, poorly performed maneuvers can result in misclassification (i.e., obstruction versus restriction versus normal). The choice of inappropriate reference equations and incorrect interpretation of results further limits the usefulness of spirometry.

The National Lung Health Education Program (NLHEP) provides recommendations for office spirometers to be used in primary care settings (Box 10-1). The goal of these recommendations is to standardize spirometry to promote early detection of chronic obstructive pulmonary disease (COPD). Office spirometers should be simple (see Figure 10-16) and designed to measure three important parameters: FEV_1, FEV_6, and the FEV_1/FEV_6 ratio. To provide accurate measurements, office spirometers should display automated messages describing the acceptability and repeatability of efforts. Automated interpretation of simple spirometry can be performed if test quality is acceptable and appropriate reference values are used. Display or printouts of spirograms are optional. Office spirometers

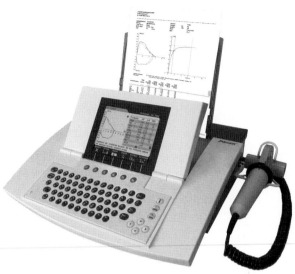

FIGURE 10-15 Portable Spirometer Using a Dedicated Microprocessor. A pneumotachometer-based portable spirometer that uses a dedicated microprocessor for data acquisition and processing. This system includes a display and a printer for hard copy results. *(Courtesy VIASYS Healthcare, Yorba Linda, Calif.)*

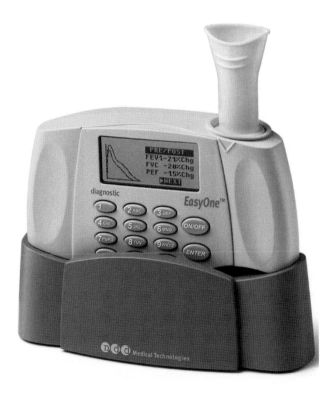

FIGURE 10-16 Handheld "Office" Spirometer. A small handheld spirometer based on the ultrasonic flow sensor principle. This type of device is designed for office screening to detect airway obstruction by measuring FEV_1, FEV_6, and the FEV_1/FEV_6 ratio according to the recommendations of the National Lung Health Education Program (NLHEP, see text). *(Courtesy ndd Medical Technologies, Inc., Andover, Mass.)*

- Office spirometers must meet or exceed current ATS/ERS minimum standards.
- Office spirometers should only report FEV_1, FEV_6, and FEV_1/FEV_6 ratio.
- Measurement end-of-test should be terminated at 6 seconds (FEV_6).
- NHANES III reference set should be used for determining lower limits of normal (LLN).
- Automated maneuver acceptability/repeatability messages should be displayed and reported.
- Airway obstruction is determined when FEV_1/FEV_6 and FEV_1 are below respective LLNs.
- Display/printout of spirograms and F-V curves is optional.
- Office spirometers should include easy-to-understand educational materials.
- Simple means of checking calibration should be included.

Adapted from Ferguson GT, Enright PL, Buist AS, et al: Office spirometry for lung health assessment in adults; a consensus statement from the National Lung Health Education Program, *Chest* 2000; 117:1146-1161.

should meet the accuracy recommendations of the ATS/ERS (see Chapter 11).

PEAK FLOW METERS

PEF can be measured easily with most spirometers, particularly the flow-sensing types. Many devices are available that measure PEF exclusively. PEF has become a recognized means of monitoring patients who have asthma. By incorporating a simple measurement into an inexpensive package, portable peak flow meters allow monitoring of airway status in a variety of settings.

Most **peak flow meters** use similar designs. The patient expires forcefully through a resistor or flow tube that has a movable indicator attached (Figure 10-17). An orifice provides the resistance in most devices. The movable indicator is deflected in proportion to the velocity of air flowing through the device. PEF is then read directly from a calibrated scale. Because these devices are nonlinear, different flow ranges are usually available. High-range peak

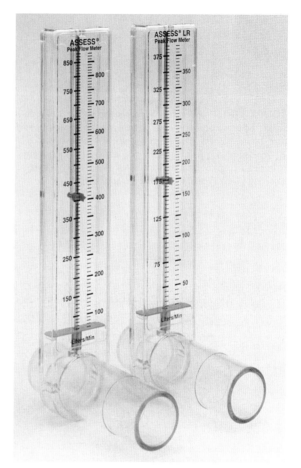

FIGURE 10-17 **Portable Peak Flow Meters.** Portable peak flow meters for measuring peak expiratory flow (PEF) outside of the pulmonary function laboratory. The patient exhales forcefully through the mouthpiece at the bottom. Pressure generated by the flow of gas deflects the movable indicator up the scale. Two flow ranges are available, for normal and reduced peak flows. *(Courtesy Respironics, Inc., Murrysville, Pa.)*

flow meters typically measure flows as high as 850 L/min. Low-range meters measure up to 400 L/min (Table 10-1). Low-range peak flow meters are useful for small children or for patients who have marked obstruction.

The absolute accuracy of portable peak flow meters is less important than their precision (i.e., repeatability of measurements). Within-instrument variability should be less than 5% or 0.15 L/sec (10 L/min), whichever is greater. Between-instrument

TABLE 10-1		
Peak Flow Meter Recommended Ranges		
	Children	Adults
National Asthma Education Program	100–400 L/min ± 10%	100–700 L/min ± 10%
American Thoracic Society (1994)	60–400 L/min ± 10% or 20 L/min, whichever is greater	100–850 L/min ± 10% or 20 L/min, whichever is greater

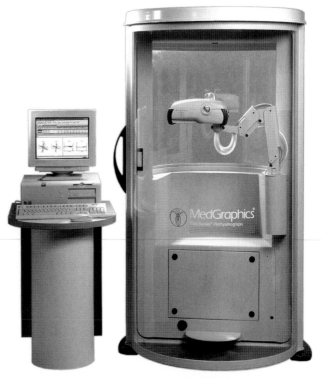

FIGURE 10-18 **Body Plethysmograph.** A modern plethysmograph setup, with a highly transparent box, self-contained calibration equipment, and computerized data reduction and display. *(Courtesy Medical Graphics, Inc., St. Paul, Minn.)*

variability should be less than 10% or 0.3 L/sec (20 L/min), whichever is greater. These devices are intended to provide serial measurements of peak flow as a guide to treatment. Patients who are carefully instructed should be able to reproduce their peak flow measurements within 0.67 L/sec (40 L/min). However, asthmatics may have difficulty repeating their PEF, particularly during exacerbations. PEF meters must be easy to use and easy to read. Scale divisions of 5 L/min for low-range devices and 10 L/min for high-range devices allow small changes in PEF to be detected. The scale should be calibrated to read flow in BTPS units. Corrections for altitude should be included because PEF meters tend to underestimate flow as altitude increases (i.e., approximately 7% per 100 mm Hg change in barometric pressure).

Although the simple design of portable peak flow meters allows them to be used repeatedly, moisture or other debris can cause sticking of the movable parts. This can be problematic because it may suggest that the patient's asthma has worsened. Some instruments can be cleaned, but may need to be replaced periodically. Because portable peak flow meters may have a limited life span, variability between same-model instruments should be 10% or 20 L/min as noted. This allows the patient to continue monitoring with a new device. Clear instructions on how to use and maintain the peak flow meter should come with each device. Most peak flow meters comply with the National Asthma Education Program's "color zone" scheme for identifying clinically significant changes (see Chapter 2).

BODY PLETHYSMOGRAPHS

Body plethysmographs (Figure 10-18) are used in many pulmonary function laboratories. Body plethysmographs are also called body boxes. Two types of plethysmographs are available: the constant-volume, variable-pressure plethysmograph and the flow or variable-volume plethysmograph. These are sometimes called the **pressure plethysmograph** and **flow plethysmograph**, respectively. Pressure-type plethysmographs are more commonly used than flow types. Both designs are used to measure thoracic gas volume (V_{TG}) (see Chapter 3) and airway resistance (Raw) and its derivatives (see Chapter 2). Both types of box use some type of pneumotachometer to measure flow, as well as a mouth pressure transducer with a shutter to measure alveolar pressure. They differ in the method used to measure volume change in the box, and hence in the lungs.

Pressure Plethysmographs

The pressure plethysmograph is based on an adaptation of Boyle's law (see Appendix E). Volume changes in a sealed box are inversely related to pressure changes if temperature is constant. A sensitive pressure transducer monitors box pressure changes. Pressure change is related to volume change by calibration (see Chapter 11 for calibration techniques). Pressure changes result from compression and decompression of gas within both the patient's chest and the box. If box temperature remains constant, each unit of pressure change equals a specific volume change. For example, a volume change of 15 ml may result in a pressure change of 1 cm H_2O. After the box has been calibrated empty, the calibration factor changes slightly when a patient enters the plethysmograph. This change is easily corrected using an estimate of the volume displaced by the patient (based on the patient's weight).

The pressure plethysmograph must be essentially leak free. Most pressure boxes use a solenoid to vent the box and maintain thermal equilibrium. In some implementations, the vent remains open until the pressure measurement begins, so that the box is continually being vented. Making V_{TG} and Raw measurements with the patient panting reduces unwanted pressure changes caused by thermal drift, leaks, or background noise. Some pressure plethysmograph systems use a controlled leak to facilitate thermal equilibrium. The leak allows gas to escape as the interior of the box warms but does not interfere with high-frequency changes such as those that occur with panting. Similarly, connecting the atmospheric side of the box pressure transducer to a container within the box dampens the effects of thermal drift. Both methods reduce the effect of temperature changes within the box and maintain good frequency response. Pressure plethysmographs are best suited to maneuvers that measure small volume changes (i.e., 100 ml or less). Measurements of VC or FVC can usually be made only with the door open or the box adequately vented to the atmosphere.

Flow Plethysmographs

The flow plethysmograph uses a flow transducer in the box wall to measure volume changes in the box. Gas in the box is compressed or decompressed, causing flow through the opening in the box wall. Flow through the wall is integrated, corrections are applied, and volume change is recorded as the sum of the volume passing through the wall and the volume compressed. In one implementation, the patient breathes through a pneumotachometer connected to the room (transmural breathing). The transmural pneumotachometer allows larger gas volumes (i.e., the VC or flow-volume curves) to be measured while the patient is enclosed in the plethysmograph. The transmural flow is redirected to the plethysmograph for Raw measurements so that the ratio of flow to box volume can be plotted. For V_{TG} measurements, the flow transducer in the plethysmograph wall is occluded so that the device works like a pressure box. The flow-type plethysmograph requires that the pressure, volume, and flow signals be measured in phase. Although thermal changes must be accounted for, the flow plethysmograph does not need to be rigorously airtight. The flow box's primary advantage is the ability to measure flows at absolute lung volumes (i.e., corrected for gas compression).

In both types of plethysmograph, a flow sensor (i.e., pneumotachometer) is needed to measure airflow at the mouth (Figure 10-19). Flow measurement is required to compute Raw. The flow signal is also used to determine end-expiration for shutter closure in V_{TG} measurements. The pneumotachometer must be linear across the range of flows encountered in spontaneous breathing and panting (±2 L/sec) and should meet all ATS/ERS requirements for spirometers (e.g., range, accuracy, frequency response) for measurement of VC and/or

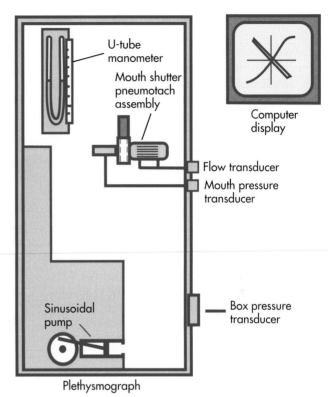

FIGURE 10-19   Diagram of a Pressure Plethysmograph. A pneumotachometer (flow sensor) with an automatic shutter mechanism is mounted at a height that is comfortable for a patient sitting in the plethysmograph. Pressure transducers for flow, mouth pressure, and box pressure provide signals that are digitized and processed by a computer. A sinusoidal pump allows calibration of the box pressure signal; a small, known volume change can be repeatedly generated. A pressure manometer (U-tube) or similar device is used to calibrate the mouth pressure transducer. A 3-L syringe is used to calibrate the pneumotachometer. Flow plethysmographs are arranged similarly, with an additional pneumotachometer in the wall of the box so that volume changes in the box are measured as gas flows through wall (see text).

FVC. Heated Fleisch or Silverman types of pressure-differential pneumotachometers are often used in the plethysmograph. Pitot tube or heated-wire flow transducers can also be used.

A mouth pressure transducer is normally coupled to a shutter mechanism. The shutter can be an electric solenoid, a scissors-type valve, or a balloon valve. The mouth pressure transducer records pressures in the range of -20 to $+20$ cm H_2O when the airway is occluded but should be able to measure pressures of more than ±50 cm H_2O, with a flat frequency response greater than 8 Hz. Some systems require the technologist to close the shutter by remote control at end-expiration. This may be accomplished by observing the tidal breathing maneuver on a display and actuating the shutter at end-expiration. However, most systems automatically close the shutter at a preselected point in the breathing cycle. The technologist initiates a sequence in which the computer monitors flow and closes the shutter when expiratory flow becomes

zero. Automated shutters allow the airway to be occluded for a fixed length of time or for a specified number of panting breaths.

Plethysmograph or box pressure is recorded by a sensitive pressure transducer connected to the box chamber. This transducer needs to be able to accurately measure pressure changes as small as ±0.2 cm H_2O with a flat frequency response that accommodates the panting rates that are commonly encountered (e.g., >8 Hz). The box pressure transducer should have a range that can accommodate the pressures typically encountered because of thermal drift, tidal breathing, and so forth. If a slow leak is incorporated into the box to promote thermal stability, it should have a time constant of approximately 10 seconds.

Recording of plethysmographic maneuvers is usually performed by a computer. Breathing efforts are displayed in real time, allowing the technologist to elicit proper maneuvers from the patient. The **real-time display** assists in ensuring that panting maneuvers are performed correctly; some systems display prompts or flags so that the patient can be coached to pant at the correct frequency. The computer then stores the data and performs the necessary calculations to compute thoracic gas volume and airway resistance. Because the computer can track volume changes in the body box, V_{TG} and airway resistance are sometimes measured from the same maneuver. The patient breathes normally to establish the end-expiratory level and then pants. When an appropriate pattern of panting is obtained (e.g., correct frequency and volume), the shutter closes at end-expiration and the thoracic gas volume is measured. The volume change between the established end-expiratory level and the point at which the shutter was closed is then used to "correct" the measured V_{TG} so that it equals the patient's FRC. If V_{TG} is measured at lung volumes other than FRC, the alveolar pressure should also be corrected for any difference from ambient pressure (i.e., P_B).

Computerized plethysmographs compute a "best-fit" line to determine the slope (i.e., tangent) for both the open-shutter (flow versus box pressure) and closed-shutter (mouth pressure versus box pressure) panting maneuvers. The technologist can also manipulate the tangent by means of the computer keyboard or mouse. This allows some degree of correction for efforts in which the patient panted incorrectly or noise was introduced into the recorded signal. Plethysmography software provides lung volume and airway resistance data immediately after completion of the maneuver. This aids in selecting acceptable maneuvers to report. The test can also be repeated as required when questionable values are obtained. Using computer-displayed panting frequency, the technologist can coach the patient to maintain a desired rate.

Most plethysmographs include the necessary signal-generating devices to perform physical calibration (see Chapter 11). A pressure manometer (or fluid filled U-tube) may be mounted on the box for calibration of the mouth pressure transducer. Some systems provide a fixed pressure signal for mouth pressure calibration. A small syringe (30–50 ml) driven by an electric motor allows calibration of the box pressure transducer. The motorized syringe usually produces a sine-wave flow with frequency

that can be varied. This allows checking of box pressure calibration at various frequencies. Most computerized plethysmographs use a standard 3-L syringe to calibrate the pneumotachometer or flow sensor. However, a flow generator and rotameter (i.e., a flowmeter) may be included for flow calibration. Computerized plethysmograph systems provide automated calibration of transducers. The output of the transducer (i.e., its amplified signal) is measured, and the computer generates a software correction factor. This correction is then applied to every measurement made with the transducer. Some manufacturers also supply quality control (QC) devices such as an isothermal lung analog (see Chapter 11). These devices provide QC to verify calibration of transducers and appropriateness of software correction factors.

PF TIP

Most patients can perform plethysmographic measurements acceptably, even if they experience some claustrophobia. Modern body plethysmographs use Plexiglas or similar transparent material so that the subject feels less confined. Plethysmographic measurements can usually be made quickly, reducing the length of time spent with the door closed. Plethysmography may not be practical for some patients, such as those who have orthopedic impairments.

The ease with which a patient can enter the plethysmograph and perform the required maneuvers is an important feature. Some patients may experience claustrophobia when inside the plethysmograph. Older boxes used a plywood cabinet to provide the necessary rigidity so that pressure changes were not attenuated. Boxes made of durable plastics are largely transparent and less confining for the patient (see Figure 10-18) while maintaining the necessary rigidity. Most plethysmographs contain 500–700 L of volume and can accommodate even large patients. Careful design allows the patient to easily enter the box. Some plethysmographs are large enough to accommodate patients in wheelchairs. Others use a clamshell design so that the patient may be seated and the box closed around him or her. Most plethysmographs provide an internal switch or mechanism that allows patients to open the box from inside if they become uncomfortable.

Equally important is a communication system that allows both voice and visual contact with the patient. Panting against a closed shutter may be difficult for some individuals, and continuous coaching is often necessary to elicit valid maneuvers. An intercom system that provides continuous two-way communication is essential.

BREATHING VALVES

Various types of valves are commonly used for pulmonary function tests, particularly for dilutional lung volume, DLCO, and exercise tests. These valves direct inspired or expired gas through the spirometer or provide a means of sampling for gas analysis.

Free Breathing and Demand Valves

The simplest type of valve allows the patient to be switched from breathing room air to breathing gas contained in a spirometer or special breathing circuit. **Free breathing valves** are often used in both open-circuit and closed-circuit FRC determinations. The free breathing valve is designed so that the patient can be "switched in" to the system either manually or by computer controls at a specific point in the breathing cycle.

The typical free breathing valve consists of a body with two or more ports. A drum in the valve body rotates to connect different combinations of ports. Because these valves are used mainly for tidal breathing or slow vital capacity (SVC) maneuvers, resistance to flow is usually not critical. Most have ports with diameters of 1.5–3 cm. For studies involving gas analysis, such as FRC determination, the valve must be free of leaks. The dead space of valves used in measurements of FRC should be less than 100 ml.

Some systems use a "breathing manifold" that consists of multiple ports and valves all connected to the patient mouthpiece. The different ports allow inspired or expired gas to be directed to the spirometer or gas-sampling devices. The valves may be electric or gas-powered **solenoids**, balloon valves that inflate with compressed air, or scissors-type valves that pinch flexible tubing to control flow. Under computer control, different combinations of valves and ports are opened and closed. This type of manifold permits spirometry, dilutional lung volumes, and DLCO tests to be performed with the same breathing circuit. A similar manifold is used in many body plethysmograph systems to permit measurement of V_{TG} and Raw along with DLCO.

Infection control of free breathing valves and multiple-port manifolds involves disassembly, cleaning, and disinfection or sterilization. Because cleaning between patients may not be practical, in-line filters may be used to prevent contamination of these devices.

PF TIP

The most common problem encountered in breathing circuits that use valves is failure of the valves to operate correctly. Balloon-type valves often develop leaks. Demand valves sometimes stick or require excessive inspiratory pressure to open. Solenoid-type valves have O-rings that must be properly lubricated to prevent leaks. Directional valves (one-way and two-way) may have leaflets that stick or have been assembled incorrectly.

Demand valves (also sometimes referred to as demand-flow regulators) are used in many circuits in which the patient inspires a test gas (e.g., DLCO, FRC_{N2}). The primary considerations for demand valves are the pressure required to trigger gas flow and the adequacy of flow once the valve opens. Most demand valves consist of a valve body that contains a sensitive diaphragm. The diaphragm moves in response to the patient's inspiratory effort, opening the valve and allowing gas to flow from a high-pressure source. Maximal flow is controlled by the valve and usually depends on the driving pressure (typically 20–50 psi). Demand valves are often adjustable, allowing the sensitivity to be set so that minimal pressure is needed to trigger gas flow. Problems typically encountered with demand valves include inadequate source pressure (turned off or not connected) and sticking or incorrectly adjusted diaphragms. Demand valves used in DLCO circuits should be able to deliver 6 L/sec flow with less than 10 cm H_2O pressure.

Directional Valves

Directional (one-way and two-way) valves are used in many types of breathing circuits. The simplest type consists of a flap or diaphragm that opens in only one direction. The valve is then mounted in a rigid tube that can be inserted in a breathing circuit. Because gas is only permitted to flow in one direction, these valves are called one-way valves.

Another common valve design is that used to separate inspired from expired gas, often called a two-way nonrebreathing valve. This type of directional valve consists of a T-shaped body with three ports and two separate diaphragms (Figure 10-20). The diaphragms allow gas to flow in only one direction. The patient connection is between the diaphragms, effectively separating inspired from expired gas. Two-way nonrebreathing valves are used in exercise testing, metabolic studies, or any procedure requiring collection, measurement, or analysis of exhaled gas. The valve body may contain a tap for connection of gas sample tubing. This tap is typically placed between the diaphragms so that both inspired and expired gas can be sampled.

Two factors must be considered in the selection of appropriate directional valves: dead space volume and flow resistance. For one-way valves, only flow resistance is a concern. In two-way nonrebreathing valves, dead space is the volume contained between the two diaphragms along with the volume of any connectors (e.g., a mouthpiece). Most manufacturers supply information about the dead space of individual valves. Sometimes the dead space value is printed on the valve body. Unknown dead space

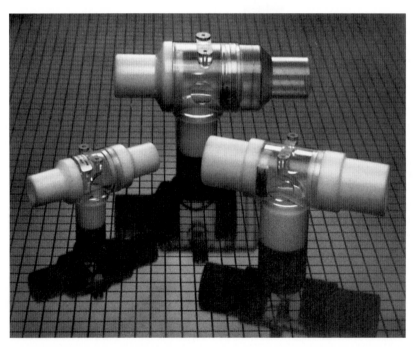

FIGURE 10-20 Two-way Nonrebreathing Valves. Three differently sized valves used for measurement of expired gas are shown. Each valve consists of a T-shaped body containing two diaphragms that separate inspired and expired gas. The smaller valves have less dead space but higher resistance to flow; the large valve has low flow resistance but more dead space. The small and medium valves are used for studies in which low flows are encountered, such as metabolic measurements. The large valve is appropriate for high flow rates such as those occurring during maximal exercise testing. *(Courtesy Hans Rudolph, Inc., Kansas City, Mo.)*

can be determined by blocking two of the three ports and measuring the water volume required to fill the dead space portion of the valve.

Low dead space valves (<50 ml) may be required for children or if the patient already has increased dead space, particularly if only tidal breathing is being assessed. Valves with large-bore ports and low-resistance diaphragms usually have larger dead space volumes. For exercise testing, large-bore nonrebreathing valves are used to minimize resistance at high flows. These valves may have a dead space volume of 100–200 ml. Selection of an appropriate-sized nonrebreathing valve should be based on the maximal flow anticipated during the test. For example, a maximal exercise test for a healthy adult patient may include flows greater than 100 L/min. A large-bore valve would be selected to accommodate the high flow. Valve dead space would be less of a concern because large tidal volumes are necessary to generate the increased flow. Mechanical (i.e., valve) dead space must be accurately determined for use in calculations involving gas analysis, such as physiologic dead space measurements.

Low resistance to flow is also a critical characteristic of one-way and two-way valves. Resistance to flow through most valves is nonlinear and depends on the cross-sectional area of valve leaflets or diaphragms (Figure 10-21). Resistance is usually not critical for tests in which flows of less than 1 L/sec occur. Small-bore (15–22 mm) directional valves can be selected based on an appropriate dead space volume. Most small-bore nonrebreathing valves have a resistance in the range of 1–2 cm H_2O/L/sec at flows of up to 1 L/sec (60 L/min). However, if the patient breathes through the valve for long intervals, even a small resistance may result in respiratory muscle fatigue and changes in the ventilatory pattern. Applications such as exercise testing typically involve increased flows. Large-bore two-way valves are indicated when flows greater than 1 L/sec (60 L/min) can be expected to develop. Pressures less than 3 cm H_2O can be maintained even at flows of 5 L/sec (300 L/min) with large-bore valves. Saliva and moisture may collect in valves during prolonged tests (e.g., exercise or eucapnic hyperventilation). Valves with "saliva traps" may be needed for these procedures. If a valve is used in a spirometry circuit, it must have very low resistance to meet the ATS/ERS recommendation of less than 1.5 cm H_2O/L/sec at flows of 12 L/sec. Valves used in a

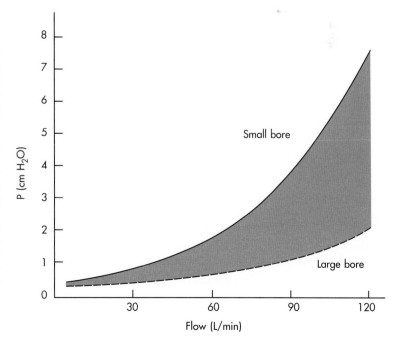

FIGURE 10-21 Breathing Valve Resistance. A graph plotting pressure developed across two different-sized valves in relation to gas flow through the valves. For small-bore valves (see Figure 10-20), pressures of less than 1 cm H_2O are generated up to approximately 60 L/min (1 L/sec). Large-bore valves have less resistance (pressure per unit of flow) and are typically used for studies in which the patient has high flow rates. Other factors affecting resistance include the design and material used for the diaphragms in the valve and whether the diaphragms move freely. Resistance increases nonlinearly in all types of valves; high resistance can occur even in large-bore valves at very high flows.

DLCO circuit should produce a total resistance of less than 1.5 cm H_2O/L/sec at flows of 6 L/sec.

Any valve can cause increased resistance if not properly maintained. Rubber, plastic, or silicon leaflets and diaphragms can stick or become rigid with age. Valves should be disassembled and cleaned after each use according to the manufacturer's directions and allowed to dry thoroughly before reassembly. Care must be taken when reassembling valves to ensure that all diaphragms are oriented properly. Valves should be visually inspected to make sure that diaphragms are mounted correctly and that they open and close properly before being used.

Gas-Sampling Valves

Specialized valves (valve manifolds) may be used to sample gas during tests such as the single-breath DLCO. These valves open and close during the breathing maneuver to allow the patient to inspire test gas and expire to a gas collection device. The same mechanisms are often used to occlude the airway near the patient's mouth for breath-holding maneuvers or to measure mouth pressure. Many of these valves use electrically or pneumatically powered solenoids to direct flow to a spirometer or sample collection device. Other systems employ scissors valves to pinch compressible tubing. The primary concern with gas-sampling valves is smooth operation with appropriate direction of the gas to be sampled. Electrically activated solenoids may deteriorate with age, particularly if exposed to high humidity conditions (e.g., expired air). Replacement of O-rings or similar types of seals may be necessary to ensure uncontaminated gas samples. Some sampling valves use balloons that inflate to block or direct the flow of gas. These balloons require periodic replacement because small leaks can prevent the balloon from occluding flow. When this occurs, gas may not be directed to the appropriate device, or the gas itself may be contaminated. Scissors-type valves offer an advantage in that the compressible tubing can be changed easily between patients.

Infection control for sampling valves usually requires disassembly and cleaning. Some complex valve manifolds may be difficult or impossible to disassemble. In such devices, an in-line filter may be needed to avoid cross-contamination.

PULMONARY GAS ANALYZERS

Various types of gas analyzers are used in pulmonary function testing. O_2 and CO_2 analyzers are used for metabolic studies and exercise testing. Helium analysis is used for closed-circuit functional residual capacity (FRC) determinations and for several types of DLCO tests. N_2 analysis is used in the open-circuit FRC method. CO measurements are integral to all of the diffusion capacity methods currently used. Analyses of neon, argon, methane, and acetylene are used in specialized tests for diffusion, lung volume measurements, and cardiac output determination. NO (nitric oxide) analyzers are used to assess airway inflammation in the diagnosis and treatment of asthma.

How rapidly a gas analyzer can detect and display a change in gas concentration is termed **response time**. Response time is commonly measured in seconds or milliseconds (thousandths of a second). Manufacturers of gas analyzers list response time as the interval required for an analyzer to measure some fraction of a given step change in gas concentration. For example, an O_2 analyzer might require 2 seconds to respond to an increase in O_2 concentration from 21% – 100%. The response time may be listed as the time required for 90% of the total change to be detected. Response time of an analyzer often depends on the size of the step change in gas concentration. A related factor in gas analysis is transport time. **Transport time** is how long it takes to move the gas from the sample site to the analyzer itself. How rapidly a gas (e.g., O_2) can be analyzed depends on both the response time and the transport time of the instrument. A third consideration is phase delay (or phase shift) in the gas analyzer signal. When the gas analyzer signal is integrated with a flow signal, the two signals may be out of phase; that is, the flow signal may be considered instantaneous while the gas analyzer signal lags slightly behind (because of transport and response time). The two signals can be aligned by measuring the phase delay (or shift) and offsetting one of the signals; this is usually done in software. In breath-by-breath gas analysis, response time, transport time, and phase delay are critical, and rapidly responding analyzers are required. Tests such as the DLCO or FRC measurement by He dilution require very accurate gas analysis, but rapid response is not necessary.

Oxygen Analyzers

Oxygen analysis can be performed by several different methods. Table 10-2 lists some types of O_2 analyzers available. Two types are used for rapid analysis of O_2 such as breath-by-breath exercise tests: the **polarographic electrode** and **zirconium fuel cell**. The other O_2 analyzers listed are used for specialized applications, including patient monitoring.

Polarographic Electrodes

The polarographic electrode is similar to the blood gas O_2 electrode (see the section on blood gas analyzers, oximeters, and related devices). For gas analysis, a platinum cathode is used without a membrane covering the tip. A gas pump draws the sample past the polarized electrode at a constant flow. Oxygen is reduced in proportion to its partial pressure. The electrode is calibrated by exposing it to known fractional concentrations of O_2 at a known barometric pressure. Response times of approximately 200 msec

can be attained by using special electronic circuitry. Rapid response allows continuous analysis for breath-by-breath measurements. Contamination of the electrode can degrade its response time and cause difficulty with calibration.

Zirconium Fuel Cells

An electrode is formed by coating a zirconium element with platinum. The zirconium, when heated to 700°–800°C, acts as a solid electrolyte between the platinum coating on either side. When the two sides of the electrode are exposed to different partial pressures of O_2, gas traverses the electrode, creating a voltage proportional to the difference in concentrations. Sample gas is drawn past the element at a constant low flow. This allows rapid, continuous analysis without altering the temperature of the electrode. Electrode temperature must be held constant, so the electrode requires adequate insulation. A warm-up period of 10–30 minutes is typically required to reach thermal equilibrium at the elevated temperature. Response times of less than 200 msec are possible with the zirconium fuel cell, making it useful for breath-by-breath measurements.

The zirconium fuel cell and the polarographic electrode each measure the partial pressure of oxygen. Pressure changes in the sampling circuit can affect the concentration measurement. Such pressure changes can be caused by gas flow in a breathing circuit or by positive pressure in a

TABLE 10-2		
Oxygen Analyzers		
Type	Applications	Advantages/Disadvantages
Paramagnetic	Monitoring	Discrete sampling only
Polarographic electrode	Monitoring, exercise testing, metabolic studies	Discrete or continuous sampling; requires special electronic circuitry for fast response (200 msec)
Galvanic cell (fuel cell)	Monitoring	Continuous sampling; similar to polarographic but does not require polarizing voltage
Zirconium cell	Breath-by-breath exercise and metabolic studies	Heated (650°–800°C) electrochemical sensor; fast response useful for continuous sampling; thermal stabilization required
Gas chromatograph	Exercise testing, monitoring, metabolic measurements	Discrete sampling; response time ~30 sec; very accurate; multiple gas analysis

mechanical ventilator circuit. The presence of water vapor in the sample affects both electrodes similarly. Oxygen concentration is measured accurately but is diluted in proportion to the water vapor pressure present in the sample. Zirconium fuel cells eventually degrade in relation to the volume of O_2 analyzed. The cell may be refreshed by passing a current through it, thus reversing the oxygen uptake process.

Infrared Absorption (CO_2, CO) Analyzers

Several types of respiratory gas analyzers are based on absorption of infrared radiation to measure gas concentrations. Infrared absorption is used in CO analyzers for DLCO tests. Infrared CO_2 analyzers are used for exercise testing, metabolic studies, and bedside monitoring (capnography) in critical care (Figure 10-22).

Certain gases (e.g., CO_2 and CO) absorb infrared radiation. A common type of infrared analyzer uses two beams of infrared radiation directed through parallel cells. One cell contains sample gas, while the other contains a reference gas. The two beams converge on a single infrared detector (Figure 10-23). A small motor rotates an interrupter or "chopper" between the infrared source and the cells. The chopper blades alternately interrupt the infrared radiation passing through the sample and reference cells. If the sample and reference gases have the same concentration, the radiation reaching the detector is constant. However, when a sample with

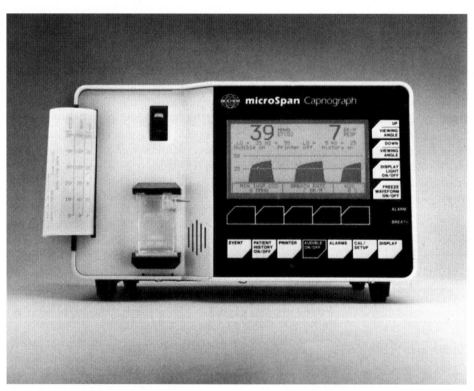

FIGURE 10-22 **Infrared CO_2 Monitor.** A microprocessor-controlled infrared CO_2 analyzer as used for critical care monitoring. A liquid crystal display (LCD) allows presentation of end-tidal CO_2 values, breathing rate, and CO_2 waveforms. This capnograph includes a printer and alarms, along with a water trap to remove condensation from the sample line. *(Courtesy BCI, Inc., Waukesha, Wis.)*

a different gas concentration is introduced, the radiation reaching the detector varies in a rhythmic fashion. This causes a vibration in the detector that is translated into a pulsatile signal proportional to the difference between the two beams.

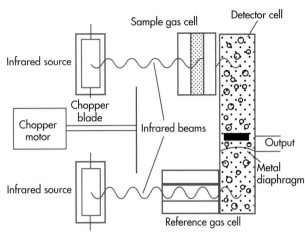

FIGURE 10-23 Infrared Absorption Gas Analyzer. Components of an infrared analyzer used to measure CO_2 are depicted. Infrared sources emit beams that pass through parallel cells. One cell contains a reference gas; the other contains a gas sample to be analyzed. A rotating blade "chops" the infrared beams in a rhythmic fashion. When both reference and sample cells contain the same gas, the radiation reaching each half of the detector cell is the same. When a gas sample is introduced, it absorbs some infrared radiation. Different amounts of radiation reach the two halves of the detector cell, causing the diaphragm separating the compartments of the detector to oscillate. This oscillation is transformed into a signal proportional to the difference in gas concentrations. The infrared analyzer is ideal for determining small changes in concentration in gas samples. *(From Beckman Instruments, Inc., Medical gas analyzer LB-2: operating instructions, FM-149997-301, Schiller Park, Ill.)*

Infrared analyzers can measure small changes in gas concentrations such as the difference between inspired and expired CO in DLCO tests. Infrared analyzers respond rapidly once the gas has been transported to the measuring chamber. Gas can be sampled either continuously or discretely with infrared analyzers. For continuous sampling, the gas flow must be constant. The analyzer must be calibrated using the same flow at which measurements are made. Pump settings and the sample line should not be altered after calibration. Water condensation or other debris in the sample line can significantly alter the flow and affect the accuracy of the measurement. Water vapor in the sample will dilute the gas being analyzed. Water vapor can be removed if response time is not critical. For rapid response times, as required for breath-by-breath analysis, the effects of water vapor can be corrected mathematically by assuming that expired gas is fully saturated, or by using semi-permeable tubing that equilibrates the sample with ambient saturation (see Gas-Conditioning Devices, this chapter).

Infrared analyzers used to measure CO (and in some cases tracer gas) during the DLCO test need to have a linear output because the calculation of DLCO commonly uses the ratio of CO to tracer gas (see Chapter 5). The analyzer should display nonlinearity of 0.5% or less of full scale across the range of gas concentrations typically used (~0.3% for CO). Although the output of the infrared detector may be nonlinear, it can be easily corrected electronically or by means of a look-up table in software. For measuring CO and tracer gases during DLCO tests, the analyzer needs to be stable (i.e., no drift) for at least as long as the test may last (typically 30 seconds). Because water vapor and CO_2 affect the measurement of CO, these gases need to be removed ("scrubbed") before reaching the infrared detector.

Manual of Pulmonary Function Testing

Common problems occurring with infrared analyzers involve the chopper motor, sample cell, and infrared detector. Motors turning the chopper blades may wear out or work intermittently. Some analyzers use a nonmechanical means of alternating the infrared beams, thus eliminating the problem. The sample cell can easily become contaminated. Water or other debris can be aspirated into the analyzer and contaminate the cell "window," interfering with transmission of the infrared beam. Infrared detector cells degrade over time and become less sensitive. Both contamination of the sample cell and detector aging can alter response time or make the analyzer impossible to calibrate.

Emission Spectroscopy Analyzers

The single-breath and multiple-breath N_2-washout tests (open-circuit FRC determination) use N_2 analysis. The Giesler tube ionizer is an N_2 analyzer based on the principle of **emission spectroscopy** (Figure 10-24). This instrument consists of an enclosed ionization chamber that contains two electrodes and a photo cell. A vacuum pump creates a constant low pressure in the ionization chamber by bleeding gas through a needle valve. The needle valve draws gas to be sampled from the breathing circuit. When current is supplied to the electrodes, the N_2 between them is ionized and emits light.

After being filtered, this light is monitored by a photo detector. The intensity of the light is directly proportional to the concentration of N_2 in the sample. The current, distance between electrodes and gas pressure must remain constant. The photo detector converts the light signal into a DC voltage. This analog signal is then amplified, linearized, and directed to an appropriate meter or analog-to-digital converter. The Giesler tube ionizer allows continuous and rapid analysis of N_2 with response times typically less than 100 msec.

Emission spectroscopy analyzers used for measuring FRC by N_2 washout should have a range of 0–80% and should be linear ($\leq 0.2\%$ error) across this range. N_2 analyzers need to have a resolution of 0.01% or less with a 95% response time of 60 msec or less. Because these analyzers measure rapidly changing concentrations of N_2, correction for phase delay in the N_2 signal may be required.

Analyzers using emission spectroscopy usually require a vacuum pump. Vacuum pressure must be maintained at a stable level to ensure accuracy and linearity. Leaks in the seals around the needle valve or in the pump itself may occur. Inability to zero or span the analyzer (i.e., adjust the gain) often indicates a leak or faulty vacuum source. The photo detector, ionizing electrodes, and light filter may all degrade over time. Periodic linearity checks allow adjustment for small changes in these components.

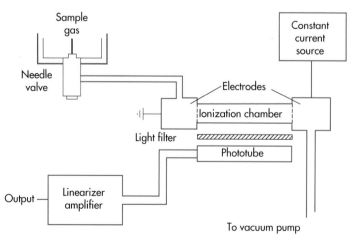

FIGURE 10-24 **Emission Spectroscopy-Type Gas Analyzer.** The optical emission analyzer (Giesler tube) is commonly used for N_2 analysis. A vacuum pump draws a small gas sample through a needle valve (usually in the breathing circuit). The gas sample passes through an ionization chamber, where the ionized gas emits light. All light except that from the desired gas is filtered out, and the remaining light is monitored by a phototube or similar detector. The detector transmits a signal proportional to the intensity of the light, allowing rapid gas analysis. *(From Hewlett-Packard, Application Note AN 729, San Diego, Calif.)*

Thermal Conductivity Analyzers

Measurement of FRC by the closed-circuit method requires He analysis. Some DLCO systems also analyze helium as the tracer gas. **Thermal conductivity analyzers** measure gas concentrations in a sample by detecting the rate at which different gases conduct heat. Heated wires or beads (thermistors) are exposed to the gas sample. The concentration of a specific gas can be detected by measuring the change in electrical resistance of the thermistors. Two glass-coated thermistors serve as sensing elements connected by a Wheatstone bridge circuit (Figure 10-25). Thermistors change temperature and electrical resistance as a function of the molecular weight of the gases surrounding them. One thermistor serves as a reference. A difference in the concentration of gases between two thermistors can be detected because differences in heat conducted away alter the electrical resistance in the circuit. He analyzers use a reference cell containing no helium (He). Other gases can be analyzed by means of thermal conductivity if no interfering gases are present. Thermal conductivity analyzers are used in conjunction with gas chromatography (see the section on gas chromatography). Water vapor and CO_2 must be removed before He analysis. Thermal conductivity analyzers can be used for continuous or discrete measurements but have response times in the range of 10–20 seconds. Thermal conductivity analyzers cannot be used to detect rapid changes in gas concentration.

When a thermal conductivity analyzer is used for FRC_{He} measurements, a range of 0–10% full scale is required, with a resolution of 0.01% or less over this range. The 95% response time should be 15 seconds or less for step changes in He concentration of 2%. The analyzer should show minimal drift ($\leq 0.02\%$) for as long as the test may last (up to 10 minutes).

Thermal conductivity analyzers are very stable. Other than the pump used to draw gas into the analyzer, there are no moving parts. Unless the thermistor in the sampling chamber is contaminated or physically damaged, the analyzer remains accurate for an extended period. Gas pressure and temperature should be maintained at levels similar to those used during calibration in order for the analyzer to produce accurate results. Water vapor or CO_2 in the sample circuit (caused by malfunctioning absorbers) is a common cause of errors with

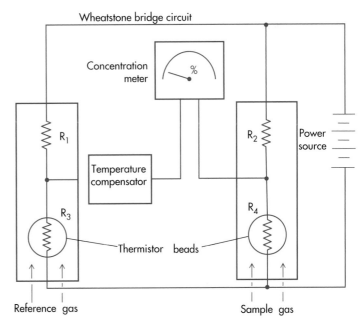

FIGURE 10-25 **Thermal Conductivity Analyzer.** A thermal conductivity gas analyzer, as used for helium (He) analysis or gas chromatography, is shown. Two thermistor beads (temperature-sensitive electrical resistors) are connected in a Wheatstone bridge circuit. When the thermistors are subjected to the same gas concentrations, their electrical resistances are equal and the meter registers zero (by calibration). When a gas is applied to the sample thermistor (R_4) and the reference thermistor submitted to a reference gas, an electrical potential occurs. This deflects the meter (i.e., a voltmeter) by an amount proportional to the difference in gas concentrations.

this type of analyzer. Some He analyzers also use a water absorber in line with the reference thermistor. This allows dry room air to be used to zero the analyzer. Exhaustion of this absorber can result in calibration errors.

Gas Chromatography

Gas chromatography combines a means of separating a sample into component gases and a detector for measuring concentrations of the components. The detector is usually a thermal conductivity analyzer as previously described. Most chromatographs use the principle of column separation to segregate the component gases of the sample (Figure 10-26). The chromatograph column contains a packing material that impedes movement of gas molecules, depending on their size. The material is usually a high-surface-area inorganic or polymer packing. Some columns also use materials that combine chemically with specific gases. A combination of

columns allows a wide range of gases to be analyzed with a single detector. He is used as a carrier gas because of its high thermal conductivity. The sample gas, along with the He carrier gas, is injected into the column. Component gases exit the column at varying rates and are detected by a thermal conductivity analyzer. The concentrations of each gas can be determined by comparing the output of the thermal conductivity analyzer with a known calibration gas. When He is used as the carrier gas, it cannot be used as an inert indicator for lung volume determinations or diffusing capacity measurements. Neon, which is relatively insoluble, may be substituted for He in these tests. Water vapor and CO_2 are usually removed from the sample to prevent contamination of the separator column.

Gas chromatographs are well suited to applications requiring analysis of multiple gases, such as DLCO determinations. If gas chromatography is used for DLCO measurements, the linearity of the device should be 0.5% of full scale for both CO and the tracer gas. As for infrared analyzers, gas

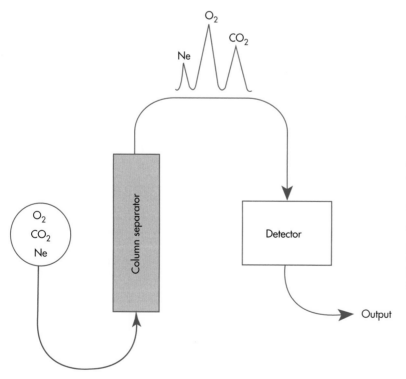

FIGURE 10-26 **Gas Chromatograph.** Diagram of the components of a gas chromatograph for analyzing respiratory gases. The gas sample moves through a separator column via a carrier gas, usually helium (He). Gases of different molecular sizes pass through the column at different rates and are monitored sequentially by a thermal conductivity detector. The output of the detector is proportional to the concentration of the gases in the sample. Gases can be analyzed accurately by using appropriate separator columns.

chromatographs in DLCO systems need to be stable (i.e., no drift) for the interval between calibration and test gas analysis. Gas chromatograph response times are typically from 15–90 seconds, depending on the gas to be detected and the flow of carrier gas.

Chromatography is very accurate and is widely used for analysis of certified reference gases. Column material must be replaced when exhausted to maintain accuracy. Some chromatographs heat the column to enhance separation. Failure of the heating mechanism can lead to inaccurate analyses. Exhaustion of water or CO_2 absorbers can also cause the column to become contaminated.

Chemoluminescence Analyzers

Chemoluminescence analyzers are based on the principle that when two reactants are mixed to form an excited intermediate state, the intermediate may emit light as it decays back to a lower energy level. Chemoluminescence is routinely used to measure nitric oxide (see FE_{NO} in Chapter 9) to assess airway inflammation. Ozone may be combined with NO to form NO_2 (nitrogen dioxide) in an excited state:

$$NO + O_3 \rightarrow NO_2[\lozenge] + O_2$$

where:
NO = nitric oxide
O_3 = ozone
NO_2 = nitrogen dioxide

$[\lozenge]$ = represents decay to a lower energy state
O_2 = oxygen

The activated NO_2 luminesces (i.e., emits light) in visible and infrared wavelengths as it decays to a lower energy state. A photomultiplier or charge-coupled device (CCD) counts photons emitted at a specific wavelength, which are proportional to the amount of NO in the sample. Figure 10-27 shows an example of one commercially available chemoluminescence analyzer for measurement of NO.

Specific recommendations for chemoluminescence NO analyzers have been published by the ATS/ERS (Table 10-3). Calibration of NO analyzers is critical because of the small gas concentrations typically involved (parts per billion [ppb]). Chemoluminescence analyzers used to measure FE_{NO} should be calibrated with gases that span the range of values encountered in clinical practice. These ranges differ depending on whether airway or nasal NO is being measured. In addition to appropriate calibration gases, a zero gas that is free of NO is also required. Ambient air can be drawn through an NO scrubber to provide the zero gas. Chemoluminescence analyzers are sensitive to changes in ambient conditions, especially temperature, and may require recalibration if conditions change. Sample inlet flow also affects the temperature of the reaction chamber and must be carefully controlled.

Gas-Conditioning Devices

Interference from water vapor or CO_2 in expired gas is common to many types of gas analyzers.

TABLE 10-3		
Specifications for Nitric Oxide Analyzers		
	FE_{NO}	Nasal NO
Range	1–500 ppb	10 ppb–50 ppm
Sensitivity	1 ppb	10 ppb
Accuracy	Better than 1 ppb	Better than 10 ppb
Response time (90%)	<500 msec	<500 msec
Drift	<1% full scale/24 hours	<1% full scale/24 hours
Reproducibility	Better than 1 ppb	Better than 10 ppb

Modified from ATS/ERS Recommendations for Standardized Procedures for the Online and Offline Measurement of Exhaled Lower Respiratory Nitric Oxide and Nasal Nitric Oxide, 2005, *Am J Respir Crit Care Med* 2005; 171:912-930.

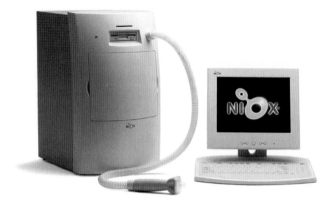

FIGURE 10-27 **Chemoluminescent Gas Analyzer for Nitric Oxide (NO).** A commercially available analyzer designed to measure trace amounts of NO in the exhaled breath. The monitor includes an NO scrubbing device so that the subject can inhale NO-free gas and immediately exhale into the sampler. The analyzer uses the chemoluminescence effect to measure NO (see text). The computer display also serves as a feedback device so that the patient can exhale against a slight resistance and maintain a controlled flow to the analyzer. *(Courtesy Aerocrine Inc., New York, N.Y.)*

These two gases are usually removed by chemical "scrubbers."

CO_2 may be absorbed by passing the sample through granules containing either barium hydroxide ($Ba[OH]_2$) or sodium hydroxide (NaOH). Granules containing NaOH usually have a light brown appearance that changes to white when saturated with CO_2. $Ba(OH)_2$ (Baralyme) is usually supplied with an indicator (ethyl violet), which changes from white to purple when saturated with CO_2. Both NaOH and $Ba(OH)_2$ are mildly corrosive and may generate heat if exposed to high concentrations of CO_2. Both generate water as a product of combination with CO_2. Therefore they should be placed upstream of any water vapor absorber used in the same circuit.

Water vapor is absorbed by passing the humidified gas over granules of anhydrous calcium sulfate ($CaSO_4$ [Drierite]) or silica gel. These substances are termed desiccants. $CaSO_4$ usually contains an indicator that changes from blue to pink when saturated with water vapor. Some analyzers use silica gel to remove water vapor.

Conditioning of gas that contains water vapor may also be accomplished with special sample tubing (Nafion). This tubing is permeable to water vapor. Sample gas passing through the tubing equilibrates its water vapor pressure with that of the surrounding atmosphere. Water vapor is not removed; it remains constant at a known level. If wet gas (e.g., expired air) is passed through the tubing, the sample falls to ambient humidity. If dry gas (e.g., calibration gas) is passed through the tubing, the sample rises to ambient humidity. This allows corrections for water vapor pressure to be accurately applied, as long as the ambient humidity level is known.

Failure to adequately remove water vapor or CO_2 from a gas sample usually results in dilution of the remaining gases. Dilution lowers the fractional concentration of the gas being analyzed. In some types of analyzers (e.g., thermal conductivity) CO_2 or water vapor may also directly alter the output of the analyzer. Chemical scrubbers or permeable tubing should always be replaced according to the manufacturer's recommendations.

BLOOD GAS ANALYZERS, OXIMETERS, AND RELATED DEVICES

Measurements of arterial or mixed venous blood gases include determination of PO_2, PCO_2, and pH. Calculation of arterial oxygen concentration (SaO_2), bicarbonate (HCO_3^-), total CO_2, base excess, and other variables depends on measurements derived from one or more of the three primary electrodes. Oxyhemoglobin saturation, as well as other forms of Hb, is measured with a multiwavelength oximeter. Oxyhemoglobin saturation may also be estimated with a pulse oximeter. Other methods of assessing blood gases and oxygen saturation rely on transcutaneous electrodes and reflective spectro-photometry.

pH Electrodes

The traditional glass pH electrode contains a solution of constant pH on one side of a glass membrane. The sample to be analyzed is brought into contact with the other side of the pH-sensitive glass (Figure 10-28). The difference in pH on either side of the glass causes a potential difference, or voltage. To measure this potential, two half-cells are used: one for the constant solution and one for the sample. The constant solution half-cell (i.e., the measuring electrode) is usually a silver–silver chloride wire. The external half-cell is usually a saturated calomel (i.e., approximately 20% KCl) electrode called the **reference electrode**. The reference electrode makes contact with the unknown solution by means of a permeable membrane or a liquid junction. These half-cells are connected to a voltmeter calibrated in pH units. The voltage difference between the two electrodes is proportional to the pH difference of the solutions. Because the pH of one solution is constant, the developed potential is a measure of the pH of the sample. This type of analysis is thus referred to as a **potentiometric** because a potential is measured. Potentiometric electrodes are widely used in instruments with permanent electrodes as well as in some disposable cartridge–based systems.

pH can also be measured by an optical pH indicator. The indicator is an azo-dye substance in a cellulose membrane; the indicator exists in an acidic and basic form. Each of the two forms absorbs light in different regions of the spectrum (i.e., blue and red). The acidic form absorbs blue light while the basic form absorbs red light. Light is passed through the blood sample and analyzed at different wavelengths. Increased absorbance in the blue wavelength indicates a lower pH, while increased absorbance in the red portion of the spectrum indicates a higher pH. By analyzing the absorptions at multiple wavelengths, the actual pH can be determined. This method is used in some cartridge-based blood gas analyzers.

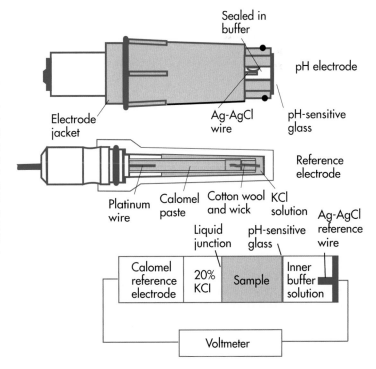

FIGURE 10-28 pH and Reference Electrodes. The pH electrode is a microelectrode, shown here with its plastic jacket *(top)*. At the tip is a silver–silver chloride wire in a sealed-in buffer behind pH-sensitive quartz glass. The reference electrode *(center)* contains a platinum wire in calomel paste that rests in a 20% KCl solution. The blood sample is introduced in such a way that it contacts the measuring electrode tip and the KCl. A voltmeter measures the potential difference across the sample, which is proportional to the pH.

A third method used for measuring pH in blood gas analysis uses a fluorescent chemosensor or optode. The optode has a pH-sensitive fluorescent indicator dye that exists in two forms (protonated and deprotonated). The deprotonated form fluoresces (emits light), but the protonated form (higher H^+ concentration) does not. By measuring the fluorescence, the pH can be measured.

Protein contamination of the pH-sensitive glass is a common problem that increases with the number of specimens analyzed. Routine cleaning with a proteolytic agent (e.g., bleach) reduces buildup of protein on the electrode tip. KCl depletion or blockage of the reference junction can also cause pH electrode malfunction. Contamination of reagents used for pH electrode calibration may also result in measurement errors. Daily (or more frequent) use of suitable quality control (QC) materials can detect these and other problems (see Chapter 11). pH measurements made with optical methods are dependent on how well the sample is mixed. Poorly mixed specimens may result in absorbances that do not accurately reflect the acid-base status of the patient. Fluorescent optodes are designed to separate the blood specimen from the sensor itself using an isolation layer to prevent contaminants from affecting the sensor.

$$CO_2 + H_2O \leftrightarrow H_2CO_3 \leftrightarrow H^+ + HCO_3^-$$

The higher the P_{CO_2}, the more the equation is driven to the right. The change in H+ concentration is proportional to the change in P_{CO_2}. The electrode detects the change in P_{CO_2} as a change in pH of the electrolyte (i.e., a potentiometric measurement). The voltage developed is exponentially related to P_{CO_2}. A tenfold increase in P_{CO_2} is approximately equal to a decrease of 1 pH unit. Partial pressure of CO_2 can be determined by calibrating the pH change when the electrode is exposed to gases with known P_{CO_2} values.

PF TIP

Computerized blood gas analyzers do an excellent job of monitoring analyzer function and detecting problems. Automated calibration allows tracking of electrode or sensor performance. The function of traditional electrodes is monitored by evaluating drift or trends during calibration. Optical sensors can be checked before and during measurements to detect abnormal responses. If either electrode or sensor errors are discovered, an alert is displayed.

Pco₂ Electrodes

Traditional P_{CO_2} electrodes (Severinghaus electrodes) measure P_{CO_2} potentiometrically using an adaptation of the pH electrode (Figure 10-29). A combined pH-reference electrode is placed inside of a membrane-tipped plastic jacket. The jacket is filled with a bicarbonate electrolyte. The membrane is usually Teflon or a similar material permeable to CO_2 molecules. A spacer or wick made of nylon is sometimes placed between the pH-sensitive glass and the membrane. The spacer ensures that a thin layer of bicarbonate electrolyte is in contact with the electrode. When the blood sample is introduced at the tip of the electrode, CO_2 diffuses across the membrane. CO_2 is hydrated in the electrolyte according to the following equation:

Another method of measuring P_{CO_2} uses infrared absorption of dissolved CO_2 at three different wavelengths. By modulating the length of the light path through the specimen, absorption due to factors other than the blood itself can be factored out. Once the concentration of CO_2 has been determined (solving for three different wavelengths) the P_{CO_2} can be calculated by dividing the concentration by the solubility factor for CO_2.

P_{CO_2} can also be measured with optical fluorescence. An optode similar to that used for pH measurements (see the preceding section) is covered by a membrane that is permeable to CO_2. CO_2 diffuses into the optode where it forms carbonic acid and lowers the pH. As the pH decreases (more H+) there is less fluorescence, and P_{CO_2} can be measured indirectly in much the same way as in the traditional electrode.

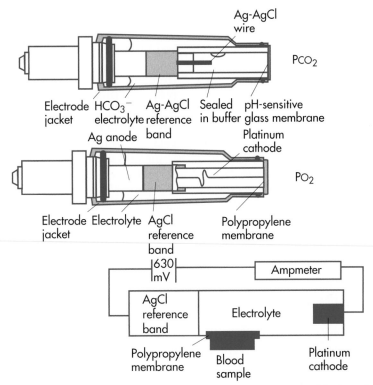

FIGURE 10-29 P_{CO_2} and P_{O_2} Electrodes. The P_{CO_2} (Severinghaus) electrode is a modified pH electrode. The electrode has a sealed-in buffer; an Ag-AgCl reference band is the other half-cell. The entire electrode is encased in a Lucite jacket filled with a bicarbonate electrolyte. The jacket is capped with a Teflon membrane that is permeable to CO_2. A nylon mesh (not shown) covers the pH-sensitive glass, acting as a spacer to maintain contact with the electrolyte. CO_2 diffuses through the Teflon membrane, combines with the electrolyte, and alters the pH (see text). The change in pH is displayed as partial pressure of CO_2. The P_{O_2} (polarographic or Clark) electrode contains a platinum cathode and a silver anode. The electrode is polarized by applying a slightly negative voltage of approximately 630 mV. The tip is protected by a polypropylene membrane that allows O_2 molecules to diffuse but prevents contamination of the platinum wire. O_2 migrates to the cathode and is reduced, picking up free electrons that have come from the anode through a phosphate–potassium chloride electrolyte. Changes in the current flowing between the anode and cathode result from the amount of O_2 reduced in the electrolyte and are proportional to partial pressure of O_2.

The most common problem with traditional P_{CO_2} electrodes is degradation or contamination of the permeable membrane. Protein or debris deposited on the membrane slows diffusion of CO_2. Equilibrium between the sample and electrode may not be achieved. Electrolyte depletion or exhaustion in the jacket around the electrode may also occur with extended use. Careful attention to shifts in electrode performance, during either calibration or control runs, can detect these common problems. Routine maintenance includes replacing the membrane and refilling the electrode with fresh electro-

lyte. Most manufacturers provide a kit that contains a disposable jacket with a membrane and fresh electrolyte. Analyzers that use single-use electrodes eliminate most of the listed problems related to the membrane and electrolyte in the electrode.

Analyzers that use the infrared photometric methodology typically use single-use measurement cuvettes, eliminating problems of contamination of the measuring chamber. However, photometric absorption measurements require that the specimen be well mixed. Fluorescent optode analyzers utilize an optical isolation layer to prevent contaminants and stray light from entering the optode. Guidelines for QC of blood gas electrodes are included in Chapter 11.

PO₂ Electrodes

The standard PO₂ electrode (Clark electrode) consists of a platinum cathode that is usually a thin wire encased in plastic or glass, together with a silver–silver chloride (Ag-AgCl) anode (see Figure 10-29). Both anode and cathode are placed inside a plastic jacket that is tipped with a polypropylene or polyethylene membrane. This membrane is semipermeable and allows diffusion of oxygen molecules. The jacket is filled with phosphate–potassium chloride buffer. A polarizing voltage of approximately 630 mV is applied to the electrode. The cathode is slightly negative with respect to the anode. Because the electrode is polarized, it is referred to as a *polarographic* electrode. Oxygen is reduced (i.e., takes up electrons) at the cathode according to the following equation:

$$O_2 + 2H_2O + 4e^- \rightarrow 4OH^-$$

Electrons (*e* in the preceding equation) are supplied by the Ag-AgCl anode. Electrons flow from the anode to the cathode with a current proportional to the number of molecules of O_2 reduced. Each O_2 molecule can take up four electrons, and the greater the number of O_2 molecules present, the greater the current. The membrane causes a diffusion limitation to the number of molecules reaching the electrode. The greater the partial pressure on the sample side of the membrane, the higher the rate of diffusion. The measurement of the current (**amperometric**) developed within the electrode is therefore proportional to PO₂.

Optical methods of measuring PO₂ include phosphorescence and **fluorescence quenching**. In each of these methods a dye that emits light and is sensitive to the presence of O_2 is used (Figure 10-30). The higher the PO₂ is in the sensor or optode, the lower the phosphorescence or fluorescence (i.e., increased quenching of emitted light).

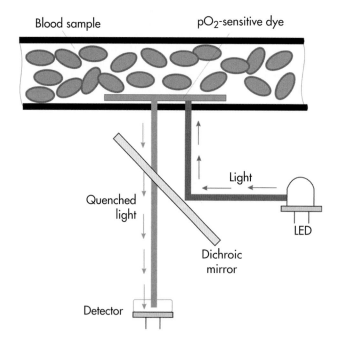

FIGURE 10-30 Phosphorescence and Luminescence Quenching. Quenching of light emitted either by phosphorescence or luminescence can be used to measure the concentration of an analyte such as the partial pressure of oxygen in blood. Light from an LED bounces off a dichroic mirror and is directed toward an indicator (e.g., dye) that fluoresces. In the case of oxygen, the higher the PO₂ the more the emitted light is quenched. The emitted light then passes through the dichroic mirror and strikes a detector (e.g., a photocell or CCD) that provides a measure of the PO₂.

As with the P_{CO_2} electrode, contamination or degradation of the membrane alters diffusion of O_2 and can result in erratic measurements. Depletion of the phosphate buffer can also cause a change in electrode sensitivity. Most polarographic electrodes use a platinum wire of small diameter to reduce the actual consumption of O_2 at the tip of the electrode. The exposed surface of the platinum cathode gradually becomes plated with metal ions and must be periodically polished to maintain its sensitivity. Alternatively, the entire electrode can be replaced.

Because the membrane causes a diffusion limit to O_2 molecules reaching the cathode, the electrode performs differently when exposed to liquid versus gas samples. Many blood gas systems use gas to calibrate the P_{O_2} electrode. Noticeable differences may result when the electrode is then used to analyze the tension of O_2 dissolved in a liquid (e.g., blood). These differences are usually compensated for by correcting the P_{O_2} with an empirically determined gas-to-liquid factor.

Laboratory Analyzers

Although the gas-measuring (P_{O_2} and P_{CO_2}) electrodes and the pH electrode system can each be used separately, all three are usually implemented together in a blood gas analyzer (Figure 10-31). The three electrodes are mounted in a single measuring chamber. This allows a small blood sample ($\leq 200\,\mu l$) to be analyzed. Most blood gas analyzers are microprocessor controlled. Sample aspiration, rinsing, and calibration can all be done automatically with program control. Standardization of these functions, especially calibration, reduces measurement error and improves precision. The microprocessor can calculate other blood gas values derived from pH, P_{CO_2}, and P_{O_2}, including HCO_3^-, total CO_2, and base excess (BE). In addition to pH, P_{CO_2}, and P_{O_2}, most modern laboratory analyzers incorporate a hemoximeter to provide total Hb and its derivatives (e.g., O_2Hb, COHb). Computerized analyzers can monitor

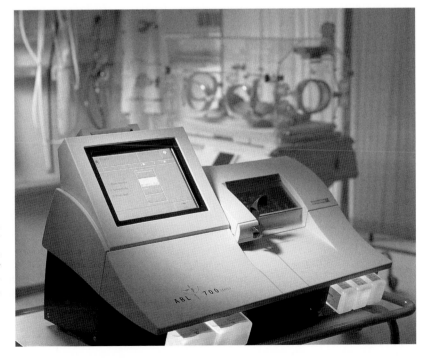

FIGURE 10-31 Automated Blood Gas Analyzer, Including Spectrophotometric Oximeter. This system provides automatic sample handling, flushing, and calibration. Results of sample analysis and calibrations are displayed using an integrated computer and display terminal. pH, P_{CO_2}, and P_{O_2} are measured; HCO_3^-, total CO_2, standard bicarbonate, and other variables are calculated. This system also incorporates a spectrophotometric oximeter for analysis of Hb, O_2Hb, COHb, and MetHb. Base excess is calculated with HCO_3^- calculated from the blood gas analysis and Hb measured by the oximeter. Additional parameters can include bilirubin, electrolytes, glucose, and lactate. *(Courtesy Radiometer America, Westlake, Ohio.)*

automated calibrations and electrode performance to alert the technologist of existing or impending problems. The computer can monitor the level of reagents and calibrating solutions/gases as well. Some analyzers automatically perform quality control runs (i.e., auto QC) and monitor the results.

Point-of-Care Analyzers

To provide rapid results of critical analytes (e.g., blood gases and electrolytes), portable or bedside analyzers (i.e., point-of-care [POC]) have become widely available (Figure 10-32). These devices are typically designed for use in the emergency department, critical care unit, or outpatient clinic. Most can be battery-operated, but some POC instruments require standard power. Blood gas measurement techniques differ slightly among models. Some POC blood gas analyzers use microelectrodes similar to those described previously, whereas others use spectrophotometry, infrared spectroscopy, or fluorescence quenching methods. Reagents, calibration materials, and waste containers are usually contained in disposable cartridges. Some POC systems use cartridges that allow a fixed number of analyses, whereas others use a single-patient sample chamber. Calibrations for POC systems that use multiple-specimen cartridges are usually performed in the traditional manner (see Chapter 11). These POC instruments use aqueous buffers in the single-patient chamber to perform calibration immediately before sample analysis. Single-use devices often have the sample chamber precalibrated by the manufacturer. Many POC instruments include ion-specific electrodes for analysis of electrolytes (e.g., K^+, Na^+, and Ca^+) along with other metabolites and hematocrit. A few POC analyzers also incorporate hemoximetry in addition to pH, P_{CO_2}, and P_{O_2}.

The accuracy and precision of most POC blood gas analyzers appear comparable to that obtained with standard laboratory instruments. Routine analysis of multiple levels of quality control (QC) material is required to assess precision. However, because of the design of the sensors and the fact that reagents and reference electrodes may not be

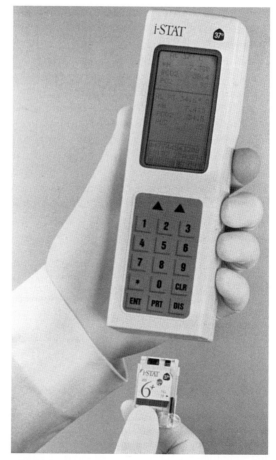

FIGURE 10-32   Point-of-Care (POC) Blood Gas Analyzer. This handheld POC blood gas analyzer uses microelectrodes. It is battery powered, so it can be used in a variety of clinical settings. *(Courtesy i-Stat Corp., East Windsor, N.J.)*

required, some cartridge-based systems require QC only when the cartridge is changed. Analysis of unknown specimens and comparison with other instruments or laboratories (proficiency testing) is required to determine accuracy.

Transcutaneous P_{O_2} and P_{CO_2} Electrodes

The transcutaneous O_2 electrode (tcP_{O_2}) operates on a principle similar to that of the polarographic electrode. The $tcPO_2$ electrode typically consists of a ring-shaped silver anode heated by a coil to increase blood flow at the skin placement site. Inside the circular anode is a platinum cathode (Figure 10-33). All elements are enclosed in a plastic case. The face of the sensor is covered by a Teflon membrane. Electrolyte (KCl) is placed between the membrane and the sensor. A second layer of electrolyte and a cellophane membrane are added to form a double membrane. The current between the silver anode and platinum cathode is proportional to the PO_2 diffusing through the skin and membrane. A feedback controller keeps the temperature constant at the skin site. This also compensates for changes in capillary blood flow and stabilizes the measurement.

The gradient between $tcPO_2$ and PaO_2 is relatively constant in patients with normal cardiac output. In neonates there is a close correlation between transcutaneous and PaO_2. In hemodynamically stable adults, $tcPO_2$ is approximately 80% of PaO_2. Measurement of $tcPO_2$ can trend oxygenation when this gradient has been established. In patients with reduced cardiac output, the gradient between $tcPO_2$ and PaO_2 widens. Conditions that affect perfusion to the skin may also alter the gradient between arterial and $tcPO_2$.

Transcutaneous measurements of PCO_2 are possible with a sensor that uses a CO_2-permeable membrane like that in the traditional blood gas electrode. CO_2 diffuses through the skin and into the sensor. $tcPCO_2$ and $tcPO_2$ sensors typically require calibration. This is usually accomplished by attaching the sensor to a port that exposes it to a calibration gas. Several types of transcutaneous monitors combine $tcPCO_2$ with $tcPO_2$ or pulse oximetry (SpO_2).

Most transcutaneous monitors heat the skin site from $40°-45°C$. The increased temperature "arterializes" capillary blood flow. The fastest response times are usually attained at the highest temperature setting. However, this necessitates moving the electrode every 3-4 hours to prevent burns. Changing sensor sites is particularly important in neonates because of the reduced thickness of their epidermis. Periodic recalibration of the electrode is necessary even if the sensor site has not been changed. After placement of the sensor, an interval of 5-30 minutes may be required for equilibration to be reached.

Spectrophotometric Oximeters

The **spectrophotometric oximeter** uses light absorption to analyze saturation of hemoglobin (Hb) with O_2. The concentration of carboxyhemoglobin (COHb) or other forms of Hb (e.g., methemoglobin, sulfhemoglobin) can also be determined.

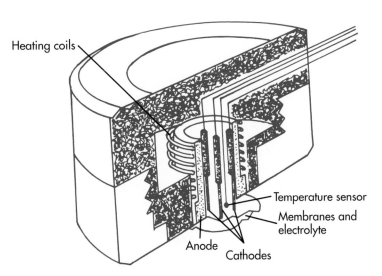

FIGURE 10-33 Transcutaneous PO_2 ($tcPO_2$) Electrode. Cross-sectional diagram of a $tcPO_2$ electrode showing a circular anode around a series of cathodes and a temperature sensor. A heating coil causes local hyperemia so that skin PO_2 closely resembles PaO_2. A double membrane separates the electrode proper from the skin. Because the electrode warms the skin, it must be moved periodically. A similar design uses a modified PCO_2 electrode to provide $tcPCO_2$.

Heating coils

Temperature sensor

Membranes and electrolyte

Anode

Cathodes

This type of spectrophotometer is sometimes called a **co-oximeter** or **hemoximeter.** In addition to various forms of Hb, spectrophotometric measurement principles (absorption of light) can be used to measure pH and P_{CO_2}, as described previously.

The hemoximeter analyzes the absorption of light in a blood sample at multiple wavelengths. At certain wavelengths, two or more forms of Hb have similar absorbances (Figure 10-34). These common wavelengths are termed **isobestic points**. An isobestic point for oxyhemoglobin (O_2Hb), reduced Hb (RHb), and COHb is 548 nm. At this wavelength, the absorbance of a mixture of the three pigments is directly proportional to the total concentration of Hb. An isobestic point for O_2Hb and RHb is 568 nm. The absorbance of COHb at this point is considerably higher. A change in absorbance at 568 nm compared with 548 nm indicates a change in the concentration of COHb relative to the sum of the concentrations of the other two species. The isobestic point for RHb and COHb is 578 nm, with O_2Hb absorbance being considerably greater. The difference in absorbance at 578 nm indicates the concentration of O_2Hb relative to the other two pigments. The total Hb concentration, O_2Hb, COHb, and methemoglobin (MetHb) saturation can be determined by analyzing absorbances and solving simultaneous equations.

The hemoximeter provides the true O_2Hb saturation (see the section on oxygen saturation in Chapter 6). This is particularly important if increased concentrations of COHb, MetHb, or other abnormal hemoglobins are present. Some automated blood gas analyzers calculate O_2Hb saturation. Calculated saturation is based on the measured P_{O_2} and pH at 37° C. This calculation assumes

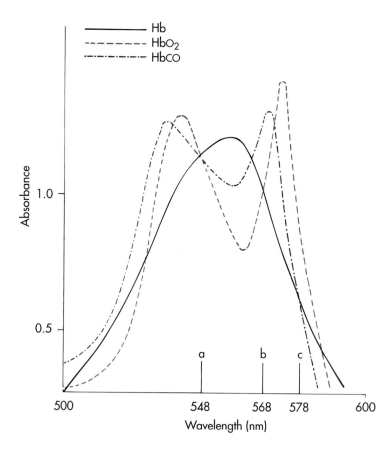

FIGURE 10-34 **Principle of Spectrophotometric Oximetry.** Absorbance measurements are made at three or more distinct wavelengths (548, 568, 578 nm) as light passes through a sample of hemolyzed blood. At 548 nm, all three forms of Hb (Hb, O_2Hb, and COHb) have identical absorbances. At 568 nm, only Hb and HbO_2 coincide, whereas at 578 nm, Hb and COHb coincide. The solution of simultaneous equations provides the relative proportions of each species, as well as total Hb (see text).

that the Hb has a normal P_{50} (see Chapter 6). Calculated O_2Hb may significantly overestimate true saturation in the presence of increased levels of COHb or methemoglobin. The hemoximeter provides the most accurate estimate of the actual O_2 saturation. Most laboratory blood gas analyzers and some POC analyzers combine blood gases and hemoximetry. These instruments provide pH, PCO_2, PO_2 and spectrophotometric measurements of Hb saturation, all performed with the same blood sample.

Hemoximeters may give erroneous Hb, O_2Hb, or COHb readings if forms of hemoglobin are present that the instrument does not recognize. For example, blood from a newborn (e.g., containing fetal Hb) will give erroneous values if analyzed by an oximeter set up for adult blood. Substances that cause light scattering in the specimen (e.g., lipids resulting from lipid therapy) may also cause false readings. To function properly, the hemoximeter must hemolyze the sample so that Hb molecules are suspended in solution rather than contained within the red cells. Hemolysis is accomplished by chemical or mechanical disruption of red cell membranes. Incomplete hemolysis results in light scattering within the sample rather than simple absorption. Sickle cells are not easily disrupted, particularly by chemical lysis, and may result in false readings for O_2Hb and COHb. Incomplete hemolysis may be difficult to detect unless whole-blood QC or proficiency testing is performed (see Chapter 11). Blood specimens used for hemoximetry must be well mixed or the concentration of Hb (i.e., total Hb) may be incorrect. Most hemoximeters report errors such as incomplete hemolysis or light scattering.

In addition to measurements of O_2Hb, COHb, and MetHb saturations, the hemoximeter can calculate oxygen content and P_{50}. P_{50} can be estimated by measuring the actual saturation of a specimen (usually a venous sample with a saturation of less than 90%) and comparing this value with the calculated saturation based on PO_2 and pH of the same blood. This simplified method compares favorably with tonometering of the blood sample with various low-oxygen concentrations and constructing a dissociation curve.

Pulse Oximeter

Pulse oximeters (Figure 10-35) are commonly used to assess oxygenation noninvasively. Pulse oximeters treat Hb as a filter that allows only red and near-infrared light to pass. The **Lambert-Beer law** relates total absorption in a system of absorbers to the sum of their individual absorptions:

$$A_{total} = E_1C_1L_1 + E_2C_2L_2 + \ldots E_nC_nL_n$$

where:

A_{total} = absorbance of a mixture of substances $1 \ldots n$ at a specific wavelength

E_n = molar extinction of substance n

C_n = concentration of substance n

L_n = length of light path through substance n

In principle, the standard pulse oximeter measures absorption of a mixture of just two substances, O_2Hb and RHb. The concentration of either one can be determined if their extinction is measured while the path length stays constant. The wavelengths of light used in standard pulse oximetry are near 660 nm in the red region of the spectrum and near 940 nm in the near-infrared region. Extinction curves for O_2Hb and RHb show that reduced Hb has absorption 10 times higher than oxyhemoglobin at 660 nm, whereas O_2Hb has a higher absorbance (two to three times) at 940 nm. Calculating all possible combinations of the two forms of Hb (i.e., varying the saturation from 0%–100%) allows the ratio of absorbances at the two wavelengths to be determined. As a result, a calibration curve can be constructed. The capillary bed does not follow the optical principles exactly as described by the Lambert-Beer law, so the calibration curve is derived empirically. The ratio of absorbances at the two distinct wavelengths is expressed as follows:

$$R = A_{660nm}/A_{940nm}$$

A series of R values (e.g., the calibration curve) is determined by relating this ratio to actual saturation measurements. Unlike the hemoximeter, which measures absorption in a hemolyzed blood sample, the pulse oximeter measures light passing through living tissue. The transmitted light is not only

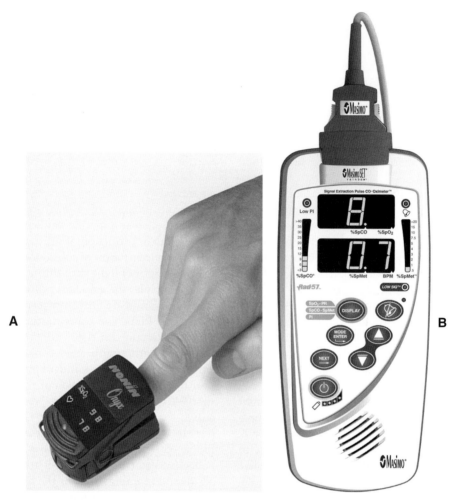

FIGURE 10-35 **Pulse Oximeters.** Most pulse oximeters provide a digital display of oxygen saturation and pulse rate. **A,** A small, portable pulse oximeter that fits over the patient's finger. Miniaturized components allow a device of this size to be easily transported. **B,** A sophisticated multiwavelength pulse oximeter that is capable of measuring COHb and MetHb in addition to O_2Hb and pulse rate. (*A courtesy Nonin Medical, Inc., Plymouth, Minn.; B courtesy Masimo Corporation, Irvine, Calif.*)

absorbed but also refracted and scattered. This causes the absolute accuracy of the pulse oximeter to be less than the accuracy of a hemoximeter.

The transmitted light at each wavelength consists of two components, the AC and DC components (see Figure 10-36). The AC component varies with the pulsation of blood. The DC component represents light absorbed by tissue and venous blood. The DC component is larger than the AC

and is relatively constant. The amplitude of both AC and DC levels depends on the intensity of the incident light. The AC component represents the arterial blood because the arterioles pulsate in the light path. By dividing the AC level by the DC level at each of the two wavelengths, the AC component is effectively corrected. The AC component then becomes a function of the extinction of O_2Hb and RHb. The ratio just described then becomes:

$$R = \frac{(AC_1/DC_1)}{(AC_2/DC_2)}$$

where:

1 = red wavelength (660 nm)

2 = near-infrared wavelength (940 nm)

Correcting the pulsatile component (AC) in this manner allows the pulse oximeter to "ignore" absorbances caused by venous blood, tissue, and skin pigmentation.

The light source used in pulse oximetry is the **light-emitting diode (LED)**. LEDs are capable of emitting a very bright light near the 660-nm and 940-nm wavelengths required for analysis of Hb saturation. Light intensity is controlled by a feedback circuit that regulates the driving current to the LED. The greater the DC component resulting from pigmentation or venous blood, the greater the current supplied to the LED. One problem with LEDs is that the exact wavelength of light emitted varies with individual diodes. Each LED has its own center wavelength that may differ from 660 nm or 940 nm by as much as 15 nm. To overcome this variation, each oximeter must have a series of calibration curves programmed into it so that it can accommodate a range of LEDs. The extinction curves for RHb and O_2Hb are steep and different at 660 nm, so 10 or more calibration curves are typically required for the red-light range. Slight variations in center wavelength are less critical in the 940-nm region because the extinction characteristics of O_2Hb and RHb are the same from 800–1000 nm.

A photo diode detects transmitted light in the pulse oximeter. A single photo diode senses both red and near-infrared light. The microprocessor that controls the oximeter cycles the LEDs on and off separately 400–500 times per second. The oximeter also turns both LEDs off during each cycle. This allows the photo diode to detect ambient light caused by scattering and to offset the LED signals.

Pulse oximeter accuracy tends to decrease at low saturations. Low saturations occur as the concentration of RHb increases. RHb has a much higher absorbance at 660 nm than does O_2Hb. Therefore slight variations in the center wavelength of the red LED (as described) exaggerate the error in measured saturation. This is one reason pulse oximeters exhibit decreasing accuracy at lower saturations.

PF TIP

The standard pulse oximeter measures the saturation of available hemoglobin at two wavelengths. In these devices, the presence of COHb causes absorption at wavelengths similar to O_2Hb, and the pulse oximeter tends to read higher than the true saturation. MetHb causes increased absorption at both red and infrared wavelengths. This causes the ratio of the absorptions to be close to unity, and the pulse oximeter tends to read 85%. However, some pulse oximeters are capable of multiwavelength analysis and can detect COHb and MetHb, as well as O_2Hb (see text).

Because the AC, or pulsatile component, is usually much smaller than the DC component, detecting it can sometimes cause problems. Low perfusion or poor vascularity can cause the oximeter to be unable to measure the pulsatile component. Most oximeters display a warning message if the photo detector senses inadequate light levels. Motion artifact can also cause inaccuracy with pulse oximeters. Movement, especially shivering, often occurs in the same frequency range as the signal to be detected (i.e., arterial pulsations). If the motion is consistent and lasts long enough, it introduces a signal of approximately the same amplitude into both red and infrared channels. The pulse oximeter senses motion artifact as part of the DC component. This adds a large value to both the numerator and denominator of the ratio (R). The motion signal forces R toward a value of 1, which is equal to a saturation of 85% on the typical oximeter calibration curve. Some oximeters use multiple digital filters to discriminate motion artifact and produce a more reliable signal.

Most pulse oximeters use the AC signal from one channel (660 nm or 940 nm) to calculate pulse rate. An algorithm implemented by the microprocessor locates peaks in the waveform of the AC signal and counts them (Figure 10-36). Some oximeters use

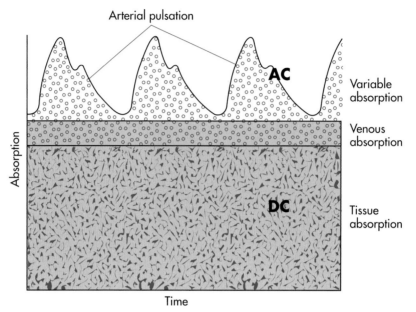

FIGURE 10-36 Measurement Principle of Standard Pulse Oximetry. Transmitted light (at wavelengths of 660 and 940 nm) consists of two components. A large fixed component, the DC component, represents light passing through tissue and venous blood without being absorbed. A smaller portion is pulsatile in nature and changes absorption as blood pulses through the arterioles; this is represented as the AC component. The pulse oximeter divides the AC signal by the DC signal at each wavelength, effectively canceling the DC component. The ratio of the AC signals at the two wavelengths is then a function of the relative absorptions of O_2Hb and RHb (see text). Modern pulse oximeters include sophisticated digital filters to better distinguish the AC and DC components of the signal. Some oximeters operate with additional wavelengths and can detect other forms of Hb (e.g., COHb and MetHb).

this signal to display graphic representations of pulse waveforms. Pulse oximeters that measure absorption at multiple wavelengths (see Figure 10-35, *B*) can detect COHb (SpCO) and MetHb (SpMet) in addition to the standard SpO_2.

Reflective Spectrophotometers

Reflective spectrophotometry is based on the variable reflection of light by O_2Hb and RHb at different wavelengths. Just as the light absorbed by O_2Hb and RHb is a function of wavelength, so is the intensity of reflected or back-scattered light. Carefully spaced optical fibers can be used as transmitting and receiving paths for light. Reflective spectrophotometry can be used to monitor arterial saturation in a manner similar to that of pulse oximetry. Reflective spectrophotometry can also be

incorporated into a pulmonary artery catheter to measure mixed venous oxygen saturation ($S\bar{v}O_2$).

A reflective sensor can be placed at a site where a thin layer of tissue covers bone, such as the forehead. The oximeter then measures O_2Hb in a manner similar to that used for pulse oximetry but uses reflected rather than absorbed light. Pulse oximeters are available that can use either the regular sensor (i.e., absorption) or a reflective sensor.

A specially designed pulmonary artery (Swan-Ganz) catheter contains fiber optic bundles (Figure 10-37). This catheter has regular pressure-sensing ports, a balloon tip for flotation through the right side of the heart, and capability for cardiac output determinations. Three LEDs similar to those used in pulse oximeters illuminate blood flowing past the tip of the catheter via one of the optical fibers. A photodetector senses the reflected light and con-

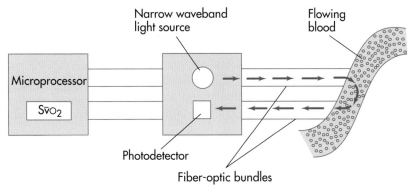

FIGURE 10-37 Principle of Reflective Spectrophotometry. A diagrammatic representation of the components of an optical pulmonary artery catheter. This type of catheter (Swan-Ganz) is used for continuous monitoring of $S\bar{v}O_2$. LEDs provide a narrow-waveband light source. Light is transmitted along one fiber optic filament to blood flowing past the tip of the catheter. Light reflected from the blood is transmitted back to a photodiode by the second fiber optic bundle. The light intensity signals are then evaluated by a microprocessor to calculate light intensity ratios. These ratios (usually two ratios are determined from three wavelengths) determine the $S\bar{v}O_2$. The principle of reflective absorption can also be used for pulse oximetry.

verts its intensity into a signal. A microprocessor calculates two independent ratios of reflected light intensities from the three wavelengths. Combining two reflected light intensity ratios reduces the instrument's sensitivity to pulsatile blood flow or changing hematocrit. This design also minimizes changes caused by light scattering from red cell surfaces and the walls of the blood vessel. $S\bar{v}O_2$ is calculated from the light ratios using programmed calibration curves, similar to those used for a pulse oximeter. As in a pulse oximeter, saturation measured is the saturation of functional Hb (see Chapter 6). $S\bar{v}O_2$ determination by this method tends to be higher than that measured by a hemoximeter, especially if large amounts of COHb or MetHb are present. $S\bar{v}O_2$ is then displayed and may be printed using a trend recorder (Figure 10-38).

The reflective spectrophotometer must be routinely calibrated to ensure that observed changes in $S\bar{v}O_2$ are the result of physiologic phenomena rather than instrument drift. The catheter is usually standardized by calibrating it against an absolute color reference before insertion. After the catheter is in place, calibration is accomplished by adjusting the output to match saturation measured by a

co-oximeter. This type of calibration is accurate at the time it is performed but may change if there are shifts in pH or hematocrit. Because reflective spectrophotometers measure reflected light in whole blood that is flowing rather than transmitted light in a hemolyzed blood sample, their absolute accuracy is less than that of a hemoximeter.

COMPUTERS FOR PULMONARY FUNCTION TESTING

All modern pulmonary function equipment uses computers in one form or another. Many spirometers use either a dedicated microprocessor (see Figure 10-16) or are interfaced to a desktop or laptop (Figure 10-39). Computerized pulmonary function systems allow sophisticated data handling and storage, accurate calculations, graphic display of maneuvers, and enhanced reporting capabilities. Some laboratories use networked computers in which each pulmonary function system has a dedicated workstation. Networked systems allow rapid exchange of information and centralized data storage and retrieval.

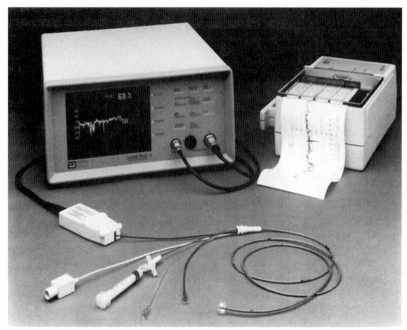

FIGURE 10-38 Reflective Spectrophotometer and Pulmonary Artery Catheter. A microprocessor-controlled reflective spectrophotometer. The pulmonary artery catheter contains fiber optic bundles for continuous measurement of $S\bar{v}O_2$, as well as the usual pressure-measuring ports and sensors for both continuous cardiac output determinations and thermodilution cardiac output. The instrument displays mixed venous saturation digitally and as a trend graph that can be printed. High and low saturation alarms are included along with a "light intensity" alarm to detect artifact caused by catheter motion or problems with the fiber optics. *(Courtesy Abbott Critical Care Systems, Mountain View, Calif.)*

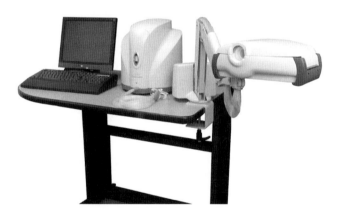

FIGURE 10-39 Computerized Pulmonary Function System. Modern laboratory systems use personal computers (PCs) interfaced to spirometers, gas analyzers, body plethysmographs, and associated breathing circuitry. This automated system includes flow sensing spirometer, gas analyzers, and a computer-controlled breathing circuit. The PC allows rapid and accurate processing of data, including calculation of test variables, calibration, BTPS and STPD corrections, and graphic display. Data can be stored locally on a high capacity hard disk or on a networked server. *(Courtesy Medical Graphics, St. Paul, Minn.)*

Data Acquisition and Instrument Control

Computerized pulmonary function systems process analog signals from spirometers, plethysmographs, and gas analyzers. Equally important is the computer's capacity to control instrument functions, such as switching valves or recording signals. Computer control allows the technologist to manage complex test maneuvers. Data acquisition and instrument control are implemented with an interface (Figure 10-40) between the computer and pulmonary function equipment. Similar principles are applied in large laboratory systems and in small handheld spirometers.

An important component of the pulmonary equipment interface is the analog-to-digital (A/D) converter. The A/D converter senses an analog signal (such as pressure or flow) and transforms it into a digital value. The analog signal is usually a

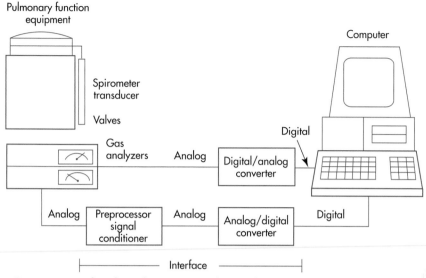

FIGURE 10-40   Computer Interface for Pulmonary Function Equipment. Components of a typical interface between a spirometer, gas analyzers, and a personal computer (PC) are shown. Analog signals from the pulmonary function equipment are preprocessed and then passed to an A/D converter. The A/D converter transforms a voltage (usually DC) into digital form. Digital data are then processed by the computer for calculations, display, and storage. Some systems use digital transducers that combine all of these functions and can communicate directly with the PC. For the computer to control various instrument functions, a D/A converter transforms digital data into appropriate analog signals to control system functions, such as opening valves in the breathing circuit.

DC voltage in the range of either 0–10V or ±5V. A/D converters are classified by the number of bits (binary digits) into which they convert the signal. The higher the number of bits, the greater the resolution of the input signals. A 12-bit converter can transform a voltage into a number represented by 000000000000 to 111111111111 as a binary number. In the decimal notation, this corresponds to a range of 0–4096, or 2^{12}. For example, a 10-L spirometer may produce an analog signal ranging from 0–10V (i.e., 1 V = 1 L). If the spirometer is connected to a 12-bit converter, the signal can be divided into 4096 parts. This provides a resolution of approximately 0.0024V or 2.4ml. The smallest volume change that can be detected would be 2.4ml for this spirometer system. For most volume and flow sampling applications, 12-bit converters are adequate. For greater resolution, a 16-bit A/D converter may be used. Some systems use transducers (i.e., pressure or flow) that directly produce a digital output. These transducers do not require an A/D converter, simplifying the measurement.

The rate at which data are sampled also affects accuracy. High-speed A/D converters can perform more than 20,000 conversions per second on a single channel. Most computerized pulmonary function systems sample data 100 times/sec (i.e., 100 Hz) or greater. These high rates exceed the frequency bandwidth of breathing maneuvers by a factor of more than two. Accuracy is attained by matching analog output of a device (e.g., a spirometer) to an A/D converter with appropriate sampling rate and voltage resolution.

Another means of sampling volume or flow signals is measuring the time required for a known change in volume or flow. For example, the number of clock ticks that occur for a volume change of 100 ml can be counted and flow calculated. This technique requires a spirometer that uses a position encoder or generates pulses for each volume increment. The accuracy of encoder-pulse systems depends on clock resolution and volume increment, especially when measuring high flows.

Most devices (e.g., pulse oximeters or capnographs) use dedicated microprocessors and A/D boards to process data. These instruments often include a communication port so that data can be sent to a PC or printer. Most computers have serial ports (USB or conventional) that can be used to interface various instruments. Some instruments (e.g., monitors) include Ethernet ports so that the device can communicate as a network device.

Pulmonary Function Data Storage and Programs

Computerized pulmonary function systems, even small, portable spirometers, generate large volumes of patient data. Managing these large amounts of data is relatively easy via computer networks. Almost all PC-based systems support networking to some extent. Networked computers allow multiple users to share data, as well as peripheral devices such as printers. The network typically consists of a primary computer or server. Other computers are then linked by one of several types of networks. Data can be transferred between any two computers linked by the system. The server usually maintains programs and data that all of the networked users need.

The format in which test data are stored is determined by (1) complexity of the data, (2) volume of data (i.e., number of tests done per month or year), and (3) how data will be accessed. Three methods for data management are used with computerized pulmonary function systems.

Temporary Storage or No Data Storage

Some portable spirometers provide only temporary storage of patient data. In these devices, a microprocessor performs calculations and then displays or prints the results, but patient data are not stored. Some spirometers store tests in RAM (random access memory) for viewing and printing. These instruments permit tests from multiple patients to be stored; data can be recalled whenever the system is operating. Data can usually be transferred to a host computer or to a printer. Some monitoring devices (e.g., pulse oximeters) also provide limited data storage with interfaces for computers or printers.

Permanent Individual Patient Data Files

Patient data records are stored by creating individual files, usually on the PC's hard drive. The volume of data stored in files of this type is limited only by the computer's operating system and the physical capacity of the storage device. Tabular and graphic data (e.g., flow-volume curves) may be stored in a single file or in separate files. Graphic data often require more disk space than tabular data, depending on the format in which they are stored. Modern systems support large hard drives, so a large volume of test data can be stored on a desktop or laptop PC. Because so much data can be stored on a single physical device, an appropriate backup mechanism is required.

Database Storage

Many pulmonary function systems use a relational database format. Tests from different patients are stored as individual records in a file. Files (sometimes called tables) are then "linked" to form a database. One table may contain all spirometry records, a second all lung volume records, a third table DLCO measurements, and so on. Complete tests are linked across files by an index using patient number or test date. A database structure allows sorting, selecting, searching, and editing of patient data. Some applications of a database system for pulmonary function data include the following:
- Serial comparisons of multiple tests on a single patient may be extracted to plot a trend.
- Data from longitudinal studies on groups of patients may be extracted for statistical analysis or export to an external program.
- Queries may be performed to extract data that match selected criteria.
- An unlimited number of report formats may be generated.

- Reference equations may be stored in a database format. This structure allows input of user-defined equations for predicting normal values.

Relational database systems support a special command language called Structured Query Language (SQL). SQL databases (or similar) provide a standardized means for the user to enter and retrieve data, generate reports, and perform functions such as importing or exporting records. SQL databases can be easily restructured, so that additional information can be added to existing databases.

Pulmonary function software often includes interpretation programs. Interpretation programs use algorithms for identifying obstructive, restrictive, combined, or normal patterns of pulmonary function. Spirometers designed for detecting obstruction in the primary care setting (i.e., office spirometers) typically include a computerized interpretation. More sophisticated algorithms can evaluate spirometry, lung volumes, and $D_{L}CO$, comparing measured and reference values. Although algorithms use logic similar to that of a clinician, they are usually not able to consider the patient's clinical history or other laboratory findings. Some programs are very sophisticated and can diagnose obstruction or restriction reasonably well. An incorrect computer interpretation may occur if test data are not acceptable or repeatable because of poor patient effort or technical problems. However, most spirometers include software functions that assess acceptability and repeatability of efforts. If the computerized interpretation considers data quality, an accurate interpretation is possible. Even if computerized interpretation is not implemented, computer-generated statements regarding test quality can be useful for traditional interpretation. Computer interpretation in no way substitutes for evaluation by a qualified clinician. It may be helpful when an immediate report of abnormalities is necessary, such as for screening purposes. If a computerized interpretation is included in the final report, it should be clearly labeled as such.

Summary

- Spirometers that use either volume-displacement or flow-sensing principles are used for many different pulmonary function tests.
- Small computerized spirometers (office spirometers) are often used for testing in many areas outside of the traditional pulmonary function laboratory.
- Small, portable peak flow devices have been developed and are widely used in clinical and home settings.
- Body plethysmography, using either a pressure box or flow box, is commonly used for measuring lung volumes and airway resistance. Its design and ease of use have benefited from advances in electronics and computerization.
- Various types of pulmonary gas analyzers and their principles of operation are discussed along with how they are used for pulmonary function testing.
- Breathing valves and gas conditioning devices are described, with particular attention to selection and maintenance.
- Blood gas electrodes, along with other technologies used for blood gas analysis, are reviewed. Spectrophotometric oximeters, pulse oximeters, and related monitors are illustrated.
- Information on the components of computer systems, data acquisition and storage, and specific interfaces to pulmonary function equipment are presented.

SELF-ASSESSMENT QUESTIONS

Entry-level

1. Which of the following are true in regard to a dry, rolling-seal spirometer?
   I. It cannot be used to measure D_{LCO} by the single-breath method
   II. Measured volumes need to be corrected to BTPS
   III. Inspiratory and expiratory flows can be measured
   IV. Leaks do not affect spirometric measurements
      a. I and III
      b. II and IV
      c. II and III
      d. I and IV

2. A 3-L syringe is used to check a wedge bellows spirometer, and the following results are observed:

Trial	Volume
1	2.78
2	2.55
3	2.92

   Which of the following best explains these findings?
      a. Automatic BTPS correction was turned off
      b. The calibration syringe has a leak
      c. The spirometer has a leak
      d. The 3-L volume was injected too rapidly

3. Flow integration is used to measure volume in which of the following?
      a. Water-seal spirometer
      b. Pressure differential pneumotachometer
      c. Turbine respirometer
      d. Dry rolling-seal spirometer

4. Which of the following principles are used in flow sensing spirometers?
   I. Paired heated wires to detect temperature change
   II. Ultrasonic sound waves passing through a gas stream
   III. Molecular impaction on a gel membrane
   IV. Pressure drop across a resistive element
      a. I and IV only
      b. II and III only
      c. I, II, and IV
      d. II, III, and IV

5. A demand flow valve used to supply test gas for single breath D_{LCO} testing should provide:
      a. A dead space less than 10 ml
      b. 6 L/sec flow at less than 10 cm H_2O
      c. Less than 5 cm H_2O flow resistance at 1 L/sec
      d. A built-in high-efficiency bacteria filter

6. Which of the following are commonly used to measure carbon monoxide concentration for the $D_{LCO}sb$?
   I. Emission spectroscopy-type analyzer
   II. Gas chromatograph
   III. Fuel cell analyzer
   IV. Infrared analyzer
      a. I and II
      b. III and IV
      c. I and III
      d. II and IV

7. Which of the following is commonly used to measure He concentration in dilutional lung volume determinations?
      a. Thermal conductivity analyzer
      b. Emission spectroscopy analyzer
      c. Infrared absorption analyzer
      d. Chemoluminescence analyzer

8. A gas analyzer circuit uses chemical absorbers to remove water vapor and CO_2 from exhaled gases. Which of the following describe how these should be used?
      a. Both chemical absorbers should contain granules with the same color
      b. The water vapor absorber should be placed before the CO_2 absorber
      c. The CO_2 absorber should be placed before the water vapor absorber
      d. The order of the absorbers is not important

Advanced

9. Some plethysmographs have a built-in "slow" leak; the purpose of this leak is to:
      a. Allow oxygen to slowly enter the box while the door is closed
      b. Compensate for differences in the size of patients
      c. Prevent excessive pressure that may cause ear discomfort
      d. Help maintain thermal equilibrium when a patient is in the box

10. Which of the following principles can be used to measure the pH in a blood gas analyzer?
    I.   Molecular resonance spectroscopy
    II. Potential difference across pH-sensitive glass
    III. Optical absorption in a dye-indicator at multiple wavelengths
    IV. Chemoluminescent optodes sensitive to pH
        a. I and III only
        b. II and IV only
        c. I, II, and III
        d. II, III, and IV

11. A patient in the emergency department has his O_2 saturation measured by standard pulse oximetry, and SpO_2 of 85% is recorded. Blood gases are drawn immediately, and the SaO_2 (by hemoximetry) is reported as 98%. A possible explanation of these findings is that the patient:
    a. Had polycythemia (increased hemoglobin)
    b. Was shivering
    c. Was hyperventilating
    d. Had an elevated level of COHb

12. Some pulse oximeters use sensors that can be placed on the forehead rather than on a finger or ear lobe; these types of sensors:
    a. Are based on the principle of reflective spectrophotometry
    b. Measure absorption at five to eight distinct wavelengths
    c. Use the chemoluminescent quenching principle
    d. Can measure total Hb concentration in addition to SpO_2

13. Office spirometers used to screen for chronic obstructive lung disease should:
    I.   Incorporate automated interpretation of acceptable spirometry
    II. Measure the FEV_1, FEV_6, and FEV_1/FEV_6 ratio
    III. Provide feedback concerning test acceptability and repeatability
    IV. Calculate the $FEF_{25\%-75\%}$ based on the largest FVC
        a. I and III only
        b II and IV only
        c. I, II, and III
        d. I, III, and IV

14. When selecting a body plethysmograph, the box pressure transducer should be:
    a. Able to measure pressures of ± 50 cm H_2O at 8 Hz
    b. Calibrated with a 3-L volume injected at 1–2 Hz
    c. Connected to a "slow" leak with a time constant of 30–60 seconds
    d. Capable of measure pressure changes as small as ± 0.2 cm H_2O at 8 Hz

15. A pulmonary function laboratory wants to screen a large number of healthy subjects at multiple locations to establish reference values for spirometry. Which of the following methods would be the most appropriate?
    a. Office spirometers capable of producing printed reports
    b. Several volume-based spirometers interfaced to laptop computers
    c. Different types of flow-based spirometers to provide comparative values
    d. Portable spirometers communicating with an SQL database

Selected Bibliography

SPIROMETERS
Banks DE, Wang ML, McCabe L et al: Improvement in lung function measurements using a flow spirometer that emphasizes computer assessment of test quality, *J Occup Environ Med* 1996; 38:270-283.

Enright PL, Hyatt RE, editors: *Office spirometry: a practical guide to the selection and use of spirometers,* Philadelphia, 2003, Lea & Febiger.

Ferguson GT, Enright PL, Buist AS et al: Office spirometry for lung health assessment in adults: a consensus statement from the National Lung Health Education Program, *Chest* 2000; 117:1146-1161.

Hankinson JL: Instrumentation for spirometry. In Eisen JE, ed: *Occupational medicine: state of the art reviews,* Philadelphia, 1993, Hanley and Belfus.

Johns DP, Ingram C, Booth H et al: Effect of a microaerosol barrier filter on the measurement of lung function, *Chest* 1995; 107:1045-1048.

Kendrick AH, Johns DP, Leeming JP: Infection control of lung function equipment: a practical approach, *Respir Med* 2003; 97:1163-1179.

Miller MR, Hankinson J, Brusasco V et al: Standardisation of spirometry, *Eur Respir J* 2005; 26:319-338.

Porszaz J, Barstow TJ, Wasserman K: Evaluation of a symmetrically disposed Pitot-tube flowmeter for measuring gas flow during exercise, *J Appl Physiol* 1994; 77:2651-2665.

Pulmonary Function Standards for Cotton Dust, 29 Code of Federal Regulations; 1910.1043 Cotton Dust, Appendix D, Occupational Safety and Health Administration, 1980.

Ruppel GL: Spirometry, *Respir Care Clin North Am* 1997; 3:155-181.

Townsend MC, Hankinson JL, Lindesmith LA et al: Is my lung function really that good? Flow-type spirometer problems that elevate test results, *Chest* 2004; 125:1902-1909.

Townsend MC: ACOEM position statement: spirometry in the occupational setting. American College of Occupational and Environmental Medicine, *J Occup Environ Med* 2000; 42:228-245.

PEAK FLOW METERS

Bongers T, O'Driscoll BR: Effects of equipment and technique on peak flow measurements, *BMC Pulm Med* 2006; 6:14.

Folgering H, vander Brink W, van Heeswijk O et al: Eleven peak flow meters: a clinical evaluation, *Eur Respir J* 1998; 11:188-193.

Fonseca JA, Costa-Pereira A, Delgado L et al: Pulmonary function electronic monitoring devices: a randomized agreement study, *Chest* 2005; 128:1258-1265.

Irvin CG, Martin RJ, Chinchilli VM et al: Quality control of peak flow meters for multicenter clinical trials. The Asthma Clinical Research Network (ACRN), *Am J Respir Crit Care Med* 1997; 156:396-402.

Jackson AC: Accuracy, reproducibility, and variability of portable peak-flow meters, *Chest* 1995; 107:648-651.

Jensen RL, Crapo RO, Berlin SL: Effect of altitude on hand-held peak flowmeters, *Chest* 1996; 109:475-479.

Koyama H, Nishimura K, Ikeda A et al: Comparison of four types of portable peak flow meters (Mini-Wright, Assess, Pulmo-graph and Wright Pocket meters), *Respir Med* 1998; 92:505-511.

PLETHYSMOGRAPHS

American Association for Respiratory Care: Clinical practice guideline: body plethysmography—2001 update, *Respir Care* 2001; 46:506-513.

Bargeton D, Barres G: Time characteristics and frequency response of body plethysmographs. International Symposium on Body Plethysmography, Nijmegen, *Prog Respir Res* 1969; 4:2.

Coates AL, Peslin R, Rodenstein D, Stocks J: Measurement of lung volumes by plethysmography, *Eur Respir J* 1997; 10:1415-1427.

DuBois AB, Bothello SY, Bedell GN et al: A rapid plethysmographic method for measuring thoracic gas volume: a comparison with nitrogen-washout method for measuring functional residual capacity in normal subjects, *J Clin Invest* 1956; 35:322-326.

DuBois AB, Bothello SY, Comroe JH: A new method for measuring airway resistance in man using a body plethysmograph: values in normal subjects and in patients with respiratory disease, *J Clin Invest* 1956; 35:327-331.

Quanjer PH, Tammeling GJ, Cotes JE et al: Lung volumes and forced ventilatory flows: report of the Working Party for Standardization of Lung Function Tests, European Community for Steel and Coal, *Eur Respir J* 1993; 16 (suppl):5-40.

Wanger J, Clausen JL, Coates A., Pedersen OF: Standardisation of the measurement of lung volumes, *Eur Respir J* 2005; 26: 511-522.

GAS ANALYZERS

Macfarlane DJ: Automated metabolic gas analysis systems: a review, *Sports Med* 2001; 31:841-861.

Müllera KC, Jörres RA, Magnussen H et al: Comparison of exhaled nitric oxide analysers, *Respir Med* 2005; 99:631-637.

Norton AC: Accuracy in pulmonary measurements, *Respir Care* 1979; 24:131-147.

Rebuck AS, Chapman KR: Measurement and monitoring of exhaled carbon dioxide. In Nochomovitz ML, Cherniack NS, eds: *Non-invasive respiratory monitoring,* New York, 1986, Churchill Livingstone.

Zar HA, Noe FE, Szalados JE et al: Monitoring pulmonary function with superimposed pulmonary gas exchange curves from standard analyzers, *J Clin Monit Comput* 2002; 17:241-247.

BLOOD GAS ELECTRODES, OXIMETERS, AND RELATED DEVICES

Barker SJ, Curry J, Redford D et al: Measurement of carboxyhemoglobin and methemoglobin by pulse oximetry: a human volunteer study, *Anesthesiology* 2006; 105:892-897.

Barker SJ, Shah NK: The effects of motion on the performance of pulse oximeters in volunteers (revised publication), *Anesthesiology* 1997; 86:101-108.

Berkenbosch JW, Tobias JD: Comparison of a new forehead reflectance pulse oximeter sensor with a conventional digit sensor in pediatric patients, *Respir Care* 2006; 51:726-731.

Cariou A, Monchi M, Dhainaut JF: Continuous cardiac output and mixed venous oxygen saturation monitoring, *J Crit Care* 1998; 13:198-213.

Franklin ML: Transcutaneous measurement of partial pressure of oxygen and carbon dioxide, *Respir Care Clin North Am* 1995; 1:119-131.

Gehring H, Hornberger C, Matz H et al: The effects of motion artifact and low perfusion on the performance of a new generation of pulse oximeters in volunteers undergoing hypoxia, *Respir Care* 2002; 47:48-60.

Kozlowski-Templin R: Blood gas analyzers, *Respir Care Clin North Am* 1995; 1:35-46.

Nishiyama T, Nakamura S, Yamashita K: Effects of the electrode temperature of a new monitor, TCM4, on the measurement of transcutaneous oxygen and carbon dioxide tension, *J Anesth* 2006; 20:331-334.

Peruzzi WT, Shapiro BA, eds: Blood gas measurements, *Respir Care Clin North Am* 1995; 1:1-157.

Severinghaus JW: The invention and development of blood gas analysis apparatus, *Anesthesiology* 2002; 97:253-256.

Severinghaus JW, Bradley AF: Electrodes for blood PO_2 and PCO_2 determination, *J Appl Physiol* 1958; 13:515-523.

Tremper KK, Waxman KS: Transcutaneous monitoring of respiratory gases. In Nochomovitz ML, Cherniack NS, editors: *Noninvasive respiratory monitoring*, New York, 1986, Churchill Livingstone.

Townshend J, Taylor BJ, Galland B et al: Comparison of new generation motion-resistant pulse oximeters, *J Paediatr Child Health* 2006; 42:359-365.

Tusa JK, He H: Critical care analyzer with fluorescent optical chemosensors for blood analytes, *J Mater Chem* 2005; 125:2640-2647.

Villanueva R, Bell C, Kain ZN et al: Effect of peripheral perfusion on accuracy of pulse oximetry in children, *J Clin Anesth* 1999; 11:317-322.

COMPUTERS

American Thoracic Society, Committee on Proficiency Standards for Clinical Pulmonary Laboratories: Computer guidelines for pulmonary laboratories, *Am Rev Respir Dis* 1986; 134:628-632.

Beardsmore CS, Paton JY, Thompson JR et al: Standardizing lung function laboratories for multicenter trials, *Pediatr Pulmonol* 2007; 42:51-59.

Ellis JH, Perera SP, Levin DC: A computer program for the interpretation of pulmonary function studies, *Chest* 1975; 68:209-215.

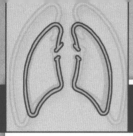

Chapter 11

Quality Assurance in the Pulmonary Function Laboratory

OBJECTIVES

After studying this chapter you will be able to:

Entry-level
1. Describe how to calibrate a spirometer using a 3-L syringe
2. Determine whether a blood gas analyzer is "in control" using a control chart
3. Describe standard precautions to be applied during blood gas specimen collection and analysis
4. Compose technologist's comments to describe acceptable and unacceptable spirometry

Advanced
1. List the necessary calibrations required for body plethysmographs
2. Apply results obtained from biologic control subjects to troubleshoot pulmonary function equipment
3. Describe two methods for performing quality control of a DLCO system
4. Identify potential sources of cross-contamination in pulmonary function equipment

KEY TERMS

accuracy
back-pressure
biologic control

calibration factor
coefficient of repeatability (CR)
coefficient of variation (CV)

computerized syringe
control
DLCO simulator

drift	multiple-rule method	shift
isothermal lung analog	proficiency testing (PT)	sine-wave rotary pump
leak check	random error	tonometry
lung analog	serial dilution	two-point calibration

This final chapter discusses issues related to quality assurance. General concepts include equipment standards for spirometers, plethysmographs, gas analyzers (including DLCO systems), and blood gas analyzers. Proper instrument maintenance and calibration are bases for obtaining acceptable and repeatable data. The chapter also deals with specific quality control (QC) methods for equipment used in pulmonary function testing and blood gas analysis. Problems commonly encountered with various types of equipment are listed to guide in troubleshooting.

Personnel who perform pulmonary function tests often must make decisions during testing that determine the quality of data obtained. Special attention is given to methods by which the pulmonary function technologist can assess data quality. Documentation of pulmonary function data quality (e.g., acceptability, repeatability, and reproducibility) is discussed.

Safety and infection control are discussed as they relate to patients and to those performing pulmonary function tests. As in previous chapters, case studies and self-assessment questions are included.

ELEMENTS OF LABORATORY QUALITY CONTROL

Quality control (QC) is one aspect of quality assurance. QC is essential in the operation of a pulmonary function laboratory to obtain valid and reproducible data. There are four general elements to consider in regard to a quality assurance program.

Methodology

The type of equipment used (e.g., volume-based versus flow-based spirometer) often determines the specific procedures that are required for calibration and QC. For example, both flow-based and volume-based spirometers require calibration with a 3-L syringe, but only volumetric spirometers need to be checked for leaks. The number and complexity of the tests performed may also dictate which equipment and methods are used. Methods and equipment that have been validated in the scientific literature should be used whenever possible. QC is usually easier to perform when standardized techniques are used.

Equipment Maintenance

The type and complexity of instrumentation for a specific test determine the long-term and short-term maintenance that will be required. Daily maintenance includes replacing disposable items such as filters and gas conditioning devices. Preventive maintenance is scheduled in anticipation of equipment malfunction to reduce the possibility of equipment failure. Corrective maintenance or repair is unscheduled service that is required to correct equipment failure. These types of failures are often detected by QC procedures or unusual test results. Familiarity with the operating characteristics of spirometers, gas analyzers, plethysmographs, and application software requires manufacturer support and thorough documentation. A procedure manual (Box 11-1) and accurate records are essential to a comprehensive maintenance program. Documentation of procedures and repairs is required by most accrediting organizations. Upgrades to application

BOX 11-1   Pulmonary Function Procedure Manual

Items to be included in a typical procedure manual for a pulmonary function laboratory. For each procedure performed, the following should be present:

1. Description of each test performed in the laboratory and its purpose
2. Indications for ordering the test and contraindications, if any
3. Description of the general method(s) and any specific equipment required, including disposable supplies
4. Calibration of equipment required before testing (manufacturer's documentation may be referenced)
5. Patient preparation for the test, if any (e.g., withholding medication) and patient assessment before beginning the test
6. Step-by-step procedure for measurement/ calculation of results; how to perform the measurement or calculation manually is useful for quality monitoring
7. Quality control guidelines with acceptable limits of performance and corrective actions to be taken when control values are outside of their limits
8. Safety precautions related to the procedure (e.g., infection control, hazards) and alert values that require physician notification with read-back of critical results
9. Description of results reporting
10. References for all equations used for calculating results and for predicted normals, including a bibliography
11. Documentation of computer protocols for calculations and data storage; guidelines for computer downtime and software upgrades
12. Dated signatures of medical and technical directors (may be electronic)

Adapted from American Thoracic Society: *Pulmonary function laboratory management manual,* ed 2, 2005, New York, American Thoracic Society.

Control Methods

A **control** is any known test signal for an instrument that can be used to determine its accuracy and precision. Controls or control materials must be available for spirometers, gas analyzers, plethysmographs, blood gas analyzers, and other instruments. Because many laboratories use computerized pulmonary function or blood gas analyzers, controls are required to ensure that both software and hardware are functioning within acceptable limits. In many instances, application software is used to record and evaluate control runs (e.g., automated blood gas analyzers). Control methods may vary from use of 3-L syringes for spirometers to commercially prepared materials for blood gas analyzers. **Biologic controls** are test subjects for whom specific variables have been determined.

Testing Technique

A primary means of ensuring data quality is to rigidly control the procedures by which data are obtained. For many pulmonary function tests, how the data are obtained depends on the technologist's ability to conduct the procedure and to elicit subject cooperation in the test maneuvers. Technologist and subject performance, as well as proper equipment function, must be evaluated for each test completed. This may be accomplished by using appropriate criteria to judge the acceptability of results. Recommendations for testing procedures published by the American Thoracic Society and European Respiratory Society (ATS/ERS) are widely recognized as standards for test performance.

Each pulmonary function laboratory should have a written quality assurance program that includes the following:

- Methods used for specific tests
- Specific guidelines as to how tests are to be performed
- Limitations of each procedure (if any)
- Indications or schedules for maintenance
- QC materials or signals to be used
- Action to be taken if controls exceed specified limits

The quality assurance program should be included as part of the laboratory procedure manual (see Box 11-1).

Two concepts that are central to quality assurance are accuracy and precision. **Accuracy** may be

software should be considered an essential component of equipment maintenance in the pulmonary function laboratory.

defined as the extent to which measurement of a known quantity results in a value approximating that quantity. For most laboratory tests, repeated measurements of a control are made and the mean, or average, is calculated. If the mean value approximates the known value of the control, the instrument is considered accurate.

Precision may be defined as the extent to which repeated measurements of the same quantity can be reproduced. If a control is measured repeatedly and the results are similar, the instrument may be considered precise. Precision is often defined in terms of variability based on the standard deviation (SD) of a series of measurements (see Appendix G for a sample calculation).

Accuracy and precision are desirable but may not always be present together in the same instrument. For example, a spirometer that consistently measures a 3-L test volume as 2.5 L is precise but not very accurate. A spirometer that evaluates a 3-L test volume as 2.5, 3.0, and 3.5 L on repeated maneuvers produces an accurate mean of 3.0 L, but the measurements are not precise. Determining both the accuracy and precision of instruments such as spirometers is critical because many pulmonary function variables are effort dependent. The largest observed value, rather than the mean, is often reported as the best test (see Chapter 2). Reporting the largest result observed is based on the rationale that the subject cannot overshoot on a test that is effort dependent. Other pulmonary function tests, such as the DLCO, are reported as an average of two or more acceptable maneuvers; in these instances precision of the measuring devices (e.g., gas analyzers) needs to exceed the normal physiologic variability of the parameter being measured.

For instruments such as blood gas analyzers, accuracy is determined by measuring an unknown control and comparing the results with a large number of laboratories using similar equipment and methods. This is commonly referred to as **proficiency testing (PT)**. Precision for blood gas analyzers is determined by checking the day-to-day variability of controls and expressing the variability in terms of the standard deviation. These general principles for assessing accuracy and precision can be applied to most types of pulmonary function equipment.

CALIBRATION AND QUALITY CONTROL OF PULMONARY FUNCTION EQUIPMENT

Calibration is the process in which the output signal from an instrument is adjusted to match a known input. This may be accomplished by one of several methods:

1. Adjustment of the analog output signal from the primary transducer (e.g., spirometer bell, flow sensor, gas analyzer)
2. Adjustment of the sensitivity of the recording device (specifically mechanical recorders)
3. Software correction or compensation

Calibration involves adjustment of the instrument (or its signal). It should not be confused with verification or QC. QC assesses function of the instrument after it has been calibrated. Most pulmonary function systems use software-based calibration but allow for adjustment of analog outputs as well.

Spirometers

Spirometers that produce a voltage signal by means of a potentiometer (see Chapter 10) normally allow some form of "gain" adjustment so that the analog output can be matched to a known input of either volume or flow. For example, a 10-L volume-displacement spirometer may be equipped with a 10-V potentiometer. The potentiometer amplifier would be adjusted so that 0 V equals 0 L (zero), and 10 V equals 10 L (gain). The calibration could be verified by setting the spirometer at a specific volume and noting the analog signal (e.g., 5 L should equal 5 V).

A second technique is adjustment of the sensitivity of the recording device. This method is used for older spirometers equipped with mechanical recorders (e.g., kymographs, X-Y plotters, or strip chart recorders). In these devices, a known volume is injected into the spirometer and deflection of the recording device is adjusted to match the volume. For example, a strip chart recorder is turned on and has its pen adjusted to read 0 L when the spirometer is empty. A 3-L volume is then injected. The gain of the recorder is adjusted so that the tracing deflects to the 3-L mark on the graph paper. This method is appropriate when the recorded tracing is to be manually measured but is seldom used because most modern spirometers use computerized output (display or printer). The ability to evaluate a spirometer's accuracy with a mechanical recorder may be useful for checking a computerized system.

Most spirometer systems are computerized. In computerized systems, the signal produced by the spirometer is often corrected by applying a software **calibration factor**. A known volume or flow is injected into the spirometer with a large-volume (usually 3-L) syringe. A correction (i.e., calibration) factor is calculated based on the measured versus expected values:

$$\text{Correction factor} = \frac{\text{Expected volume}}{\text{Measured volume}}$$

The correction factor derived by this method is then stored in memory and applied to all subsequent volume measurements. For example, if a syringe with a volume of 3.00 L were injected into a spirometer and a volume of 2.97 L recorded, the correction factor would be as follows:

$$1.010 = \frac{3.00\,\text{L}}{2.97\,\text{L}}$$

The correction factor 1.010 would then be used to adjust subsequent measured volumes. This method assumes that the spirometer's output is linear and that the same factor would be correct for any volume, large or small. Most automated spirometers allow the correction factor to be verified by re-injecting a known volume, usually 3 L. Taking into account the accuracy of the syringe, after calibration the spirometer should display a volume of 3.0 L ±3.5%. Three and one-half percent of a standard 3-L volume means that the spirometer should read 3.00 ±0.105 L (range, 2.895 – 3.105 L).

Care should be taken that the gas in the syringe, which is at ambient temperature (ATPS) is not "temperature corrected" by the software. Many computerized spirometers provide software functions specifically for calibration and verification. This allows the use of a 3-L syringe without applying corrections that are necessary when patients are tested. Inaccurate temperature corrections produce an erroneous correction factor. Ambient temperature should be available from an accurate thermometer, both for calibration and for testing. If the ambient temperature changes significantly, the temperature used by the software should be updated, or recalibration may be needed. Many spirometers automatically measure ambient temperature. These devices should be checked regularly to verify that appropriate temperature corrections are being applied. The calibration syringe should be maintained at the same environmental conditions as the spirometer.

PF TIP

Most spirometers provide a means of verifying the volume calibration. This step typically uses the 3-L calibration syringe. After calibration, additional injections and withdrawals of a known volume (usually 3 L, but other volumes may be used) can be used to verify that the spirometer produces a known output. The verification step should include a range of flows to demonstrate volume accuracy that is independent of flow.

Other factors that may influence establishment of the software correction value include the accuracy of the large-volume syringe and the speed with which injections are performed. An inaccurate syringe or leaks in the connection to the spirometer may produce erroneous software corrections. Syringes used for calibration should be accurate to within ±15 ml or ±0.5% of the stated volume (i.e., 15 ml for a 3-L syringe). Accuracy of calibration syringes should be verified annually. Syringes can be checked for leaks simply by occluding the port and trying to empty the syringe. Some laboratories use two syringes: one to calibrate and another to verify volume accuracy.

Some spirometers, particularly those that are flow-based, may require that the calibration volume be injected within certain flow limits. Flow-based spirometers that measure both inspiratory and expiratory volumes require the syringe volume to be injected and withdrawn. This allows separate correction factors for inspired and expired gas to be generated. Many flow-sensing spirometers also require a "zero" before measuring exhaled volume. This means that the flow sensor must be held motionless (so there is no flow through it) while the software adjusts the output of the sensor to equal zero. If an in-line bacteria filter will be used for testing, calibration should be performed with the device in place.

Spirometers that use disposable flow sensors may or may not allow calibration. Many disposable sensors are calibrated during manufacture and are coded so that the spirometer software applies appropriate correction factors (see Chapter 10). If these types of spirometers provide for user calibration, they should be calibrated at least daily. At a minimum, a daily calibration check (see the following paragraphs) should be performed with a sensor from the lot used for patient testing.

Quality control of spirometers is closely related to calibration, and the two are sometimes confused. An important distinction is that calibration (i.e., adjustment) may or may not be needed, but QC should be performed on a routine basis. Calibration, whether it includes the output of the spirometer, recorder sensitivity, or generation of a software correction factor, involves adjustment of the device to perform within certain limits. QC is a test performed to determine the accuracy, precision, or both of the device with a known standard or signal. Various control methods (e.g., signal generators) are available for spirometers.

Simple Large-Volume Syringe

A syringe of at least 3-L volume (Figure 11-1) should be used to generate a control signal for checking spirometers. A 3-L syringe can be used to verify volume-displacement spirometers and associated deflection of mechanical recorders. A large-volume syringe may also be used to check the volume accuracy of flow-based spirometers. Computerized systems often have the user inject (or withdraw) a 3-L volume to calibrate the spirometer, and then immediately perform additional injections to verify the calibration. Some portable flow-based spirometers (i.e., those using disposable flow sensors) do not provide for calibration, but do allow checking or verification of a stored calibration.

QC for spirometer volume measurements should be performed at least once each day that the device is to be used. For field studies, accuracy may need to be checked more often. Frequent checks are recommended for industrial applications or epidemiologic research, especially if the spirometer is moved or used for a large number of tests or if the ambient temperature and humidity change

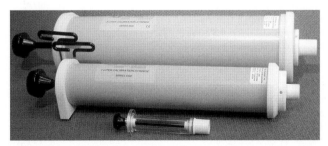

FIGURE 11-1   Calibration Syringes. Standard 3-L syringe *(top)* is used for volume calibration of volume-based and flow-based spirometers for testing of adults and adolescents. The same type syringe may be used for FRC and DLCO quality control (see text). Smaller calibration syringes may be used for calibration and verification of pulmonary function equipment used for small children and infants. *(Courtesy Hans Rudolph, Inc., Kansas City, Mo.).*

rapidly. The accuracy of any spirometer can be calculated as follows:

$$\% \, Error = \frac{Expected \, volume - Measured \, volume}{Expected \, volume} \times 100$$

where:

Expected volume = known syringe volume (usually 3 L)

Measured volume = volume recorded for the test

The maximum acceptable error for spirometers, according to American Thoracic Society/European Respiratory Society (ATS/ERS) recommendations, is ±3.5% or ±65 ml, whichever is larger. Table 11-1 lists the minimal requirements for spirometers (excluding the accuracy of the 3-L syringe). If the error exceeds these limits, careful examination of the spirometer, recording device, software, most recent calibration, and testing technique should be performed (Quality Assurance 11-1).

Flow-based spirometers should have their accuracy checked using at least three different flows ranging from 0.5 – 12.0 L/sec. This can be accomplished easily by injecting the 3-L volume over intervals of 0.5 seconds up to about 6 seconds. At each flow the volume accuracy of ±3.5% should be maintained.

Linearity of volume-based spirometers should be verified at least quarterly. Volume-displacement spirometers should be checked in 1-L increments across their volume range (i.e., 0 – 8 L). A 3-L syringe injection performed when the spirometer is nearly empty or nearly full should yield accurate results. The linearity of flow-sensing spirometers should be tested weekly by injecting a series of 3-L volumes at low, moderate, and high flows. Different flows can

TABLE 11-1

Minimal Recommendations for Spirometers
A 3-L calibration syringe is recommended for testing VC and FVC. Twenty-four standardized waveforms are available for validating FVC, FEV_1, and $FEF_{25\%-75\%}$. Twenty-six standard flow waveforms are available for validating PEF. Other flows require manufacturer's proof of performance. A sine-wave pump is recommended for MVV validation.

Test	Range/Accuracy (BTPS)	Flow Range (L/sec)	Time (sec)	Resistance / Back-Pressure
VC	0.5 – 8 L ±3% of reading or ±0.05 L, whichever is greater	0 – 14	30	N/A
FVC	0.5 – 8 L ±3% of reading or ±0.05 L, whichever is greater	0 – 14	15	<1.5 cm H_2O/L/sec (0.15 kPa/L/sec)
FEV_1	0.5 – 8 L ±3% of reading or ±0.05 L, whichever is greater	0 – 14	1	<1.5 cm H_2O/L/sec (0.15 kPa/L/sec)
Time zero	Time point for calculating all FEV_T values	N/A	N/A	Back extrapolation
PEF	Accuracy: ±10% of reading or ±0.3 L/sec (20 L/min), whichever is greater; repeatability: ±5% of reading or ±0.15L/sec (10 L/min), whichever is greater	0–14	N/A	Mean resistance at 200, 400, 600 L/min (3.3, 6.7, 10 L/sec) <2.5 cm H_2O/L/sec (0.25 kPa/L/sec)
$\dot{V}$ (except PEF)	±5% of reading or ±0.2 L/sec, whichever is greater	0–14	N/A	<1.5 cm H_2O/L/sec (0.15 kPa/L/sec)
$FEF_{25\%-75\%}$	7.0 L/sec ±5% of reading or ±0.2 L/sec, whichever is greater	±14	15	<1.5 cm H_2O/L/sec (0.15 kPa/L/sec)
MVV	250 L/min at V_T of 2 L ±10% of reading or ±15 L/min, whichever is greater	±14 (±3%)	12 – 15	<1.5 cm H_2O/L/sec (0.15 kPa/L/sec)

Adapted from Miller MR, Hankinson J, Brusasco V, et al: Standardisation of spirometry, *Eur Resp J* 2005; 26:319-338.

be generated by varying the speed at which the syringe is emptied. Applying different flows and measuring the resulting volumes may indicate if the spirometer (and its software) is accurate across the range of flows. For example, three different injection times, 0.5–1.0 seconds, 1.0–1.5 seconds, and 5.0–6.0 seconds, may be used with a 3-L syringe to simulate a wide range of flows.

Computerized syringes are also available for assessing the accuracy of commonly measured parameters such as forced expiratory volume (FEV_1) and $FEF_{25\%-75\%}$. These syringes use a built-in microprocessor to time the volume injection and calculate the flows. The microprocessor displays volume and flows for comparison with those produced by the spirometer. A computerized syringe provides a 3-L volume for calibration or volume checks, and tests accuracy for commonly reported flows.

QC for spirometers should be performed as if a patient were being tested. The 3-L syringe should be connected to the patient port, with the circuitry used for the actual test. Spirometer temperature correction may need to be set to 37° C (i.e., no correction applied). Most computerized spirometers provide a specific routine for volume checks or calibration that disables temperature corrections. In some systems, temperature correction cannot be disabled. In these spirometers, injection of 3 L at

ATPS results in a reading greater than 3 L because the system attempts to "correct" the volume to body temperature (BTPS). For water-seal spirometers, the syringe should be filled and emptied several times to allow equilibration with the humidified air in the device. Some flow-sensing spirometers require a length of tubing between the flow sensor and syringe to reduce artifact caused by turbulent flow in the syringe. If an in-line bacteria filter is used, volume verification should be performed with it in place.

Biologic Controls

Biologic controls are healthy subjects who are available for repeated tests. These controls can be laboratory personnel or other individuals who can be tested repeatedly. Using biologic controls does not eliminate other control devices such as large-volume syringes. Although a 3-L syringe can verify volume and flow accuracy of a spirometer, biologic controls can evaluate an entire system, including spirometers, gas analyzers, plethysmographs, and software. A disadvantage of using biologic controls is that pulmonary function varies from day to day. However, by establishing means and measures of variability from repeated tests, real problems with most pulmonary function equipment can be identified (Quality Assurance 11-2).

Control subjects should have normal lung function (i.e., no asthma or other respiratory symptoms) and, ideally, span a range of values. For example, a 64-inch-tall female and a 72-inch-tall male will provide a wide range of values for most pulmonary function parameters. Pulmonary function studies on controls should be performed on a regular basis (weekly or monthly). All tests should use the same protocols applied to the patient population. Control measurements should meet all criteria for acceptability and repeatability. Tests should be performed at the same time of day to minimize the effects of diurnal variation. If the laboratory has multiple pulmonary function systems, controls may be tested on each instrument on the same day to provide a check of interinstrument bias.

To provide useful statistics, 10–20 sets of measurements should be recorded. However, means

QUALITY ASSURANCE 11-2

HOW TO USE BIOLOGIC CONTROLS

1. *Performance of a single instrument.* Test biologic controls on a regular basis. Compare variables (e.g., FEV$_1$) to the established mean. Control values should fall within a range of ±2 SDs of the mean (at least 95% of the time). If the value is outside of this range, the cause of the change should be identified. Was the last calibration performed correctly? Have any modifications been made to the spirometer hardware? Have any software upgrades or modifications been made? If the source of the problem is found and corrected, the control should be retested to confirm that the instrument performs as expected.

2. *Establish precision of the system.* Include data in the control database that falls within the 2-SD limit. Data outside of 2 SDs may be included if it is clearly caused by variability and not an equipment problem. This may be verified by repeating the test. If the second test produces another result more than 2 SDs from the mean, there is likely an equipment or procedural error. By calculating SDs from repeated measures, the precision of a particular instrument or system can be established.

3. *Use CV to reduce variability.* The coefficient of variation (CV) for most pulmonary function variables should be approximately 5% or less. Some parameters, such as FEF$_{25\%-75\%}$ are more variable in healthy subjects and may show CV values closer to 10%. If the CV is greater than 10%, calibration and testing procedures should be reviewed to see if sources of error can be eliminated.

4. *Compare instruments or laboratories.* Biologic controls can be used to perform interinstrument or interlaboratory evaluation. Similar devices should produce similar control results. However, if different instruments (e.g., a flow-based and a volume-based spirometer) are compared, slightly different values for the same control may be obtained. This difference is the bias between the two systems. The true value for a particular variable (e.g., FVC, DLCO) may be considered the average of the means for the two instruments or laboratories. Alternatively, one instrument may be considered the "gold standard"; the other instrument can be described as having a negative or positive bias, depending on whether its measurement is less than or greater than the gold standard.

5. *Compare methods.* Biologic controls may also be used to compare different methods within the same laboratory. For example, FRC might be measured with a gas dilution technique and by plethysmography. The means, SDs, and CVs of each method can then be compared.

6. *Troubleshooting.* Biologic controls can be used to troubleshoot a problem instrument. For example, if a system produces low DLCO values in several otherwise healthy patients, a problem might exist. Test a biologic control; if the control value is within expected limits, the low DLCO values may be valid.

and standard deviations (SDs) from controls with fewer sets may be used. Pulmonary function variables that are not derived from other measurements should be recorded. These include FVC, FEV$_1$, FRC, and DLCO. Calculated values such as TLC or DL/V$_A$ can also be used; however, if subsequent control tests show significant differences, it may be unclear which component test is at fault. A calculator or a computer spreadsheet may be used to perform the simple statistics required (Table 11-2). Most spreadsheets have built-in functions to calculate mean and SD and to allow data to be graphed. The **coefficient of variation (CV)** may be calculated by dividing the SD by the mean. The **coefficient of repeatability (CR)** may also be calculated. Separate statistics should be calculated for each control and for separate instruments. Data more than 1 or 2 years old should be replaced with more recent measurements to account for small normal changes in pulmonary function that occur over time.

Other Calibration/Quality Control Tools

Sine-Wave Rotary Pump. **Sine-wave rotary pumps** produce a biphasic volume signal. A biphasic or sine-

TABLE 11-2				
Example Spreadsheet for a Biologic Control* **Control subject: J.S.**				
Date	FVC	FEV$_1$	FRC	D$_{LCO}$
2/1/07	4.51	3.93	3.51	25.1
2/15/07	4.61	3.99	3.55	26.2
3/14/07	4.49	3.95	3.65	27.2
3/19/07	4.40	3.90	3.50	25.5
4/21/07	4.57	3.89	3.60	26.0
5/1/07	4.50	3.94	3.66	27.2
5/15/07	4.55	3.95	3.65	27.0
Mean	4.52	3.94	3.59	26.31
SD	0.07	0.03	0.07	0.85
CV	1.49%	0.85%	1.91%	3.21%

*Most spreadsheet programs have built-in functions to calculate means and standard deviations; additional calculations, such as coefficient of variation, can be entered by the user. Quality control charts may be constructed with mean and standard deviation data for each variable.

wave signal may be useful for checking volume and flow accuracy for both inspiration and expiration. A rotary-drive syringe may be useful for checking the frequency response of a spirometer, or to evaluate a spirometer's ability to adequately record tests such as the MVV. Sine-wave pumps are also commonly used in the calibration of body plethysmographs (see Figure 10-19).

Computer-Driven Syringes. These devices incorporate large-volume syringes with a computer-controlled motor drive. Computerized syringes are usually used only by equipment manufacturers or for research applications. The ATS has developed a series of standard waveforms that may be used to drive a computer-controlled syringe. These waveforms are used to validate spirometers and peak flow meters.

Explosive Decompression Devices. Explosive decompression simulates the exponential flow pattern of a forced expiratory maneuver. Such devices use compressed gas, such as carbon dioxide (CO_2), released through an orifice. The gas from the device is injected into a spirometer to generate a simulated forced exhalation. The primary advantage of these devices is that they allow flow and volume signals to be reproduced. When the control signal can be reproduced, both accuracy and precision can be assessed. Using a gas other than air may

not work properly with certain types of flow-sensing spirometers.

In addition to checking the volume and flow accuracy of spirometers, several other important aspects of QC require routine evaluation.

Leak Checks. **Leak checks** should also be performed on volume-based spirometers daily before assessing volume accuracy. The spirometer should be filled with air to approximately half of its capacity and 3 cm H_2O pressure applied with the breathing port occluded. The pressure may be generated by a weight or spring. Any volume loss greater than 30 ml/min is a significant leak and should be corrected before calibration or patient testing.

Flow Resistance. The **back-pressure** from a spirometer should be less than 1.5 cm H_2O up to flows of 14 L/sec. Resistance to flow is measured by placing an accurate manometer or pressure transducer at the patient connection and applying a known flow. This is easily accomplished with flow-sensing devices but somewhat difficult with volume-displacement devices. Measurement of flow resistance is normally performed only when there is some reason to suspect that the spirometer is causing undue resistance. The total resistance requirement must be met with all tubing, valves, and filters in place.

Frequency Response. Frequency response refers to the spirometer's ability to produce accurate volume and flow measurements across a wide range of frequencies. Frequency response is most critical for peak expiratory flow (PEF) and maximal voluntary ventilation (MVV) maneuvers. Frequency response is usually evaluated by means of a sine-wave pump or computer-driven syringe. It should be measured as part of the manufacturer's validation and rechecked if the spirometer is suspect.

Flow. Flow-sensing spirometers directly measure flow and indirectly calculate volume by integration or counting volume pulses. It may be necessary to assess the flow accuracy of such devices. Inaccurate measurement of flow usually results in inaccurate volume determinations. A rotameter (a large calibrated flow-metering device) may be used in conjunction with an adjustable compressed gas source to supply a gas at a known flow to the device. A weighted volume-displacement spirometer, such as a water-seal type, can also be used to generate a known flow. Most commercial flow-sensing spirometers use a volume signal (e.g., a 3-L syringe) to perform software calibration/verification as previously described. It may be useful to check the flow signal from the spirometer at different known flows if the volume accuracy is observed to vary with flow.

Recorder/Displays. Printed records or computer-generated displays of spirometry signals are required for diagnostic functions, validation, or when waveforms are to be measured manually. Table 11-3 lists recommended scale factors and resolutions for both printed graphs and computer displays. Printed copies of volume-time or flow-volume graphs should be available for diagnostic spirometry. Flow-volume curves should be plotted with expired flow in the positive direction on the vertical (y) axis and expired volume from left to right on the horizontal (x) axis. A flow-to-volume aspect ratio of 2:1 should be maintained (i.e., 2 L/sec flow for each 1 L of volume). Accurate recorder speed and volume sensitivity are particularly important if FEV_1 or other flows are calculated manually. Recorder accuracy should be checked at least quarterly, and the accuracy of the timer should be within 2% of the stated value. Paper speed of strip chart recorders can be easily checked with a stopwatch. Mechanical recording devices (e.g., kymographs, strip-chart recorders) may require repair or replacement of drive motors if paper speed is determined to be inaccurate. Most pulmonary function systems are computerized, and printed tracings are generated by ink-jet, thermal, or laser printers. The output of these devices should adhere to the recommended scale factors but often do not. In effect, it may be difficult or impossible to check the timing during forced spirometry using computer-generated tracings.

Gas Analyzers and DLCO Systems

Accurate analysis of inspired and expired gases is required to measure lung volumes, DLCO, and gas exchange during exercise or metabolic testing. The validity of these tests depends on accuracy of both the spirometer and gas analyzers used. Various types of gas analyzers are commonly used in pulmonary function testing (see Chapter 10). Calibration refers to the process of adjusting analyzer output to match the input of a known concentration of gas. QC refers to a method for routinely checking the accuracy and/or precision of the gas analyzer. Important factors related to calibration techniques for gas analyzers include the following.

Physiologic Range

Many gas analyzers are not linear or exhibit poor accuracy over a wide range of gas concentrations. Analyzers should be calibrated to match the physiologic range over which measurements will be made. For example, an oxygen (O_2) analyzer may be used to measure fractional concentrations from 0.00–1.00, representing a wide physiologic range. If the O_2 analyzer is to be used for exercise tests in subjects who are breathing air, an appropriate calibration range might be from 0.12–0.21. This

TABLE 11-3				
Minimum Recommended Scale Factors for Recorders and Displays				
	INSTRUMENT DISPLAY		**PRINTED GRAPHS**	
	Resolution	Scale factor*	Resolution	Scale factor*
Volume	0.05 L	5 mm/L	0.025 L	10 mm/L
Flow	0.20 L/sec	2.5 mm/L/sec	0.10 L/sec	5 mm/L/sec
Time	0.2 sec	10 mm/sec	0.2 sec	20 mm/sec

*Scale factors for flow and volume produce an aspect ratio of 2:1.
Adapted from Miller MR, Hankinson J, Brusasco V, et al: Standardisation of spirometry, *Eur Resp J* 2005; 26:319-338.

narrow interval represents the physiologic range of expired O_2 likely to be encountered during an exercise test in a patient breathing air. Reducing the physiologic range of an analyzer generally allows better accuracy and precision. Some types of analyzers provide range adjustments for this purpose. Calibration gases should represent the extremes of the physiologic range. In the example of the O_2 analyzer described, air and a gas containing 12% O_2 would be appropriate.

Sampling Conditions

Gas analyzers should be calibrated under the same conditions that will be encountered during the test. Analyzers that are sensitive to the partial pressure of gas may be affected by the sample flow rate. For some tests, gas is sampled continuously from the breathing circuit using a pump (e.g., breath-by-breath gas analysis during exercise). Sample flow through the pump must be adjusted before calibration, and then left unchanged during sampling. If gas flow stops before analysis is actually performed (e.g., some types of DLCO systems), sample flow is usually not critical. A gas analyzer in this type of system should be calibrated under conditions of zero flow. Measurement errors may occur if an analyzer is calibrated and then configuration of the sampling circuit is changed. This may happen if tubing, valves, or stopcocks are added or changed. Any gas conditioning devices, such as those used for CO_2, H_2O vapor, or dust, should be in place during calibration as well. If a CO_2 or H_2O absorber is changed, calibration should be repeated.

Two-Point Calibration

The most common technique for analyzer calibration, **two-point calibration**, involves introducing two known gases. One gas is typically used to "zero" or adjust the low end of the range, whereas the second gas is used to "span" or adjust the high end of the range. Adjusting the span is actually setting the gain of the analyzer so that a known input produces a known output. For some pulmonary function tests, the gas to be analyzed is not normally present in expired air (e.g., helium [He], CO, or

neon [Ne]). For such tests, air may be used to zero the analyzer. Calibration gas (cal gas) representing the other end of the physiologic range may be used to span the analyzer. He dilution FRC and DLCOsb are examples of such tests. He and carbon monoxide (CO) analyzers are zeroed by drawing ambient air into the measuring chambers. He and CO are assumed to be absent from the atmosphere. Compressed air from a cylinder or other source may be used instead if there is concern about trace amounts of other gases (e.g., CO_2, CO, argon) in the ambient air. Then calibration gas containing a known concentration of the gas to be analyzed is introduced. The analyzer gain is adjusted to match the known concentration. The calibration gas approximates the concentration to be analyzed during the test. The analyzer may then be rezeroed, and the entire process repeated to verify the calibration. A similar technique may be used with two gases of known concentration if the expirate normally contains varying concentrations of the gas. For example, air and 12% O_2 may be used to perform a two-point calibration of an O_2 analyzer for exercise testing. Depending on the stability of the analyzer, calibration may need to be repeated before (and after) each test or measurement. Gas analyzers should be calibrated before each patient for gas dilution lung volumes, DLCO, exercise tests, and metabolic studies. Gas analyzers used for monitoring (e.g., capnographs) should be calibrated on a schedule appropriate for the extent of use. Calibration should be performed according to the manufacturer's recommendations. The accuracy of the calibration gas should reflect the necessary accuracy of the measurements involved. For exercise or metabolic studies, calibration gases should be accurate to at least two decimal places (i.e., hundredth of a percent). Calibration gases may require verification by an independent method.

Multiple-Point (Linearity) Calibration

An assumption made by a two-point calibration is that analyzer output is linear between the points used. To verify linearity or to determine the pattern of nonlinearity, three or more calibration points

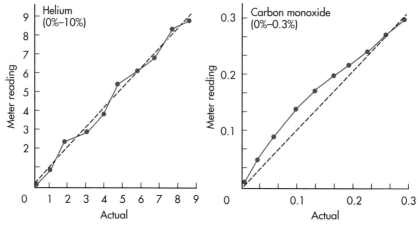

FIGURE 11-2   Calibration and Linearity Check of Gas Analyzers. Two plots of varying gas concentrations (for helium [He] and carbon monoxide [CO]) are shown. Each graph plots the meter reading of the analyzers against the actual concentration of the gas. Different dilutions of each gas are prepared and then analyzed. The He analyzer shows good linearity in the comparison of measured versus expected concentrations. The CO analyzer shows a nonlinear pattern, typical of an infrared analyzer. If enough points are determined, a calibration curve can be generated to correct meter readings. Computerized systems often use an equation or a table of points representing a calibration curve. This allows an analyzer to be calibrated using only two points. Three or more points (gas concentrations) are required to demonstrate linearity.

must be determined (Figure 11-2). A multiple-point calibration is performed in a manner similar to the two-point calibration except that concentrations of known gases across the range to be analyzed are checked and plotted. If multiple points are determined, regression analysis may be used to determine the slope (or type of curve) relating the measured gas concentrations to the expected gas concentrations. A spreadsheet or graphing calculator can be used to analyze the data points. If the analyzer is linear, the points plotted will approximate a straight line. A minimum of three points (i.e., gases) is required to demonstrate linearity. If the analyzer is nonlinear, a calibration curve must be constructed to correct the results. In most instances, an equation describing a nonlinear curve can be generated. This equation can then be used either manually or by software to correct analyzer readings. Most nonlinear analyzers incorporate electronics that linearize their output. Linearity of analyzers used for Dlco, lung volumes, exercise, and metabolic studies should be assessed at least quarterly.

PF TIP

The 3-L calibration syringe can often be used as a lung model to evaluate the accuracy of gas analyzers used for lung volumes or Dlco tests. For example, a Dlco test can be simulated by setting the calibration syringe to a volume of 1 L and then connecting it to the patient port of the pulmonary function system. The syringe is then withdrawn to "inspire" 2 L of test gas. After a 10-second breath hold, the syringe is emptied. This simulates a lung with a total volume (TLC) of 3 L and an inspired volume (VC) of 2 L. With this technique, the Dlco should be close to zero because no diffusion occurred in the syringe.

Dlco Systems

Gas analyzer accuracy and linearity is particularly important in pulmonary function systems that measure Dlco. For measurement of Dlco by the single-breath method, analyzer linearity is more critical than the absolute measurement of gas concentrations. Small errors in which the analyzer outputs for CO and tracer gas are not linear with respect to one another can result in significant errors in the calculation of DLCO. The nonlinearity of each of the analyzers should be 0.5% or less of the full scale. Analyzers used for DLCO tests also need to be stable, with minimal drift (<±0.5% of full scale) between calibration and testing. To detect drift or similar problems during testing, the actual readings of the analyzers should be displayed. Removal of water vapor and CO_2 is usually accomplished by chemical absorbers or related devices (see Chapter 10). Some analyzers use software corrections for the effects of water vapor and CO_2 rather than physically removing or altering the interfering gases.

Quality Control of Gas Analyzers and DLCO Systems. Quality control of gas analyzers can be performed by submitting known concentrations of gases to the analyzer, by testing a lung analog, or by using biologic controls. Several gases with concentrations that span the range of the analyzer can be maintained. This can be a costly means of QC for pulmonary function laboratories. A simpler technique is to prepare **serial dilutions** of a known gas using a large-volume syringe. The syringe may be the type used for volume calibration. For example, 100 ml of He and 900 ml of air may be mixed in a syringe to produce a 10% He mixture which is then injected into the analyzer. Subsequently, 100 ml of He may be diluted in 1000 ml, then 1100 ml, and so on, with the expected concentrations calculated as follows:

$$\text{Expected \% test gas} = \frac{\text{Volume of test gas}}{\text{Total volume of gas}} \times 100$$

where:

Total volume of gas =

test gas + added air + syringe dead space

As each dilution is analyzed, the meter reading is recorded and plotted against the expected percentage (see Figure 11-2). This method is simple and available in most laboratories. Care must be taken when preparing samples so that air does not

leak into the syringe, further diluting the test gas. The volume of air in the syringe connectors (i.e., dead space) must be included when calculating the dilution of the test gas. Some calibrated syringes include their dead space volume.

A second method of verifying analyzer performance involves simulating either lung volume or DLCO tests. This may be accomplished using a lung analog. A **lung analog** is simply an airtight container of known volume. The lung volume simulator is attached at the patient connection with the system set up for a lung volume or DLCO test. A large-volume syringe is used to "ventilate" the lung analog, mimicking the patient's breathing. The resulting lung volume (e.g., FRC) is compared with the known volume of the analog system. A calibration syringe may also be used by itself as the lung analog. Many calibration syringes feature a locking collar that can be adjusted so that only a portion of the syringe's volume can be emptied. With a known volume of air in the syringe, the test is performed by filling and emptying the syringe to the starting volume.

Simulation of the DLCOsb maneuver with a calibration syringe can be used to check analyzer linearity. Both the tracer gas (He, Ne, CH_4) and CO are diluted equally in the syringe, and their relative concentrations should be identical if the two analyzers used are linear with respect to one another. This causes the calculated DLCOsb to be near zero (approximately ±0.3 ml CO/min/mm Hg with a 3-L syringe). If the two analyzers are not linear in relation to one another, the ratio of tracer gas to CO will not equal 1. Calculated DLCOsb may be either slightly above or below zero. This method tests not only the gas analyzers, but also the volume transducer, breathing circuit, and software. Temperature or gas corrections should be disabled. A linearity check at different dilutions can be performed by varying the volume of the calibration syringe. For each different syringe volume, however, the calculated DLCOsb should be close to zero.

A **DLCO simulator** is commercially available (Figure 11-3). This simulator uses precision gas mixtures to allow repeatable DLCO measurements at different levels (e.g., high DLCO, low DLCO). Two large-volume syringes are included; an adjustable

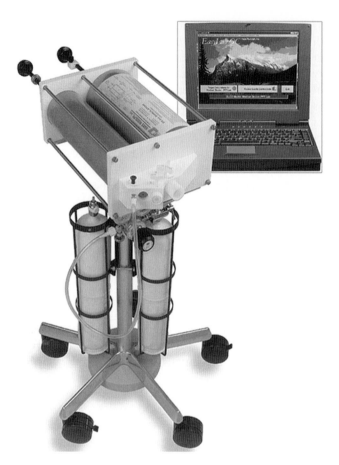

FIGURE 11-3 **DLCO Simulator.** A DLCO simulator that incorporates two large volume syringes and multiple precision gas mixtures provides quality control for DLCO systems. The simulator attaches to the patient port of the DLCO system. Gas is inspired using the large adjustable syringe; this provides a measurement of inspired volume. After a 10-second breath hold, a precision gas that has been loaded into the smaller syringe is emptied into the system for gas analysis. Application software calculates the expected DLCO and compares this to the measured value from the system (see text). *(Courtesy Hans Rudolph, Inc., Kansas City, Mo.).*

5-L syringe provides measured inspiratory volumes. A smaller second syringe is loaded with one of the precision gases; this gas is "exhaled" at the end of the breath-hold interval and sampled by the gas analyzers. Application software calculates the expected DLCO with the known gas concentrations (inspired and expired) along with the inspired volume, breath-hold time, and environmental conditions. The measured DLCO is then compared with the expected value and the percent error reported. By using different precision gases and varying the inspired volume, a range of expected DLCO values can be generated. This type of simulator is most useful for large laboratories with multiple DLCO systems, or for multicenter research applications in which accurate DLCO measurements are critical.

Some computerized pulmonary function systems may make lung simulators difficult to use. The software may be designed to make all necessary corrections for human subjects, giving erroneous results when a simulator is used. However, if the software reports gas analyzer values, the accuracy and linearity of various dilutions can usually be checked.

Testing biologic controls (see Quality Assurance 11-2) is a fourth means of evaluating gas analyzers. This method may not detect small changes in analyzer performance because of day-to-day variability of lung volumes, DLCO, or resting energy expenditure. Despite variability as high as 10% for DLCO or exercise parameters in healthy patients, gas analyzer malfunctions can be detected. Biologic controls may be the simplest means of checking automated exercise/metabolic systems that depend on accurate gas analysis. Abnormal results from biologic controls can suggest which component of the gas analyzer may be faulty (Quality Assurance 11-3).

Body Plethysmographs

The calibration techniques described here apply primarily to variable-pressure, constant-volume plethysmographs. Flow-based plethysmographs may require slightly different calibration procedures for the box transducer. Mouth pressure and pneumotachometer calibrations are similar for both types of plethysmographs.

Mouth Pressure Transducer

Calibration is done by connecting the pressure transducer to a water manometer or a similar device that can generate an accurate pressure. The manometer is a fluid-filled, U-shaped tube with a

---

QUALITY ASSURANCE 11-3

COMMON GAS ANALYZER PROBLEMS

Some problems detected by routine calibration or quality control of gas analyzers include the following:
- Leaks in sample lines or connectors
- Blockage of sample lines
- Exhausted water vapor or CO_2 absorbers
- Exhausted water vapor permeable tubing (Nafion)
- Contamination of photocells or electrodes
- Inadequate warm-up time
- Unstable ambient conditions (chemoluminescence analyzers)
- Deterioration or contamination of column packing material (gas chromatographs)
- Poor vacuum pump performance (emission spectroscopy analyzers)
- Chopper motor malfunction (infrared analyzers)
- Electrolyte or fuel cell exhaustion (O_2 analyzers)
- Aging of detector cells (infrared analyzers)
- Poor optical balance (infrared analyzers)

---

calibration scale that allows very accurate pressures to be generated (see Figure 10-19). Some plethysmographs use a weighted piston to produce a calibration pressure signal. The mouth pressure transducer should be able to accurately record pressures greater than ±50 cm H_2O at frequencies of 8 Hz or more. The actual mouth pressures encountered are often less than this level. Air is injected into one port of the U-tube manometer. For example, a small volume of air may be introduced to cause a deflection of 5 cm. In effect, this creates a difference of 10 cm between the two columns of the manometer. The gain of the mouth pressure amplifier is then adjusted so that its signal display deflects by an amount equivalent to 10 cm H_2O/cm. The display device is most commonly a computer screen. The deflection then equals the calibration factor for the mouth pressure transducer. In the previous example, if a pressure change of 10 cm H_2O resulted in a 1-cm deflection on the display, the calibration "factor" would be 10 cm H_2O/cm. Because almost all plethysmograph systems are computerized, the analog output of the transducers is measured and a software correction factor is determined. The correction (or calibration) factor is calculated in a manner similar to that used for spirometer output (see the section on spirometers). The correction factor is then applied by the software as the mouth pressure signals are acquired.

Box Pressure Transducer

Calibration of the box pressure transducer is accomplished by closing the door of the plethysmograph and applying a volume signal comparable to what occurs during patient testing. In a plethysmograph of 500–700 L, a volume signal of 25–50 ml is typical. The box pressure transducer should be capable of accurately measuring pressures as small as ±0.2 cm H_2O. The box pressure transducer typically requires a range of up to 5–10 cm H_2O to accommodate large changes in box pressure (e.g., thermal drift) An adjustable sine-wave pump connected to a small syringe is ideal for box calibration. A small volume is pumped into and out of the box. With the pump operating, the gain of the box pressure transducer is adjusted so that volume change in the box causes a specific pressure change. For example, if the pressure signal generated by a 30-ml volume change is adjusted to cause a 2-cm deflection on the display, the box pressure calibration factor would be 15 ml/cm. For computerized systems (most plethysmographs), a software calibration factor is derived rather than an actual adjustment of the displayed signal. In other words, no actual adjustment of the output of the box pressure transducer is necessary; the software correction is simply applied to all signals generated during measurements. The calibration procedure may be repeated by adjusting the pump speed from 0.5–8.0 cycles/sec (Hz). Varying the frequency allows the frequency response of the box and transducer to be checked. The volume deflection or calibration factor should not change at frequencies up to 8.0 Hz. Flow-based plethysmographs may be calibrated similarly. The output of the box flow transducer is adjusted (instead of a pressure transducer) to correspond to a known volume change within the plethysmograph chamber. Flow boxes can be used as pressure boxes simply by occluding the flow sensor in the box wall. For plethysmographs that use this method, a box pressure transducer may need calibration as well.

Plethysmographs are normally calibrated empty. A volume correction for the displacement of gas by the patient can be calculated from the patient's weight. This correction is then applied in the calculation of results (see Appendix F).

Flow Transducer

The pneumotachometer (flow sensor) may be calibrated by applying either a known flow or a known volume. A precise flow may be generated with a rotameter or similar calibrated flow meter. Most systems, however, calibrate the pneumotachometer with a 3-L syringe. The flow is integrated, and the gain of the flow signal is then adjusted until the output of the integrator matches the 3-L volume, just as is done for most flow-based spirometers. The flow sensor used in the plethysmograph should meet the volume range and accuracy requirements for spirometers (see Table 11-1). Just as for the box and mouth pressure transducers, a software calibration

factor may be computed rather than physically adjusting the output of the flow sensor. Pressure-differential, heated-wire, or Pitot tube flow sensors may be used (see Chapter 10). Once the flow sensor is calibrated, both volumes and flows (as needed for measurement of Raw) can be measured.

QC of body plethysmographs may be accomplished with one or more of the following: an **isothermal lung analog**, fixed resistors, biologic controls, or comparison with gas dilution or radiologic lung volumes.

An isothermal volume analog can be constructed from a glass bottle or jar of 4–5 L (for adult-size plethysmographs). The jar is filled with metal wool, usually copper or steel. The metal wool acts as a heat sink (Figure 11-4) so that small pressure changes within the jar can be measured with minimal temperature change. The mouth of the bottle is fitted with two connectors. One connector attaches to the mouth shutter (or the patient connection). The other is attached to a rubber bulb with a volume of 50–100 ml (e.g., the bulb from a blood pressure cuff). The actual volume of the lung analog can be determined by subtracting the volume of the metal wool from the volume of the bottle. The volume occupied by metal wool is calculated from its weight times its density. The gas volume of the empty bottle may be measured by filling it with water from a volumetric source. The volume of the connectors and rubber bulb should be added to the total volume.

The accuracy check is performed with an assistant seated in the sealed plethysmograph. The isothermal volume device is connected to the mouthpiece. The mouth shutter is then closed. While the assistant holds his or her breath, the bulb is squeezed at a rate of 1–2 times per second. A P_{MOUTH}/P_{BOX} tangent is recorded just as would be done when testing a patient. Thoracic gas volume (V_{TG}) is calculated as usual, except that PH_2O is not subtracted. The V_{TG} calculated should equal the volume of the isothermal lung analog (as determined previously) within 50 ml or ±3%, whichever is greater. Correction should be made for the assistant's volume (based on body weight) plus the known volume of the isothermal lung analog. The procedure may be repeated by squeezing the bulb

FIGURE 11-4 Isothermal Lung Analog. A schematic of an isothermal lung analog for quality control of the body plethysmograph. A 3-L to 4-L jar or flask is fitted with a stopper with two openings. One opening connects to the mouthpiece shutter apparatus; the other is connected to a rubber hand bulb with an extension tube to the bottom of the jar. Copper or steel wool is used to fill the container. The metal wool acts as a heat sink so that pressure changes in the bottle cause only minimal changes in gas temperature. A patient sits in the plethysmograph, holds his or her breath, and squeezes the bulb. This simulates a VTG maneuver. The P_{MOUTH}/P_{BOX} angle may be recorded, and the volume of the jar calculated. The measured volume should be within 5% of the actual volume. The true volume is determined by filling the container with water and subtracting the volume of the metal wool. The volume of metal wool may be calculated by multiplying its density and its weight. The volumes of the connectors and rubber bulb should be considered as well.

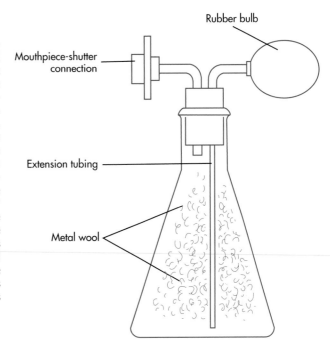

at 0.5–5.0 cycles/sec to check the frequency response of the box. If the box's frequency response is "flat," tangents should not change when the bulb is squeezed at different rates. The lung analog must contain a sufficient mass of metal wool to act as a heat sink (i.e., isothermal). The metal wool "absorbs" changes in temperature that would result from the compression and decompression of gas in the bottle. If there is not enough metal wool, small temperature changes may affect the volume determination. Some manufacturers provide an automated isothermal lung analog that can be placed in the plethysmograph and operated under software control.

The accuracy of the box for measuring airway resistance (Raw) can be assessed with known resistances. A resistor can be made using a plug with a small-diameter orifice. Alternatively, a resistor can be constructed from capillary tubes arranged lengthwise in a flow tube. In either case, the pressure drop across the resistor must be measured at a known flow rate. Some manufacturers supply resistors with known resistances. The resistor is then inserted between the pneumotachometer/

mouth shutter assembly and a test subject. The subject, whose Raw has been previously measured, then has Raw measured with the resistor in place. The increase in measured Raw should approximate that of the resistor.

A simple but effective means of checking plethysmograph function is to measure V_{TG}, Raw, or both from biologic control subjects (see Quality Assurance 11-2). A series of 10–20 box measurements (usually done over a period of days or weeks) provides an appropriate mean value for comparison with subsequent results. Day-to-day variability in trained subjects is usually less than 10%, so changes in FRC_{pleth} that are greater than 10% suggest a problem with the box. This method allows checking of the box, the transducers, the recording devices (if any), as well as the software. A discrepancy between the established mean and an individual QC measurement will detect a problem but may not indicate which component is causing the problem. For example, a control with an established FRC_{pleth} of 3 L is measured again, and the FRC_{pleth} is calculated to be 2 L. The biologic control establishes that there is a problem, but the cause of the discrepancy requires further investigation. In this example, either incorrect calibration of box or mouth pressure transducers or a leaky door seal may be the cause (Quality Assurance 11-4).

A third method of checking plethysmograph accuracy is to compare the V_{TG} with FRC determined by gas dilution. Correlations greater than 0.90 have been demonstrated between gas dilution and plethysmograph lung volumes in healthy individuals. Differences greater than 10% (in healthy individuals) for volumes measured by plethysmograph and gas dilution are not specific but may indicate equipment malfunction. This method, as well as use of biologic controls, is based on measurements of healthy individuals with normal day-to-day variability. It is important that control subjects perform the breathing maneuvers correctly (see Chapter 3).

CALIBRATION AND QUALITY CONTROL OF BLOOD GAS ANALYZERS

Modern blood gas analyzers rely on a microprocessor or computer to control functions such as calibration. The user selects a "calibration sched-

ule" appropriate for the complexity and number of tests performed. For example, in a laboratory that performs many blood gas analyses, automated one-point calibration may be performed every 30 minutes with two-point calibration every 2 hours. Government agencies and some voluntary credentialing organizations have specific schedules for the frequency and type of calibrations that must be performed. Different calibration schedules may be required for different types of blood gas analyzer (e.g., point-of-care devices versus laboratory instruments).

For traditional blood gas electrodes, calibration involves exposing the gas electrodes (i.e., PO_2, PCO_2) to one or two gases (or liquids) with known partial pressures of O_2 and CO_2. If only one gas is used, the calibration is termed a "one-point calibration"; if two gases are used, it is called a "two-point calibration." Similarly, one or two known buffers may be used to calibrate the pH electrode. Calibration gases spanning the physiologic ranges of the PO_2 and PCO_2 electrodes are used, just as for gas analyzers. Typical combinations include one calibration gas with a fractional O_2 concentration of 0.20 (20%) and a fractional CO_2 concentration of 0.05 (5%). A second calibration gas may have a CO_2 concentration of 0.10 (10%) with an O_2 concentration close to zero.

As for gas analyzers, a "low" gas (or buffer solution) is used to zero or balance each electrode. A "high" gas (or buffer) is used to adjust the gain (also called the slope) of the electrode's amplifier. "Electronic" zeroing may be done without exposing the electrode to a gas with a partial pressure of zero. Some blood gas analyzers use this method to zero the PO_2 electrode. Computerized systems allow the user to select how frequently and what type of calibration is performed on the gas and pH electrodes. The PO_2 electrode is usually calibrated over a range of 0–150 mm Hg. The PCO_2 electrode is typically calibrated for the range of 40–80 mm Hg. The pH electrode is usually calibrated using buffers with pH values of 6.840 (low) and 7.384 (high).

Most blood gas analyzers use precision gases to calibrate the gas electrodes, even though gas tensions are measured in liquid (i.e., blood). Some difference may exist when partial pressure of gas is analyzed in gaseous versus liquid medium, especially for O_2. The reduction of O_2 at the tip of the polarographic electrode occurs more rapidly in a gaseous medium than in a liquid. If the electrode is calibrated with a gas, its response when measuring a liquid will be to read slightly lower. This difference is termed the gas-liquid factor. Gas-liquid corrections may be clinically important when measuring high partial pressures of O_2, particularly above 400 mm Hg.

Computerized calibration brings calibration gases or buffers into contact with the electrodes. Electrode responses to the calibration gas or buffer are then stored. The microprocessor compares the measured responses to expected calibration values. The computer then "corrects" the zero and gain (for a two-point calibration) so that measured and expected values match. Most computerized blood gas analyzers compare the current calibration results with the previous calibration. The difference between calibrations is termed **drift** and indicates an electrode's stability.

Automatic calibrations can be programmed to occur at predetermined intervals. Adjustments are performed automatically, based on the response of the electrodes. Because of this, all conditions for an acceptable calibration must be met before the procedure actually begins. Automated blood gas analyzers check most conditions that may affect accurate results, such as temperature of the measuring chamber. During automatic calibration, inadequate buffer or the wrong calibration gas may cause the microprocessor to correct inappropriately for a properly functioning electrode. A similar problem arises if protein contaminates the electrode tip, altering its sensitivity. The microprocessor adjusts the electrode's output in an attempt to bring it into range. This process works well for minor changes in electrode sensitivity. However, electrodes cannot be properly calibrated if they are contaminated with protein, if membranes are damaged, or if the electrolyte is depleted. The user must maintain reagents, calibration gases, and electrodes so that automatic calibration can occur successfully. Systematic errors can sometimes be masked by automatic calibration. Contamination of the calibration gases or buffers is a common example. If the microprocessor adjusts

electrodes to match a contaminated calibration standard, the calibrations appear normal but analysis of control samples will show differences. Detection of these errors usually requires appropriate QC and proficiency testing (described later in this section). Automated blood gas analyzers reduce variability by controlling calibration as well as sample analysis but require careful attention to function appropriately.

Many blood gas analyzers (such as point-of-care devices) use electronic checks of the function of the various sensors (e.g., PO_2, PCO_2). Some analyzers use a combination of electronic checks and traditional calibration methods. Electronic checks are typically performed immediately before sample processing, and some checks are performed during analysis to detect bubbles, clots, and so forth. Electronic checks are sufficient for ensuring proper functioning of sensors such as optodes, spectrophotometers, or fluorescence quenching devices. The adequacy of electronic sensor checks and traditional calibration methods must be demonstrated by appropriate quality controls and calibration verification.

Two methods of QC for blood gas analysis may be used: **tonometry** of whole blood and commercially prepared controls. Although tonometry is no longer commonly used in blood gas laboratories, the method is the basis for commercially prepared controls. Interpretation of blood gas QC is the same for either method.

Tonometry

A tonometer allows precision gas mixtures to be equilibrated with either whole blood or a buffer solution. One type of tonometer creates a thin film of blood or buffer by spinning it in a chamber flooded with precision gas. A second type bubbles gas through the blood or buffer; the bubbles create a large surface for gas exchange. In both types, the tonometer is maintained at 37° C and the gas is humidified. The equilibration time is determined by gas flow and volume of control material. A portion of the blood or buffer is then injected into the blood gas analyzer. The expected gas tensions are calculated from fractional concentrations of the precision gas. If whole blood is used as the control material, only PO_2 and PCO_2 can be checked because pH cannot be easily calculated. Blood is ideal for QC of the gas electrodes because its viscosity and gas exchange properties are the same as those of patient samples. For the most precise control of the PO_2 electrode, tonometry is the method of choice. However, pH cannot be accurately calculated for whole blood because its buffering capacity is usually unknown. Tonometry of a bicarbonate-based buffer using a known fractional concentration of CO_2 allows both gas and pH electrodes to be quality controlled. The gas exchange characteristics of this type of buffer make it less useful than whole blood for QC of PO_2 and PCO_2.

Tonometry can be performed inexpensively with pooled waste blood and small amounts of precision gas. Using pooled blood requires special care. All blood specimens must be handled using standard precautions (see the section on infection control and safety section). QC of the pH electrode requires additional tonometry of a buffer. Three levels of control materials spanning the measuring range of the electrode are recommended. Three precision gas mixtures are therefore required.

Accuracy of tonometry is highly dependent on a standardized technique. Sampling syringes should be lubricated and then flushed with the precision gas. Careful attention to the preparation and sampling from the tonometer is required to obtain reproducible results. The values obtained using tonometry may depend on individual technique. Problems that occur with tonometry include contamination of the precision gas resulting from leaky connections, improper temperature control of the chamber, or inadequate gas flow to achieve equilibrium. Because of the complexity required for multilevel controls for all three electrodes, tonometry is no longer widely used.

Commercially Prepared Controls

There are two types of commercially prepared controls: aqueous and fluorocarbon-based emulsions. The aqueous material is usually a bicarbonate buffer. The fluorocarbon-based control material is a perfluorinated compound that has enhanced O_2-dissolving characteristics. Multiple levels (e.g., acidosis, alkalosis, normal) of these materials provide control over the range of blood gases seen clinically. Aqueous and fluorocarbon-based controls usually contain dyes that generate known absorptions when injected into hemoximeters designed for blood. These dyes allow the materials to be used for QC of blood gases and hemoximetry at the same time.

Both types of controls are packaged in sealed glass ampoules of 2–3 ml volume. They require minimum preparation for use. Aqueous and fluorocarbon-based controls can be stored under refrigeration for long periods or at room temperature for day-to-day use. Most aqueous and fluorocarbon-based controls have shelf lives of 1 year or longer. Each requires agitation for 10–15 seconds before use to ensure equilibration with the gas sealed in the ampoule. Care must be taken when handling the glass ampoules because temperature changes (from the hands) can affect the amount of gas dissolved in the liquid, particularly for O_2. If the ampoules are stored at a temperature significantly different from 25° C, the control values for PO_2 may need to be adjusted. Commercially prepared controls may cost more than samples prepared with tonometry. They are convenient to use, however, and may be less susceptible to handling errors than tonometered materials.

PF TIP

Most laboratories use commercially prepared controls. These controls should be prepared according to the manufacturer's instructions. This usually involves shaking the contents to mix the liquid and gaseous contents of the ampoule. Once opened, the contents should be immediately injected (or aspirated) into the analyzer. Delay in injecting blood gas controls results in PO_2 values drifting toward 150 mm Hg and PCO_2 values drifting toward zero. The temperature at which the ampoule is stored may be needed to correct for small differences in the PO_2 of the control.

One problem with aqueous controls (and to a lesser extent with fluorocarbon solutions) is poor precision of PO_2. The O_2-carrying capacity of these materials is much lower than that of whole blood. Consequently, the PO_2 in the control material changes rapidly on exposure to air. Controls with low PO_2 values (50–60 mm Hg) become quickly contaminated after opening. Aqueous or fluorocarbon controls may produce a wide range of "expected" PO_2 values, limiting their usefulness in detecting an out-of-control device. Some of these difficulties may be overcome by careful statistical evaluation of PO_2 control data as described in this section.

Some analyzers provide automatic measurement of QC materials. In these devices, control materials are contained in cartridges, similar to cartridge-based reagents. Controls are then run on a predetermined schedule with little operator intervention. In most instruments, the auto-QC software can be set to "lock out" the analyzer for those analytes (e.g., pH, PO_2) that fail QC. This prevents the analyzer from being used to report values that might be inaccurate.

A sound statistical method of interpreting "control runs" is necessary to detect blood gas analyzer malfunctions (Quality Assurance 11-5). The most commonly used method for detecting out-of-control situations is calculating the control mean ±2 SDs. A series of runs of the same control material is performed. Twenty to 30 runs provide an adequate base for calculation of the mean and SD (see Appendix F for a sample calculation). One SD on either side of the mean in a normal distribution includes approximately 67% of the data points. Two SDs include 95% of the data points in a normal distribution. Three SDs include 99% of the data points in a normal series. A QC value that falls within ±2 SDs of the mean is usually considered to be "in control." If the control value falls between 2 and 3 SDs from the mean, there is only a 5% chance that the run is in control. The normal variability that occurs when multiple measurements are performed is called **random error**. One of 20 control runs (i.e., 5%) can be expected to produce a result in the 2–3 SD range and still be acceptable. In practice, if a control run shows a value that is more than 2 SDs above or below the mean, the control is

---

QUALITY ASSURANCE 11-5

COMMON BLOOD GAS ANALYZER PROBLEMS

Some problems detected by routine quality control or proficiency testing of blood gas analyzers include the following:

- *Electrode or sensor malfunction.* Protein deposited on membranes or sensors is common and can usually be remedied by cleaning. Leaks in membranes, electrolyte depletion, or sensor failure can cause drift or shifts in performance.
- *Temperature control.* Failure to maintain 37° C in the measuring compartment or thermometer inaccuracy causes QC results to be out of control.
- *Improper calibration.* Problems during calibration are almost always related to inadequate or contaminated buffer or calibration gas. QC data that are consistently high or low may indicate a problem with reagents.
- *Mechanical problems.* Leaks in pump tubing or poorly functioning pumps allow calibrating solutions, controls, and patient samples to be contaminated. Air bubbles introduced during analysis may cause gas tensions to be in error. Inadequate rinsing may also occur with pump problems or improperly functioning valves. This usually results in blood clotting in the transport tubing or measuring chamber.
- *Improper sampling technique.* Failure to anaerobically collect arterial specimens or improperly storing samples (e.g., plastic syringes in ice water), excessive or incorrect anticoagulant, or bubbles in the specimen all may result in questionable results. Another common problem related to sampling is inadvertently obtaining a venous specimen. Adequately functioning electrodes or sensors, as demonstrated by good QC, can distinguish poor sampling from actual clinical abnormalities.

---

usually repeated. If the second run shows a value within 2 SDs of the mean, the first value was probably a random error. Conversely, if the second run produces a result that is similar to the first run (>2 SDs on the same side of the mean), the instrument is probably "out of control." This simple approach works very well for detecting most types of errors that occur in analytical instruments like blood gas analyzers.

More complex sets of rules have been developed to distinguish true out-of-control situations from random errors. A widely used set of rules is that proposed by Westgard (see Selected Bibliography). The rules are selected to provide the greatest probability for detecting real errors and rejecting false errors. This approach to QC is termed the **multiple-rule method**. An example of the multiple-rule method may be applied as follows:

1. When one control observation exceeds the mean ±2 SDs, a "warning" condition exists.
2. When one control observation exceeds the mean ±3 SDs, an out-of-control condition exists.
3. When two consecutive control observations exceed the mean +2 SDs or the mean −2 SDs, an out-of-control condition exists.
4. When the range of differences between consecutive control runs exceeds 4 SDs, an out-of-control condition exists.
5. When four consecutive control observations exceed the mean +1 SD or the mean −1 SD, an out-of-control condition exists.
6. When 10 consecutive control observations fall on the same side of the mean (±), an out-of-control condition exists.

These are just some of the rules that may be applied; not all rules have to be used at all times. Rules 1 and 2 detect marked changes in electrode performance, sometimes called a **shift**, by examining how far from the mean a single control value falls. Rule 3 looks for a shift by comparing two consecutive control runs. Rule 4 looks for shifts in electrode performance by noting excessive variability between consecutive runs. Rules 5 and 6 look for "trends" in instrument response by evaluating an unexpected pattern (i.e., multiple consecutive values on the same side of the mean) in the recent history of control runs.

The multiple-rule method can also be applied when two or more levels of controls are evaluated on the same measurement device (electrode). The rules may be applied by linking multiple levels (e.g., high, normal, low) of control material. For example, if three levels of controls all show values greater

than 2 SDs above their respective means, it is likely that the electrode (sensor) is out of control.

One problem with a strict statistical approach is that if outliers (i.e., values more than 2 SDs from the mean) are sometimes excluded, the SD becomes smaller with repeated calculations. Eventually, valid control data may be rejected. This situation can be managed by including data in the calculations that are clinically acceptable, although they may be more than 2 SDs above or below the mean.

When using the multiple-rule method, it is necessary not only to evaluate the mean and SD of the current control run, but to keep a control history as well. This is often accomplished by means of a control chart (Figure 11-5), also called a Levey-Jennings plot. A graph for each control is created with the mean ±2 SDs on the y-axis and control run number (or time) on the x-axis. Individual controls are then plotted as they are run to track electrode performance.

To provide adequate QC for a blood gas analyzer, three levels of control materials are normally used. Three levels of control for each of the three electrodes (i.e., pH, PCO_2, and PO_2) require that 9 means and 9 SDs must be calculated for each instrument. Controls may also be used for blood oximeters, and this adds more control histories to be managed. When controls are run several times daily, tracking multiple runs can become complex. To simplify this task, computerized QC programs are often used. Such programs are usually included in the software for automated blood gas analyzers. Many laboratory computer systems also support statistical databases for control data. The chief advantages of computerized QC are simplified data storage and maintenance of necessary statistics. Multiple rules can be applied easily to each new control run to detect problems. Computerized records and control charts can be printed. These types of routine QC records are required by many accrediting agencies. (See Appendix D for a list of regulatory agencies.)

QC of blood gas analyzers should be performed on a schedule appropriate for the number of specimens analyzed. In most laboratories, controls must be performed daily or more often. In busy laboratories, multiple levels of controls may be required

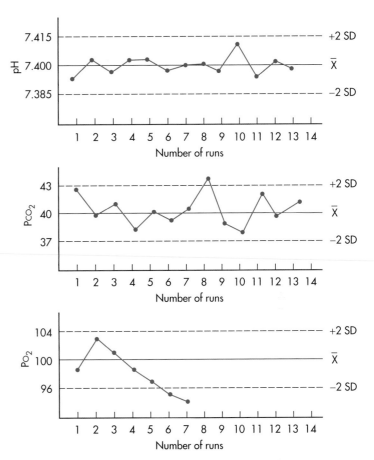

FIGURE 11-5 Blood Gas Quality Control Charts. Three examples of Levey-Jennings charts for pH, P_{CO_2} and P_{O_2}. The mean for each control material is plotted as a solid line, and the ±2 SD lines are dashed. The left y-axis on each graph is labeled with the actual mean and ±2 SD values. Consecutive control runs are plotted on the x-axis. On the pH control chart *(top)* all values vary about the mean in a regular fashion; the electrode appears in control (all values within ±2 SDs) for the 13 measurements plotted. The P_{CO_2} chart *(middle)* shows somewhat more variability. Control run 8 shows a value outside of the ±2 SD range. This may be considered a random error because subsequent controls show normal variability about the mean. The P_{O_2} chart *(bottom)* shows a trend of decreasing control values. Runs 6 and 7 both produce values of more than 2 SDs below the mean. This pattern suggests that the electrode or sensor is malfunctioning and needs to be serviced. By applying multiple rules (see text) to the interpretation of consecutive control runs, with or without charts, most out-of-control situations can be detected.

on each shift. QC is also usually required after any significant maintenance is performed in order to verify proper function of the instrument.

In addition to providing regular checks of acceptable instrument performance, routine QC establishes the precision (variability) of each measurement. Instrument precision must be determined so that blood gas interpretation can be related to a range of values. For example, the variability of the P_{O_2} measurement for a specific analyzer may be determined to be ±6 mm Hg (i.e., 2 SDs) around a mean of 50 mm Hg. Each P_{O_2} result (near 50 mm Hg) can then be interpreted with some certainty that it is within 6 mm Hg of the reported value.

Several other techniques related to QC of blood gas analyzers are commonly used. Interlaboratory comparison of control results can compare the performance of similar instruments for measuring the same lot of control materials. Manufacturers of control materials and some voluntary credentialing agencies provide such interlaboratory databases. Each laboratory submits its control values for a specific period, usually once per month. The laboratory then receives a report showing its performance related to all participating laboratories. This type of comparison is useful for detecting systematic errors that may go unnoticed when running daily controls.

Interlaboratory proficiency testing (PT) consists of comparing unknown control specimens from a single source in multiple laboratories. This allows an individual laboratory to compare its results with other laboratories using similar methods. Results from laboratories that used different methods (e.g., analyzers) may also be compared. Results of proficiency testing are usually reported as means and SDs for each instrument participating in the program. Proficiency testing does not measure day-to-day precision, as does daily QC. However, it provides a measure of the absolute accuracy of the individual laboratory. An analyzer may have acceptable precision as determined by daily QC but be inaccurate when compared with analyzers from other laboratories. Proficiency testing often detects systematic errors that occur because of improper calibration, contaminated reagents, or procedural problems. Multiple levels of unknowns (for PT) are usually provided to check the range of values seen in clinical practice. Proficiency testing programs are available from professional organizations such as the College of American Pathologists, as well as from commercial vendors. Satisfactory performance on interlaboratory proficiency testing has been mandated by the U.S. Department of Health and Human Services under the Clinical Laboratory Improvement Amendment of 1988 (see Appendix D).

CRITERIA FOR ACCEPTABILITY AND REPEATABILITY OF PULMONARY FUNCTION STUDIES

Quality assurance in the pulmonary function laboratory requires not only appropriate calibration, verification, and QC, but also careful attention to how the data are obtained (i.e., testing techniques). Testing technique may be compared with "sampling" technique in other laboratory sciences. In pulmonary function testing, sampling refers to procedures used to obtain patient data. How the data are obtained becomes extremely important because many of the tests performed are effort dependent. Eliciting maximal effort and cooperation from the patient is often just as critical as correct performance of the equipment. Applying objective criteria to determine the validity of data is one means of providing high-quality results.

Using Criteria for Acceptability/Repeatability

Criteria for assessing the validity of various tests have been described in Chapters 2 through 9.

Standards for pulmonary function testing have been published by the American Thoracic Society (ATS) in conjunction with the European Respiratory Society (ERS). Clinical practice guidelines for pulmonary function testing have also been developed by the American Association for Respiratory Care (AARC).

Criteria for acceptability have three primary uses:

1. To provide a basis for decision making during testing. Standards or guidelines can be used to decide whether equipment is functioning properly, whether the patient is giving maximal effort, or whether testing should be continued or repeated. Standardized criteria also help to characterize the types of problems known to occur during specific tests (e.g., poor effort during spirometry).
2. To evaluate validity of pulmonary function data from an individual patient. Criteria may be applied by the technologist performing the test, by computer software, or by the clinician responsible for interpretation. This may consist of assigning a letter grade or a code to individual efforts or tests.
3. To score or evaluate the performance of the technologist. Many pulmonary function tests, especially spirometry, depend on the interaction between technologist and patient. Criteria for acceptability can be used to gauge the performance of individual technologists and to provide objective feedback.

Implementation of a quality assurance program in the pulmonary function laboratory should use acceptability and repeatability criteria during and after testing, both to evaluate individual tests and to provide feedback for technologists. For each of these, certain procedures will be similar.

Examine Printed Tracings or Displayed Graphics Whenever Available

Compare the observed tracing with the characteristics of an acceptable curve or pattern. Computer graphic displays make this particularly easy and can usually display tracings in real time. Graphics may be superimposed or displayed side-by-side to assess patient effort and cooperation. Similarly, expected values can be displayed graphically along with each individual effort. The user should be able to modify the graphic display (e.g., change graphing scale) to allow for extremes such as very low flows or volumes. During testing, graphs of multiple efforts should be available. Storage of graphic data (all acceptable maneuvers) may be useful for assessing data quality after testing has been completed. Some portable (office) spirometers may not display graphics of volume-time or flow-volume curves during testing, but are able to print graphics. In these cases the printed graphs may be used to assess test quality.

Look at Numerical Data

Are the largest values from multiple efforts within the accepted range of repeatability? The decision to perform additional maneuvers is usually based on repeatability. Most manufacturers provide software that applies current standard guidelines for repeatability. Data from multiple efforts should be maintained during testing to allow selection of appropriate results for the final report. Storage of all efforts may be necessary for subsequent review or editing. Data that are not repeatable may be valid (i.e., usable) but need to be identified as such.

Evaluate Key Indicators

Most pulmonary function tests have one or two features that determine whether the test was performed acceptably. For spirometry, the start-of-test and duration of effort are key indicators. For gas dilution lung volumes, absence of leaks and test duration are key indicators. For DLCOsb, inspired volumes and breath-hold times are important. Key indicators vary with the method used for specific tests. In each instance, the important indicator should be assessed in relation to an accepted standard. During testing, these indicators help to determine whether additional patient instruction or tests are needed. Key indicators are also useful in assessing what factors might influence the interpretation of the test (e.g., the patient was unable to blow out for 6 seconds).

Check for Consistent Results

The results of various tests should be consistent with the clinical history and presentation of the patient. Spirometry, lung volumes, DLCO, and blood gas values should all suggest a similar interpretation for a specific diagnosis. Discrepancies among tests may indicate a technical problem rather than a clinical condition.

Technologist's Comments

Scoring or grading the quality of a patient's test is an important component of quality assurance for pulmonary function testing. The technologist administering the test can accomplish this by adding notes. Some automated spirometers use software that grades test performance or that includes codes denoting problems with the test. Evaluation of spirometry, lung volumes, DLCO, and any other tests performed should be included.

The technologist's comments or notes can usually be added to the test results. The commentary should be based on standardized criteria. If a particular test meets all criteria, that fact should be stated. Failure to meet any of the laboratory's criteria should be documented as well. The reason the patient was unable to perform the test acceptably should be explained whenever possible. Failure to meet criteria for acceptability does not necessarily invalidate a test. For some patients, their best performance may fail one or more of the criteria. Table 11-4 lists examples of statements that may be used to document test quality.

The technologist's comments can be included in the final report. Many automated systems provide for "free text" comments to be included with tabular data. Some software supports "canned text" functions that allow predetermined statements (see Table 11-4) to be entered with a single keystroke. The technologist's name or initials should be included. The technologist's comments should be clearly identified to avoid confusion with the physician's interpretation.

Some computerized spirometer systems automatically score FVC maneuvers. The score may be

TABLE 11-4	

Technologist's Comments (Examples)*

Test	Comments
Spirometry	Meets all ATS/ERS recommendations.
	Poor start of test or patient effort.
	Expiration did not last 6 seconds, or no obvious plateau.
	Back-extrapolated volume was >5% of FVC.
	Patient was unable to continue to exhale because of _____.
	Two best FVC maneuvers were not within 150 ml.
	Two best FEV_1 maneuvers were not within 150 ml.
	MVV does not correlate with FEV_1.
Lung volumes (gas dilution)	Lung volumes by _ (method) _ meet ATS/ERS recommendations.
	Lung volumes reported were the average of (n) FRC determinations.
	Slow VC was (greater/less) than FVC (____ %).
	Lung volumes were unacceptable because of a leak.
	Equilibration not reached within 7 minutes—He dilution.
	Alveolar N_2 > 1.5% after 7 minutes—N_2 washout.
Plethysmography	All plethysmographic measurements met ATS/ERS recommendations.
	FRC_{pleth} measurements were variable.
	Raw measurements were variable.
	Patient was unable to pant at the correct frequency.
DLCOsb	Meets all ATS/ERS recommendations.
	DLCO reported is average of (n) maneuvers.
	Predicted DLCO corrected for an Hb of _____.
	Inspired volume < 85% of best VC (_____ %).
	Breath-hold time not within 8–12 seconds (_____ seconds).
	DLCO values not within 3 ml CO/min/mm Hg or 10%.
	DLCO not corrected for Hb or COHb.

*Values in parentheses may be filled in with appropriate values from the patient's data.

indicated by a letter or numeric code that is attached to each maneuver. For example, an FVC maneuver that meets all criteria (e.g., start-of-test) might be scored with an "A." Other systems allow the technologist to select a user-defined code to attach to individual maneuvers. Both techniques can be used to provide feedback that enhances quality assurance.

Technologist's Feedback

A well-trained and highly motivated technologist is a key component for obtaining valid data, particularly in tests that require patient instruction and encouragement. A quality assurance program based on established criteria for acceptability and repeatability can be used to provide feedback on test performance to individuals conducting the tests.

Routine review of tests performed by each technologist is recommended. If criteria for acceptability and repeatability have been recorded (as described in this section), these can be used to grade the performance of the technologist. This information forms the basis for reinforcing superior performance or correcting identified problems. Feedback should include the type and extent of unacceptable or nonrepeatable tests. Feedback should also include what corrective action can be taken to improve performance. Feedback needs to be ongoing to maintain a high level of proficiency. For research applications or in clinical trials, review of test data and performance, along with feedback to the personnel conducting the tests, may be necessary to provide the highest quality results.

INFECTION CONTROL AND SAFETY

Pulmonary function tests, including blood gas analysis, often involve patients with blood-borne or respiratory pathogens. Reasonable precautions applied to testing techniques and equipment handling can prevent cross-contamination among patients. Similar techniques can prevent infection of the technologist performing the tests.

Policies and Procedures

Each laboratory should have written guidelines defining safety and infection control practices. The guidelines should be part of a policy and procedure manual (see Box 11-1). Procedures should include, but not be limited to, handwashing techniques, use of protective equipment such as laboratory coats and gloves, and guidelines for equipment cleaning. The handling of contaminated materials (e.g., waste blood) should be clearly described. Policies and procedures should include education of technologists regarding proper handling of biologic hazards. Department policies and procedures should be consistent with those mandated by individual hospitals or institutions. Most accrediting agencies require written plans for safety, waste management, and chemical hygiene. In the United States, the Occupational Safety and Health Administration (OSHA) has published strict guidelines regarding handling of blood and other medical waste (see Appendix D).

Pulmonary Function Tests

Pulmonary function testing does not present a significant risk of infection for patients or technologists. However, some potential hazards are involved. Most respiratory pathogens are spread by either direct contact with contaminated equipment or by an airborne route. Airborne organisms may be contained in droplet nuclei, on epithelial cells that have been shed, or in dust particles. The following guidelines can help reduce the possibility of cross-contamination or infection:

1. Disposable mouthpieces and nose clips should be used for spirometry. Reusable mouthpieces should be disinfected or sterilized after each use. Proper handwashing should be done immediately after direct contact with mouthpieces or valves. Gloves should be worn when handling potentially contaminated equipment. Hands should always be washed between patients, and after removing gloves.

2. Tubing or valves through which subjects rebreathe should be changed after each test. Any equipment that shows visual condensation from expired gas should be disinfected before reuse. This is particularly important for maneuvers such as the FVC, where there is a potential for mucus, saliva, or droplet nuclei to contaminate the device. Breathing circuit components should be stored in sealed containers (e.g., plastic bags) after disinfection.

3. Spirometers should be cleaned according to the manufacturer's recommendations. The frequency of cleaning should be appropriate for the number of tests performed. For open-circuit systems, only that part of the circuit through which air is rebreathed needs to be decontaminated between patients. Some flow-based systems offer pneumotachometers that can be changed between patients. These may be advantageous if patients with known respiratory infections must be tested. Pneumotachometers not located proximal to the patient are less likely to be contaminated by mucus, saliva, or droplet nuclei. Disposable flow sensors should not be reused. Volume-displacement spirometers should be flushed using their full volume at least five times between patients. Flushing with room air helps clear droplet nuclei or similar airborne particulates. Water-sealed spirometers should be drained at least weekly, allowed to dry completely, and refilled only with distilled water. Bellows and rolling-seal spirometers may be more difficult to disassemble but should be disinfected on a

routine basis. After disassembly and disinfection, the spirometer may require recalibration.

4. Bacteria filters may be used in some circuits to prevent equipment contamination. Systems used for spirometry, lung volumes, and diffusing capacity tests often use breathing manifolds that are susceptible to contamination. Bacteria filters may be used to prevent contamination of these devices. Filters may impose increased resistance, affecting measurement of maximal flows as well as airway resistance or conductance. Some types of filters show increased resistance after continued use in expired gas. Spirometers with bacteria filters should be calibrated with the filter in line; the spirometer should meet the minimal recommendations in Table 11-1 with the filter in place. If filters are used for procedures such as lung volume determinations, their volumes must be included in the calculations. Filters may be useful in protecting equipment from contamination when patients with known respiratory pathogens must be tested.

5. Small-volume nebulizers, such as those used for bronchodilator administration or bronchial challenge, offer the greatest potential for cross-contamination. These devices, if reused, should be sterilized to destroy vegetative microorganisms, fungal spores, tubercle bacilli, and some viruses. Disposable single-use nebulizers are preferable but may not be practical for routines such as inhalation challenges. Metered-dose devices may be used for bronchodilator studies by using disposable mouthpieces or "spacers" to prevent colonization of the device.

6. Gloves or other barrier devices minimize the risk of infection for the technologist who must handle mouthpieces, tubing, or valves. The risk of transmission from subjects with hepatitis B, human immunodeficiency virus (HIV), or acquired immunodeficiency syndrome (AIDS) through respiratory secretions is slight. Special precautions should be taken whenever there is evidence of blood on mouthpieces or tubing. There is a risk of acquiring infections such as tuberculosis or pneumonia caused by *Pneumocystis carinii* from infected patients. The technologist should wear a mask when testing subjects who have active tuberculosis or other diseases that can be transmitted by coughing. Masks may be required for "reverse isolation" when testing immunocompromised patients.

7. Patients with respiratory diseases such as tuberculosis may warrant specially ventilated rooms, particularly if many individuals need testing. Risk of cross-contamination or infection can be greatly reduced by filtering and increasing the exchange rate of air in the testing room. Equipment can be reserved for testing only infected patients. Patients with known pathogens can also be tested in their own rooms or at the end of the day (to facilitate equipment decontamination).

8. Surveillance may include cultures of reusable components, such as mouthpieces, tubing, and valves, after disinfection.

Blood Gases

The Centers for Disease Control and Prevention (CDC) has established standard precautions that apply to personnel handling blood or other body fluids containing blood. Standard precautions apply to blood, semen, vaginal secretions, cerebrospinal fluid, synovial fluid, pleural fluid, pericardial fluid, and amniotic fluid. Some of these fluids (i.e., blood) are commonly encountered in the blood gas or pulmonary function laboratory. These fluids present a significant risk to the health care worker. Hepatitis B, HIV, and other blood-borne pathogens must be assumed to be present in these fluids.

PF TIP

The two most important practices for infection control in the pulmonary function laboratory are proper use of gloves and handwashing. Gloves should be worn any time blood is handled or drawn, including handling of blood-tinged mouthpieces. Handwashing is essential to prevent cross-contamination. Hands should be washed between patient contacts; any time mouthpieces, tubing, or nebulizers are handled; and when gloves are removed.

Body fluids to which the standard precautions do NOT apply include feces, nasal secretions, sputum, sweat, tears, urine, and vomitus, unless they contain visible blood. Some of these fluids may be encountered in the pulmonary function laboratory. These fluids present an extremely low or nonexistent risk for HIV or hepatitis B. However, they are potential sources for nosocomial infections from other non–blood-borne pathogens. Standard precautions do not apply to saliva, but infection control practices such as use of gloves and handwashing further minimize the risk involved in contact with mucous membranes of the mouth.

These standard precautions should be applied in the pulmonary function and/or blood gas laboratory:

1. Treat *all* blood and body fluid specimens as potentially contaminated.
2. Exercise care to prevent injuries from needles, scalpels, or other sharp instruments. Do not resheath used needles by hand. If a needle must be resheathed, use a one-handed technique or a device that holds the sheath. Do not remove used, unprotected needles from disposable syringes by hand. Do not bend, break, or otherwise manipulate used needles by hand. Use a rubber block or cork to obstruct used needles after arterial punctures. Use needle safety devices (now used in almost all blood gas kits) as described by the manufacturer. Place used syringes and needles, scalpel blades, and other sharp items in puncture-resistant containers. Locate the containers as close as possible to the area of use.
3. Use protective barriers to prevent exposure to blood, body fluids containing visible blood, and other fluids to which standard precautions apply. Examples of protective barriers include gloves, gowns, laboratory coats, masks, and protective eyewear. Gloves should be worn when drawing blood samples, whether from a needle puncture or an indwelling catheter. Gloves cannot prevent penetrating injuries caused by needles or sharp objects. Gloves are also indicated if the technologist has cuts, scratches, or other breaks in the skin. Protective barriers should be used in situations where contamination with blood may occur. These situations include obtaining blood samples from an uncooperative patient, performing finger-heel sticks on infants, and receiving training in blood drawing. Examination gloves should be worn for procedures involving contact with mucous membranes. Masks, gowns, and protective goggles may be indicated for procedures that present a possibility of blood splashing. Blood splashing may occur during arterial line placement or when drawing samples from arterial catheters.
4. Wear gloves while performing blood gas analysis. Laboratory coats or aprons that are resistant to liquids should also be worn. Protective eyewear may be necessary if there is risk of blood splashing during specimen handling. Maintenance of blood gas analyzers, such as repair of electrodes and emptying of waste containers, should be performed wearing similar protective gear. Laboratory coats or aprons should be left in the specimen handling area. Blood waste products (e.g., blood gas syringes) should be discarded in clearly marked biohazard containers.
5. Immediately and thoroughly wash hands and other skin surfaces that are contaminated with blood or other fluids to which the standard precautions apply. Hands should be washed after removing gloves. Blood spills should be cleaned up using a solution of 1 part 5% sodium hypochlorite (bleach) in 9 parts of water. Bleach should also be used to rinse sinks used for blood disposal.

Summary

- Calibration and verification of spirometers, gas analyzers, and body plethysmographs is discussed. Special emphasis is placed on techniques to ensure that pulmonary function equipment meets established standards of accuracy. QC methods are reviewed, including the use of large-volume syringes, biologic controls, and lung simulators.
- Calibration and QC of blood gas analyzers are discussed, as well as advantages and disadvantages of automated calibration.

- Basic statistical concepts commonly used in laboratory situations are covered, including the application of multiple control rules.
- Testing technique is a key element in ensuring the validity of pulmonary function data. Some guidelines for applying acceptability and repeatability criteria (as listed throughout the text) are given. These include decision making during testing, assessing test quality for interpretive purposes,

and providing feedback on technologist performance.
- Infection control and safety issues are presented. Cleaning of spirometers and related equipment, along with techniques to avoid cross-contamination, are listed. Standard precautions applicable to blood gas analysis and pulmonary function testing are reviewed. Case studies and self-assessment questions are also included.

CASE 11-1

Case Studies

 This case describes the use of blood gas QC to detect analytical errors.

HISTORY

F.F. is a 30-year-old man who works as a firefighter. He is referred for pulmonary function testing and arterial blood gas analysis as part of a 5-year physical examination required by the fire district for which he works. He has no symptoms or history suggestive of pulmonary disease. He has never smoked. He performed all portions of the spirometry, lung volumes, and D_{LCO} maneuvers acceptably. All results were within normal limits for his age and height. Arterial blood gases were drawn for analysis.

Blood Gases

FIO_2	0.21
pH	7.41
$PaCO_2$ (mm Hg)	39
PaO_2 (mm Hg)	54
HCO_3^- (mEq/L)	24.1
Hb (g/dl)	15.1
SaO_2 (%)	96.0
COHb (%)	1.4
MetHb (%)	0.2

Because of the low PaO_2 in an otherwise normal patient and because SaO_2 measured independently

by hemoximetry showed normal saturation, the PO_2 measurement of the automated blood gas analyzer was questioned.

A review of the two most recent automatic calibrations revealed the following:

	Calibration	Expected	Drift
9 AM			
pH	7.387	7.384	0.003
PCO_2 (mm Hg)	39.1	38.6	0.5
PO_2 (mm Hg)	132.0	140.1	−8.1
10 AM			
pH	7.383	7.384	−0.001
PCO_2 (mm Hg)	38.4	38.6	−0.2
PO_2 (mm Hg)	151.2	140.1	11.1

For each automatic calibration, the instrument analyzes a calibration gas or buffer and compares the measured value with an expected value based on the local barometric pressure. Drift is the amount of adjustment applied to a particular electrode to bring it within the expected calibration limits. The drift exhibited by the PO_2 electrode prompted a review of the most recent QC runs performed on the analyzer.

Blood Gas Quality Control (Five Most Recent Runs)

Control	Mean (mm Hg)	SD	Runs* 1	2	3	4	5
Level A	45	±2.1	46	47	49	42	50
Level B	100	±2.0	101	99	97	96	105
Level C	150	±3.1	147	151	151	149	143

*Control runs performed every 8 hours.

QUESTIONS

1. What are the possible explanations for the patient's low P_{O_2}?
2. What is the significance of the 9 AM and 10 AM automated calibrations for the blood gas analyzer?
3. What do the routine QC runs show?
4. What corrective action, if any, might be necessary?

DISCUSSION

Explanation of the Low P_{O_2}

The low P_{O_2} might be caused by lung disease or might be an erroneous reading from the automated blood gas analyzer. An abnormally low Pa_{O_2} in an otherwise healthy person with normal lung function suggests that an analytical error might have occurred. The findings in this case regarding the P_{O_2} electrode function are not unusual. The P_{O_2} is the sole abnormal value; even the Sa_{O_2} measured from the same specimen (but using hemoximetry) shows a normal result. If the patient had been seen with evidence of lung disease or abnormalities in his pulmonary function test, the inaccuracy of the Pa_{O_2} might not have been questioned, resulting in inappropriate O_2 therapy.

Automatic Blood Gas Analyzer Calibrations

Excessive drift of the O_2 electrode should have prompted the immediate attention of the technologist performing the blood gas analyses. A common problem with automated analyzers is their apparent simplicity. Because calibrations are performed automatically, corrections that the analyzer makes may be overlooked. Automated analyzers adjust the zero and gain of each electrode or sensor to correct for small changes that occur in electrode performance. These small changes may be caused by a buildup of protein on the electrode, electrolyte depletion, or slight temperature alterations. If there is a large change in electrode performance, the instrument attempts to "correct" the electrode's output just as it would for small changes that occur normally. Some automated analyzers flag a large drift in electrode performance as an error, whereas others simply report the drift. In this case, the reported drifts indicated that the P_{O_2} electrode seemed to be fluctuating markedly. One calibration reading was high, and the next one read lower than the expected value.

Quality Controls

The change in electrode performance should have been detected by the routine QC run before the excessive drift was observed during automatic calibration. Blood gas QC used in this laboratory consisted of multiple levels of control materials. Means and SDs had been determined for each level.

Examination of control runs 1 through 4 reveal acceptable electrode performance. All values are within ±2 SDs of the mean. Run 5 (the most recent run) shows values that are all 2 SDs or more away from the mean. These control results may be expected to occur 5% of the time simply because of the random error associated with sampling. If run 5 is compared with the previous 4 runs and multiple rules are applied (see the section on calibration and quality control of blood gas analyzers), the electrode is clearly out of control. When multiple levels of controls are evaluated, more than one control value outside of the 2-SD limit suggests an out-of-control situation. For both levels A and B, there is a change of 4 SDs from run 4 to run 5. Changes of this magnitude are not consistent with random error and are detected only when a control history is kept. Similarly, there are inconsistencies within run 5 across the three levels of controls. Levels A and B both show control values that are more than 2 SDs above their respective means, but level C shows a value that is more than 2 SDs below its mean. This pattern suggests fluctuating electrode performance, as displayed during the automatic calibrations that followed.

Corrective Action

The P_{O_2} electrode was removed and inspected. A new membrane was installed and the electrode was refilled with fresh electrolyte. The instrument was recalibrated, and multiple levels of controls were repeated. All P_{O_2} values fell within 2 SDs of the established mean. Another specimen was drawn from the patient, and a Pa_{O_2} value of 89 mm Hg was obtained.

CASE 11-2

Case Studies

 This case addresses the use of biologic controls in the pulmonary function laboratory.

HISTORY

Pulmonary function studies are performed on three consecutive patients, each of whom has a chief complaint of shortness of breath. The following data are obtained:

	Patient 1	Patient 2	Patient 3
FVC	4.04 (101%)	5.22 (97%)	3.90 (83%)
FEV$_1$	3.51 (99%)	4.10 (103%)	3.12 (82%)
FEV$_{1\%}$	87%	79%	80%
TLC	5.11 (98%)	6.96 (100%)	5.01 (81%)
DLCO*	14.3 (69%)	18.2 (65%)	10.2 (50%)

*Percent of predicted values corrected for Hb.

The pulmonary function technologist notices that each patient has apparently normal spirometry and lung volumes, but their DLCO values are reduced.

QUESTIONS

1. Is the reduction in DLCO representative of the actual lung function of each patient, or has a technical problem occurred?
2. What can be done to evaluate the accuracy of the DLCO system?
3. What (if anything) needs to be done to correct the problem?

DISCUSSION

Has a Technical Problem Occurred?

This type of situation arises frequently in the pulmonary function laboratory when patients with possible pulmonary disease are being evaluated. The technologist is this case noticed a pattern in which three patients all had apparently normal results from spirometry and lung volume measurements but displayed reduced DLCO values. Careful attention to inconsistencies in different categories of tests can often point to technical problems with spirometers, gas analyzers, or software. In this case, it is difficult to determine whether the low DLCO values may be due to a physiologic abnormality or a technical problem with the DLCO system.

Evaluating the DLCO System

The first step in assessing a possible technical error would be to look for problems with the DLCO measurement system. In this case, pretest calibrations and all other system functions appeared to be acceptable. This facility used a monthly program of testing laboratory personnel as biologic controls. Each of three technologists performed spirometry, lung volumes, and DLCO measurements on one another to establish representative means and standard deviations. The technologist in this case tested one of the biologic controls before performing any further tests on patients and obtained the following values:

	Control Subject	Expected Value (Control History)
DLCO mlCO/min/mm Hg	18.5	27.1 ± 1.5

The biologic control's DLCO had been established from a series of 22 previous measurements. The measured value from the control subject is lower than 3 SDs below the expected value (i.e., $27.1 - 4.5 = 22.6$). This simple comparison suggests that the DLCO system is malfunctioning and that the results obtained from the three patients in question were most likely erroneous.

What Needs to Be Done?

The use of a biologic control in this case demonstrated that the DLCO system was not functioning properly. This suggests that the low DLCO values obtained from three apparently normal patients do not represent real disease. Although the comparison with a biologic control subject showed that there was a problem, it did not define exactly what was causing the low values.

This laboratory was fortunate to have access to a DLCO simulator (see Figure 11-3) as described previously. Simulations were performed with two different levels of precision gases. The simulator showed DLCO values that were similarly reduced in comparison to the expected values. Examination of the measured CO and tracer gas concentrations with the simulator revealed that the CO values were significantly larger than expected, resulting in low calculated DLCO. The faulty gas analyzer was replaced before any further patient testing was conducted. Both biologic controls and simulations showed acceptable DLCO values after replacement of the analyzer.

SELF-ASSESSMENT QUESTIONS

Entry-level

1. A pulmonary function technologist is checking a small portable spirometer that uses disposable flow sensors. Repeated injections from a 3-L syringe produce the following results:

   3.24 L
   3.30 L
   3.29 L

   Which of the following best describes these results?
   a. The flow sensor is defective
   b. Spirometer shows excessive drift
   c. Volume is being corrected to BTPS
   d. Volumes were injected too rapidly

2. QC is performed on a blood gas analyzer. The PCO_2 electrode shows the following results when plotted on a QC chart (Levey-Jennings):

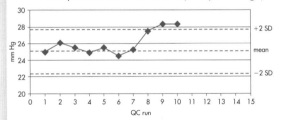

   Which of the following best describes the result of control run 10?
   a. An out-of-control situation
   b. A trend
   c. A random error
   d. Normal electrode performance

3. A 3-L syringe is used to check the calibration of a dry rolling-seal spirometer and the following values are obtained:

Injection	Result
1	2.90
2	3.03
3	2.95
4	3.06

   These results indicate that the spirometer
   a. Is functioning properly
   b. Shows excessive drift
   c. Has a significant leak
   d. Has a seal that is sticking

4. Which of the following should the pulmonary function technologist do when drawing an arterial blood sample?
   I. Use eye protection if there is a possibility of blood splashing
   II. Check the patient history to see if protective barriers are needed
   III. Wear gloves while drawing and analyzing the specimen
   IV. Dispose of needles and syringes in red plastic bags marked "Biohazard"
   a. I and III
   b. II and IV
   c. I, II, and III
   d. I, III, and IV

5. After performing eight FVC maneuvers these results are recorded from the three best efforts:

	Trial 2	Trial 5	Trial 7
FVC (L)	4.90	5.41	4.79
FEV₁ (L)	1.91	2.01	1.88
PEF (L/sec)	4.90	4.41	4.67

   Which of the following comments should the pulmonary function technologist use to describe the patient's spirometry?
   a. "Spirometry meets all ATS/ERS criteria"
   b. "FVC is not repeatable"
   c. "FEV_1 is not repeatable"
   d. "Peak flow is not repeatable"

Advanced

6. Daily maintenance of a body plethysmograph should include which of the following:
   I. Calibration of the box pressure transducer
   II. Calibration of the flow sensor (pneumotachometer)
   III. Checking the mouth pressure transducer against a known standard
   IV. Quality control using an isothermal lung analog
   a. I and III only
   b. II and IV only
   c. I and II only
   d. I, III, and IV

7. A biologic control subject performs multiple FRC_{pleth} maneuvers to check the accuracy of a variable-pressure body box. The control subject's established FRC is 3.60 L with an SD of 0.15 L. The following FRC values are obtained from the control:
4.55 L
4.45 L
4.49 L
Based on these findings, the pulmonary function technologist should conclude that:
   a. The plethysmograph is functioning within acceptable limits
   b. The plethysmograph door seal has a small leak
   c. The mouth pressure transducer has not been calibrated correctly
   d. The flow sensor has not been calibrated correctly

8. Which of the following can be used to verify the function of an automated D_{LCO} system?
   I. D_{LCO} simulator
   II. Biologic control subjects
   III. Isothermal lung analog
   IV. 3-L syringe
      a. I, II, and III
      b. II, III, and IV
      c. I, II, and IV
      d. I and III only

9. Which of the following are most likely to cause cross-contamination in the pulmonary function laboratory?
   a. Disposable mouthpieces and nose clips
   b. Volume-displacement spirometers
   c. Flow-sensing spirometers
   d. Nebulizers used for bronchial challenge

10. A pulmonary function technologist simulates D_{LCO}sb maneuvers using a 3-L calibration syringe. She turns the BTPS correction off but all other settings are configured as for patient testing. Three maneuvers produce the following results:
Trial 1: 0.13 mlCO/min/mm Hg
Trial 2: −0.20 mlCO/min/mm Hg
Trial 3: 0.11 mlCO/min/mm Hg
On the basis of these results the technologist should conclude that
   a. BTPS corrections should have been on to simulate D_{LCO}
   b. The CO analyzer is malfunctioning
   c. The signal from the tracer gas analyzer is not linear
   d. The gas analyzers are functioning properly

Selected Bibliography

GENERAL REFERENCES

American Thoracic Society: *Pulmonary function laboratory management manual,* ed 2, New York, 2005, American Thoracic Society.

Wanger J: Quality assurance, *Respir Care Clin North Am* 1997; 3:273-289.

CALIBRATION AND QUALITY CONTROL

Enright PL: How to make sure your spirometry tests are of good quality, *Respir Care* 2003; 48:773-776.

Ferguson GT, Enright PL, Buist AS et al: Office spirometry for lung health assessment in adults: a consensus statement from the National Lung Health Education Program, *Respir Care* 2000; 45:513-530.

Kozlowski-Templin R: Blood gas analyzers, *Respir Care Clin North Am* 1995; 1:35-46.

Krarup T: New QC process validates new blood gas technology at each measurement, *Clin Chim Acta* 2001; 307:75-85.

Leith DE, Mead J: *Principles of body plethysmography,* Bethesda, Md, 1974, National Heart, Lung, and Blood Institute, Division of Lung Diseases.

Liistro G, Vanwelde C, Vincken W et al: Technical and functional assessment of 10 office spirometers; a multicenter comparative study, *Chest* 2006; 130:657-665.

Multiple and Westgard rules. http://www.westgard.com/mltirule.htm. Accessed February 17, 2007.

Olafsdottir E, Westgard JO, Ehrmeyer SS et al: Matrix effects and the performance and selection of quality-control procedures to monitor PO_2 measurements, *Clin Chem* 1996; 42:392-396.

Townsend MC, Hankinson JL, Lindesmith LA et al: Is my lung function really that good? Flow-type spirometer problems that elevate test results. *Chest* 2004; 125:1902-1909.

Westgard JO, Groth T, Aronsson T et al: Performance characteristics of rules for internal quality control: probabilities for false rejection and error detection, *Clin Chem* 1977; 23:1857.

CRITERIA FOR ACCEPTABILITY OF PULMONARY FUNCTION STUDIES

Enright PL, Johnson LJ, Connett JE et al: Spirometry in the Lung Health Study: methods and quality control, *Am Rev Respir Dis* 1991; 143:1215-1223.

Ferris BG, ed: Epidemiology standardization project: recommended standardized procedures for pulmonary function testing, *Am Rev Respir Dis* 1978; 118 (suppl 2):55.

Gardner RM, Clausen JL, Crapo RO et al: Quality assurance in pulmonary function laboratories, *Am Rev Respir Dis* 1986; 134:626-627.

Gardner RM, Clausen JL, Epler GR et al: Pulmonary function laboratory personnel qualifications, *Am Rev Respir Dis* 1986; 134:623-624.

INFECTION CONTROL

Canakis A-M, Ho S, Kovack D, Ho B et al: Does the in-line filter on the spirometer protect the patient? Comparing cross-infection risks of six respiratory filters, *Am J Respir Crit Care Med* 2001; 163:A373.

Centers for Disease Control and Prevention: Guidelines for preventing the transmission of *Mycobacterium tuberculosis* in health care facilities, *MMWR Morb Mortal Wkly Rep* 1994; 43:1-132.

Centers for Disease Control and Prevention: Recommendations for preventing transmission of human immunodeficiency virus and hepatitis B virus to patients during exposure-prone invasive procedures, *MMWR Recomm Rep* 1991; 40:1-9.

Johns DP, Ingram C, Booth H et al: Effect of a microaerosol barrier filter on the measurement of lung function, *Chest* 1995; 107:1045-1048.

Kendrick AH, Johns DP, Leeming JP: Infection control of lung function equipment: a practical approach, *Respir Med* 2003; 97:1163-1179.

Rutala DR, Rutala WA, Weber DR et al: Infection risks associated with spirometry, *Infect Control Hospital Epidemiol* 1991; 12:89-92.

Standard precautions. http://www.cdc.gov/ncidod/dhqp/gl_isolation_standard.html Last updated: April 1, 2005. Accessed February 17, 2007.

STANDARDS AND GUIDELINES

American Association for Respiratory Care: Clinical practice guideline: blood gas analysis and hemoximetry: 2001 revision and update, *Respir Care* 2001; 46:498-505.

American Association for Respiratory Care: Clinical practice guideline: body plethysmography: 2001 revision and update, *Respir Care* 2001; 46:506-513.

American Association for Respiratory Care: Clinical practice guideline: sampling for arterial blood gas analysis, *Respir Care* 1992; 37:913-917.

American Association for Respiratory Care: Clinical practice guideline: spirometry, 1996 update, *Respir Care* 1996; 41:629-636.

American Association for Respiratory Care: Clinical practice guideline: static lung volumes 2001 revision and update, *Respir Care* 2001; 46:531-539.

American Association for Respiratory Care: Single-breath carbon monoxide diffusing capacity, 1999 update, *Respir Care* 1999; 44:539-546.

Clinical Laboratory Standards Institute: *C46-A blood gas and pH analysis and related measurements,* Approved guideline, 2001, Wayne, PA.

Clinical Laboratory Standards Institute: *H11-A4 Percutaneous collection of arterial blood for laboratory analysis,* ed 4, Approved standard, 2004, Wayne, PA.

Clinical Laboratory Standards Institute: *HS4-A, Application of a quality system model for respiratory services: approved guideline,* Wayne, PA, NCCLS, 2002.

Clinical Laboratory Standards Institute: *M29-A2 Protection of laboratory workers from occupationally acquired infection,* ed 2, 2001, Wayne, PA.

MacIntyre N, Crapo RO, Viegi G et al: Standardisation of the single-breath determination of carbon monoxide uptake in the lung, *Eur Respir J* 2005; 26:720-735.

Miller MR, Crapo RO, Hankinson J et al: General considerations for lung function testing, *Eur Respir J* 2005; 26:153-161.

Miller MR, Hankinson J, Brusasco V et al: Standardisation of spirometry, *Eur Respir J* 2005; 26:319-338.

Wanger J, Clausen JL, Coates A et al: Standardisation of the measurement of lung volumes, *Eur Respir J* 2005; 26:511-522.

Answers to Self-Assessment Questions

Chapter 1

1. c
2. b
3. c
4. b
5. b
6. a
7. c
8. c
9. b
10. d
11. d
12. b
13. a
14. b

Chapter 2

1. b
2. c
3. c
4. b
5. b
6. d
7. b
8. c
9. b
10. c
11. d

12. c
13. a
14. c

Chapter 3

1. a
2. c
3. b
4. c
5. c
6. c
7. c
8. c
9. c
10. b
11. d
12. d

Chapter 4

1. b
2. c
3. c
4. b
5. a
6. d
7. d
8. a

9. c
10. a

Chapter 5

1. b
2. d
3. d
4. b
5. c
6. c
7. d
8. b
9. a
10. c

Chapter 6

1. a
2. c
3. c
4. c
5. b
6. c
7. b
8. d
9. c
10. a

Chapter 7

1. c
2. b
3. c
4. b
5. c
6. d
7. a
8. c
9. c
10. d
11. c
12. a

Chapter 8

1. b
2. b
3. b
4. a
5. d
6. b
7. c

8. d
9. c
10. d

Chapter 9

1. a
2. c
3. d
4. c
5. c
6. d
7. c
8. d
9. a
10. d

Chapter 10

1. c
2. c
3. b
4. c

5. b
6. d
7. a
8. c
9. d
10. d
11. b
12. a
13. c
14. d
15. d

Chapter 11

1. c
2. a
3. a
4. a
5. b
6. c
7. c
8. c
9. d
10. d

Reference Values

TYPICAL VALUES FOR PULMONARY FUNCTION TESTS

Values are for a healthy young male, $1.7\,m^2$ body surface area.

Test	Value
Lung Volumes (BTPS)	
IC	3.60 L
ERV	1.20 L
VC	4.80 L
RV	1.20 L
FRC	2.40 L
VTG	2.40 L
TLC	6.00 L
(RV/TLC) × 100	20%
Resting Ventilation (BTPS)	
V_T	0.50 L
Frequency	12 breaths/min
$\dot{V}_E$	6.00 L/min
V_D	0.15 L
$\dot{V}_A$	4.20 L/min
V_D/V_T	0.30
Spirometry and Pulmonary Mechanics	
FVC	4.80 L
FEV_1	4.00 L
$FEV_{1\%}$	83%
$FEF_{25\%-75\%}$	4.7 L/sec
$Vmax_{50}$	5.0 L/sec
PEF	10.0 L/sec
MVV	160 L/min
C_L	0.2 L/cm H_2O
C_{LT}	0.1 L/cm H_2O
Raw	1.5 cm H_2O/L/sec
sGaw	0.25 L/sec/cm H_2O
MIP	130 cm H_2O
MEP	250 cm H_2O

Test	Value
Gas Distribution	
$\Delta N2_{750-1250}$	<1.5% N_2
7-minute N_2	<2.5% N_2
Diffusion	
DLCOsb	25 ml CO/min/mm Hg
DL/V_A	4.2 ml CO/min/mm Hg/L
Blood Gases and Related Tests	
pH	7.40
$PaCO_2$	40 mm Hg
HCO_3^-	24.0 mEq/L
PaO_2	95 mm Hg
SaO_2	97%
COHb	<1.5%
MetHb	<1.5%
$\dot{Q}_S/\dot{Q}_T$	<7%

SELECTING AND USING REFERENCE VALUES

Reference values for pulmonary function tests are derived by statistical analysis of a population of healthy subjects. These subjects are classified as healthy because they have no history of lung disease in themselves or their families. Minimal exposure to risk factors, such as smoking or environmental pollution, is usually considered in selecting these individuals.

All lung function measurements vary in healthy individuals. Some tests vary much more than others. Arterial pH and $PaCO_2$ have a very narrow range in healthy individuals. However, $FEF_{25\%-75\%}$ may vary by as much as ±2 L/sec. This variability becomes important when measured values are compared with reference values. Most measurements regress; that is, they vary in a predictable way in relation to one or more physical factors. The physical characteristics that most influence pulmonary function are as follows:

- Age
- Sex
- Height (standing/sitting)
- Race or ethnic origin
- Weight or body surface area

The altitude at which individuals reside may also influence their lung function. By analyzing each pulmonary function variable in regard to the individual's physical characteristics, regression equations can be generated to predict the expected value. For many pulmonary function variables, lung function is linearly related to physical characteristics such as age and height. This may not be true in individuals who are very old or young, or very tall or short. Adolescents during the "growth spurt" display changing lung function that does not fit a linear model.

Race or ethnic origin influences stature and body proportions. Lung function, particularly lung volumes and diffusing capacity (DLCO), differs significantly among races. Some computerized pulmonary function systems apply a "correction factor" to reference values for whites to adjust for different races. Although differences in lung function among races are well documented, no single correction factor is applicable to all measurements. Some laboratories reduce reference values for volumes (e.g., FVC, TLC) by factors of 10%–15% for African Americans. Separate regression equations derived from healthy individuals of each race tested are preferred. Race-specific reference values should be used if they are representative of the population the laboratory tests. In the United States, the NHANES III reference set is recommended for whites, African Americans, and Hispanic Americans.

Several methods for applying reference values are used:

- Tables of reference values
- Nomograms
- Graphs
- Regression equations used in calculators or software

Tables, nomograms, and graphs are used infrequently because of the widespread availability of computerized systems. Peak flow meters and other simple devices designed for use outside the clinic or laboratory sometimes use a nomogram or printed graph to allow the user to look up a predicted value. The use of computers (or calculators) allows regression equations to be available in software. In most automated systems, the user selects sets of prediction equations best suited to the population being tested. Some software allows users to enter their own equations or modify published equations. This provides a means of adding new reference equations as they become available.

Establishing the lower limit of normal (LLN) should be done by analyzing some measure (e.g., FVC, FEV_1) in healthy subjects and then determining the variability of that measurement. In clinical medicine, the fifth percentile is often defined as the LLN because it represents the segment of healthy subjects farthest below the average. Even though subjects in the fifth percentile are healthy, they are arbitrarily defined as "abnormal" for clinical purposes. Figure B-1 depicts the predicted and the lower limit of normal (LLN) for white females from ages 8–80 years (NHANES III). It is noteworthy that the statistical LLN is approximately the same across the adult age range.

Some clinicians use a fixed percentage (measured value divided by the reference value × 100) of the reference value to determine the degree of abnormality. Eighty percent (80%) is often used as the limit of normal. Unfortunately, this method leads to errors because the variability around the predicted value is relatively constant in adults. In other words, the scatter of normal values does not vary with the size of the predicted value. Figure B-2 illustrates why using fixed percentages, such as 80% of the predicted, can lead to misclassification. In tall, young subjects 80% of the predicted is often less than the fifth percentile; using 80% as the limit can allow a patient who really does have decreased lung function (in the fifth percentile or lower) to be misclassified as normal. This situation is a false-negative result; the patient has disease but the test does not indicate abnormality. Similarly, an elderly patient who is short may have a lung function

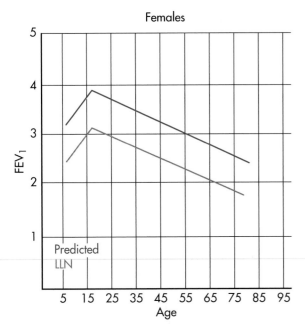

FIGURE B-1   Predicted and Lower Limit of Normal.
The predicted FEV$_1$ for females aged 8 – 80 years is shown by the upper line *(blue)* based on the third National Health and Nutrition Evaluation Survey (NHANES III) regression equations for white adults. The lower line *(gray)* represents the statistical lower limit of normal (LLN) for the same group. FEV$_1$ increases from age 8 years to age 18 years in females and then declines from ages 18–80 years, with the LLN showing a similar pattern. The LLN line represents the 95th percentile.

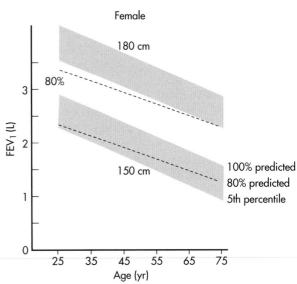

FIGURE B-2   Bias Introduced by Using Percents of Predicted. The graph illustrates the fall in predicted FEV$_1$ for tall (180 cm) and short (150 cm) females with age. The shaded areas represent the "normal" range from 100% of the predicted value down to the fifth percentile. The *dashed line* shows a fixed percentage of the predicted— in this case 80%, as is sometimes used to represent the lower limit of normal. For a young tall female, 80% is less than the statistical lower limit. A subject with a low FEV$_1$ (below the fifth percentile) might still be above 80% of predicted; this would result in a false-negative finding on spirometry. Similarly, a short, older female might have an FEV$_1$ below 80% of predicted and be considered to have disease when her FEV$_1$ is actually above the fifth percentile. In this instance the result is false-positive. Similar bias occurs when percents of predicted are used from adult males because the variability of FEV$_1$ (and other pulmonary function parameters) does not tend to vary with the size of the predicted value. Clinical decisions should be based on well-defined lower limits of normal rather than fixed percents of predicted (in adults).

parameter that is less than 80% of predicted but well within the statistically normal range (above the fifth percentile). This short elderly subject would be misclassified as having lung disease when in fact she is within the "normal" range (i.e., a false-positive result). Using percents of predicted introduces both age and height biases. The situation is slightly different in children because the variability of lung function measures tends to change proportionately with the size of the predicted value. For this reason, percents of predicted may be appropriate for classifying lung function in children.

A more statistically sound approach for classifying abnormality is to compute the z-score or standard deviation score (SDS). If lung function varies in a normal fashion (a Gaussian or bell-shaped distribution curve), the mean ±1.96 standard deviations (SDs) defines the 95% confidence interval. Statistically, 95% of the healthy population falls within approximately 2 SDs of the mean. The remaining subjects fall into either the highest or lowest 2.5% of the distribution. The z-score or SDS can be calculated easily if the variability (residual standard deviation) of the reference population is known:

$$z\text{-score} = \frac{(\text{measured} - \text{predicted})}{\text{RSD}}$$

where:

RSD = residual standard deviation

The RSD is the normal variability that remains when all other sources of variability have been accounted for in the regression. If an individual's z-score is less than −1.65, there is only a 5% chance that the test result is normal. If the z-score is less than −1.96, the measured value is found in only 2.5% of healthy subjects.

For example, consider a male subject who is 70 years old and 69 inches (175 cm) tall. His FEV_1 is measured as 2.40 L; his predicted FEV_1 is 3.12 L. His FEV_1 is 77% of predicted; is this abnormal? Using 80% as the cut-off suggests that this patient has mild lung disease. However, if the patient's z-score is calculated as:

$$z\text{-score} = \frac{(2.40 - 3.12)}{0.468}$$
$$= \frac{-0.72}{0.468}$$
$$= -1.53$$

where 0.468 is the residual standard deviation from the reference population, the z-score of −1.53 suggests that this subject is above the fifth percentile and likely has normal lung function. The advantage of z-scores is that they can be used for any index that is normally distributed. Because the z-score accounts for the variability occurring in healthy subjects, it tells how common, or uncommon, the finding may be in the patient being studied.

For many pulmonary function variables, only the lower limit of normal (i.e., below the mean) is significant. For example, it is not usually clinically significant if FVC is greater than predicted, only if it is lower. For normally distributed variables, 1.645 × RSD can be considered the LLN. Variables that can be abnormally high or low (e.g., RV, TLC, $PaCO_2$) must consider the upper limit of normal (ULN) in a similar manner.

The lower limit of normal can be easily calculated when the variable of interest (e.g., FEV_1, FVC) is normally distributed in the population. Using the fifth percentile to define the LLN, however, does not require the pulmonary function variable to be normally distributed in the population. Simple counts can determine the level for a specific variable that separates the lowest 5% of the subjects from the remainder. Lower limits of normal using the fifth percentile are sometimes defined for specific groupings of age or gender.

There are several areas in which the definition of lung function abnormality may have important clinical consequences. One such area is the use of a fixed ratio to define airway obstruction, as is frequently done with the FEV_1/FVC (FEV_1/VC). Some clinicians use 70% as a cut-off, with ratios less than this value defining the presence of airway obstruction. However, because the FEV_1/FVC ratio falls with age (sex, height, and ethnicity also may play a role), using a fixed ratio may misclassify younger subjects as normal and older subjects as obstructed. Similarly, using fixed percentages of predicted (e.g., 80%, 50%) to categorize the severity of obstruction may misclassify subjects who are young and tall or old and short (as discussed in a preceding paragraph). These misapplications of fixed ratios and fixed percents of predicted can have serious consequences for individual patients and for large groups of subjects when research is involved. Misclassifying an elderly subject as having COPD may mean inappropriate prescription of drugs that can have serious side effects. Using an inappropriate classification, such as an FEV_1/FVC ratio of 70%, to exclude subjects from a clinical trial (because they are incorrectly classified as "obstructed") means that otherwise healthy subjects are not exposed to the treatment or drug being evaluated.

Pulmonary function laboratories should try to choose reference studies from a population similar to the patients they test. The following factors may be considerations in selecting reference values:

1. *Type of equipment used for the reference study:* Does equipment comply with the most recent recommendations of the American Thoracic Society and European Respiratory Society? (See Chapter 11.)
2. *Methodology:* Were standardized procedures used in the reference study similar to those to be used, particularly for spirometry, lung volumes, and D_{LCO}?
3. *Reference population:* What were the ranges of ages of the individuals in the reference population?

Were both males and females tested? Did the study generate different regressions for different ethnic origins? Did the study include smokers or other "at-risk" individuals as healthy individuals? If a specific group of subjects was studied, are the results applicable to the population in general?

4. *Statistical analysis:* Are lower limits of normal specifically defined (e.g., fifth percentile, 1.645 × RSD)? Are adequate measures of variability available (RSD, SEE) so that upper or lower limits of normal can be calculated along with the predicted values?

5. *Conditions of the study:* Was the study performed at a different altitude or under significantly different environmental conditions?

6. *Published reference equations:* Do reference values generated using the study's regressions differ markedly from other published references?

Individual laboratories may wish to perform measurements on subjects who represent a healthy cross-section of the population that the laboratory usually tests. Doing this in a statistically meaningful way may require testing a large number of subjects. However, measured values from these individuals can then be compared with expected values using various reference equations. Equations that produce the smallest average differences (measured – predicted) may be preferable. Evaluation of a small number of individuals may not show much difference between equations for FVC and FEV_1. However, there may be noticeable discrepancies for DLCO or maximal flows. Equations for spirometry, lung volumes, and DLCO should be taken from a single reference, if possible. If healthy individuals fall outside the limits of normal, the laboratory should examine its test methods, how the individuals were selected, and the prediction equations being used.

There are no universally accepted reference values. Several excellent studies are available that address most of the considerations listed previously. In the United States, the NHANES III reference equations (Hankinson) are recommended for subjects between the ages of 8 and 80 years for spirometry, and the equations of Wang et al. for children ages 6–8 years. References for lung volumes and DLCO must be selected based on the criteria listed in the preceding paragraphs. The reference sets included here are widely used and compare favorably with other published studies. Other acceptable studies are included in the Selected Bibliography. Laboratories are encouraged to evaluate these and other equations in selecting references.

PREDICTION REGRESSIONS FOR PULMONARY FUNCTION TESTS

Values are BTPS unless otherwise noted.

- Tables B-1 and B-2 show coefficients for calculating predicted values and lower limits of normal (LLN) for commonly used spirometric variables. Table B-3 includes the coefficients for calculating the FEV_1/FVC ratio and the FEV_6/FVC ratio, as well as their lower limits of normal. The format of the equations is included at the bottom of each table.

- Tables B-4 and B-5 show regression equations for calculating lung volumes, DLCOsb, and other pulmonary function parameters; height is in inches and age is in years unless otherwise noted.

- Tables B-6 and B-7 include regression equations for spirometry, lung volumes, and DLCO in children.

TABLE B-1

NHANES III[1] Prediction and Lower Limit of Normal Equations for Spirometric Parameters for Males*
(Height in centimeters and age in years)

Males	Intercept	Age	Age^2	Ht$_{PRD}$(cm)^2	Ht$_{LLN}$(cm)^2	R^2
White < 20 Years of Age						
FEV$_1$	−0.7453	−0.04106	0.004477	0.00014098	0.00011607	0.8510
FEV$_6$	−0.3119	−0.18612	0.009717	0.00018188	0.00015323	0.8692
FVC	−0.2584	−0.20415	0.010133	0.00018642	0.00015695	0.8668
PEF	−0.5962	−0.12357	0.013135	0.00024962	0.00017635	0.7808
FEF$_{25\%-75\%}$	−1.0863	0.13939		0.00010345	0.00005294	0.5601
White 20 Years of Age						
FEV$_1$	0.5536	−0.01303	−0.000172	0.00014098	0.00011607	0.8510
FEV$_6$	0.1102	−0.00842	−0.000223	0.00018188	0.00015323	0.8692
FVC	−0.1933	0.00064	−0.000269	0.00018642	0.00015695	0.8668
PEF	1.0523	0.08272	−0.001301	0.00024962	0.00017635	0.7808
FEF$_{25\%-75\%}$	2.7006	−0.04995		0.00010345	0.00005294	0.5601
African American < 20 Years of Age						
FEV$_1$	−0.7048	−0.05711	0.004316	0.00013194	0.00010561	0.8080
FEV$_6$	−0.5525	−0.14107	0.007241	0.00016429	0.00013499	0.8297
FVC	−0.4971	−0.15497	0.007701	0.00016643	0.00013670	0.8303
PEF	−0.2684	−0.28016	0.018202	0.00027333	0.00018938	0.7299
FEF$_{25\%-75\%}$	−1.1627	0.12314		0.00010461	0.00004819	0.4724
African American 20 Years of Age						
FEV$_1$	0.3411	−0.02309		0.00013194	0.00010561	0.8080
FEV$_6$	−0.0547	−0.02114		0.00016429	0.00013499	0.8297
FVC	−0.1517	−0.01821		0.00016643	0.00013670	0.8303
PEF	2.2257	−0.04082		0.00027333	0.00018938	0.7299
FEF$_{25\%-75\%}$	2.1477	−0.04238		0.00010461	0.00004819	0.4724
Mexican American < 20 Years of Age						
FEV$_1$	−0.8218	−0.04248	0.004291	0.00015104	0.00012670	0.8536
FEV$_6$	−0.6646	−0.11270	0.007306	0.00017840	0.00015029	0.8657
FVC	−0.7571	−0.09520	0.006619	0.00017823	0.00014947	0.8641
PEF	−0.9537	−0.19602	0.014497	0.00030243	0.00021833	0.7530
FEF$_{25\%-75\%}$	−1.3592	0.10529		0.00014473	0.00009020	0.5482
Mexican American 20 Years of Age						
FEV$_1$	0.6306	−0.02928		0.00015104	0.00012670	0.8536
FEV$_6$	0.5757	−0.02860		0.00017840	0.00015029	0.8657
FVC	0.2376	−0.00891	−0.000182	0.00017823	0.00014947	0.8641
PEF	0.0870	0.06580	−0.001195	0.00030243	0.00021833	0.7530
FEF$_{25\%-75\%}$	1.7503	−0.05018		0.00014473	0.00009020	0.5482

*Ht$_{PRD}$ coefficient is used for prediction equation, and Ht$_{LLN}$ is used (replaces Ht$_{PRD}$) for the lower limit of normal equation.
Lung function parameter = $b_0 + b_1 \times$ age + $b_2 \times$ age^2 + $b_3 \times$ height^2.

TABLE B-2

NHANES III[1] Prediction and Lower Limit of Normal Equations for Spirometric Parameters for Females* (Height in centimeters and age in years)

Females	Intercept	Age	Age^2	Ht$_{PRD}$(cm)^2	Ht$_{LLN}$(cm)^2	R^2
White < 18 Years of Age						
FEV$_1$	−0.8710	0.06537		0.00011496	0.00009283	0.7494
FEV$_6$	−1.1925	0.06544		0.00014395	0.00011827	0.7457
FVC	−1.2082	0.05916		0.00014815	0.00012198	0.7344
PEF	−3.6181	0.60644	−0.016846	0.00018623	0.00012148	0.5559
FEF$_{25\%-75\%}$	−2.5824	0.52490	−0.015309	0.00006982	0.00002302	0.5005
White 18 Years of Age						
FEV$_1$	0.4333	−0.00361	0.000194	0.00011496	0.00009283	0.7494
FEV$_6$	−0.1373	0.01317	−0.000352	0.00014395	0.00011827	0.7457
FVC	−0.3560	0.01870	−0.000382	0.00014815	0.00012198	0.7344
PEF	0.9267	0.06929	−0.001031	0.00018623	0.00012148	0.5559
FEF$_{25\%-75\%}$	2.3670	−0.01904	−0.000200	0.00006982	0.00002302	0.5005
African American < 18 Years of Age						
FEV$_1$	−0.9630	0.05799		0.00010846	0.00008546	0.6687
FEV$_6$	−0.6370	−0.04243	0.003508	0.00013497	0.00010848	0.6615
FVC	−0.6166	−0.04687	0.003602	0.00013606	0.00010916	0.6536
PEF	−1.2398	0.16375		0.00019746	0.00012160	0.4736
FEF$_{25\%-75\%}$	−2.5379	0.43755	−0.012154	0.00008572	0.00003380	0.3787
African American 18 Years of Age						
FEV$_1$	0.3433	−0.01283	−0.000097	0.00010846	0.00008546	0.6687
FEV$_6$	−0.1981	0.00047	−0.000230	0.00013497	0.00010848	0.6615
FVC	−0.3039	0.00536	−0.000265	0.00013606	0.00010916	0.6536
PEF	1.3597	0.03458	−0.000847	0.00019746	0.00012160	0.4736
FEF$_{25\%-75\%}$	2.0828	−0.03793		0.00008572	0.00003380	0.3787
Mexican American < 18 Years of Age						
FEV$_1$	−0.9641	0.06490		0.00012154	0.00009890	0.7268
FEV$_6$	−1.2410	0.07625		0.00014106	0.00011480	0.7208
FVC	−1.2507	0.07501		0.00014246	0.00011570	0.7103
PEF	−3.2549	0.47495	−0.013193	0.00022203	0.00014611	0.4669
FEF$_{25\%-75\%}$	−2.1825	0.42451	−0.012415	0.00009610	0.00004594	0.4305
Mexican American 18 Years of Age						
FEV$_1$	0.4529	−0.01178	−0.000113	0.00012154	0.00009890	0.7268
FEV$_6$	0.2033	0.00020	−0.000232	0.00014106	0.00011480	0.7208
FVC	0.1210	0.00307	−0.000237	0.00014246	0.00011570	0.7103
PEF	0.2401	0.06174	−0.001023	0.00022203	0.00014611	0.4669
FEF$_{25\%-75\%}$	1.7456	−0.01195	−0.000291	0.00009610	0.00004594	4.4305

*Ht$_{PRD}$ coefficient is used for prediction equation, and Ht$_{LLN}$ is used (replaces Ht$_{PRD}$) for the lower limit of normal equation.
Lung function parameter = $b_0 + b_1 \times age + b_2 \times age^2 + b_3 \times height^2$.

TABLE B-3

NHANES III[1] Prediction and Lower Limit of Normal Equations for $FEV_1/FEV_6\%$ and $FEV_1/FVC\%$ for Male and Females* (Age in years)

	Intercept$_{PRD}$	Age	Intercept$_{LLN}$	R^2
Males				
White				
$FEV_1/FEV_6\%$	87.340	−0.1382	78.372	0.2151
$FEV_1/FVC\%$	88.066	−0.2066	78.388	0.3448
African American				
$FEV_1/FEV_6\%$	88.841	−0.1305	78.979	0.0937
$FEV_1/FVC\%$	89.239	−0.1828	78.822	0.1538
Mexican American				
$FEV_1/FEV_6\%$	89.388	−0.1534	80.810	0.1711
$FEV_1/FVC\%$	90.024	−0.2186	80.925	0.2713
Females				
White				
$FEV_1/FEV_6\%$	90.107	−0.1563	81.307	0.3048
$FEV_1/FVC\%$	90.809	−0.2125	81.015	0.3955
African American				
$FEV_1/FEV_6\%$	91.229	−0.1558	81.396	0.1693
$FEV_1/FVC\%$	91.655	−0.2039	80.978	0.2284
Mexican American				
$FEV_1/FEV_6\%$	91.664	−0.1670	83.034	0.2449
$FEV_1/FVC\%$	93.360	−0.2248	83.044	0.3352

*Intercept$_{PRD}$ coefficient is used for prediction equation, and intercept$_{LLN}$ is used (replaces intercept$_{PRD}$) for the lower limit of normal equation.
Lung function parameter = $b_0 + b_1 \times$ age.

TABLE B-4

Lung Volume Regression Equations (Height in inches and age in years, unless otherwise noted)

Test		Regression Equation	SD	Source
VC (L)				
	Males	(Same as for FVC)		1
	Females	(Same as for FVC)		1
FRC (L)				
	Males	0.130H − 5.16	—	2
	Females	0.119H − 4.85	—	2
RV (L)				
	Males	0.069H + 0.017A − 3.45	—	3
	Females	0.081H + 0.009A − 3.90	—	3
Derived Lung Volumes				
		TLC (L) = VC + RV or		
		TLC (L) = FRC + IC		

TABLE B-5

Other Pulmonary Function Regression Equations (Height in inches and age in years, unless otherwise noted)

Test		Regression Equation	SD	Source
$\dot{V}max_{75}$ (L/sec)				
	Males	$0.090H - 0.020A + 2.726$	—	4
	Females	$0.069H - 0.019A + 2.147$	—	4
$\dot{V}max_{50}$ (L/sec)				
	Males	$0.065H - 0.030A + 2.403$	—	4
	Females	$0.062H - 0.035A + 1.426$	—	4
$\dot{V}max_{25}$ (L/sec)				
	Males	$0.036H - 0.041A + 1.984$	—	4
	Females	$0.023H - 0.035A + 2.216$	—	4
MVV (L/min)				
	Males	$3.03H - 0.816A - 37.9$	—	4
	Females	$2.14H - 0.685A - 4.87$	—	4
CV/VC (%)				
	Males	$0.357A + 0.562$	4.15	5
	Females	$0.293A + 2.812$	4.90	5
CC/TLC (%)				
	Males	$0.496A + 14.878$	4.09	5
	Females	$0.536A + 14.420$	4.43	5
$D_{LCO}sb$ (ml CO/ min/ mm Hg STPD)				
	Males	$0.250H - 0.177A + 19.93$	—	6
	Females	$0.284H - 0.177A + 7.72$	—	6
Maximal Expiratory Pressure (cm H_2O)				
	Males	$268 - 1.03A$	—	7
	Females	$170 - 0.53A$	—	7
Maximal Inspiratory Pressure (cm H_2O)				
	Males	$143 - 0.55A$	—	7
	Females	$104 - 0.51A$	—	7
$\dot{V}o_2max$ (L/min STPD)				
	Males	$4.2 - 0.032A$	0.4	8
	Females	$2.6 - 0.014A$	0.4	8
HRmax (beats/min)				
	Males and females	$210 - 0.65A$	10–15	8
Pao_2 (mm Hg)				
	Males and females	$-0.279A + 0.113PB + 14.632$	—	9

TABLE B-6

Reference Values for Spirometry in Children (All values BTPS unless otherwise noted. Height in centimeters and age in years unless otherwise noted.)

Test		Regression Equation	SD	Source
Children, Males 8–20 Years of Age, Females 8–18 Years of Age				
FEV_1 (L)				
	Males	See Table B-1		10
	Females	See Table B-2		10
FEV_6 (L)				
	Males	See Table B-1		
	Females	See Table B-2		
FVC (L)				
	Males	See Table B-1		10
	Females	See Table B-2		10
PEF (L/sec)				
	Males	See Table B-1		10
	Females	See Table B-2		10
$FEF_{25\%-75\%}$(L)				
	Males	See Table B-1		10
	Females	See Table B-2		10
FEV_1/FVC				
	Males	See Table B-3		10
	Females	See Table B-3		10
MVV (L/min)				
Children 42–78 Inches, 5–17 Years of Age				
	Males and females	$3.81H_{in}-134$	—	11

TABLE B-7

Lung Volumes,* RV/TLC%[†] and DLCO* in Children. (All values BTPS unless otherwise noted. Height in centimeter and age in years unless otherwise noted.)

	a	b	SD[‡]	Source
Male Subjects, 5–18 Years of Age				
VC (ml)		Same as FVC		
FRC_{BOX} (ml)	−2.4915	+2.6523	0.0381	12
RV_{BOX} (ml)	−1.2720	+1.9427	0.838	12
TLC_{BOX} (ml)	−2.0018	+2.5698	0.0276	12
Female Subjects, 5–18 Years of Age				
VC (ml)		Same as FVC		
FRC_{BOX} (ml)	−2.4314	+2.6149	0.0538	12
RV_{BOX} (ml)	−2.0493	+2.3062	0.0819	12
TLC_{BOX} (ml)	−2.0377	+2.5755	0.0361	12
Males and Females				
RV/TLC$_{BOX}$ (%)	−34.6549	−0.0673	3.91	12
DLCOsb (ml CO/min/mm Hg STPD)	−3.2292	+2.0876	0.09	12

*Log(lung function parameter) = a + b(log height [cm]).
[†]Lung function parameter = a + b(height [cm]).
[‡]Upper/lower limit = antilog(a + [b±SD] [log height (cm)]).

Selected Bibliography

PREDICTION REGRESSIONS FOR ADULTS (TABLES B-1 THROUGH B-5)

1. Hankinson JL, Odencrantz JR, Fedan KB: Spirometric reference values from a sample of the general U.S. population, *Am J Respir Crit Care Med* 1999; 159: 179-187.
2. Bates DV, Macklem PT, Christie RV: *Respiratory function in disease,* ed 2, Philadelphia, 1971, WB Saunders.
3. Goldman HI, Becklake MR: Respiratory function tests: normal values at median altitudes and the prediction of normal results, *Am Rev Tuberculosis* 1959; 79: 457-471.
4. Cherniack RM, Raber MD: Normal standards for ventilatory function using an automated wedge spirometer, *Am Rev Respir Dis* 1972; 106:38.
5. Buist SA, Ross BB: Predicted values for closing volumes using a modified single-breath nitrogen test, *Am Rev Respir Dis* 1975; 111:405-411.
6. Gaensler EA, Wright GW: Evaluation of respiratory impairment, *Arch Environ Health* 1966; 12:146-167.
7. Black LF, Hyatt RE: Maximal respiratory pressures: normal values and relationships to age and sex, *Am Rev Respir Dis* 1969; 99:696-707.
8. Jones NL, Campbell EJM, Edwards RHT et al: *Clinical exercise testing,* ed 2, Philadelphia, 1983, WB Saunders.
9. Morris AH, Kanner RE, Crapo RO et al: *Clinical pulmonary function testing,* ed 2, Salt Lake City, 1984, Intermountain Thoracic Society.

SOURCES FOR NORMAL VALUES IN CHILDREN (TABLES B-6 AND B-7)

1. Hankinson JL, Odencrantz JR, Fedan KB: Spirometric reference values from a sample of the general U.S. population, *Am J Respir Crit Care Med* 1999; 159:179-187.
2. Dickman ML, Schmidt CD, Gardner RM: Spirometric standards for normal children and adolescents (ages 5 years through 18 years), *Am Rev Respir Dis* 1971; 104:680-689.
3. Zapletal A, Samanek M, Paul T: Lung function in children and adolescents: methods, reference values. In *Progress in respiration research*, vol 22, Basel, 1987, Karger.

ADDITIONAL RECOMMENDED SOURCES FOR PULMONARY FUNCTION PREDICTED VALUES

General

American Thoracic Society: Lung function testing: selection of reference values and interpretive strategies, *Am Rev Respir Dis* 1991; 144:1202.

Pelegrino R, Viegi G, Brusasco V et al: Interpretative strategies for lung function tests, *Eur Respir J* 2005; 26:948-968.
Quanjer PH: http://www.spirxpert.com/refvalues.htm and http://www.spirxpert.com/refvalueschild.htm. Last accessed 2/25/2007.

Spirometry

Crapo RO, Morris AH, Gardner RM: Reference spirometric values using techniques and equipment that meet ATS recommendations, *Am Rev Respir Dis* 1981; 123:659-664.
Enright PL, Kronmal RA, Higgins M et al: Spirometry reference values for women and men 65 to 85 years of age, *Am Rev Respir Dis* 1993; 147:125-133.
Falaschetti E, Laiho J, Primatesta P et al: Prediction equations for normal and low lung function from the Health Survey for England, *Eur Respir J* 2004; 23: 456-463.
Knudson RJ, Lebowitz MD, Holberg CJ et al: Changes in the normal maximal expiratory flow-volume curve with growth and aging, *Am Rev Respir Dis* 1983; 127:725-734.
Quanjer PH, Tammeling GJ, Cotes JE et al: Lung volume and forced ventilatory flows. Report Working Party Standardization of lung function tests; Official Statement European Respiratory Society, *Eur Respir J* 1993; 6 (suppl 16):15-40.

Lung Volumes

Crapo RO, Morris AH, Clayton PD et al: Lung volumes in healthy nonsmoking adults, *Bull Eur Physiopathol Respir* 1982; 18:419-427.

Diffusing Capacity

Bates DV, Macklem PT, Christie RV: *Respiratory function in disease,* ed 2, Philadelphia, 1971, WB Saunders.
Crapo RO, Morris AH: Standardized single-breath normal values for carbon monoxide diffusing capacity, *Am Rev Respir Dis* 1981; 123:185-189.
Knudson RJ, Kaltenborn WT, Knudson DE et al: The single-breath carbon monoxide diffusing capacity: reference equations derived from a healthy nonsmoking population and effects of hematocrit, *Am Rev Respir Dis* 1987; 135:805-811.
Miller A, Thornton JC, Warshaw R et al: Single breath diffusing capacity in a representative sample of the population of Michigan, a large industrial state, *Am Rev Respir Dis* 1983; 127:270-277.
Paoletti P, Viegi G, Pistelli G et al: Reference equations for the single-breath diffusing capacity: a cross-sectional analysis and effect of body size and age, *Am Rev Respir Dis* 1985; 132:806-813.
Roca J, Rodriguez-Roisin R, Cobo E et al: Single-breath carbon monoxide diffusing capacity prediction equa-

tions from a Mediterranean population. *Am Rev Respir Dis* 1990; 141:1026-1032.

Children and Adolescents

Hsu KHK, Bartholomew PH, Thompson V et al: Ventilatory functions of normal children and young adults—Mexican-American, white, and black. I. Spirometry, *J Pediatr* 1979; 95:14-31.

Polgar G, Promadhat V: *Pulmonary function testing in children: techniques and standards,* Philadelphia, 1971, WB Saunders.

Wang X, Dockery DW, Wypij D et al: Pulmonary function between 6 and 18 years of age, *Pediatr Pulmonol* 1993; 15:75-88.

Conversion and Correction Factors

CONVERTING GAS VOLUMES FROM ATPS TO BTPS

$$\text{Volume (BTPS)} = \text{Volume (ATPS)} \times \frac{P_B - PH_2O}{P_B - 47} \times \frac{310}{273 + T}$$

where:

P_B = barometric pressure, mm Hg

PH_2O = vapor pressure of water at spirometer temperature

T = temperature in °C

47 = vapor pressure of water at 37°C

310 = absolute body temperature

Most factors in this equation can be combined into a single conversion factor. Local barometric pressure changes cause slight differences. The most significant differences occur with temperature changes.

Conversion Factor	Gas Temperature (°C)	PH₂O (mm Hg)
1.112	18	15.6
1.107	19	16.5
1.102	20	17.5
1.096	21	18.7
1.091	22	19.8
1.085	23	21.1
1.080	24	22.4
1.075	25	23.8
1.068	26	23.8
1.063	27	26.7
1.057	28	28.3
1.051	29	30.0
1.045	30	31.8
1.039	31	31.8
1.032	32	35.7
1.026	33	35.7
1.020	34	35.7
1.014	35	42.2
1.007	36	44.6
1.000	37	47.0

CONVERTING GAS VOLUMES FROM ATPS TO STPD

$$\text{Volume (STPD)} = \text{Volume (ATPS)} \times \frac{P_B - PH_2O}{760} \times \frac{273}{273 + T}$$

where:

P_B = barometric pressure, mm Hg

PH_2O = vapor pressure of water at spirometer temperature

T = temperature in °C

760 = standard barometric pressure at sea level

273 = absolute temperature equal to 0°C

CALCULATING WATER VAPOR PRESSURE

$$PH_2O = 47.07 \times 10^{\left[\frac{6.36(T-37)}{232+T}\right]}$$

where:

PH_2O = vapor pressure of water at spirometer temperature

T = temperature in °C (0° to 40°)

CALCULATING BAROMETRIC PRESSURE AT ALTITUDE

$$P_B = 760 \times [1 - (6.873 \times 10^{-6} \times \text{Altitude})]^{5.256}$$

where:

P_B = barometric pressure, mm Hg

Altitude = altitude, feet above sea level

CONVERTING TEMPERATURE

$$°C = (°F - 32)/1.8$$
$$°F = (1.8 \times °C) + 32$$
$$°K = °C + 273$$

SI (SYSTÈME INTERNATIONAL) UNITS

The following table shows conversion factors for units of measurement commonly used in pulmonary function testing. Except for temperature, to convert a value from conventional to SI units, multiply conventional units by the conversion factor. To convert a value from SI to conventional units, divide by the factor.

Measurement	Conventional Unit	SI Unit	Conversion Factor
Temperature	°C	K	°C + 273.15
Length	inch (in)	meter (m)	0.0254
	foot (ft)	m	0.3048
Area	in^2	cm^2	6.452
	ft^2	m^2	0.0929
Volume	ft^3	L	28.32
Pressure	cm H_2O	kilopascal (kPa)	0.09806
	mm Hg	kPa	0.1333
	pounds/in^2 (psi)	kPa	6.895
Work	kilogram meter (kg m)	joule (J)	9.807
Power	kg m/min	(J)	0.1634
Energy	kilocalorie (kcal)	(J)	4185
Compliance	L/cm H_2O	L/kPa	10.2
Resistance	cm H_2O/L/sec	kPa/L/sec	0.09806

Regulations and Regulatory Agencies

Several agencies regulate operations in pulmonary function and blood gas laboratories. These regulations typically concern laboratory procedures, infection control, safety, and reimbursement.

OCCUPATIONAL SAFETY AND HEALTH ADMINISTRATION

The Occupational Safety and Health Administration (OSHA) is a U.S. government agency that develops and implements policies to address hazards in the workplace. OSHA regulations apply to two main areas in pulmonary function and blood gas laboratories:

1. *Hazard communication* relates to all chemicals or substances used in the laboratory. Laboratories are required to maintain lists of hazardous substances. In addition, Material Safety Data Sheets (MSDSs) must be kept. Employees must be trained regarding, and kept informed of, hazardous chemicals in their workplace.
2. Training regarding *blood-borne pathogens* is mandated. Employees who may be exposed to blood or blood products must receive training regarding the transmission of blood-borne pathogens. Methods of preventing exposure, identification of tasks that cause risk of exposure, and actions to be taken must be documented. Plans for removal of blood and blood products are necessary, as are explanations of personal protective equipment, such as gloves and gowns.

Regulations mandated by OSHA are published in the *Federal Register* and are continually updated. For additional information visit http://www.osha.gov/.

NATIONAL INSTITUTE FOR OCCUPATIONAL SAFETY AND HEALTH

The National Institute for Occupational Safety and Health (NIOSH) is a U.S. government agency that enforces standards set by OSHA. NIOSH regulations concerning pulmonary function measurements are related to the "Cotton Dust Standard." Federal regulations (29 CFR: 1910.1043) describe how spirometry is to be performed in the examination of individuals exposed to cotton dust. The appendix to this statute lists standards for spirometers and recorders used, measurement techniques, interpretation of spirometry, and qualifications for personnel performing spirometry. Guidelines for minimal spirometry training are included. These NIOSH regulations regarding spirometry are often applied in areas of occupational exposure other than cotton dust, making them de facto standards.

Updates to NIOSH regulations are published in the *Federal Register*. For additional information visit http://www.cdc.gov/niosh/homepage.html.

HEALTH AND HUMAN SERVICES

Health and Human Services (HHS) is a U.S. government department. Programs affecting pulmonary function and blood gas laboratories are administered by the Centers for Medicare and Medicaid Services (CMS), formerly known as the Health Care Financing Administration (HFCA).

Clinical Laboratory Improvement Amendments of 1988

Clinical Laboratory Improvement Amendments of 1988 (CLIA 88) consist of regulations that ensure safe, accurate quality laboratory testing. Regulations 42 CFR, Part 493, HSQ-176 consist of standards regarding laboratory practices. These regulations include blood gas laboratories and may have ramifications for pulmonary function testing as well. Under CLIA 88 regulations:

1. Laboratories must register and apply for certification. Level of certification depends on the complexity of tests performed. Three categories of testing, based on complexity of the testing method, have been established:

   Waived tests: Waived tests include simple nonautomated tests such as pH measurement by dipstick method.

   Tests of moderate complexity: Tests of moderate complexity include automated tests or manual procedures with limited steps. Automated blood gas analyses that do not require operator intervention during the analytic process are included in the moderate complexity group.

   Tests of high complexity: Tests of high complexity include semi-automated or manual procedures that require multiple steps, preparation of complex reagents, and operator intervention in the analytic process.

2. Personnel requirements are linked to the complexity model for testing. For moderately complex tests, standards for laboratory directors, technical consultants, clinical consultants, and testing personnel are defined. For high-complexity tests, standards for technical and general supervisors are added to the list. The regulations list specific functions and qualifications for each position. Qualified individuals can fill more than one position in either moderate-complexity or high-complexity testing.

3. Proficiency testing is required to externally evaluate each laboratory's performance. Each laboratory performing moderate-complexity or high-complexity tests must participate in proficiency testing. Proficiency tests must be performed for each regulated analyte for which the laboratory reports results. Proficiency testing samples must include five samples for each analyte or test. The laboratory must participate in the program at least three times per year. A separate grading formula is established for each analyte. For most analytes or tests, a score of 80% (an acceptable measurement on four of five samples) is required. Laboratories that are unsuccessful (score less than 80%) on two of three tests will be subject to sanctions for the involved test.

4. Each laboratory must establish a quality control program. Regulations require that for tests of moderate complexity (e.g., blood gases) manufacturer's instructions be followed, a procedure manual be available, and calibrations be performed. Quality control runs with at least two levels must be performed daily. Instruments and test systems will be evaluated by the Food and Drug Administration (FDA) to determine the applicable levels of quality control required.

In addition to the laboratory regulations defined by CLIA 88, HHS sets standards for reimbursement under the DRG (Diagnosis Related Groups) system for Medicare inpatients and under the APC (Ambulatory Payment Classification) system for outpatients. Reimbursement requires that charges for procedures performed be correctly classified using Current Procedural Terminology (CPT) codes. HHS also lists requirements for disability according to the Social Security Administration (SSA). These regulations specify levels of pulmonary function impairment that qualify candidates for disability reimbursement (see Chapter 9).

Updates to CLIA 88 regulations are published in the *Federal Register*. Regulations related to reimbursement under CMS or SSA are published by the respective agencies. For more information visit http://www.hhs.gov/.

THE JOINT COMMISSION

The Joint Commission (TJC) is a voluntary accrediting agency that develops standards of quality for health care organizations. TJC has published standards for all areas of the health care environment. Standards that affect pulmonary function laboratories are listed primarily under Respiratory Care Services. TJC standards require the following:

1. Pulmonary function and blood gas analysis capability should be appropriate for the level of respiratory care services provided and should be readily available to meet the needs of patients. Blood gases should be available 24 hours per day.
2. The scope of diagnostic services must be defined in writing and must be related to other hospital departments by an organizational plan.
3. Services provided from outside of the hospital must meet all necessary requirements.
4. Medical direction should be provided by a physician qualified by special training or interest in respiratory problems and should be readily available for consultation.

5. Trained personnel should be available to meet the needs of the patients served. Hazardous procedures (e.g., arterial puncture) must be authorized in writing according to medical staff policy.
6. There must be written policies and procedures for pulmonary function testing and for obtaining and analyzing blood samples. Policies and procedures should address equipment maintenance, safety, infection control, and administration of medications.
7. There must be sufficient facilities (equipment, space) for performing pulmonary function studies and blood gas analysis. Requirements regarding performance of pulmonary function or blood gas studies must be met regardless of which hospital department performs them. Equipment must be calibrated and maintained according to the manufacturer's specifications.

Standards developed by TJC are published annually in its document entitled *Accreditation Manual for Hospitals*. For more information visit http://www.jointcommission.org/.

CERTIFYING AND STANDARDS ORGANIZATIONS

The following organizations offer certification or publish standards related to pulmonary function testing and blood gas analysis:

Organization and Web Address	Certification/Standards
American College of Sports Medicine (ACSM) www.acsm.org	Provides training courses and certification for exercise technologists; publishes guidelines for exercise testing and training
American Thoracic Society (ATS) www.thoracic.org	Publishes standards for spirometry, single-breath D$_{LCO}$, pulmonary function personnel qualifications, use of computers in pulmonary function testing, guidelines for quality assurance, and interpretive strategies; standards published in the *American Journal of Respiratory and Critical Care Medicine*
Centers for Disease Control and Prevention (CDC) www.cdc.gov	Promulgates standards related to infection control and disease prevention; regulations published in *Morbidity and Mortality Weekly Report*

continued

Organization and Web Address	Certification/Standards
College of American Pathologists (CAP) www.cap.org	Accredits clinical and research laboratories, including blood gas laboratories; provides quality control programs and proficiency testing survey materials
National Board for Respiratory Care (NBRC) www.nbrc.org	Provides national certification for respiratory care practitioners, including pulmonary function technologists; offers credentials of Certified Pulmonary Function Technologist (CPFT) for entry-level and Registered Pulmonary Technologist (RPFT) for advanced-level practitioners
Clinical and Laboratory Standards Institute (CLSI) www.nccls.org	Publishes standards for all areas of laboratory medicine, including blood gas laboratories

Appendix E

Some Useful Equations

ALVEOLAR AIR EQUATION

It is often necessary to calculate the partial pressure of O_2 in alveolar gas. One practical application of the alveolar air equation is determination of PaO_2 for calculation of the present shunt. The alveolar air equation is as follows:

$$PaO_2 = (FIO_2 \times (P_B - 47)) - \left(PaCO_2\left(FIO_2 + \frac{1 - FIO_2}{R}\right)\right)$$

where:

FIO_2 = fractional concentration of inspired O_2
P_B = barometric pressure
47   = partial pressure of water vapor at 37° C
$PaCO_2$ = arterial CO_2 tension, presumed equal to alveolar CO_2 tension
R   = respiratory exchange ratio ($\dot{V}CO_2/\dot{V}O_2$)

If the fraction of inspired O_2 is 1.0, the factor in the parentheses on the right equals 1 and can be deleted. R varies, especially during exercise; it is often assumed to be 0.80.

POISEUILLE'S LAW

Poiseuille's law relates variables that affect gas flow through a tube. The law has many applications in pulmonary physiology. It describes laminar gas flow through the conducting airways. It is also used in pneumotachography to relate flow and pressure changes within a tube. The law is stated as follows:

$$\Delta P \frac{\dot{V}8\eta l}{\pi r^4}$$

where:

ΔP = change in pressure from one end of the tube to the other
$\dot{V}$ = flow through the tube
η = coefficient of viscosity of the gas
l   = length of the tube
r   = radius of the tube

The equation can be rearranged as follows:

$$\Delta P\dot{V} = 8\eta l\pi r^4$$

The ratio of pressure differences at the end of the tube (ΔP) to flow through the tube ($\dot{V}$) defines resistance. Resistance varies directly with the length (l) of the conducting tube. It varies inversely with the fourth power of the radius (r^4). A twofold increase in the length of the tube doubles resistance. A reduction of the radius by half increases the pressure difference 16 times. In the airways, narrowing caused by secretions or other lesions can significantly increase airway resistance. Poiseuille's law applies to any round tube in which laminar flow is possible. Pressure differential pneumotachography is based directly on this law (see the section on pressure-differential flow sensors in Chapter 10). The length and radius of a pressure differential flow sensor remain constant. The viscosity of respiratory gases varies only slightly. The variables in Poiseuille's equation, except for ΔP and $\dot{V}$, can be reduced to a single constant. Flow can then be defined as follows:

441

$$\dot{V} = \frac{\Delta P}{K_R}$$

where:

K_R = resistance constant determined by length and radius of the flow tube

Using this equation, $\dot{V}$ can be measured by determining the pressure differential. This is easily accomplished by means of pressure transducers.

THORACIC GAS VOLUME EQUATION

Measurement of V_{TG} with the body plethysmograph is based on Boyle's law:

$$P_1 V_1 = P_2 V_2$$

or by expanding:

$$P_1 V_1 = (P_1 + \Delta P)(V_1 + \Delta V)$$

where:

P_1 = initial dry pressure in the lungs (713 mm Hg or 970 cm H_2O)
V_1 = V_{TG} or volume of gas in the thorax
ΔV = change in lung volume
ΔP = change in lung pressure

Then by rearranging:

$$P_1 \Delta P + V_1 \Delta P + \Delta V \Delta P = 0$$

Solving for V_1:

$$V_1 = -\frac{\Delta V}{\Delta P}(P_1 + \Delta P)$$

Because ΔP is small compared with P_1, $P_1 + \Delta P \approx P_1$; therefore:

$$V_1 = -\frac{P_1(\Delta V)}{\Delta P}$$

In terms of the plethysmographic method (and disregarding the sign):

$$V_{TG} = 970 \frac{\Delta V}{\Delta P}$$

$\Delta V/\Delta P$ is represented as a sloping line recorded on a computer screen or an oscilloscope. The slope represents the change in mouth pressure per unit change in box volume ($\Delta P/\Delta V$), or λV_{TG}, as the patient pants against an occluded airway. The equation then becomes:

$$V_{TG} = \frac{970}{\lambda V_{TG}}$$

This is the working form of the equation. Box pressure and mouth pressure calibration factors are also required to complete the calculation (see Appendix F). Water vapor pressure must be subtracted from all pressure measurements in subjects. Measurement of the slope of the tracing allows rapid calculation of V_{TG}. If the inspiration against the occlusion is rapid the full form of the equation must be used:

$$V_{TG} = -(\Delta V/\Delta P) \times P_2 \times (P_1/P_B)$$

where:

P_2 = $P_1 + \Delta P$
P_1/P_B = correction when alveolar pressure is above or below ambient

If airway occlusion occurs at a volume other than FRC, a volume correction is required.

FICK'S LAW OF DIFFUSION (MODIFIED)

In reference to gas exchange across a membrane, Fick's law states that:

$$\dot{V}_{GAS} = \frac{A}{T} \times D \times (P_1 - P_2)$$

where:

A   = area of the membrane
T   = thickness of the membrane
$P_1 - P_2$ = pressure gradient across the membrane
D   = diffusion constant for a specific gas

D is related to the molecular weight and solubility of the gas to which it refers by:

$$D \propto \frac{\dot{V}_{GAS}}{\sqrt{\text{Molecular weight}}}$$

Because A and T remain relatively constant in the lungs:

$$D_L \propto \frac{\dot{V}_{GAS}}{P_A - P_C}$$

where:
D_L = diffusion constant for the lung
P_A = alveolar gas pressure
P_C = capillary gas pressure

When D_L is measured with carbon monoxide (CO), the capillary partial pressure is assumed zero, thus:

$$D_L = \frac{\dot{V}CO}{P_A CO}$$

All CO methods of measuring D_L use this basic equation. The single-breath and steady-state methods differ in that the former measures $\dot{V}CO$ during breath holding, whereas the latter measures it during normal breathing. The steady-state methods vary by the way in which they measure $P_A CO$.

FICK PRINCIPLE (CARDIAC OUTPUT DETERMINATION)

The Fick principle relates $\dot{V}O_2$ to arterial-mixed venous $\dot{V}O_2$ content difference $(Ca\text{-}\bar{v}O_2)$ to determine cardiac output $(\dot{Q}_T)$:

$$\dot{Q}_T = \frac{\dot{V}O_2}{CaO_2 - C\bar{v}O_2}$$

This equation forms the basis for determining various fractions of the cardiac output, namely, the shunt fraction $(\dot{Q}_S)$ and the fraction participating in ideal gas exchange $(\dot{Q}_C)$. The relationship between $\dot{Q}_S$ and the total cardiac output $\dot{Q}_T$ can be expressed as a ratio using the concept of O_2 content differences:

$$\frac{\dot{Q}_S}{\dot{Q}_T} = \frac{CcO_2 - CaO_2}{CcO_2 - C\bar{v}O_2}$$

where:
$CcO_2 - CaO_2$ = content difference between pulmonary end capillary blood, CcO_2, and arterial blood, CaO_2, which increases when blood passes through the pulmonary system without coming into contact with alveolar gas (a shunt)
$CcO_2 - C\bar{v}O_2$ = content difference between blood returning to the lungs by way of the pulmonary artery and the pulmonary end-capillary blood; the total change reflects the arterialization of mixed venous blood

If all pulmonary capillary blood equilibrates with alveolar gas, CcO_2 and CaO_2 become identical, no matter what the value of the denominator, so the ratio becomes zero and the shunt must be zero. If some blood does not equilibrate, the numerator becomes larger in relation to the denominator and an increased $\dot{Q}_S/\dot{Q}_T$ results.

Pulmonary end-capillary O_2 content (CcO_2) is impossible to sample and represents a mathematical entity rather than an actual phenomenon. A modified form of the equation is used clinically (as described in Chapter 6):

$$\frac{\dot{Q}_S}{\dot{Q}_T} = \frac{(P_A O_2 - PaO_2)(0.0031)}{(C[a-\bar{v}]O_2) + (P_A O_2 - PaO_2)(0.0031)}$$

where:
$P_A O_2 - PaO_2$ = difference in O_2 tension between alveoli and arterial blood
0.0031 = solubility factor to convert O_2 tension to volume percent

The equation is applied after the patient has breathed 100% O_2 long enough to completely saturate Hb ($PaO_2 > 150$ mm Hg). The only difference between pulmonary end-capillary blood (assumed to be in equilibrium with PaO_2) and arterial blood exists in the difference in O_2 content in the dissolved form. This difference is related to the normal $a - \bar{v}$ content difference ($C[a - \bar{v}]O_2$) plus the actual dissolved content difference, denoted by the same term in both numerator and denominator. A ratio between the content difference of shunted blood and the total difference is derived using dissolved O_2 differences. PaO_2 is determined by the alveolar air equation outlined previously in this appendix.

CALCULATED BICARBONATE (HCO_3^-)

The bicarbonate concentration in plasma can be calculated with the Henderson-Hasselbalch equation if pH and PCO_2 are known:

$$pH = pK + \log\frac{HCO_3^-}{H_2CO_3}$$

The working form of the equation becomes as follows:

$$(HCO_3^-) = 0.0306 \times PCO_2 \times 10^{([pH-6.161]/[0.9524])}$$

where:
HCO_3^- = bicarbonate concentration, mEq/L
0.0306 = solubility coefficient for CO_2
6.161 = pK of carbonic acid
0.9524 = an empirically determined constant

Total CO_2 concentration can then be determined by summing HCO_3^- and dissolved CO_2:

$$TCO_2 = 0.0306 \times PCO_2 + HCO_3^-$$

CALCULATED OXYGEN SATURATION

Although it is preferable to measure oxygen saturation (see Chapter 10), saturation of Hb with O_2 can be calculated if pH and PO_2 are known. Assuming that oxygen binding capacity of the Hb is normal (P_{50} of 26.6), saturation may be calculated as follows:

$$HbO_2 = \frac{Z^{2.60}}{(26.6)^{2.60} + Z^{2.60}} \times 100$$

where:

$$Z = PO_2 \times 10^{(-0.48[7.40-pH])}$$

where:
PO_2 = partial pressure of O_2 in the sample
pH = negative log of the hydrogen ion concentration in the sample
-0.48 = the Bohr factor (normal blood)

Because Hb is assumed to be normal, calculated saturation may be in error if the O_2 binding capacity of Hb is altered (see Chapter 6).

Appendix F

Sample Calculations

SAMPLE CALCULATIONS

Open-Circuit Multiple-Breath FRC Determination (N_2 Washout) (See Chapter 3)

(This example uses data from a test in which the volume of N_2 expired on each breath is summed.)

FRC_{N2}:	Unknown
N_2 Volume:	1.71 L (sum of FN_2 (V_T for all breaths collected during testing)
$F_A N_{2alveolar\ 1}$:	0.76 ($F_E N_2$ at beginning of the washout)
$F_A N_{2alveolar\ 2}$:	0.01 ($F_E N_2$ of the last breath at end of the washout)
BSA:	1.70 m^2
N_2 Tissue:	Unknown
V_{Dsys}:	0.06 L (system dead space)
Spirometer temperature:	24° C

1. N_2 Tissue $= ((BSA \times 96.5) + 35)/0.8$
    $= (1.70 \times 96.5) + 35)/0.8$
    $= ((164) + 35)/0.8$
    $= 199/0.8$
    $= 249\,ml = 0.249\,L$

2. $FRC_{N2} = \dfrac{(N_2\ Volume - N_2\ Tissue)}{(F_A N_{2alveolar1} - F_A N_{2alveolar2})} - V_{Dsys}$

    $= \dfrac{(1.71 - 0.249)}{(0.76 - 0.01)} - 0.06\,L$

    $= \dfrac{(1.461\,L)}{0.75} - 0.06\,L$

    $= 1.948 - 0.06\,L$

    $= 1.888\,L$

3. $FRC_{N2} = 1.888\,L$ (ATPS)
    This value is ATPS and must be corrected to BTPS. The spirometer temperature was 24°C. Using the appropriate correction factor from Appendix C:
4. FRC_{N2} (BTPS) $= 1.888\,L \times 1.080$
5. FRC_{N2} (BTPS) $= 2.04\,L$

Closed-Circuit Multiple-Breath FRC Determination (Helium Dilution) (See Chapter 3)

FRC_{He}:	Unknown
He_{added}:	0.5 L
F_{He1}:	9.5% (0.095 as a fraction)
F_{He2}:	5.5% (0.055 as a fraction)
Spirometer temperature:	24°C
V_{Dsys}:	0.075 L (system dead space)
Vsys:	Unknown (system volume at beginning of He breathing)

1. $FRC_{He} = [Vsys(F_{He1} - F_{He2})/F_{He2}] - V_{Dsys}$

2. $Vsys = \dfrac{He_{added}}{F_{He1}}$

    $= \dfrac{0.5\,L}{0.095}$

    $= 5.26\,L$

3. $FRC_{He} = [5.26\,L(0.095 - 0.055)/0.055] - 0.075\,L$
    $= [5.26\,L \times 0.727] - 0.075\,L$
    $= 3.825 - 0.075\,L$
    $= 3.75\,L$

4. $FRC_{He} = 3.75\,L$ (ATPS)

Correcting to BTPS with appropriate correction factor from Appendix C:

5. FRC_{He} (BTPS) $= 3.75\,L \times 1.08$
6. FRC_{He} (BTPS) $= 4.05\,L$

Single-Breath DLCO (See Chapter 5)

Volume inspired (V_I):	4.0 L (ATPS)
F_ICO:	0.003
F_ACO_{T2}:	0.00125
F_IHe:	0.10
F_EHe:	0.075
P_B:	760 mm Hg
Breath-hold time ($T_2 - T_1$):	10.0 sec
Spirometer temperature:	25°C

1. $$DLCOsb = \frac{V_A \times 60}{(P_B - 47)(T_2 - T_1)} \times Ln\left(\frac{F_ACO_{T1}}{F_ACO_{T2}}\right)$$

2. $$V_A = \frac{V_I}{F_EHe/F_IHe}$$
$$= \frac{4.0\,L}{0.075/0.10}$$
$$= 5.33\,L\,(5333\,ml)$$

3. $F_ACO_{T1} = F_ICO \times F_EHe/F_IHe$
$$= 0.003 \times \frac{0.075}{0.10}$$
$$= 0.0025$$

4. $$DLCOsb = \frac{5333\,ml \times 60\,sec}{(713\,mm\,Hg) \times (10.0\,sec)} \times Ln\left(\frac{0.0025}{0.00125}\right)$$
$$= \frac{319,980}{7130} \times Ln(1.8)$$
$$= 44.9\,ml/min/mm\,Hg \times 0.5878$$

5. $DLCOsb = 26.38\,ml\,CO/min/mm\,Hg$ (ATPS)

This value is ATPS and is normally converted to STPD (0°C), 760 mm Hg, dry. The correction factor is calculated as follows:

6. STPD correction factor $= \dfrac{273}{273 + T°C} \times \dfrac{P_B - PH_2OT°C}{760}$

where:

$T°C$ = spirometer temperature

$PH_2O\,T°C$ = partial pressure of water vapor at the spirometer temperature, in this case 24 mm Hg at 25°C

7. STPD correction factor $= \dfrac{273}{273 + 25} \times \dfrac{760 - 24}{760}$
$= 0.916 \times 0.968 = 0.887$
$= 0.887$

8. $DLCOsb = (26.38\,ml\,CO/min/mm\,Hg) \times (0.887)$
$= 23.4\,ml\,CO/min/mm\,Hg$ (STPD)

FRC (V_{TG}) Determination (Body Plethysmography) (See Chapter 3)

Data for V_{TG} and Raw are from the same patient. Assume airway occlusion occurs at FRC.

FRC_{pleth}:	Unknown
V_{TG} tangent (λ):	0.72 (angle 35.6)
P_B:	755 mm Hg
Patient weight:	71 kg
P_{MOUTH} calibration:	10 cm H_2O/cm
P_{BOX} calibration:	30 ml/cm
Dead space correction:	25 ml
Plethysmograph volume:	600 L

1. The barometric pressure correction (to cm H_2O) is calculated as follows:

$P_{Bcorr} = (P_B - 47) \times 1.36$
$= (755\,mm\,Hg - 47\,mm\,Hg) \times 1.36$
$= 963\,cm\,H_2O$

The patient volume correction (K) is calculated as follows:

2. $K = \dfrac{[Pleth\,volume - (Patient\,weight/1.07)]}{Pleth\,volume}$
$= \dfrac{[600\,L - (71\,kg/1.07)]}{600\,L}$
$= 0.889$

3.
$$FRC_{pleth} = \left(\frac{P_{Bcorr}}{\lambda} \times \frac{P_{BOXcal}}{P_{MOUTHcal}} \times K \right) - \text{Dead space}$$

$$= \left(\frac{963\,cm\,H_2O}{0.72} \times \frac{30\,ml/cm}{10\,cm\,H_2O/cm} \times 0.889 \right) - 25\,ml$$

After canceling like terms in the numerator and denominator (cm, cm H_2O):

4. $= (1338 \times 3\,ml \times 0.889) - 25\,ml$

$FRC_{pleth} = 3542\,ml\,(3.54\,L)$

Airway Resistance (Raw) and Conductance (sGaw) (See Chapter 2)

Raw:	Unknown
P_{MOUTH}/P_{BOX} TAN:	0.61 (angle = 31)
$\dot{V}/P_{BOX}$ TAN:	3.0 (angle = 72)
P_{MOUTH} calibration:	10 cm H_2O/cm
P_{BOX} calibration:	30 ml/cm
$\dot{V}$ calibration:	1.0 L/sec/cm
R_{sys}:	0.25 cm H_2O/L/sec

1.
$$Raw = \left(\frac{P_{MOUTH}/P_{BOX}\,TAN}{\dot{V}/P_{BOX}\,TAN} \times \frac{P_{MOUTHcal}}{V_{cal}} \right) - R_{sys}$$

$$= \left(\frac{0.61}{3.0} \times \frac{10\,cm\,H_2O/cm}{1.0\,L/sec/cm} \right) - 0.25$$

$$= (0.203 \times 10) - 0.25$$

2. Raw = 1.78 cm H_2O/L/sec

Several repetitions of the panting maneuver are usually performed. Unlike the FRC_{pleth} maneuver, however, tangents are not averaged. Because flow and volume tangents influence each other, Raw is calculated and then averaged. To calculate sGaw (specific airway conductance), the volume (V_{TG}) at which each Raw maneuver was performed is calculated as for FRC_{pleth}, with the P_{MOUTH}/P_{BOX} tangent from the specific maneuver. In this example:

1. sGaw = $(1/Raw)/V_{TG}$

2.
$$V_{TG} = \left(\frac{963\,cm\,H_2O}{0.61} \times \frac{30\,ml/cm}{10\,cm\,H_2O/cm} \times 0.874 \right) - 100$$

$$= (1579 \times 3\,ml \times 0.874) - 100$$

$$= 4040\,ml\,(4.04\,L)$$

Calculating the sGaw:

3. $sGaw = \dfrac{1/1.78\,cm\,H_2O/L/sec}{4.04\,L}$

4. $= 0.14\,cm\,H_2O/L/sec/L$

The average of three to five maneuvers is usually reported, after the sGaw for individual efforts has been calculated.

Exercise Study (See Chapter 7)

Volume exhaled (V):	20.0 L (ATPS)
Collection time (sec):	60 sec
Temperature (T):	24° C
F_EO_2:	0.17
F_ECO_2:	0.03
f_b:	25/min
HR:	100/min
PaO_2:	95 mm Hg
$PaCO_2$:	35 mm Hg
P_B:	750 mg Hg
Mechanical V_D:	18 ml (0.018 L)
Patient's weight:	55 kg

The first step is to calculate conversion factors to correct ventilation and gas exchange measurements to BTPS and STPD, respectively. This STPD factor is for conversion from BTPS:

1. $BTPS\ factor = \dfrac{P_B - PH_2O}{P_B - 47} \times \dfrac{273 + 37}{273 + T}$

$$= \frac{721}{703} \times \frac{310}{297}$$

$$= 1.07$$

2. $STPD\ factor = \dfrac{P_B - 47}{760} \times \dfrac{273}{273 + 37}$

$$= \frac{703}{760} \times 0.881$$

$$= 0.815$$

Next, parameters of ventilation are calculated as follows:

3. $\dot{V}_E(BTPS) = \dfrac{V_{exhaled} \times 60}{\text{Collection time in seconds}} \times BTPS\ factor$

$$= \frac{20.0\,L \times 60}{60} \times 1.07$$

$$= 21.4\,L\,(BTPS)$$

4. $V_T(BTPS) = \dfrac{\dot{V}_E(BTPS)}{f_b}$

$= \dfrac{21.4}{25}$

$= 0.856\,L\,(BTPS)$

5. $V_D(BTPS) = V_T(BTPS) \times \left[1 - \dfrac{F_ECO_2 \times (P_B - 47)}{PaCO_2}\right] - V_{Dmech}$

$= 0.856 \times \left[1 - \dfrac{0.03 \times 703}{35}\right] - 0.018$

$= (0.856 \times 0.397) - 0.018$

$= 0.340 - 0.018$

$= 0.322\,L$

6. $\dot{V}_A(BTPS) = \dot{V}_E(BTPS) - [f_b \times V_D(BTPS)]$

$= 21.4 - [25 \times 0.322]$

$= 21.4 - 8.05$

$= 13.4\,L$

7. $V_D/V_T = \dfrac{0.322}{0.856}$

$= 0.38$

Next, gas exchange parameters are calculated as follows:

8. $\dot{V}_E(STPD) = \dot{V}_E(BTPS) \times STPD\ factor$

$= 21.4 \times 0.815$

$= 17.4\,L$

9. $\dot{V}O_2(STPD)$

$= \left[\left(\dfrac{1 - F_EO_2 - F_ECO_2}{1 - F_IO_2} \times F_IO_2\right) - F_EO_2\right] \times \dot{V}_E(STPD)$

$= \left[\left(\dfrac{1 - 0.17 - 0.03}{1 - 0.2093} \times 0.2093\right) - 0.17\right] \times 17.4$

$= \left[\left(\dfrac{0.80}{0.79} \times 0.2093\right) - 0.17\right] \times 17.4$

$= [(1.01 \times 0.2093) - 0.17] \times 17.4$

$= [0.212 - 0.17] \times 17.4$

$= 0.042 \times 17.4$

$\dot{V}O_2(STPD) = 0.731\,L$

10. $\dot{V}CO_2(STPD) = (F_ECO_2 - 0.0003) \times \dot{V}_E(STPD)$

$= (0.03 - 0.0003) \times 17.4$

$= 0.297 \times 17.4$

$= 0.517\,L$

11. $R = \dfrac{\dot{V}CO_2(STPD)}{\dot{V}O_2(STPD)}$

$= \dfrac{0.517}{0.731}$

$= 0.71$

12. $\dot{V}_E/\dot{V}O_2 = \dfrac{\dot{V}_E(BTPS)}{\dot{V}O_2(STPD)}$

$= \dfrac{21.4}{0.731}$

$= 29.3\,L/L\ \dot{V}O_2$

13. $\dot{V}O_2/HR = \dfrac{\dot{V}O_2(STPD)}{HR} \times 1000$

$= \dfrac{0.731\,L/min}{100\,beats/min} \times 1000$

$= 7.31\,ml\ O_2/beat$

The calculation of energy expenditure at any particular workload is described by the term METS, for multiples of the resting $\dot{V}O_2$. The MET level for any workload is calculated by one of two methods. In each method:

14. $METS = \dfrac{\dot{V}O_2(STPD)\ exercise}{\dot{V}O_2(STPD)\ rest}$

but the means of estimating $\dot{V}O_2$ (STPD) at rest differs. $\dot{V}O_2$ (STPD) at rest can be measured, or it may be estimated as $0.0035\,L/min/kg$ ($3.5\,ml/kg$). Using the second method in this example:

$METS = \dfrac{0.731\,L/min}{0.0035\,L/min/kg \times 55\,kg}$

$= 3.80$

If the patient's measured $\dot{V}O_2$ at rest had been $0.225\,L/min$ (STPD), then:

$METS = \dfrac{0.731\,L/min}{0.225\,L/min}$

$= 3.25$

The Mean and the Standard Deviation

CALCULATION OF THE MEAN AND THE STANDARD DEVIATION

The mean ($\bar{X}$) and standard deviation (SD) are computed to determine the variability of a series of values. The SD is affected by every value in the series, especially extreme values. If the values are normally distributed, that is, each value has an equal chance of appearing, the SD may be used to relate any subsequent value to the population of values already obtained. In the laboratory setting, this concept is often applied to determine the variability of blood gas controls or biologic controls. Performing multiple measurements of the same quantity (i.e., the "control") allows the mean to be determined and precision to be expressed by the SD of the measurements. Assuming that all of the values sampled are normally distributed, 68.3% of them will be within ±1 SD of the mean, 95.5% will be within ±2 SDs, and 99.7% within ±3 SDs. When the mean and standard deviation have been determined for a series of measurements, subsequent values may be checked to see if they are "in control." Values between ±2 and ±3 SDs from the mean should occur only 5% of the time (i.e., random error), and values more than ±3 SDs from the mean should occur less than 1% of the time.

The mean ($\bar{X}$) may calculated as follows:

$$\bar{X} = \frac{\sum (X)}{N}$$

where:

Σ = a symbol meaning "the sum of"
X = individual data values
N = number of items sampled

The SD is calculated as follows:

$$SD = \sqrt{\frac{\sum (X^2)}{N}}$$

where:

X^2 = deviations from the mean $(X - \bar{X})$ squared
N = number of items sampled

If the SD is computed from a sample of 30 data points or less, N − 1 is usually substituted for N.

Example calculation of the mean and SD for a series of PCO_2 values:

Sample	PCO_2 (mm Hg)	Deviation from Mean (X)	Deviation Squared (X^2)
1	39	−0.9	0.81
2	40	0.1	0.01
3	43	3.1	9.61
4	42	2.1	4.41
5	39	−0.9	0.81
6	38	−1.9	3.61
7	40	0.1	0.01
8	41	1.1	1.21
9	38	−1.9	3.61
10	39	−0.9	0.81
Total	399		24.90
Mean	39.9		

$$SD = \sqrt{\frac{24.9}{(10-1)}}$$

$$= \sqrt{2.77}$$

$$= 1.66$$

The range of PCO_2 values (in this example) within 2 SDs of the mean is $39.9 \pm (2 \times 1.66)$, or from $36.6 - 43.2$ mm Hg.

Glossary

(See also Symbols and Abbreviations Used in Pulmonary Function Testing for pulmonary function abbreviations.)

$\Delta\%N_{2\ 750-1250}$ The 750 to 1250 ml portion of the SB_{N2} test

2-minute tidal breathing method A method of delivering methacholine to the airway where only a nebulizer is used; normal relaxed breathing is used as the patient inhales aerosol

5th (fifth) percentile The lower limit of normal (or LLN) in which the lowest 5% of healthy subjects are considered "abnormal" for clinical purposes

5-breath dosimeter method A quantitative challenge test activated during inspiration to deliver a consistent volume of drug, either automatically (by a flow sensor) or manually for an optimum output of 0.009 ml for each 0.6-second actuation of the dosimeter

6-minute walk test Test used to assess response to a medical or surgical intervention; assess functional capacity; and estimate morbidity and mortality

A-aO_2 gradient Difference in partial pressure of oxygen between the alveoli (A) and arterial blood (a)

Absorbance Change in the intensity of light passing through arterial or mixed venous blood without producing reflection

Accuracy The extent to which a measurement is close to the true value

acetylene technique Method for calculating cardiac output (CO) during exercise with closed-circuit or open-circuit methods; technique depends on the rate of uptake of a soluble gas (acetylene) with a very low diffusion coefficient

acid-base disorder Any condition in which the normal pH of the body or blood is disrupted

acidosis An increase in hydrogen ion concentration in in the body

air contamination Corruption of arterial or mixed venous blood specimens by atmospheric gas that can seriously alter blood gas values

air trapping Condition in which air spaces distal to the terminal bronchioles are abnormally increased in size, alveolar walls undergo destructive changes, resulting in overinflation of lung units; frequently occurs as a result of emphysematous changes or obstruction caused by asthma or bronchitis

airway inflammation Localized protective response to pathogens occurring within the routes for passage of air into and out of the lungs and involving the release of mediators including mast cells, eosinophils, macrophages, epithelial cells, and T lymphocytes, which results in recurrent exacerbations that manifest as wheezing, progressive shortness of breath, chest tightness, and coughing

airway resistance (Raw) The pressure drop across the airways related to flow at the mouth

alkalosis A decrease in hydrogen ion concentration in the body

Allen's test Momentary occlusion of the radial and ulnar arteries to establish adequacy of collateral circulation

allergic rhinitis Chronic inflammatory response to allergens in contact with the mucous membranes of the nose

alveolar dead space Alveoli that are ventilated but not perfused

alveolar plateau Breathing phase in which, in healthy patients, CO_2 rises to a plateau as alveolar gas is expired; if all lung units empty CO_2 evenly, the plateau appears flat

alveolar pressure Gas pressures within the alveoli at any given time

alveolar sample Gas collected from alveoli in a small bag (~500 ml or less) or by continually aspirating a sample of the exhaled gas

alveolar ventilation ($\dot{V}_A$) That part of the total ventilation that participates in gas exchange at the alveolar level

alveolar volume (V_A) Measure of alveolar capacity

alveolitis Inflammation of the alveoli, often allergic in origin

alveolocapillary Refers to the membrane of the lung that separates the gas exchange units (alveoli) from the pulmonary capillaries

ambient temperature Surrounding level of heat or cold

amperometric Measurement of the current

amyotrophic lateral sclerosis (ALS) Disease of the anterior horn cells of the spinal cord

anaerobic Without oxygen; in metabolism, the production of energy without oxidative phosphorylation

anaerobic threshold (AT) This occurs when the energy demands of the exercising muscles exceed the body's ability to produce energy by aerobic metabolism

analog A representation of numerical quantities by an output signal that measures continuous physical variables (such as voltage, length, pressure, flow) proportionate to the input

analog-to-digital converter An instrument measuring an analog signal and converting it to digital form, thus enabling the data to be fed to a computer

analog signal A signal that is proportionate to something else; a measurable quantity

anatomic dead space That part of the lung volume that is not part of the gas exchange units; the upper airway, trachea, and bronchi down to the level of respiratory bronchioles

anode The electrode to which anions migrate in an electrolic reaction; the positive electrode

anticoagulant Drug used to prevent or slow blood coagulation, such as heparin, coumadin, or streptokinase

aqueous control A bicarbonate buffer that contains a known partial pressure of O_2 and CO_2 and a known pH, used for quality control of blood gas analyzers

asbestosis Fibrotic lung disease caused by inhalation of asbestos fibers

asthma Obstructive airway disease characterized by reversible airway narrowing, mucus hypersecretion, inflammation, and episodic shortness of breath

asynchronous movement Lack of simultaneous rise and fall of the rib cage and abdomen, seen in paradoxical breathing

atelectasis A state of fluid-filled or collapsed alveoli

atopic Pertaining to a genetic predisposition toward hypersensitivity to certain substances, causing development of immediate allergic reactions

ATPS Ambient temperature, pressure, and saturation (water vapor)

a-v̄ content difference Difference in O_2 content between arterial and mixed venous blood

back-extrapolated volume A "time zero" error that can result during adult spirometry in particular as a result of hesitation prior to the forced expiratory maneuver

back-extrapolation Process of correcting for small leaks at the beginning of an FVC maneuver

back-pressure Pressure caused by resistance to flow in a tube or vessel, or across a membrane

bacteria filter A device designed to remove particles and bacteria; usually rated in pore size or in microns

Baralyme (Ba[OH]₂) Commonly used chemical "scrubber" agent used to aid removal of CO_2 from gas analyzers and breathing circuits

barrier device A device to minimize the risk of contamination, such as gloves or face masks

basal metabolic rate (BMR) Original term for Harris-Benedict equations; the metabolic rate (i.e., oxygen consumption) of a healthy individual at rest

base deficit Condition in which the buffering capacity is less than the expected value; a negative value

base excess (BE) The difference between the actual buffering capacity of the blood and the expected value

bell factor In volume displacement spirometers, a measure of the vertical distance moved to a specific volume (milliliters or liters); the number of milliliters of gas that must be displaced to cause a recording pen to move 1 ml

beta- (β-) adrenergic bronchodilator Type of bronchodilator commonly used in spirometry; also sometimes called a beta- (β-) agonist

bicarbonate buffer Substance used in conjunction with a modified pH electrode to construct a P_{CO_2} electrode in a blood gas analyzer

biologic control Use of healthy human individuals as a standard for measuring actual performance of an instrument or procedure

black lung Legal term describing chronic respiratory disease in a coal miner

body plethysmograph Instrument used to measure lung volumes (FRC_{pleth}) and airway resistance (Raw); consists of an enclosed booth or chamber in which the patients sits to measure changes in lung volume indirectly.

Bohr equation A method for calculating dead space ventilation from the relationship between arterial P_{CO_2} and mixed expired P_{CO_2}

Borg scale One of several numeric scales used to rate perceived exertion during exercise testing

Boyle's law Observation credited to Robert Boyle, early in the 18th century, that predicts the relation of a volume of a fixed mass of gas to a pressure change

braking Adduction of vocal cords during exhalation that creates a physiologic positive end-expiratory pressure (PEEP)

breath-by-breath Refers to measurement of respiratory variables during each breathing cycle

breath hold Suspension of breathing, used as an aid in various diffusing capacity tests

breathing strategy The change or adaptation in respiratory rate and/or tidal volume, usually during exercise; also called breathing kinetics

bronchial challenge Bronchial provocation test; used to assess airway response after a challenge to the airways, particularly useful in measuring response to bronchodilator medications; also known as bronchochallenge

bronchial hyperresponsiveness Abnormal (increased) reactions of the airways when exposed to irritants or other triggers, commonly seen in asthma, but also present in other disorders such as COPD and allergic rhinitis

bronchiectasis A pulmonary obstructive disease characterized by destruction of the bronchial walls

bronchiolitis obliterans An obstructive lung disease in which small airways are almost completely destroyed; also called bronchiolitis obliterans syndrome (BOS)

bronchoconstriction Spasm of the airways causing a narrowing of the lumen

bronchodilator Any drug or agent that opens the airways to promote increased airflow

bronchospasm Constriction of the smooth muscle surrounding the airways, resulting in obstruction

BTPS Body temperature, pressure, and saturation; most lung volumes and flows are expressed in BTPS terms

calibration curve An equation describing the relationship between input and output signals that can then be used to correct instruments such as gas analyzers or spirometers

calibration factor A software correction tool for computerized spirometry systems that makes an accuracy calculation based on the measured versus expected values of volume; the correction factor is then stored in memory and applied to all subsequent volume measurements

calibration syringe Quality-control instrument used to calibrate both volume-based and flow-based spirometers

calorimetry Measurement of the heat produced by an object; also measurement of metabolic requirements

capillary tube Heparinized glass tube for collecting arterialized capillary blood when arterial puncture is impractical

capnography The measurement and/or recording of exhaled carbon dioxide (CO_2)

carbon dioxide (CO_2) absorber A device for removing carbon dioxide from a breathing circuit; usually a chemical absorber

carbon dioxide (CO_2) rebreathing A noninvasive method for testing cardiac output during exercise

carboxyhemoglobin (COHb) Compound resulting from the combination of carbon monoxide (CO) gas and hemoglobin (Hb)

cardiac output The volume of blood pumped by the heart each minute

cardiomyopathy Chronic disease of the heart muscle that may involve hypertrophy and obstructive disease of the heart

cathode The negative pole of an electrolytic cell or electrode

chemoluminescence A method for measuring the presence or concentration of a gas such as nitric oxide, using a dye or material that emits lights in the presence of the substance to be measured.

chloral hydrate An oral sedating agent

chronic bronchitis Obstructive lung disease characterized by chronic cough and mucus production on most days for at least 3 months for 2 consecutive years

chronic obstructive pulmonary disease (COPD) Progressive, irreversible condition characterized by dypsnea, difficulty exhaling, and sometimes including chronic cough

Clark electrode A platinum electrode covered with a thin polypropylene membrane; see also *polarographic*

claustrophobia Fear of being in a small enclosed space or area

closed-circuit or rebreathing technique Technique in which the patient rebreathes from a reservoir (usually an anesthesia bag) of 7% CO_2 in O_2; used most often for pressure monitoring (P_{100}) and for extracting gas samples ($PETCO_2$)

closing capacity (CC) The volume (as a portion of total lung capacity) remaining in the lungs when airways begin to close

coal worker's pneumoconiosis (CWP) Lung disorder caused by an accumulation of coal dust in the lungs

coefficient of repeatability (CR) Calculation or measure of an instrument's or test's precision

coefficient of variation (CV) The standard deviation divided by the mean for a sample measurement

compliance The distensibility of the lungs; volume change with each unit of pressure change

computerized syringe Syringe using a built-in microprocessor to time the volume injection and calculate flows; provides a known volume for calibration or volume checks, and tests accuracy for commonly reported flows

computerized tomography (CT) Imaging technique used to record transverse planes within the body; can be used to provide an estimate of lung volume

congestive heart failure (CHF) Loss of left ventricular efficiency so that the heart becomes inefficient and overloaded; may be caused by systemic hypertension, coronary artery disease, or aortic insufficiency

conscious sedation Administration of a sedative that can be easily reversed by stimulation or a reversal agent, and in which a state of general wakefulness and responsiveness to environment is maintained

continuous-flow canopy Head hood device used to determine resting energy expenditure (REE) without direct connection to the patient's airway by measuring the change in flow into and out of the hood during breathing ("bias" flow)

control A system or device for establishing standards and measuring actual performance or comparing results

control run Testing in which a series of runs of the same control material is performed

co-oximeter A spectrophotometer designed for analyzing the various forms and states of hemoglobin, especially carboxyhemoglobinemia (COHb)

cor pulmonale Right-sided heart failure caused by lung disease

correction factor Calibration measure in which the degree of an instrument's accuracy is determined by calculating the measured versus expected values; this resultant correction factor is then stored in memory and applied to all subsequent measurements

corticosteroid Any of various adrenal cortex steroids

cross-contamination Contamination that spreads from one patient to another (or from health care worker to patient) because of infected equipment, air filters, or lack of barrier devices

cyanosis Bluish coloration of the nailbeds or skin associated with hypoxemia; caused by elevated levels of reduced hemoglobin

cycle ergometer A stationary bicycle designed specifically for exercise testing; ergometers allow work to be estimated

cystic fibrosis (CF) A hereditary disorder of the exocrine glands characterized by deficiency in pancreatic enzymes and respiratory symptoms

dead space The volume of the lung that is ventilated but not perfused by pulmonary capillary blood flow

deconditioning Dysfunction characterized by reduced SV and poor O_2 extraction by the muscles from lack of use

defibrillator A device used to shock the heart when fibrillation is present

demand valve A device that opens in response to volume, flow, or pressure changes

desaturation Reduction of oxygen level caused by dissociation of O_2 from Hb

diffusing capacity Measure of the uptake of small volumes of carbon monoxide (CO); referred to as DLCO or DCO

diffusion Movement of a gas through a gaseous or liquid medium, dependent on the molecular weight and solubility of the gas

diluent A diluting agent

dilutional lung volume Either of two measurement methods (helium [He] dilution and nitrogen [N_2] washout) involving the breathing of gases or gas concentrations not normally present in the lungs: He or 100% oxygen (O_2)

disability A patient's inability to perform certain tasks

distribution of ventilation An estimate of the evenness of ventilation obtained by recording the time to reach equilibrium and plotting the dilution curve

DLCO simulator Device that uses precision gas mixtures to allow repeatable DLCO measurements at different levels (e.g., high DLCO, low DLCO)

DLCOsb Single breath diffusing capacity test

DL/V$_A$ The ratio of DLCO to lung volume

Drierite ($CaSO_4$) Substance that removes water vapor from gas, including an indicator that changes color when the substance is exhausted

drift In electronics, to vary or deviate from a set adjustment; variation in the output of an instrument

dry rolling-seal A type of volume-displacement spirometer that consists of a lightweight piston mounted horizontally in a cylinder

dry seal A rubberized seal that connects a bell to the internal wall of a spirometer well; this rubber seal then "rolls" over itself, much the same as the dry rolling-seal spirometer

dynamic compression Collapse of airways caused by a pressure gradient that occurs with breathing or forced breathing

dynamic FRC A positive end-expiratory pressure (PEEP)–like effect that can appear in infants suffering from hypoxia

dynamic hyperinflation Increased lung volume that occurs during breathing or forced breathing, as with exercise

dyspnea Shortness of breath; difficult or labored respiration

edema Leakage of fluids from blood vessels caused by imbalance in pressures

effort-dependent Pertaining to a requirement for optimal patient effort for a maneuver's success; for example, in spirometry, optimal patient effort is vital for analyzing the inspiratory loop

Eisenmenger's syndrome A congenital abnormality involving the heart and great vessels; pulmonary hypertension is usually severe

elastance (E) Stiffness factor of the lung as measured in forced oscillation technique

electrocardiogram (ECG) A recording of the heart's electrical activity

electrode A device used to establish electrical contact with a nonmetallic part of a circuit; in electrochemistry, a device to measure current or voltage during chemical analysis

emission spectroscopy Method of measuring gas concentrations by analyzing light emitted when the gas is excited or ionized

emphysema Obstructive airway disease characterized by destruction of alveolar walls and collapse of small airways; may be accompanied by air trapping and hyperinflation of the lungs

end-expiratory level The volume of gas remaining in the lungs at the end of a quiet breath on a simple spirogram

end-expiratory lung volume (EELV) The volume of gas in the lungs at the end of a quiet (tidal) breath

end-tidal Refers to gas collected at the end of a quiet breath, usually assumed to represent alveolar gas

end-tidal CO$_2$ The concentration or partial pressure of CO$_2$ measured at the end of a tidal breath

energy Quantity expressed by oxygen consumption ($\dot{V}O_2$), in liters or milliliters each minute (STPD), or in kilocalories, or in terms of multiples of the resting O$_2$ uptake (METs)

enteral Passing through the stomach and intestines

eosinophilic inflammation Inflammatory response characterized by the presence of a specific type of white blood cells (eosinophils) in the tissue or blood

equipment dead space The wasted volume that must be ventilated in breathing circuits; this volume usually needs to be subtracted from patient volumes in various tests.

esophageal balloon A small-volume elastic device used to measure lung compliance by insertion into the esophagus; the volume of gas compressed in the patient's lungs is related to the observed pressure changes measured in the esophagus

eucapnic voluntary hyperventilation Technique in which the patient breathes at a high level of ventilation. Heat or water loss from the upper airways provokes bronchospasm in susceptible individuals, particularly when the patient inhales cold, dry gas

exercise-induced asthma (EIA) Respiratory disorder typified by bronchospasm during or immediately after vigorous exercise

exercise-induced bronchospasm (EIB) See *exercise-induced asthma*

exhaled nitric oxide (eNO or F$_E$NO) Normally occurring substance found in reproducible levels in exhaled air, but whose measurement is a useful indicator of eosinophilic inflammation of the airways, as with asthma

expiratory reserve volume (ERV) Largest volume of gas that can be expired from the resting endexpiratory level; a subdivision of volume capacity

explosive decompression A process or device that uses rapid expansion of gas to generate a known flow

extrathoracic obstruction Condition that usually shows normal expiratory flow but diminished inspiratory flow

fast Fourier transformation A mathematical function that breaks down the output into unique sine waves, each of its own frequency

FEF$_{25\%-75\%}$ The average flow during the middle half (from the 25%–75% points) of an FVC

FEV$_{0.5}$ Forced expiratory volume in the first half-second of an FVC maneuver; used more commonly in pediatric patients than in adults

FEV$_1$/VC The most standardized index of airway obstructive disease, related to ability to work and function in daily life

fibrosis Scarring of tissue caused by chemical or biologic agents, repeated infection, or inflammation, as in pulmonary fibrosis

Fick method A means of determining cardiac output by measuring oxygen consumption and arteriovenous oxygen content difference

Fleisch-type pneumotachometer A device that operates on the principle that the flow of the gas through the device is proportional to the pressure drop that occurs as the gas flows across a known resistance (a bundle of brass capillary tubes arranged in parallel)

flow at FRC ($\dot{V}$max FRC) The maximal flow at FRC identified on the x-axis (volume) of the F-V loop; commonly used to assess airways in neonates or very young children

flow limitation The characteristic of gas movement in the airways when increases in driving pressure do not result in further increases in flow

flow plethysmograph A type of body box that uses a flow sensor mounted in its wall to register variations in pulmonary volume

flow-sensing Designation for a type of pneumotachometer that produces a signal proportional to gas flow, which is then integrated to measure volume in addition to flow

flow-volume loop A plot of maximal inspiratory and expiratory flows versus FVC and FIVC on a single graph or display

fluorescence quenching Increased quenching of emitted light, commonly used to measure the presence or partial pressure of gases

fluorocarbon-based control A perfluorinated compound that has enhanced oxygen-dissolving characteristics. Multiple levels (e.g., acidosis, alkalosis, normal) of these materials provide control over the range of blood gases seen clinically

forced deflation technique Method used to produce maximal expiratory F-V curves (MEFV); opposite to the positive pressure generated during the RTC method

forced expiratory volume (FEV$_1$) Measure of the volume expired over the first second of an FVC maneuver

forced oscillation technique (FOT) Procedure in which a miniature speaker placed proximal to the device's flow sensor produces forced oscillations of flow with a range of frequencies into the airway

forced vital capacity (FVC) The maximum volume of gas that can be expired when the patient exhales as forcefully and rapidly as possible after a maximal inspiration

fractional Term used to describe the concentration of one or more gases in a mixture, expressed as a decimal fraction

FRC$_{HE}$ Functional residual capacity measured by the He dilution (closed circuit)

free breathing valve Device with two or more ports and a rotating drum to connect different combinations of ports to enable the patient to be "switched in" to the system either manually or by computer controls at a specific point in the breathing cycle

frequency response The ability of an instrument to detect a changing signal, dependent on the signal's frequency

functional residual capacity (FRC) The volume of gas remaining in the lungs at the end of a quiet breath

gag reflex Autonomic reflex to induce retching or vomiting

gain The amplification of a signal from an instrument

gas chromatography An accurate method of analyzing gases by separating them in a column that allows different gases to pass at different rates

gas-conditioning device Any chemical or physical device used to alter the composition of a gas; typically a water or CO_2 absorber included in a gas sampling circuit

gradient The difference in a quantity between two fixed points of reference

Guillain-Barré syndrome A progressive disease of the peripheral nerves

H$_2$O absorber Device in a gas analyzer that absorbs water vapor to prevent test accuracy interference

hard drive The physical device in a computer that provides permanent storage of data

Harris-Benedict equation Equations used to estimate the caloric expenditure in normal individuals under conditions of minimal activity

head hood Continuous-flow canopy that can be used for metabolic measurement systems on patients who are not intubated

heated-wire flow sensor A heated element, usually a thin, small-mass platinum wire, situated in a laminar flow tube where gas flow past the wire stimulates a drop in temperature to signal the need for an increase in current to maintain the preset temperature (the current needed to maintain the temperature is proportional to gas flow)

hemoglobin An iron-containing conjugated protein respiratory pigment occurring in the red blood cells of vertebrates

hemoglobin (Hb) affinity The degree to which Hb combines with O_2, affected by temperature, acid-base status, and other factors; usually expressed in terms of the P_{50}

hemoptysis Coughing up of blood

hemoximetry The measurement of hemoglobin (Hb) and its derivatives by spectroscopy

Henderson-Hasselbalch equation Equation that gives the pH of a buffer system

heparin A substance that inhibits blood clotting, also used to preserve blood specimens

Hering-Breuer reflex Respiratory reaction in which young infants hold their breath when their airway is occluded

histamine Chemical compound ($C_5H_9N_3$) that causes dilatation and increased permeability of blood vessels that play a role in allergic reactions

hypercapnia Higher than normal level of carbon dioxide; usually greater than 45 mm Hg in arterial blood

hyperinflation Overinflation of the lungs; usually denoted by an increased total lung capacity above the upper limit of normal (120%)

hyperpnea Rapid breathing

hyperreactivity State of being excessively responsive to stimulation

hyperventilation Ventilation in excess of CO_2 production resulting in respiratory alkalosis

hypocapnia A low level of carbon dioxide in arterial blood

hypotension Low blood pressure, usually less than 90/50

hypothermic Having a temperature below normal body temperature; usually below 37° C

hypoventilation Inadequate ventilation to remove CO_2 resulting in respiratory acidosis

hypoxemia Abnormally low level of oxygen in the blood

idiopathic fibrosis Formation of fibrous tissue that is self-originated or arises spontaneously from an unknown cause

impedance Opposition or flow resistance constituting the net force that must be overcome to move gas in and out of the respiratory system (upper airway, lungs, and chest wall)

impulse oscillometry A test that measures the resistance and impedance characteristics of the lungs and airways, usually by means of high-frequency sound waves

indirect calorimetry The determination of caloric requirements by measuring oxygen consumption and CO_2 production

inertia The tendency of objects to resist changes in position unless acted on by an outside force (from Newton's laws)

infant body box A relatively small chamber with controlled temperature and air ventilation to obtain accurate measurements of an infant's lung volumes

inflammation Complex, protective immune response of body tissues to irritation or injury in the presence of an antigen or foreign substance

informed consent Right of the patient to all information before undergoing or refusing treatments; includes the steps of disclosure, understanding, voluntary nature, competence, and permission giving

infrared absorption A type of detector of infrared radiation used in various gas analyzers

infrared analyzer Instrument using infrared radiation to measure gas concentrations; often used for exercise testing, metabolic studies, and bedside monitoring (capnography) in critical care

inspiratory capacity (IC) The largest volume of gas that can be inspired from the resting expiratory level; a subdivision of volume capacity

inspiratory reserve volume (IRV) A subdivision of vital capacity, that volume of gas measured from a slow, complete expiration after a maximal inspiration, without forced or rapid effort

interstitial lung disease A group of lung disorders characterized by infiltrates, inflammation of the alveolar walls, loss of lung volume, and exertional dyspnea

interrupter technique (Rint) A method of measuring airway resistance in the very young child; measurement involves passive tidal breathing, but with multiple interruptions in the respiratory cycle

intrabreath method A method for measuring diffusing capacity (DLCO) in which the patient inspires, then slowly exhales a test gas containing 0.3% CO, 0.3% CH_4 (methane), 21% O_2, and the balance N_2

intrathoracic airflow obstruction A condition characterized by poor ventilation due to obstructed airways

isobestic point Refers to any point on a common wavelength at which two or more chemical compounds absorb light, as measured by a spectrophotometer

isocapnia A normal level of carbon dioxide, usually in the blood

isocapnic buffering zone During exercise, that period during which increased alveolar ventilation is capable of maintaining a normal pH after the onset of anaerobic metabolism

isothermal lung analog A glass jar or container filled with copper or steel wool, used for quality control of a body plethysmograph

isovolume correction Process applied when the FVC changes by more than 10% (indicating a change in TLC or RV); requires that lung volumes be measured in conjunction with flows

Jones method Technique used to measure breath-hold time from 0.3 of the inspiratory time to the midpoint of the alveolar sample collection

kilopascal (kPa) Unit of pressure measurement in the International System; 1 mm Hg ~ 0.133 kPa

kilopond-meter (kpm) The work of moving a 1-kg mass 1 m vertically against the force of gravity

Konno-Mead loop The figures produced during a phase shift represented on an x-y graphic plot, abdominal movement on the x-axis and rib cage movement on the y-axis

kymograph A recording device, usually a rotating drum, on which a graph of motion or pressure may be traced

kyphoscoliosis A combination of anterior-posterior and lateral curvature of the spine

lactic acid An acid produced by anaerobic metabolism at high levels of work

Lambert-Beer law Principle relating total absorption in a system of absorbers to the sum of their individual absorptions

laminar airflow Streamline flow in a viscous fluid or gas near a solid boundary

large airway obstruction Any process or disease that limits flow in the upper airway, trachea, or mainstem bronchi

laryngoscopy The process of viewing the larynx endoscopically

leak check Quality control measure to assess a volume-based spirometer's accuracy; any volume loss greater than 30 ml/min is a significant leak and should be corrected before calibration or patient testing

learning effect The phenomenon in which a subject performs better after multiple attempts at a test or procedure

light-emitting diode (LED) The light source used in pulse oximetry

linear regression A statistical procedure in which an equation is computed that represents a linear (one-to-one) relationship between two variables

linearity The ability to produce a proportional output for a given input across a fixed range

lung analog Any container of known volume that can be used to simulate a lung volume measurement

lung resection Surgical removal of all or a section of the lung

lung transplantation Removal of one or both native lungs and replacement with lungs from a donor

lung volume reduction surgery (LVRS) A surgical procedure in which poorly perfused lung tissue is removed

magnetic resonance imaging (MRI) A type of scan that evaluates structures subjected to strong magnetic fields

maximal expiratory flow-volume (MEFV) A curve that shows flow as the patient exhales from maximal inspiration (TLC) to maximal expiration (RV)

maximal expiratory pressure (MEP) The highest pressure that can be developed during a forceful expiratory effort against an occluded airway at TLC

maximal heart rate (HRmax) The highest heart rate achieved during an exercise test

maximal inspiration The point at which the lungs are completely filled

maximal inspiratory flow-volume (MIFV) Measure of inspiratory flow plotted from maximal expiration (RV) to maximal inspiration (TLC)

maximal inspiratory pressure (MIP) The lowest pressure developed during a forceful inspiration against an occluded airway from RV

maximal voluntary ventilation (MVV) The volume of air that can be inspired and expired during a specific interval with rapid, forced breathing

maximum oxygen uptake ($\dot{V}O_2$max) O_2 consumption at the highest level of work attainable by normal patients; also a plateau in oxygen consumption that occurs despite further increases in external workload

mean value Average value calculated from repeated measures

medullary center Any among those areas of the medulla oblongata that are responsible for controlling the rate and depth of breathing

membrane resistance The characteristic of a membrane to impede gas diffusion; in DLCO testing it refers to the alveolar capillary membranes

metabolic measurement Any of several precise caloric need and nutritional status assessment tools, similar in method to those used in gas exchange measurements during exercise

metered-dose inhaler (MDI) A small canister containing a propellant gas to deliver reproducible doses of bronchodilator or other respiratory medications

methacholine A potent chemical that increases parasympathetic muscle tone in the airways when inhaled; used to induce bronchoconstriction to test for hyperreactivity of the airways

methemoglobin (MetHb) The fraction of hemoglobin in which the iron atoms have been oxidized to the Fe^{+++} state

METs Expression of energy in terms of metabolic equivalents based on a multiple of resting oxygen consumption; for standardization, 1 MET is considered equal to 3.5 ml O_2/min/kg

microprocessor An integrated circuit capable of performing logical and mathematical calculations; the primary component of a computer

minute ventilation The total volume of gas moved in and out of the lungs each minute; also called the minute volume

mixed venous blood Blood from the pulmonary artery; normally sampled by means of a pulmonary artery catheter

mixing chamber A container with baffles for collecting expired gas for analysis

Müller maneuver Production of negative intrathoracic pressure by closing the glottis and making a forced inspiratory effort

multigas analyzer Specialized infrared analyzer capable of detecting several gases simultaneously

multiple-rule method (Westgard) A widely used set of rules that is proposed by James Westgard; the rules are selected to provide the greatest probability for detecting real errors and rejecting false errors

myasthenia gravis A disease of the neuromuscular system characterized by progressive weakness, often episodic; neck, throat, and facial muscles may be primarily affected

Nafion Special sample tubing that is permeable to water vapor, allowing sample gas passing through the tubing to equilibrate its water vapor pressure with that of the surrounding atmosphere.

nasal NO Levels of nitric oxide in the nasal cavity, produced by the epithelial cells in the paranasal sinuses

National Lung Health Education Program (NLHEP) A leading advocate agency for the widespread use of simple office spirometry to increase the awareness and detection of COPD and other respiratory disorders

neoplasm Cancer, usually a tumor

neuromuscular Related to the nerves, muscles, or the junction of the two

nitric oxide (NO) A normally occurring gas found in exhaled air and related to inflammatory processes within cells

nutritional support Prescribed nutrition-intake program to provide for a patient's specific metabolic needs

obesity-hypoventilation syndrome A syndrome characterized by chronic respiratory acidosis in a patient who is overweight

obstruction Any process that interferes with air flow into or out of the lungs

obstructive sleep apnea (OSA) A syndrome in which an individual experiences cessation of airflow caused by blockage of the upper airway during sleep

occlusion pressure (P_{100}) The pressure generated during the first 100 msec of a breath against an occluded airway; also called P_{100} or $P_{0.1}$

office spirometer Simple spirometer that is designed to measure three important parameters: FEV_1, FEV_6, and the FEV_1/FEV_6 ratio

open-circuit calorimetry Indirect calorimetry method used to measure O_2 consumption, CO_2 production, and RER

open-circuit multiple-breath nitrogen washout (FRC_{N2}) Method of determining functional residual capacity (FRC) by washing out the N_2 from the lungs while the patient breathes 100% O_2 for several minutes

open-circuit technique Ventilatory control test in which the patient breathes increasing concentrations (1%–7%) of CO_2 in air or O_2 from a demand valve or reservoir until a steady state is reached; then measurements of $P_{ET}CO_2$, $PaCO_2$, P_{100}, and $\dot{V}_E$ may be made at each concentration

optode A fluorescent chemosensor useful in measuring pH or gas tensions in arterial or mixed venous blood

orthopnea Difficulty breathing related to body position; especially shortness of breath while lying supine

out-of-control The state or condition in which an instrument does not perform measurements accurately or precisely within specified limits

outlier Any statistical value significantly different from the mean, usually more than 2 standard deviations (SDs)

oximetry The measurement, either directly or indirectly, of the oxygen saturation of the blood

oxygen consumption Measurement of the volume of oxygen used by the tissues each minute; usually measured during exercise or metabolic studies

oxygen content Measure of blood oxygen bound to Hb and dissolved in the plasma

oxygen (O_2) desaturation Fall in the oxygen saturation of Hb as detected by pulse oximetry or hemoximetry

oxygen (O_2) prescription Flow of oxygen required to maintain a desired oxygen saturation; usually assessed by exercise testing

oxygen (O_2) pulse The volume of oxygen (ml) consumed or delivered each heartbeat; an index of stroke volume

oxygenation status A property in blood gas analysis used to assess the function of the lungs themselves in regard to oxygen transport

parenteral Nourishment occurring outside of the stomach and intestines

partial forced F-V curve A measure of an infant's maximal forced flow from a raised lung volume close to TLC, using rapid thoracoabdominal compression (RTC)

passive occlusion technique Method for measuring compliance in a quiet, relaxed infant (usually sedated), specifically an assessment in the change in volume divided by change in pressure (C = $\Delta V/\Delta P$)

P_{BOX} The pressure change within the box during body plethysmography

PC_{20} Provocative concentration of a drug at which a specified variable (such as FEV_1) changes by exactly 20%

peak expiratory flow (PEF) The maximum exhalation flow attained during an FVC maneuver

peak flow meter A device that can register PEF

personal best An individual's highest observed peak expiratory flow, usually during a period of maximum therapy

pH Negative logarithm of the hydrogen ion concentration used as a positive number

phase delay The time interval between when an event occurs and when it is registered by an instrument or analyzer; also, the delay between the response times of two separate instruments

phosphorescence Emission of light without appreciable heat

Pitot tube flow sensor Type of flow-sensing spirometer in which the pressure of gas flowing against a small tube is related to the gas's density and velocity

plethysmograph From the Greek *plethys* for pressure; any device for recording pressure. In pulmonary function testing, a booth in which the patient sits to measure pressure and volume changes in the lung

pleura The lining of the lungs and thoracic cavity

pleurisy Inflammation of the pleural surfaces

P_{MOUTH} Changes in pressure measured at the mouth with a pressure transducer during occlusion of the airway

pneumoconiosis Lung disease related to inhalation of dust or other particles

pneumotachometer Any device used to measure gas flow; in pulmonary function testing, a device used to measure flow and its integral volume

point-of-care (POC) Portable or bedside analyzer that provides rapid results of critical analytes

polarographic Refers to an electrode that is polarized by applying a voltage between an anode and cathode in order to make a measurement (see also *Clark electrode*)

postoperative complication Symptom or condition arising secondary to, or as a result of, the surgical experience

potentiometer An instrument for measuring electromotive forces

potentiometric A device for measuring electromotive force or potential difference by comparison with a known voltage; often used in blood gas electrodes (pH, P_{CO_2})

power A value in cardiopulmonary exercise testing expressed in kilopond-meters each minute (i.e., work each unit of time) or in watts

precision The extent to which an instrument measures a known value repeatedly; reproducibility

premature ventricular contraction (PVC) A common arrhythmia that occurs during exercise testing in which the ventricle contracts independently of the normal pacing mechanism of the heart

pressure differential flow sensor Device that measures gas flow using a resistive element that allows gas to flow through it but causes a pressure drop; the resultant pressure difference across the resistive element is measured by means of a sensitive pressure transducer

pressure plethysmograph Device used to measure thoracic gas volume (V_{TG}) implementing Boyle's law that volume changes in a sealed box are inversely related to pressure changes if temperature is constant

pretest probability The likelihood of a presumed diagnosis in relation to a test to confirm the diagnosis.

proficiency testing (PT) The process of comparing measurements of a known value from different sources to establish a level of accuracy

progressive multistage exercise test Tool for evaluating the effects of increasing workloads on various cardiopulmonary variables, without necessarily allowing a steady state to be achieved

protocol Written plan specifying procedures to be followed in giving a particular examination, in conducting research, or in providing care for a certain condition

provocative concentration (PC) The methacholine concentration at which a 20% decrease occurs (usually in reference to the FEV_1)

pulmonary artery occlusion pressure Measure used to estimate the effect of redirecting the entire right ventricular output to the remaining lung by measuring an induced pulmonary artery pressure increase

pulmonary compliance (C_L) Volume change per unit of pressure change for the lungs

pulmonary embolism A blood clot arising in the venous system that breaks loose and then lodges in the pulmonary vascular system

pulmonary fibrosis Scarring of lung tissue involving formation of fibrous tissue or lesions

pulmonary hypertension Elevated blood pressure in the pulmonary vascular system; usually a mean pulmonary artery pressure greater than 30–35 mm Hg

pulse oximeter Noninvasive tool for oxygenation assessment, based almost entirely on electric components

pulse oximetry Estimation of arterial saturation by analysis of light absorption of blood pulsing through a capillary bed (finger or earlobe)

quality control The process of establishing the accuracy, precision, or other desired output of a procedure or measurement

quality control (QC) material Any tool that can be used to establish the accuracy, precision, and other desired output of a procedure or measurement

radial artery Preferred site on the nondominant hand for puncture to obtain arterial blood gases

raised volume technique Method of inducing infant inspiration to total lung capacity (TLC) for effective spirometry by raising the intrathoracic pressure and volume in the child's lungs; final inflation is followed by a forced compression from an inflatable jacket

ramp test An exercise test in which the workload is increased continuously rather than incrementally

random error Variability of a measurement outside of accepted limits that occurs in a nonreproducible fashion

rapid thoracoabdominal compression (RTC) Use of a squeeze jacket to cause forced expiration in infants

rating of perceived exertion (RPE) A scale used during exercise testing that allows the patient to signal a numeric value related to his or her perception of exertion (see also *Borg scale*)

reactance (Xr) Type of pressure oscillation generated by sound waves that are out of phase with airflow

real-time display Any instrument or device that shows phenomena as they occur, in distinction to a recorded signal

rebreathing method Technique or system that allows the patient to breathe continuously while measurements are made

recruitment The increased perfusion of alveoli at the lung apices as cardiac output increases

reference electrode A saturated calomel electrode used in blood gas analysis to measure pH in a sample for potentiometric analysis

reflective spectrophotometer Blood gas analysis tool based on the variable reflection of light by O_2Hb and RHb at different wavelengths; useful in monitoring arterial saturation or measure mixed venous oxygen saturation ($S\bar{v}O_2$)

regression equation A statistical method for estimating one variable based on the value or change of another variable

relational database Data stored in tables that can be linked in various ways so that different variables can be extracted

repeatability Consistency factor calculated by obtaining and examining 3–5 measurements (e.g., spirometry, D_{LCO}) for consistency

reproducibility Consistency of measurements made at different times or with different instruments

resection Surgical removal of part of an organ or structure

residual volume (RV) The volume of gas remaining in the lungs at the end of a maximal expiration regardless of the lung volume at which exhalation was started

resistive element Device within a pressure differential flow sensor that allows gas to flow through it while causing a measurable pressure drop

resistor Device used to quality control (QC) a pneumotachometer by causing a known pressure drop

resonant frequency The point (Hz) at which the reactance curve crosses the zero line

respiratory dead space The lung volume that is ventilated but not perfused by pulmonary capillary blood flow

respiratory exchange ratio (RER) The exchange difference CO_2 production and oxygen consumption measured at the mouth; calculated as the $\dot{V}CO_2/\dot{V}O_2$, where $\dot{V}CO_2$ is the volume of CO_2 produced and $\dot{V}O_2$ is the volume of O_2 consumed per minute

respiratory inductive plethysmography (RIP) Noninvasive method of thoracoabdominal motion analysis using respiratory tracings to monitor movement from the rib cage (RC) and abdomen (AB) simultaneously

respiratory quotient (RQ) The ratio of carbon dioxide produced to oxygen consumed at the cell level

respiratory system compliance (Crs) Change in volume divided by change in pressure ($C = \Delta V/\Delta P$)

respiratory system resistance (Rrs) Change in driving pressure divided by flow ($R = \Delta P/\dot{V}$)

resting energy expenditure (REE) The caloric needs of the body estimated from oxygen consumption and carbon dioxide production, usually expressed in kilocalories per 24 hours

rotameter A large calibrated flow-metering device that may be used in conjunction with an adjustable compressed gas source to supply a gas at a known flow to a pneumotachometer or other flow-sensing spirometer

RV/TLC ratio Measure that defines the fraction of TLC that cannot be exhaled (RV), expressed as a percentage

sample volume A quantity of gas (usually alveolar) obtained from a patient, to measure diffusing capacities or other parameters based on gas composition in the lung

sarcoidosis Chronic disease of unknown origin characterized by formation of small granulomas (nodules), especially in lymph nodes, lungs, bones, and skin

"sawtooth pattern" Visible sign (on the inspiratory and expiratory limbs of the MEFV curve) of airway obstruction associated with abnormality of the muscular control of the posterior pharynx and larynx

scleroderma A disease of connective tissue with the formation of scar tissue (fibrosis) in the skin and sometimes also in other organs of the body; often involving the lungs.

scrubber An agent or device used to aid removal of water vapor or CO_2 from gas analyzers or to maintain isocapnia in closed-circuit technique for measuring changing levels of CO_2

sedation The act of calming, especially by the administration of a sedative

serial dilution Procedure for assessing the output of a gas analyzer by blending various amounts of the test gas with air

server Computer that maintains programs and data that a network of other computers and users need

shift Marked changes in electrode performance (in blood gas analysis)

shunt A bypass; in the lungs, an area in which blood flows through the lungs without coming into contact with alveolar gas

shunt fraction The proportion of the blood passing through the lungs participating in gas exchange, expressed as a fraction of the total cardiac output

shutter A device used in a breathing circuit to occlude the airway

signal transducer Any device that converts a physiologic signal (e.g., pressure, flow, volume) into a voltage, current, or similar representation of the signal strength

silicosis Fibrotic lung disease caused by inhalation of silica dust

Silverman pneumotachometer A type of pressure differential flow sensor that measures gas flow by using one or more screens (typically three) to act as a resistive element while helping to ensure laminar flow

sine-wave flow Gas flow that occurs in a regular pattern with a fixed frequency and amplitude

sine-wave pump A pump that uses a circular motion, such as a flywheel, to produce output that varies above and below a set level in a regular fashion

single-breath nitrogen washout test (SB_{N2}) Procedure that measures the distribution of ventilation by analyzing the change in N_2 concentration during expiration of the VC after a single breath of 100% O_2

slope of phase III The change in N_2 concentration from the point at which 30% of the VC remains up to the onset of phase IV

small airway In the lungs, any airway less than 2 mm in diameter; these airways are supported by surrounding alveolar structures

Social Security Administration U.S. governmental body that, as part of its functions, sets limits for determining disability based on respiratory impairment

solenoid A cylinder containing a wire coil with a movable core; the core moves when an electrical current is applied

solubility A substance's susceptibility to being dissolved

specific airway conductance (sGaw) Airway conductance divided by the lung volume (in liters) at which the measurement is made

spectrophotometer A device for analyzing chemical composition by measuring light intensity at various wavelengths

spectrophotometric oximeter Instrument that uses light absorption to analyze saturation of hemoglobin (Hb) with O_2

standard deviation (SD) In statistics, a mathematic statement of dispersion of a set of values around the mean

standard precaution One of a set of steps to follow to guard against infection applied to the handling of blood, semen, vaginal secretions, cerebrospinal fluid, synovial fluid, pleural fluid, pericardial fluid, and amniotic fluid

start-of-test In spirometry, the baseline measure of patient effort at the beginning of the test used to monitor or detect change in flow or volume above a certain threshold

status asthmaticus A particularly severe episode of asthma that does not respond adequately to therapy

steady-state condition Established condition of constant metabolic demand used in steady-state tests and usually defined in terms of HR, oxygen consumption ($\dot{V}O_2$), or ventilation ($\dot{V}_E$)

steady-state test In exercise testing, refers to tests conducted long enough for cardiopulmonary variables to reach a state of equilibrium

STPD Standard temperature, pressure, dry; measure used to report the condition of a gas; established as 0° D; 760 mm Hg, water content = 0

stridor High-pitched noise from the upper airway, usually on inspiration

strip-chart recorder Any recorder that uses paper moving at a fixed speed to record physiologic signals.

stroke volume (SV) Absolute volume of blood ejected during a single contraction of a ventricle

Structured Query Language (SQL) A special computer command language that provides a standardized means for the user to enter and retrieve data, generate reports, and perform functions such as importing or exporting records

ST-segment A portion of the electrical conduction pattern of the ECG; used to assess cardiac ischemia

subglottic stenosis Lesion or group of lesions of the laryngeal-tracheal airway that are important causes of large airway obstruction, especially in the pediatric population

submaximal Pertaining to below the maximum level of function or performance

suppurative To form or discharge mucus or pus

Swan-Ganz catheter A balloon-tipped catheter that can be floated through the right atrium and ventricle into the pulmonary artery

"switch-in" error An instrument dysfunction that must be calculated for when determining FRC with gas dilution techniques

systemic lupus erythematosus (SLE) Chronic inflammatory disease affecting the lungs, heart, kidneys, nervous system, joints, and skin

tangent A number that describes the slope of a line

tension pneumothorax A pneumothorax in which the pressure within the chest exceeds atmospheric pressure

thermal conductivity Measure of gas concentrations in a sample calculated by detecting the rate at which different gases conduct heat

thermal equilibrium Condition in which temperature is balanced, with no net gain or loss of heat

thermodilution method Technique for determining cardiac output by measuring temperature change of a solution injected into the right atrium and passing into the pulmonary artery

three-equation method Technique that uses separate equations for the three phases of the breathing maneuver (inspiration, breath hold, expiration) during a diffusing capacity test

tidal flow-volume loop Graphic representation of flow versus volume during tidal breathing

tidal volume (V_T) The volume of gas moved in and out of the lung with each breath

time constant (Trs) A fixed measure of the time required for a specific physiologic event such as the emptying of the lung; calculated as compliance times resistance (Trs = Crs × Rrs)

tonometry The process of measuring or establishing pressure of a gas in a liquid

total lung capacity (TLC) The volume of gas contained in the lungs after maximal inspiration

tracer gas An insoluble, inert gas such as helium (He), methane (CH_4), or neon (Ne)

tracheal malacia Degeneration of elastic and connective tissue of the trachea; also tracheomalacia

tracheal stenosis Tightening or stricture of the trachea

transcutaneous Refers to a measurement made through the skin

transducer Any device that produces a signal (electrical voltage or current) in response to a physiologic phenomenon such as pressure or sound

transfer factor (DLCO) Diffusing capacity expressed as conductance

transmural Across a wall or boundary

transport time Amount of time required to move the gas from a sample site to the analyzer itself

transpulmonary pressure (Ptp) Pressure across the lung from alveoli to pleural space

treadmill A device that incorporates a motor-driven belt on which walking, jogging, or running can be performed

tuberculosis A chronic granulomatous infection caused by an acid-fast bacillus, *Mycobacterium tuberculosis,* usually affecting the lungs and transmitted by droplet nuclei

turbine A device to measure flow by the pressure of air against the curved vanes of a wheel or set of wheels fastened to a driving shaft

T wave Measurement on an electrocardiogram that reflects deflections due to recovery of the ventricles in repolarization after excitation

two-point calibration Technique for adjusting the electronic output of an instrument to two known standards

ultrasonic flow sensor Type of flow-sensing spirometer that detects and measures gas flow by passing high-frequency sound waves across the stream of gas

universal precautions Standards for handling blood or specimens containing blood when there is possibility of infection

U-tube A pressure manometer that is used to calibrate a pressure transducer

V-slope method The use of regression analysis to determine the "breakpoint" at which $\dot{V}CO_2$ changes abruptly in relation to $\dot{V}O_2$ to measure the onset of anaerobic metabolism during exercise

Valsalva maneuver High intrathoracic pressure caused by closing the glottis and constricting the abdominal and chest muscles

V_D/V_T ratio The fraction of a tidal breath that is wasted (ventilation without perfusion) expressed in relation to the tidal breath

ventilation-perfusion scan ($\dot{V}/\dot{Q}$ scan) A nuclear medicine procedure in which radioisotopes are used to measure the relation between lung ventilation and blood flow

ventilatory equivalent for carbon dioxide ($\dot{V}_E/\dot{V}CO_2$) A measurement of relationship between breathing and CO_2 production, measured by dividing the minute ventilation (BTPS) by CO_2 production (STPD)

ventilatory equivalent for oxygen ($\dot{V}_E/\dot{V}O_2$) A measure of the efficiency of the ventilatory pump at various workloads, assessed as a ratio of minute ventilation during exercise to the work being performed (expressed as $\dot{V}O_2$); calculated by dividing $\dot{V}_E$ (BTPS) by $\dot{V}O_2$ (STPD) and expressing the ratio in liters of ventilation/liters of O_2 consumed per minute

ventilatory reserve The difference between maximal exercise ventilation and the MVV, sometimes expressed as a ratio or percentage, or as an absolute volume

ventilatory response Pulmonary function test that measures the change in ventilation that occurs with elevated CO_2 (hypercapnia) or decreased O_2 (hypoxemia)

ventilatory threshold The workload at which ventilation and CO_2 production increase at a more rapid rate, indicative of anaerobic metabolism

vocal cord dysfunction (VCD) Paradoxical vocal cord closure during inspiration

volume-displacement Any of three types of spirometer that that analyze respiratory gases by volumetric methods: water-seal, dry rolling-seal, and bellows-type spirometers

volume of thoracic gas (V_{TG}) The absolute volume of gas in the thorax at any point in time and any level of alveolar pressure

volume-time tracing Record created to show the forced expiratory portion of an FVC maneuver

washout volume In a diffusing capacity test, the initial exhaled sample of alveolar gas that is discarded before a true alveolar sample is collected or aspirated

water-seal Type of spirometer used to measure lung volumes and flows, using a large suspended bell in water with the open end of the bell below the surface of the water; a breathing circuit into the interior of the bell allows for accurate measurement of gas volumes, as the bell moves up during expiration and down with inspiration

watt A measure of power; 1 watt equals 6.12 kilopond meters per minute

wedge bellows A volume-displacement spirometer that folds or unfolds in response to breathing excursions

wheezing High-pitched or musical breath sounds, usually on expiration; associated with airway narrowing

workload Level of exercise being used in a given procedure

work of breathing The energy required to move a given volume into the lungs

Wright respirometer Instrument used to measure slow vital capacity at flows between 3 and 300 L/min; can also be used for ventilation testing, such as V_T and $\dot{V}_E$

zero Baseline calibration required by many devices, in which the signal to be measured is removed while the software adjusts the output of the sensor to equal zero

zirconium fuel cell An oxgen analyzer that is used for rapid analysis of O_2

z-score Statistic method for expressing the deviation from the expected value; equal to the difference between the observed and expected values divided by the standard deviation of the measurement

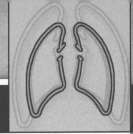

Index

Page numbers followed by f indicate figures, t, tables;
b, boxes.